Lifestyle Nur

Lifestyle medicine is an evidence-based approach to helping individuals and families adopt and sustain healthy behaviors in preventing, treating, and, oftentimes, reversing chronic diseases. This fast-growing specialty operates off of six main principles, including nutrition, physical activity, stress resilience, cessation or risk reduction of substance use, quality of sleep, and social connectivity.

Nurses are the primary providers of hospital-based patient care and deliver most of the nation's long-term care. Within healthcare, nurses are often tasked with educating patients and families and are thereby well positioned to address lifestyle intervention with patients.

Lifestyle Nursing examines the concepts of lifestyle medicine and nursing practice. It is specifically designed to help nurses introduce the concepts of lifestyle medicine to readers while also encouraging them to focus on their own wellness. This book features nutritional guidelines and supplemental materials operationalizing this basic nutrition knowledge into personal and patient wellness. It addresses evidence-based findings of chronic diseases, including heart diseases and stroke, type 2 diabetes, and cancers, which can often be prevented by lifestyle interventions.

Drawing from nursing and medical literature, this volume in the *Lifestyle Medicine* series encourages incorporation of lifestyle principles into nursing practices professionally and personally, which will lead to overall improved patient outcomes and happier, healthier nurses.

Lifestyle Medicine

Series Editor James M. Rippe
Professor of Medicine, University of Massachusetts Medical School

Led by James M. Rippe, MD, founder of the Rippe Lifestyle Institute, this series is directed to a broad range of researchers and professionals consisting of topical books with clinical applications in nutrition and health, physical activity, obesity management, and applicable subjects in lifestyle medicine.

Increasing Physical Activity: A Practical Guide, *James M. Rippe*

Manual of Lifestyle Medicine, *James M. Rippe*

Obesity Prevention and Treatment: A Practical Guide, *James M. Rippe and John P. Foreyt*

Improving Women's Health Across the Lifespan, *Michelle Tollefson, Nancy Eriksen, Neha Pathak*

Lifestyle Nursing, *Gia Merlo, Kathy Berra*

For more information, please visit: www.routledge.com/Lifestyle-Medicine/book-series/CRCLM

Lifestyle Nursing

Edited by

Gia Merlo, MD, MBA

Kathy Berra, MSN, NP, FAAN

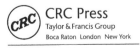

CRC Press
Taylor & Francis Group
Boca Raton London New York

CRC Press is an imprint of the
Taylor & Francis Group, an **informa** business

First edition published 2023
by CRC Press
6000 Broken Sound Parkway NW, Suite 300, Boca Raton, FL 33487-2742

and by CRC Press
4 Park Square, Milton Park, Abingdon, Oxon, OX14 4RN

CRC Press is an imprint of Taylor & Francis Group, LLC

ISBN: 9781032013688 (hbk)
ISBN: 9781032013343 (pbk)
ISBN: 9781003178330 (ebk)

DOI: 10.1201/9781003178330

Typeset in Times
by Newgen Publishing UK

Access the Support Material: https://www.routledge.com/9781032013343

Dedication

With awe and gratitude to nurses as you find the last morsel of strength to care for others at the end of the day though it feels like you have nothing left to give,

With love to your families and friends who have supported you along the way,

With joy to your spirit of giving and to all those you have helped thrive and heal every day,

With a moment of silent meditation honoring the lives we have lost that we continue to mourn every day of our lives,

With hope that you embrace self-compassion and self-care with the same gusto that you shower upon others.

Contents

PART I   *Lifestyle Medicine*

PART II The Nurses' Code of Ethics

PART III Lifestyle Medicine for Chronic Conditions

Preface

My journey as a healthcare professional began in 1989 as an intern at the University of Texas Southwestern Medical Center. On my first day, as I was introducing myself to the Emergency Room charge nurse, Jane, a patient was rushed into the room on a thumper. The thumper, an electronic CPR machine, had been keeping the patient's heart going for nearly an hour. Jane and I walked together to accept the patient from the ambulance crew. Knowing that this was my first day, Jane nodded in my direction and calmly whispered with the surety that can only come with 30 years of clinical experience, "We got this." I mentally relaxed, took a deep breath, and felt ready to serve the patient. From that moment on, she served as one of my favorite mentors, teaching me practical tips that I needed to know during my Emergency Room rotation.

Conceptualization for this book began in 2019 when I moved to New York and started teaching at New York University Rory Meyers College of Nursing. Having embraced lifestyle medicine as a physician, I was grateful for the opportunity to expand the field to nurses and nurse educators. Indeed, there are 1 million physicians in the United States and over 4 million nurses. Widely introducing lifestyle medicine into nurses' education has the potential to affect not only patient outcomes but also to improve many nurses' well-being.

Lifestyle medicine focuses on preventing, treating, and often reversing chronic illnesses. By employing a model of support that partners nurses with patients, lifestyle medicine has the capacity to improve health through prevention. Better diets, better sleep, exercising adequately, stress management, engaging in social support, and reducing the risk of substances are not new concepts to the world of healthcare but the idea of addressing them all together is. Instead of prescribing medications to treat diseases, we can prescribe 150 minutes of weekly physical movement that can be done simply by walking your dog or biking with your children. Helping patients to integrate lifestyle interventions into their day-to-day is challenging but may be easier when nurses serve as role models by focusing on their own health—mental and physical.

After spending a semester meeting with graduate NYU nursing students weekly for support and wellness at the start of the pandemic, I was encouraged to develop a curriculum focusing on nurses' wellbeing and thus began teaching lifestyle medicine to graduate and doctoral nursing students. Going into the course, I thought that I would be using my experiences as a physician to teach nursing students; however, as a repetition of my past, I learned as much from them as they learned from me. The nursing students taught me the robust history of nursing and nursing education stemming from Florence Nightingale and culminating in the creation of their core curriculum and code of ethics, which focus on health promotion. Embracing the lessons I have learned from my students, I strengthened my resolve to be a lifelong learner. I took the opportunity to continue learning and collaborating with nurses and nurse educators by writing this book. I was fortunate to be joined by Kathy Berra, a true pioneer and source of inspiration for generations of nurses, on this journey.

The literature overwhelmingly shows that nurses are struggling with their own health and well-being. One often cited problem is stress and burnout. Studies show that about 30% of new nurses leave the profession within three years due to stress and burnout. Additionally, nurses often adopt unhealthy behaviors like smoking, eating a poor, high-fat diet, and/or engaging in minimal physical activity. It is clear to me that lifestyle interventions promoting tobacco cessation, healthier diets, and daily increased physical movement should be taught and encouraged for not only our patients but also ourselves as healthcare providers. With this idea in mind, *Lifestyle Nursing* came to fruition. This book is intended to provide nurses and nursing students with a guide to help adopt lifestyle changes that will improve both their own mental and physical well-being along with their patients'.

Many of the topics presented in the book are commonly discussed in the literature, but the framing of these chapters is based on the experiences of nurses and nurse educators who generously contributed as chapter authors in hope of bringing positive changes to the nursing field. Each chapter reintroduces a topic through a nursing and lifestyle medicine lens and gives readers the necessary tools to implement lifestyle medicine in their practice.

After reading this book, I hope that practicing nurses, nurse educators, and nursing students will feel empowered to make their own lifestyle changes and begin to inspire their peers and patients to do the same. The ultimate goal of this book is to encourage incorporation of lifestyle principles into nursing practices professionally and personally that will lead to overall improved patient outcomes and happier, healthier nurses.

Gia Merlo, MD, MBA, MEd, FACLM, DipABLM

Acknowledgments

We owe a debt of gratitude to many colleagues who have contributed content and been a part of the process of conceptualizing, developing, and bringing this text to fruition. This book would not have seen the light of day without the nurse leaders who generously contributed as chapter authors. In particular, Deborah Chielli, Karen Liang, and Janine Santora served as editorial advisors and as such helped set the direction for many aspects of what is important in the book. The weekly meetings on Wednesday evening with Deborah, Karen, and Janine were spirited with laughs, support, and collaboration.

The leadership team at the American College of Lifestyle Medicine (ACLM) is a continued source of inspiration for many of us with passion towards lifestyle medicine. Ably led by the unstoppable Susan Benigas, ACLM continues to grow in numbers and impact with a vision to make lifestyle medicine the foundation of health and all healthcare. If anyone in the world can achieve this goal, it would be these resolute ACLM staff professionals working tirelessly to further these goals. Thank you all for all that you do! The ACLM RN/APRN Member Interest Group served as a sounding board and provided encouragement to move this project forward. We are especially thankful for the conversations with Josie Bidwell, Cindy Rima, Maria Grandienetti, and Nanette Morales, who served on the book planning committee early on. Many of our colleagues at New York University's Rory Meyers College of Nursing and Stanford University School of Medicine contributed to the book, and we are grateful for their ongoing support and encouragement. Especially thankful for the support of Dean Eileen M. Sullivan-Marx at NYU Rory Meyers College of Nursing and Dr. David Maron at the Prevention Research Center at Stanford Medical School.

We owe Dr. James Rippe, Lifestyle Medicine Series Editor, a debt of gratitude for believing in this project early on and providing encouragement, mentorship, and guidance with humor and friendship. Elizabeth A. Grady, managing editor of the *American Journal of Lifestyle Medicine*, and the rest of the team at Rippe Health, including Deb Adamonis and Carol Moreau, are resolute professionals who skillfully helped us navigate the publishing process from the beginning. We are thankful to the outstanding editorial team at CRC Press/Taylor & Francis, especially Randy Brehm, Senior Editor, for her support of this volume throughout the process, and Tom Connelly, Editorial Assistant, for his flexibility and organizational savvy. In addition, Vickie Liu, with her timely and thoughtful editorial assistance, was a breath of fresh air.

We received tremendous support from our families, friends, and colleagues throughout our journeys. We especially are grateful for our husbands, Rich Berra and Antonio Merlo, and daughters, Elaine Barry and Monisha Lewis, who steadfastly supported our work and career. Their love and encouragement made the impossible, possible, and every step on the path of life joyous.

Gia Merlo, MD, MBA, MEd, FACLM, DipABLM
Kathy Berra, MSN, NP-BC, FAHA, FPCNA, FAAN

About the Editors

Gia Merlo, MD, MBA, MEd, FACLM, DipABLM

Gia Merlo is Clinical Professor of Nursing and Senior Advisor on Wellness at New York University's (NYU) Rory Meyers College of Nursing. She is also a clinical professor of psychiatry in the NYU Grossman School of Medicine.

Merlo is the author of *Principles of Medical Professionalism* with Oxford University Press, in which she stresses the importance of physician wellness and addressing the social determinants of health, as well as the need to address chronic diseases with prevention. Merlo is an Associate Editor of the *American Journal of Lifestyle Medicine*. She is a contributing author of the American College of Lifestyle Medicine (ACLM) curriculum *Lifestyle Medicine 101* and its board review course, *Foundations to Lifestyle Medicine*, and was elected a fellow of ACLM in 2021. Merlo developed a novel lifestyle medicine curriculum titled Wellness in Nursing Through the Lens of Lifestyle Medicine and has been teaching this elective course to doctoral and graduate nursing students at the Rory Meyers College of Nursing at NYU since 2020.

Before joining NYU, Merlo was Associate Dean of Health Professions at Rice University. She has served on the faculty at the University of Pennsylvania School of Medicine, Baylor College of Medicine, Rice University, Texas Children's Hospital, and Children's Hospital of Philadelphia. Merlo has served on the board of directors of many nonprofits over the years and is currently on the board of directors of Plant-Powered Metro of New York (PPMNY). She has been involved in clinician care and medical education for nearly 30 years in professional development and mental health, particularly of healthcare professionals.

Kathy Berra, MSN, NP-BC, FAHA, FPCNA, FAAN

Kathy Berra graduated from Stanford University and received her master's and adult nurse practitioner degrees from the University of San Francisco. She worked in clinical research for 26 years at the Stanford Prevention Research Center, Stanford University School of Medicine. Her research activities focused on heart disease prevention, women and heart disease, and nurse case management for CVD risk reduction. She has published extensively in the medical literature, has authored two books, and speaks internationally on heart disease prevention and treatment. In 2007, Kathy started a home-based care management company—LifeCare Company. Her business is dedicated to caring for persons with complex medical problems who are living at home.

Kathy has been active in the American Heart Association for over 35 years and was awarded AHA Clinician of the Year in 2008. She is active on the AHA Council for Cardiovascular Nursing, currently serving as member of the Epidemiology and Prevention Sciences Committee. She is a founding member and past president of the American Association of Cardiovascular and Pulmonary Rehabilitation and past editor-in-chief of the *Journal of Cardiopulmonary Rehabilitation*. She is a founder and past president of the Preventive Cardiovascular Nurses Association and serves on their Board of Directors. She is a member of the Scientific Advisory Committee for WomenHeart—a national coalition of women with heart disease. WomenHeart's mission is to improve the health and quality of life of women living with or at risk of heart disease and to advocate for their benefit.

Contributor List

Sarah E. Abalos, PhD, RN
Thiel College
Greenville, PA, USA

Monica Aggarwal, MD, FACC
Division of Cardiology, University of Florida
Gainesville, Florida, USA

Susan Altman, DNP, CNM, FACNM
Rory Meyers College of Nursing
New York University
New York, New York, USA

Diana-Lyn Baptiste, DNP, RN, CNE, FAAN
Johns Hopkins School of Nursing
Baltimore, Maryland, USA

Kathy Berra, MSN, NP-BC, FAHA, FPCNA, FAAN
Stanford University School of Medicine (Ret)
Stanford, California, USA
The LifeCare Company

Steven Brady, DO
Department of Medicine, University of Florida
Gainesville, Florida, USA

Glenn S. Brassington, PhD
Department of Psychology
Sonoma State University
Rohnert Park, CA, USA

Glenn T. Brassington, PhD
Department of Psychology
Sonoma State University
Rohnert Park, CA, USA

Lynne T. Braun, PhD, ANP-BC, FAHA, FAANP, FNLA, FPCNA, FAAN
Rush University, Rush Heart Center for Women
Chicago, Illinois, USA

Samuel Byiringiro, MS, RN
Johns Hopkins School of Nursing
Baltimore, Maryland, USA

Deborah Chielli, MSN, BS Dietetics, RN, NP-C, DipACLM
Wilkes University
Wilkes-Barre, PA, USA

Jessamin Cipollina, MA
Rory Meyers College of Nursing
New York University
New York, New York, USA

Elizabeth R. Click, DNP, ND, RN, CWP
FPB School of Nursing
Case Western Reserve University
Cleveland, Ohio, USA

Lola A. Coke, PhD, ACNS-BC, FAHA, FPCNA, FNAP, FAAN
Rush University College of Nursing
Chicago, Illinois, USA

Karen Collins, MS, RDN, CDN, FAND
American Institute for Cancer Research
Arlington, Virginia, USA

Yvonne Commodore-Mensah, PhD, MHS, RN, FPCNA, FAAN
Johns Hopkins School of Nursing
Baltimore, Maryland, USA

Patricia M. Davidson, PhD, MEd, RN, FAAN
University of Wollongong
Wollongong, Australia
Johns Hopkins School of Nursing
Baltimore, Maryland, USA

Rebecca Feldman, MSN, CNM, PMHNP
Rory Meyers College of Nursing
New York University, New York, USA

Carlie M. Felion, MSN, APRN, FNP-BC, PMHNP-BC
University of Arizona College of Nursing
Mayo Clinic Phoenix, Arizona, USA

Caleb Ferguson, RN, PhD
University of Wollongong
Wollongong, Australia

Barry A. Franklin, PhD
Beaumont Hospital
Royal Oak, Michigan, USA
Oakland University William Beaumont School of Medicine
Rochester, Michigan, USA

Maria Grandinetti, PhD, RN, BSBA, CNE
Wilkes University
Wilkes-Barre, PA, USA

Bhanu Joy Harrison, LCSW, SEP
Choosing Mindfulness
Albuquerque, New Mexico, USA

Judith Haber, PhD, APRN, FAAN
Rory Meyers College of Nursing
New York University
New York, New York, USA

Susan Halli-Demeter, DNP, FNP-BC,
FPCNA, FNLA
Preventive Cardiovascular Nurses Association
Madison, Wisconsin, USA

Eileen M. Handberg, PhD, APRN-BC,
FAHA, FACC, FPCNA
Division of Cardiology, University of Florida
Gainesville, Florida, USA
One Florida PCOR.net Clinical Data Research
Network

Erin Hartnett, DNP, PNP-BC, PCPNP, FAAN
Rory Meyers College of Nursing
New York University
New York, New York, USA

Laura L. Hayman, PhD, MSN, FAAN,
FAHA, FPCNA
Robert and Donna Manning College of Nursing
and Health Sciences
University of Massachusetts
Boston, Massachusetts, USA

Nancy Houston Miller, RN, BSN, FAHA,
FPCNA
Stanford University School of Medicine (Ret)
Stanford, California, USA
The LifeCare Company

Lisa Kamsickas, MA
Northwestern University Feinberg School of
Medicine
Chicago, Illinois, USA

Michelle Knapp, DNP, PMHNP-BC
Rory Meyers College of Nursing
New York University
New York, New York, USA

Karen Laing, MS, BSN, RN, HWNC-BC,
DipACLM, CHES
All Heart Coaching, Inc.
Bon Secours Mercy Health
Cincinnati, Ohio, USA

Cindy Lamendola, BSN, MSN, NP, FAHA,
FPCNA
Stanford University
Stanford, California, USA

Jessica Landry, DNP, FNP-BC, SANE-A
School of Nursing, University of Louisiana
Lafayette, Louisiana, USA

Alexandra Lessem, FNP, DNP, DipACLM
North Colorado Family Medicine
Greeley, Colorado, USA

Donna McCabe, DNP, GNP-BC, PMHNP-BC
Rory Meyers College of Nursing
New York University
New York, New York, USA

Christy McDonald Lenahan, DNP, FNP-BC,
ENP-C, CNE
School of Nursing, University of Louisiana
Lafayette, Louisiana, USA

Mikki Meadows-Oliver, PhD, APRN, FAAN
Rory Meyers College of Nursing
New York University

Gia Merlo, MD, MBA, MEd, FACLM,
DipABLM
Rory Meyers College of Nursing
NYU Grossman School of Medicine
New York University
New York, New York, USA

Nanette Morales, DNP, NP-C, Dip-ACLM
Ochsner Hospital and Clinic
New Orleans, Louisiana, USA

Thomas F. O'Connell, MD
Department of Cardiovascular Medicine
Beaumont Hospital
Royal Oak, Michigan, USA

Oluwabunmi Ogungbe, MPN, RN
Johns Hopkins School of Nursing
Baltimore, Maryland, USA

Michelle Patch, RN PhD
Johns Hopkins School of Nursing
Baltimore, Maryland, USA

Matthew Petersen, DO, MS
Department of Medicine, University of Florida
Gainesville, Florida, USA

Demetrius J. Porche, DNS, PhD, PCC, ANEF,
FACHE, FAANP,
School of Nursing
Louisiana State University Health
Sciences Center
New Orleans, Louisiana, USA

Barbara Resnick, PhD, RN, CRNP, FAAN,
FAANP
University of Maryland School of Nursing
Baltimore, Maryland, USA

Tammy Robertson, BSN, RN
Cooking on the Veg Health and Wellness
Scottsdale, AZ, USA

Elizabeth Ann Robinson, PhD, RN, CNS
Santa Barbara Cottage Hospital
Santa Barbara, California, USA

Janine Santora, MSN, APRN, FNP-C,
SCRN, CNRN
Capital Health Institute for Neurosciences
Pennington, New Jersey, USA

Elizabeth Simkus, DNP, FNP-C, MSN, RN
Rush University College of Nursing
Chicago, Illinois, USA

Marcia L. Stefanick, PhD
Stanford Prevention Research Center
Stanford University School of Medicine
Stanford, California, USA

Cody Stubbe, MSN, RN
Wholistic Dish, LLC, Omaha, NE, USA
Physicians Committee for Responsible
Medicine's Nurses Nutrition Network

Elizabeth Johnston Taylor, PhD,
RN, FAAN
Loma Linda University
School of Nursing
Loma Linda, California, USA

Caroline Trapp, DNP, ANP-BC, CDCES,
DipACLM, FAANP
University of Michigan School of Nursing
Ann Arbor, Michigan, USA
Physicians Committee for Responsible
Medicine Scientific Advisory Board

Ruth-Alma Turkson-Ocran, PhD, MPH,
RN, FNP-BC
Johns Hopkins School of Medicine
Baltimore, Maryland, USA

Alyssa Vela, PhD, LP, DipACLM
Bluhm Cardiovascular Institute of
Northwestern, Chicago, USA
Northwestern University Feinberg School of
Medicine
Chicago, Illinois, USA

Jane Nelson Worel, MS, RN, ANP-BC,
FPCNA
Preventive Cardiovascular Nurses Association
Madison, Wisconsin, USA

Foreword

Patricia M. Davidson, RN, PhD, FAAN, FPCNA, FAHA

Gia Merlo, MD, MBA, MEd, FACLM, DipABLM, is a board-certified physician in psychiatry, child and adolescent psychiatry, and lifestyle medicine and is widely recognised for her innovative and integrated approach to healthcare. Kathy Berra, MSN, NP-BC, FAHA, FPCNA, FAAN, graduated from Stanford University, received her master's degree and adult nurse practitioner degree from the University of San Francisco, and has pioneered cardiac rehabilitation and lifestyle medicine. She has been at the Stanford University School of Medicine for over two decades. Gia and Kathy pooled together their vast experiences, expertise, and networks to produce this innovative and timely text, focussing not just on the disease and domain specific elements of lifestyle medicine, but also the critical role of nurses in the development, delivery, and evaluation of healthcare interventions. This text makes a bold and critical stance, placing nurses at the centre of the discussion of healthcare. In this text, nurses are defined and recognised as not just providers of healthcare but also consumers, and the need to take care of ourselves as nurses is clearly delineated and augmented by specific instruction in techniques, such as mindfulness and meditation.

As I write this foreword and reflect on my four plus decades as a nurse, I think about both how much has changed and also what we need to focus on moving forward to create a healthier and more just world. In my early days in coronary care, the thought of considering psychological and social factors contributing to cardiovascular disease was often met with scepticism and cynicism.

What is really gratifying as I survey the current landscape is the increasing recognition of health beyond a narrow biomedical approach to one focussing on social determinants of health—that is, the circumstances in which we are born, live, and die. Equally, we now recognise that healthcare providers are not immune to the stressors of society and the pressures of work. Even before the COVID-19 pandemic, we were shocked by the rising level of distress and burnout among clinicians. The National Academy of Medicine Action Collaborative on Clinician Well-Being and Resilience reported that 35–54% of nurses and physicians experience substantial symptoms of burnout. This distress impacts on not only health professionals but also their friends, families, and the individuals and populations they care for.

The COVID-19 pandemic has underscored many vulnerabilities in society, exacerbated many health disparities, and shone a spotlight on rising inequality. The toll of the current crisis is immensely impacting on the well-being of healthcare professionals. The release of *Lifestyle Nursing* comes at a critical juncture in the history of modern healthcare. Many of the frailties within our profession, society, and the healthcare system have been exacerbated by the pandemic. Nurses and their colleagues will need support and resources as we endure current challenges and look forward to a period of recovery, recalibration, and revival.

Lifestyle Nursing provides a roadmap to understand the professional role of nurses, our ethical obligations, and also our responsibility to ourselves. This thoughtful and provocative text not only provides information and instructions on providing care in disease-specific indications but also challenges the reader to think about its application and implementation.

Looking to the future, the information in *Lifestyle Nursing* is both inspirational and aspirational. The American Nurses' Association's first president and first superintendent of the Johns Hopkins School of Nursing, Isabel Adams Hampton Robb, said: "Nurses are trusted with the most precious thing on the earth: the life, health, and happiness of other human beings." This is a big responsibility and comes with both benefits and burdens. Recognising the importance of nurses as individuals as well as vehicles for delivery of healthcare interventions is likely to benefit not just ourselves as persons but also our profession and the individuals, families, and communities we serve.

Patricia M. Davidson, RN, PhD, FAAN, FPCNA, FAHA
Vice Chancellor and President
University of Wollongong, Australia
Dean Emerita
Johns Hopkins School of Nursing, Baltimore USA

Eileen M Sullivan-Marx, PhD, RN, FAAN, FGSA

The timing of Lifestyle Nursing edited by Gia Merlo and Kathy Berra could not be better! As we transition from a devastating pandemic that challenged our modern cure-oriented health care approach to respond with population focused solutions and compassionate care, we realized that a broader approach to well-being and health was needed. And what health providers need now is to formalize their knowledge, teaching, and practice to bring wellness to the forefront. This compendium edited by Dr. Merlo, a psychiatrist, and Kathy Berra, a nurse, brings resources to bear so that we can move forward with greater understanding and practical guidelines to address much needed wellness for all people who we serve and for ourselves.

Lifestyle as an approach to health is a new lens that encompasses systems, people, and their communities. As we have a new reckoning in social justice and the relationship of systemic racism to social determinants of health, the recent release of the American Nurses Association Foundational Report on the Commission to Address Racism in Nursing compels reflection on the part of nurses to look inwardly to being self-aware and attend to our own health and healthy lifestyles. In Chapter 13, we have an in depth global review of health disparities, cultural competence, and need for celebrating diversity that provides ways to rectify disparities with a greater awareness of lifestyle change and removing barriers that prevent such change. These barriers are rooted in social determinants of health and structural racism. Throughout the book, attention to lifestyle as it fits the individual's circumstance brings new perspectives to bear on our approach to practice, education, and research in wellness.

Readers will find Lifestyle Nursing a refreshing uplift and lens on our professional work. Moreover, the book will help us all renew ourselves to move forward with a healthy mindset that aspires compassion and conviction toward a health future for all.

Eileen M Sullivan-Marx, PhD, RN, FAAN, FGSA
Dean & Erline Perkins McGriff Professor
Rory Meyers College of Nursing
New York University, NY, USA

Part I

Lifestyle Medicine

1 The Nursing Roadmap to Lifestyle Medicine

Gia Merlo[1], Karen Laing[2], Deborah Chielli[3], and Kathy Berra[4]

[1]NYU Rory Meyers College of Nursing, NYU Grossman School of Medicine, New York, USA

[2]All Heart Coaching, Inc.

Bon Secours Mercy Health, Cincinnati, USA

[3]Wilkes University, Wilkes-Barre, PA, USA

[4]Stanford Prevention Research Center (Ret)

Stanford University School of Medicine (Ret), Stanford, USA

CONTENTS

KEY POINTS

- The impact of lifestyle on patient health has long been recognized in medicine and nursing.
- The potential benefits to the healthcare system of optimizing lifestyle factors include improved patient quality of life and financial savings.
- Nursing has an opportunity to play a vital role in the implementation of lifestyle interventions with patients.
- Lifestyle interventions support the goals of professional nursing organizations that recognize the importance of improving overall population health and the crucial role of nurse self-care.

1.1 INTRODUCTION

Thousands of years ago, Hippocrates recognized the potential power of using lifestyle as medicine when he said, "If we could give every individual the right amount of nourishment and exercise, not too little and not too much, we would have found the safest way to health" (Hippocrates, 1955). Modern lifestyle medicine is defined as the use of evidence-based lifestyle therapeutic approaches, such as a predominantly whole food, plant-based diet, regular physical activity, adequate sleep, stress management, avoidance or risk reduction of substance use, and other non-drug modalities to treat, oftentimes reverse, and prevent lifestyle-related chronic diseases that are all too prevalent. While the specific focus areas for lifestyle treatments may have expanded, the underlying concept remains the same—lifestyle habits have the potential to create a safe and effective path to health.

DOI: 10.1201/9781003178330-2

1.2   IMPROVING PATIENT QUALITY OF LIFE

The use of lifestyle interventions in nursing is not new. In her *Notes on Nursing*, Florence Nightingale addressed the need for pure water, uninterrupted sleep, and the impact of the mind upon the body (Nightingale, 1860). Lifestyle medicine has grown and is attracting many nurses. The American College of Lifestyle Medicine (ACLM), an interdisciplinary organization, has an active member interest group composed of hundreds of Registered Nurses (RN) and Advanced Practice Registered Nurses (APRN). The following chapters demonstrate that nurses can implement lifestyle interventions in many practice settings, not only in a designated Lifestyle Medicine clinic. Furthermore, these lifestyle interventions are not limited to use by APRNs.

The Centers for Medicare and Medicaid Services (CMS) report that in 2019, healthcare spending in the United States (US) reached $3.8 trillion, or $11,582 per person, increasing 4.6 percent from 2018, which increased 4.7 percent over 2017. In 2019, healthcare spending accounted for 17.7 percent of gross domestic product (GDP) in the US (CMS, 2019). The Centers for Disease Control and Prevention report that, of these nearly $4 trillion spent annually, 90 percent of the expenditures were for people with chronic physical and mental health conditions (CDC, 2021).

One of these chronic diseases is diabetes, which can lead to any or all the following: heart disease, stroke, kidney failure, blindness, and possible limb amputation. According to the World Health Organization (WHO), the number of people with diabetes increased from 108 million in 1980 to 422 million in 2014. The WHO also states that type 2 diabetes can be prevented or delayed by eating a healthy diet, being regularly physically active, and maintaining normal body weight. Diabetes can be treated and its consequences avoided by adopting these same health behaviors, screening regularly, and using medications as needed (WHO, 2021). From this example alone, significant financial savings can be easily imagined, both nationally and individually, before even considering the patient's potential improved quality of life and the possible extension of their life years.

To incorporate the lifestyle interventions previously mentioned, Healthy People 2030 resources can be used (Healthy People, 2021). The objective category of Health Behaviors includes sleep, nutrition, physical activity, drug and alcohol use, and tobacco use. Evidence-based resources are available via a link found within each specific health behavior's web page. These resources include family based physical activity interventions, internet-based tobacco use cessation interventions, and the effectiveness of brief alcohol interventions in primary care populations.

1.3   ROLE OF NURSES IN HEALTHCARE LIFESTYLE INTERVENTIONS

According to the American Nurses Association (ANA), there are currently 4 million registered nurses in the US (ANA, 2021). Nursing is the largest healthcare profession in the US, and Registered Nurses are one of the largest segments of the nation's workforce overall (AACN, 2021). Nursing is recognized as one of the most trusted professions by the public, and with this trust comes the responsibility to provide the best healthcare possible (White & O'Sullivan, 2012).

It is widely accepted that regular physical activity, daily stress management, a healthy diet, and avoidance of risky substances such as tobacco and alcohol contribute to optimal health and avoidance of disease (Heidke et al., 2020). Nurses are in an excellent position to provide an example of these behaviors as well as patient education regarding modifiable risk factors for chronic diseases. However, a nurse's own behaviors may influence the quality and amount of information shared with the patient. When nurses engage in behaviors that may be damaging to their own health, they may also be negatively impacting the health of others who consider them as role models (Heidke et al., 2020).

1.3.1   EDUCATIONAL PROGRAMS FOR NURSES AND THE IMPORTANCE OF SELF-CARE

The training for nurses begins within professional nursing education programs. The AACN's Core Competencies for professional nursing education programs include ten domains considered essential to nursing practice. Of these, three contain aspects related to lifestyle interventions. The first is Domain 2: Person-Centered Care, which includes person-centered care, built on scientific evidence guiding nursing practice in all specialties and functional areas. As noted in the definition of lifestyle medicine given previously, all lifestyle medicine interventions are evidence-based. Second, Domain 3: Population Health contains public health prevention and disease management. Returning to the definition of lifestyle medicine, the focus of these lifestyle interventions is on the prevention, reversal, and treatment of chronic disease. And, last, Domain 10: Personal, Professional, and Leadership Development supports "participation in activities and self-reflection that foster personal health, resilience, and well-being" (AACN, 2021). Domain 10 specifically addresses the importance of lifestyle activities that enhance the health and wellness of the nurse. These three AACN Essentials domains emphasize the importance of key aspects of lifestyle interventions in nursing education.

The National Academy of Medicine (NAM), in its recent report, *The Future of Nursing 2020–2030: Charting a Path to Achieve Health Equity*, made nine recommendations. Recommendation 3 states that "by 2021, nursing education programs, employers, nursing leaders, licensing boards, and nursing organizations should initiate the implementation of structures, systems, and evidence-based interventions to promote nurses' health and well-being" (NAM, 2021). Again, the power and importance of nurse self-care are being recognized by a professional healthcare organization.

The Healthy Nurse, Healthy Nation (HNHN) program launched by the American Nurses Association Enterprise in 2017 aims to empower nurses to make healthy lifestyle changes. The AACN and ANA have helped bring HNHN resources to nursing students nationwide. Participation in HNHN is open to both individuals and organizations interested in improving the health of nurses. Participants can share what they have learned with their fellow students and patients, thus expanding the reach and influence of the HNHN program (HNHN, 2021).

1.4   SOCIAL DISPARITIES IN HEALTH

Since the publication of The Code of Ethics for Nursing (The Code) in 2001, the nursing discipline has focused on health as a universal human right. The Code establishes that numerous social variables, including "poverty, access to clean water and clean air … nutritionally sound food, etc." (p. 31), contribute to health and calls upon nurses to address them (American Nurses Association, 2015). Every nursing educational institution has taught the code since its publication. Recent events around COVID-19 have magnified the necessity to continue to educate and address the nation's long-standing social disparities in healthcare.

Nursing, as defined by Florence Nightingale, is the "act of utilizing the environment of the patient to assist him [them] in his [their] recovery" (1860). In her book *Notes on Nursing: What It Is and What It Is Not* (1860), Nightingale proposed Environmental Theory, which explores the factors that impact both hospital infections and human health beyond hospital walls. Nightingale specifies five key concepts of the socio-economic drivers of health, which she termed the *health of houses*. These drivers are pure water, pure air, efficient drainage, cleanliness, and light. She observes that "without these, no house can be healthy" (Gilbert, 2020, p. 628). A person's health is so closely tied to environmental factors that researchers have determined zip code and associated factors such as income, housing, and education to be more important than genetic code when it comes to health outcomes (Graham, 2016; Slade-Sawyer, 2014).

COVID-19 amplified socio-economic disparities typically found in chronic, non-communicable diseases such as higher rates of infection and significantly worse outcomes in ethnic and racial minorities (Bambino et al., 2021). In a study by Thakur et al. (2020), COVID-19 cases consisted of approximately 30 percent Black Americans, who represent about 13 percent of the US population, and 34 percent Latinx Americans, who represent about 18 percent of the US population. At the community level, counties with the highest rates of death from COVID-19 had greater proportions of negative social determinants of health and higher percentages of Black Americans (Dalsania et al., 2021).

Krishnaswami et al. (2019) noted that "lifestyle is the most fundamental and modifiable influence on risk of disease" (p. 443). Krishnaswami determined unhealthy lifestyle factors, including limited access to healthy food and physical inactivity, are the primary causes of death inordinately affecting vulnerable and disadvantaged communities (Krishnaswami et al., 2019). The authors proposed two evidence-based solutions for improving health equity: (1) actions by health organizations building community partnerships and (2) actions by individual health professionals engaging with marginalized individuals and groups in clinical and community settings (Krishnaswami et al., 2019). These activities have included offering lifestyle-focused healthcare at a mobile Family Planning clinic for women's health and offering the "Eating for Life" program through a federally qualified health clinic (Krishnaswami et al., 2019). The individual nurse can learn community-level barriers to a healthy lifestyle from their patients and help develop strategies to overcome these potential obstacles. The nurse can also learn about the patient's cultural practices that may be impacting their dietary choices. Using that information, the nurse is better able to meet the patient partway (Krishnaswami et al., 2019).

Overall, the AACN Essentials (AACN, 2021) asserts that nurses of the future must lead initiatives to deal with systemic inequality, discrimination, and structural racism in order to provide equitable health care. To address social disparities, nurses must become aware and educated on them before taking action. Examples of actions include:

- Patient education at the bedside or in the exam room.
- Educating and organizing among colleagues.
- Participating in community walks, community gardens, or blood pressure screenings.
- Advising food banks or local leaders on the necessity for healthy food, clean drinking water, and safe recreational space.

1.5   CLIMATE CHANGE, DIET, HUMAN AND PLANETARY HEALTH

Nursing history and ethics consistently connect human health to environmental health. The Code of Ethics for Nurses with Integrative Statements (2015) clearly states that

social justice extends beyond human health and well-being to the health and well-being of the natural world. Human life and health are profoundly affected by the state of the natural world that surrounds us … social justice extends to eco-justice.

New studies carrying great urgency reaffirm climate research dating back decades. These studies connect current patterns of diet and food production with environmental and human health degradation. The landmark report, *Food in the Anthropocene: The EAT-Lancet Commission on Healthy Diets From Sustainable Food Systems* (Willett et al., 2019) provides a comprehensive scientific study with recommendations for rapidly transitioning to a diet that is healthy and derived from a sustainable food system. A key takeaway from the report is that "unhealthy and unsustainably produced food poses a global risk to people and the planet." Achieving the worldwide goal of a healthy, sustainable food system remains possible but will require dynamic shifts and implementation of targets to the full extent and in all areas (Willett et al., 2019). Strikingly, the dietary pattern healthiest for people is also best for the planet, as agreed upon by multiple health organizations. The EAT-Lancet Report (2019) recommends a diet rich in plant-based foods, stating the global consumption of fruits, vegetables, nuts, and legumes needs to double, while consumption of foods such as red meat and sugar needs to be cut in half. This plant-rich diet will offer greater human and environmental health and is the pattern supported by leading health organizations (Willett et al., 2019). The American

College of Lifestyle Medicine and the American Heart Association both recommend similar diets (Grundy et al., 2019).

Major medical organizations are speaking out with urgency about the role of human activity on climate change, the impact of climate change on human health, and the imperative to act. The American Nurses Association's Resolution on Climate Change (2008) and the American Medical Association's climate statement (2019) both agree that humans significantly contribute to climate change, which has detrimental effects on public health, and call on health professions to be part of the solution. The American College of Preventive Medicine's (ACPM) Climate Change Policy and the American College of Physicians (ACP) Position Paper share similar perspectives.

Leffers et al. (2017) recognize the lack of competent guidelines for integrating climate change into nursing education. The authors urge integration by topic area, i.e., air pollution and climate change into respiratory and cardiac pathology, along with content on vulnerable populations. The authors additionally encourage nursing education to address the environmental, social, economic, cultural, and political aspects of climate change and its relation to human health and the planet.

1.6 THE ROAD AHEAD

The healthcare landscape is constantly evolving, and this book is intended to serve as a guide for nurses interested in practicing healthcare rather than sick care. These nurses want to do more than rush past the recommended lifestyle changes noted at the beginning of many treatment guidelines. The road behind may be discouraging, with climbing numbers of patients negatively impacted by lifestyle-related chronic diseases and continually escalating healthcare costs. But, thanks to the persistence and vision of those in the nursing community, professional nurses stand on the brink of an opportunity to be a driving force in this powerful shift of focus in healthcare.

This book is organized into five sections: (1) lifestyle medicine, (2) nurse's code of ethics, (3) lifestyle medicine for chronic illness, (4) maintaining health through lifestyle medicine, and (5) application and implementation.

Lifestyle medicine begins with changes in nutrition (Chapter 2), physical activity (see Chapter 3), sleep (Chapter 4), emotional wellness and stress resilience (Chapter 5), happiness and social connectivity (Chapter 6), and avoiding harmful substances (Chapter 7) and environmental toxins (Chapter 8).

The nurse's code of ethics covers nurse self-care and the nurse's code (Chapter 9), while also addressing theories of self-promotion and self-management (Chapter 10), experiences of a nurse as the patient (Chapter 11), effects of disease on spouses and family members (Chapter 12), and health disparities (Chapter 13).

Lifestyle medicine can have profound positive effects on chronic illness, such as nutritional interventions for preventing, treating, and reversing chronic diseases (see Chapter 14), hypertension (see Chapter 15), diabetes and metabolic diseases (see Chapter 16), obesity and weight management (see Chapter 17), dyslipidemia (see Chapter 18), autoimmune disorders (see Chapter 19), cancer (see Chapter 20), cognitive disorders (see Chapter 21), psychiatric disorders (see Chapter 22), and tobacco use disorders (see Chapter 23).

Maintaining health through lifestyle medicines includes paying attention to oral health (see Chapter 24), men's health (see Chapter 25), midwifery and reproductive health (see Chapter 26), pediatric health (see Chapter 27), and optimizing function and physical health of older frail adults (see Chapter 28).

Finally, applications and implementation of lifestyle medicine consist of strategies for practicing spiritual care (see Chapter 29), coaching and empowering lifestyle changes (see Chapter 30), practicing mindfulness and meditation (see Chapter 31), promoting optimal lifestyle behaviors (see Chapter 32), and adopting digital therapeutics (see Chapter 33).

REFERENCES

American Association of Colleges of Nursing. (2021, April 6). *The essentials: Core competencies for professional nursing education.* www.aacnnursing.org/Portals/42/AcademicNursing/pdf/Essentials-2021.pdf

American Association of Colleges of Nursing. (2019). *Nursing fact sheet.* www.aacnnursing.org/news-Information/fact-sheets/nursing-fact-sheet

American College of Preventive Medicine (ACPM). (n.d.) *Climate change policy.* www.acpm.org/getmedia/fd7b5908-d204-4cc0-af79-028b9440d61f/climate_change.pdf.aspx

American Medical Association (AMA). (2019). *Global climate change and human health H-135.938.* https://policysearch.ama-assn.org/policyfinder/detail/climate%20change?uri=%2FAMADoc%2FHOD.xml-0-309.xml

American Nurses Association (2008). *2008 Resolution: Global climate change.* www.nursingworld.org/~4afb0e/globalassets/practiceandpolicy/work-environment/health--safety/global-climate-change-final.pdf

American Nurses Association. (n.d.). *About ANA.* www.nursingworld.org/ana/about-ana/

American Nurses Association. (2015). *Code of Ethics for nurses with interpretive statements.* www.nursingworld.org/practice-policy/nursing-excellence/ethics/code-of-ethics-for-nurses/coe-view-only/

Bambino, D., Tai, G., Shah, A., Doubeni, C. A., Sia, I. G., & Wieland, M. L. (2021). The disproportionate impact of COVID-19 on racial and ethnic minorities in the United States. *Clinical Infectious Diseases, 72*(4), 703–706. https://doi.org/10.1093/cid/ciaa815

Centers for Disease Control and Prevention. (n.d.). *About chronic diseases.* National Center for Chronic Disease Prevention and Health Promotion. www.cdc.gov/chronicdisease/about/costs/index.htm

Centers for Medicare & Medicaid Services. (n.d.). *National health expenditures 2019 highlights.* www.cms.gov/files/document/highlights.pdf

Dalsania, A. K., Fastiggi, M. J., Kahlam, A., Shah, R., Patel, K., Shiau, S., Rokicki, S., & DallaPiazza, M. (2021). The relationship between social determinants of health and racial disparities in COVID-19 mortality. *Journal of Racial and Ethnic Health Disparities, 1*(5), 1–8. https://doi.org/10.1007/s40615-020-00952-y

Gilbert, H. A. (2020). Florence Nightingale's Environmental Theory and its influence on contemporary infection control. *Collegian Australian College of Nursing, 27,* 626–633/ https://doi.org/10.1016/j.colegn.2020.09.006

Graham, G. N. (2016). Why your ZIP code matters more than your genetic code: Promoting healthy outcomes from mother to child. *Breastfeeding Medicine, 11*(9), 396–397. https://doi.org/10.1089/bfm.2016.0113

Grundy, S. M, Stone, N. J., Bailey, A.L., Beam, C., Birtcher, K. K., Blumenthal, R. S., Braun, L. T., de Ferranti, S., Faiella-Tommasino, J., Forman, D. E., Goldberg, R., Heidenreich, P. A., Hlatky, M. A., Jones, D. W., Lloyd-Jones, D., Lopez-Pajares, N., Ndumele, C. E., Orringer, C. E., Peralta, C. A., Saseen, J. J., Smith, S. C., Jr, Sperling, L., Virani, S. S., & Yeboah, J. (2019). AHA/ACC/AACVPR/AAPA/ABC/ACPM/ADA/AGS/APhA/ASPC/NLA/PCNA guideline on the management of blood cholesterol: a report of the American College of Cardiology/American Heart Association Task Force on Clinical Practice Guidelines. *Journal of the American College of Cardiology, 73,* e285–350. www.jacc.org/doi/full/10.1016/j.jacc.2018.11.003

Healthy Nurse, Healthy Nation Year Four Highlights: 2020–2021. (2021). *American Nurse Journal, 16*(10), 30–31.

Healthy People. (2030). *Objectives and data.* Retrieved November 29, 2021, from https://health.gov/healthypeople/objectives-and-data

Heidke, P., Madsen, W. L., & Langham, E. M. (2020). Registered nurses as role models for healthy lifestyles. *Australian Journal of Advanced Nursing, 37*(2), 11–18. https://doi.org/10.37464/2020.372.65

Hippocrates. (1955). Hippocratic writings. *Encyclopædia Britannica.*

Krishnaswami, J., Sardana, J., & Daxini, A. (2019). Community-engaged lifestyle medicine as a framework for health equity: Principles for lifestyle medicine in low-resource settings. *American Journal of Lifestyle Medicine, 13*(5), 443–450. https://doi.org/10.1177/1559827619838469

Leffers, J., Levy, R. M., Nicholas, P., & Sweeney, C. F. (2017). Mandate for the nursing profession to address climate change through nursing education. *Journal of Nursing Scholarship, 49*(6), 679–687. https://doi.org/10.1111/jnu.12331

National Academy of Medicine. (2021, May). *Recommendations: The future of nursing 2020–2030: Charting a path to achieve health equity.* www.nap.edu/resource/25982/Recommendations_Future%20of%20Nursing_final.pdf

Nightingale, F. (1860). *Notes on nursing: What it is, and what it is not.* Appleton-Century. https://digital.library. upenn.edu/women/nightingale/nursing/nursing.html

Slade-Sawyer, P. (2014). Is health determined by genetic code or zip code? Measuring the health of groups and improving population health. *North Carolina Medical Journal Nov–Dec.*, *75*(6), 394–397. https://doi. org/10.18043/ncm.75.6.394

Thakur, N., Lovinsky-Desir, S., Bime, C. Wisnivesky, J. P., & Celedon, J. C. (2020). The structural and social determinants of the racial/ethnic disparities in the U.S. COVID-19 pandemic. What's our role? *American Journal of Respiratory and Critical Care Medicine*, *202*(7). https://doi.org/10.1164/rccm.202005-1523PP

White, K. M., & O'Sullivan, A. (Eds.). (2012). *The essential guide to nursing practice: Applying ANA's scope and standards in practice and education.* Nursesbooks.org.

Willett, W., Rockstrom, J., Loken, B., Springmann, M., Lang, T., Vermeulen, S., Garnet, T., Tilman, D., DeClerck, F., Wood, A., Joneell, Ml, Clark, M., Gordon, L. J., Fanzo, J., Hawkes, C., Zurayk, R., Rivera, J. A., De Vries, W., Sibanda, L, M., … Murray, C. J. L (2019). Food in the Anthropocene: The EAT-Lancet Commission on healthy diets from sustainable food systems. *The Lancet*, *393*(10170), 447–492. https://doi.org/10.1016/S0140-6736(18)31788-4

World Health Organization. (2021, November 10). *Diabetes.* www.who.int/news-room/fact-sheets/detail/ diabetes

2 Nutrition and Nursing Practice

Deborah Chielli[1], Caroline Trapp[2], Cody Stubbe[3,4],
Tammy Robertson[4,5], and Gia Merlo[6]

[1]Wilkes University, Wilkes-Barre, PA, USA

[2]University of Michigan School of Nursing,
Ann Arbor, MI, USA

Physicians Committee for Responsible Medicine Scientific Advisory
Board

[3]Founder of Wholistic Dish, LLC, Omaha, NE, USA

[4]Physicians Committee for Responsible Medicine's Nurses Nutrition
Network Co-Leader and Certified Food for Life Instructor

[5]Cooking on the Veg Health and Wellness: Founder and Director,
Scottsdale, AZ

[6] NYU Rory Meyers College of Nursing, New York, NY, USA

NYU Grossman School of Medicine, New York, NY, USA

CONTENTS

DOI: 10.1201/9781003178330-3

2.1   WHY IS NUTRITION SO IMPORTANT?

Poor diet has been identified as the leading cause of death for Americans, ahead of tobacco use and high blood pressure (Murray et al., 2018). Diet is relevant to an individual's current state of health and has the ability to mitigate foodborne chronic diseases, such as heart disease, diabetes, and many types of cancer (Shah & Davis, 2020). Box 2.1 is a personal vignette of a nurse's journey.

BOX 2.1   PERSONAL VIGNETTE #1

My first position after graduation from the University of Michigan School of Nursing was on a Med-Surg unit at the Hospital of the University of Pennsylvania. At both of these esteemed institutions, I witnessed first-hand the failures of modern medicine, People with uncontrolled diabetes who needed dialysis or an amputation; patients with advanced colon cancer who had never been taught the importance of consuming foods that contained fiber, and people undergoing their second – or tenth – cardiac catheterization to rule out yet another blockage. Medication and procedures were prescribed, but through a nursing lens, it was easy to see that these were horribly traumatic experiences for the people experiencing these diagnoses.

Fast forward ten years to NP practice, where I specialized in the care of people with type 2 diabetes. Many of us have been taught to inform patients that it's the nature of diabetes to progress and eventually require insulin shots, and that medications are first line in all cases, with diet and exercise as adjuncts. Every continuing education conference and nursing journal emphasized the importance of tight control and avoiding clinical inertia where clinicians failed to titrate up medication. I worked in a primary care medical practice that prided itself on treating diabetes aggressively and getting blood sugars low, but to what end? My patients complained about the high cost of medications, the side effects, the fear of hypoglycemia. Worst of all, even with tight control achieved through medications, I still saw many patients develop life-altering complications– loss of eyesight, strokes, painful neuropathies, and more.

Fast forward another ten years, my clinical practice has been transformed. I'd learned about the power of nutrition, specifically a plant-based dietary pattern. People with diabetes seek me out because I have something to offer beyond more medications. I help patients reduce and even no longer need insulin injections – I see for myself that type 2 diabetes need not progress and, in fact, can be put into remission. My patients are grateful, but they should have been frustrated. What I learned about nutrition was not part of my formal education, though the research is not new. I had to seek it out on my own, and experiment with my patients until I learned how to effectively apply evidence-based nutrition in practice.

Today there is a large and growing community of nurses and other clinicians with expertise in lifestyle medicine, which recognizes plant-based nutrition as the approach that is the most effective. Many colleges of nursing and medicine build this into their curricula. Clinical practice guidelines for many chronic diseases now recommend a plant-rich dietary pattern as a first-line defense. I can't keep up with the many organizations, apps, websites, documentaries, and cookbooks providing everything from scientific studies, to comprehensive looks at the history and present state of things, to cooking demos and recipes. All of this and more, that 20 years ago, when I first began my journey, I had to work so hard to find.

Of all of the tools in my Nursing toolbox, nutrition interventions have proven to be the most powerful and the most gratifying.

Caroline Trapp, DNP, ANP-BC, CDCES, DipACLM, FAANP

2.1.1 The Burden of Chronic Disease, Non-Communicable Disease (NCD)

America has the most expensive healthcare system, yet comes in last when ranked against six comparable industrialized nations on multiple metrics including quality of life, access to care and health equity (Schneider et al., 2014). Taking a global view on the cause of death paints another important picture. According to the Global Burden of Disease (GBD) report, three-quarters of global deaths are caused by non-communicable diseases (NCD). While "suboptimal diet" is the number one cause of mortality, greater than all other risk factors including smoking, and is a factor across age, sex, and sociodemographic groups. Remarkably, though specific dietary features differ from country to country, over half of deaths and nearly two-thirds of Disability-Adjusted Life Years (DALYs) linked to diet are attributable to three nutrient groups: Suboptimal consumption of fruits, whole grains, and above-optimal intake of sodium (GBD, 2017). Seven of the ten leading causes of death in the United States are chronic diseases, and almost half of Americans live with at least one chronic disease (Murphy et al., 2020). The Academy of Nutrition and Dietetics in 2013 released a position statement stressing the role of nutrition in chronic disease prevention. The statement emphasizes the importance of beginning the prevention of disease early in life to improve health and reduce healthcare costs. It also discusses the central role that nutrition plays in obesity prevention, in addition to secondary and tertiary prevention of disease (Slawson, 2013).

2.1.2 History of Nutrition in Nursing Practice and Education

Nutrition plays a historic role in nursing. In the words of Florence Nightingale, "the most important office of the nurse, after she has taken care of the patient's air, is to take care to observe the effect of his food" (Nightingale, 1859, pp. 42–43). The first nurses were instructed in food preparation and service (Englert, Crocker, and Stotts, 1986). In the early 1900s, nutrition education for nurses expanded to include principles of nutrition and diet, culminating in 100 hours of instruction taught over three years (Hassenplug, 1960). Soon thereafter, the advent of the dietetics profession shifted nurses away from food preparation responsibilities. The period from 1950 to 1970 saw a transition from separate nutrition courses totaling about 65 classroom hours, to content that was integrated into classes throughout programs, as nursing's focus became more holistic and other academic content requirements emerged.

In 1956, many State Boards of Nursing dropped the requirement for a specific number of hours devoted to nutrition (Leitch, 1956), though nutrition was and continues to be tested on licensure exams for registered nurses (DiMaria-Ghalili et al., 2014). Topics tested include nutrition assessment and monitoring, diet therapy and enteral and parenteral nutrition, and patient education and counseling (National Council of State Boards of Nursing, 2019).

Currently, nurses have a two-fold interest in nutrition for their patients and for themselves. For patients, good nutrition promotes optimal growth and development plus freedom from diet-related diseases. As discussed in Chapter 9, chronic diseases are a public health concern for nurses as well as patients. Good nutrition is likewise critical to nurses' health and well-being. The Code (2015) states "duty to self," and further, in Provision 5, that "nurses should eat a healthy diet" (ANA, 2015, p. 19).

Nutrition science continues to evolve, as detailed in the next section, and it is important that nurses have the most up-to-date information and the skills to analyze and translate nutrition science into patient care and education. There are many lenses through which to approach diet and nutrition. This chapter focuses on optimal nutrition as a key role in all four of the Spheres of Care identified by the American Association of Colleges of Nursing: Wellness and Disease Prevention, Chronic Disease Management, Regenerative/Restorative Care, and Hospice/ Palliative Care (AACN, 2021).

2.2 THE SCIENCE OF NUTRITION

2.2.1 TREAT THE CAUSE

Many of us were taught that there is one diet for patients with heart disease (low-fat), another for diabetes (low-sugar), and yet another for certain types of cancer (high-fiber). This long-standing thinking has made the task of nutritional counseling complicated and often riddled with misinformation. Multiple studies have demonstrated that a specific healthful diet can effectively reduce risk of key chronic diseases. A landmark study in Germany, the European Prospective Investigation Into Cancer and Nutrition-Potsdam (Ford et al., 2009), found that four healthy lifestyle patterns were correlated with a significant reduction in risk of key chronic diseases, including the number one and number two causes of death, cardiovascular disease and cancer, as well as diabetes. The incidence of these chronic diseases, according to the GBD (Vos et al., 2017; Liu et al., 2020), increased by 102.9% in the 17 years from 1990 to 2017. The four healthy lifestyle factors were diet (high fruit, vegetable, whole-grain bread, and low meat), physical activity (3½ hours/week), not being obese (BMI lower than 30), and not having smoked. In fact, a dose–response relationship showed that the greater the number of an individual's healthy lifestyle factors, the lower the risk of developing one of these major chronic diseases (Ford et al., 2009).

2.2.1.1 Inflammation

Key scientific discoveries in the etiology and pathophysiology of a wide array of leading mental and physical conditions across the globe have been made possible by two decades of scientific advancements, which demonstrate a connection between a myriad of conditions and the inflammatory process and immune system. The science has come so far as to show that more than half of all deaths can now be attributed to "inflammation-related diseases such as ischemic heart disease, stroke, cancer, diabetes mellitus, chronic kidney disease, non-alcoholic fatty liver disease (NAFLD) and auto-immune and neurodegenerative conditions" (Furman et al., 2019, p. 1822). In the setting of an acute injury or infection, a natural inflammatory response occurs as the first stage in the healing process, then normally resolves. However, systemic chronic activation (SCI), although sharing some of the same processes, is "low-grade and persistent … and ultimately causes collateral damage to tissues and organs over time, such as by inducing oxidative stress" (Furman et al., 2019, p. 1823). In multiple studies examined for this report, a diet low in plant foods, fiber, and prebiotics, along with other Western lifestyle factors, correlates with SCI, and "this body of research provides converging evidence that SCI is associated with increased risk for developing a variety of chronic diseases that dominate present-day morbidity and mortality worldwide" (Furman et al., 2019, pp. 1827–1828).

These underlying biological mechanisms, including chronic inflammation, oxidative stress, immune system dysfunction, gene expression, the microbiome, and others all respond to a single, unified dietary approach, as described below.

2.2.2 Optimal Nutrition

It was T. Colin Campbell, Professor Emeritus at Cornell University, who first used the term "whole food plant-based" (WFPB) to refer to a dietary pattern of fruits, vegetables, potatoes, whole grains, legumes, nuts, and seeds that promote health, while limiting or avoiding highly processed foods and animal products – foods proven to cause harm over time, and described in the research below (Campbell & Jacobson, 2013). A whole food, plant-based dietary pattern is likewise encouraged by Ornish (2019) in his Unifying Theory as the dietary approach, with modifications for patient preferences for preventing, treating, and oftentimes reversing numerous diet-related chronic diseases. The American College of Lifestyle Medicine's (ACLM) Plate Graphic (see Figure 2.1) illustrates a whole food, plant-based eating plan. ACLM recommends eating a wide variety of nutrient-dense, antioxidant-rich, minimally processed, and fiber-filled whole plant foods at every meal (Frates et al., 2021). A WFPB dietary pattern optimizes the intake of fruits and vegetables and minimizes fat intake (Kelly, Karlsen, and Stenke, 2020). According to the Academy of Nutrition and Dietetics, a well-planned plant-based diet, free from animal products, is "appropriate for all stages of the life cycle, including pregnancy, lactation, infancy, childhood, adolescence, older adulthood and for athletes" (2016, p. 1970).

2.2.3 What Are Americans Eating?

This WFPB dietary pattern stands in sharp contrast to the typical diet of Americans and, unfortunately, of many nurses. Less than 3% of Americans who participated in the National Health and Nutrition Examination Study (NHANES) achieved a score above 60% on the Healthy Eating Index, a standardized assessment of overall diet quality (Loprinzi et al., 2016). The most common dietary

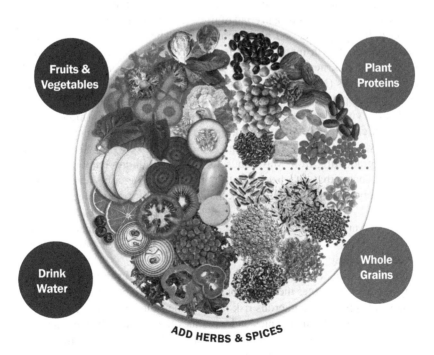

FIGURE 2.1 Whole food, plant based (WFPB) plate consisting of a variety of minimally processed vegetables, fruits, whole grains, legumes, nuts, and seeds with water

pattern in the U.S. is a diet that is high in fat and sugar and low in fiber, and is often referred to as the Standard American Diet, or "SAD."

A study by Huth et al. (2013) reports that the majority of calories come from baked sweets and bread, soft drinks, beef, snacks such as chips, cheese, milk, candy, poultry, and alcoholic beverages; together, these unhealthy, unnecessary foods account for an average of more than 51% of total daily calories. Serial data analysis from the NHANES surveys from 1990 to 2016 found that poor diet quality is observed across all age, sex, race-ethnicity, and income subgroups (Liu et al., 2020).

2.2.4 Research Support

2.2.4.1 Nurses' Health Study

Two of the largest prospective studies ever completed on non-communicable diseases in women, and the risk factors for these diseases, are the Nurses' Health Study (NHS) followed by the Nurses' Health Study II (NHS II). According to the study's website, the former Secretary of the U.S. Department of Health and Human Services Donna Shalala called the NHS "one of the most significant studies ever conducted on the health of women" (NHS, n.d.). The NHS was initially conceived by Frank Speizer in 1976 to focus on the study of smoking, heart disease, and the long-term effects of the oral birth control pills being prescribed to millions of women. The researchers selected a study population of nurses specifically for their health education and competence in fully and accurately completing the detailed medical questionnaires. In 2016, the NHS celebrated 40 years, with 275,000 participants and counting. The third-generation study had already been launched in 2010 and was underway by the time of the study's 40th anniversary. This is the Nurses' Health Study 3 (NHS3), which has as a goal inclusion of a greater diversity of nurses, including those of more diverse ethnic backgrounds, male nurses, LPNs, LVNs, and nurses from Canada, ages 19–46.

In an article titled "Nurses' Health Study: Nurses Helping Science and Themselves," Nelson (2000) applauds the hundreds of thousands of nurses who have faithfully contributed over many years, filling out detailed surveys on a myriad of lifestyle factors and medical conditions, including diet and exercise, hormone use, and health conditions. These combined efforts over more than four decades have resulted in many hundreds of articles, a vast wealth of research that is still being mined; with NHS3, new demographic groups and metrics are being researched with the next generation of nurses (Nelson, 2000). One of the exceptional qualities of the Nurses' Health Study versus other population studies, notes Nelson (2000), is that questionnaires are every two years, which is vital when tracking diet, other health practices, hormones, and other health measurements that change across time. And, importantly, notes the author, "the commitment of nurses is legendary." One subject, Lois Breen, RN of Pittsfield, MA, who was asked to participate in 1976 after graduating from Massachusetts General Nursing School, is an example of this commitment. Lois shares that "it's been great to feel that you've contributed a little bit to something. I will definitely keep on doing it. I think that everyone who does it feels very strongly about it" (Nelson 2000).

According to Harvard's JoAnn E. Manson, "The overall message is that heredity isn't destiny. We largely control our risk of these major diseases through our lifestyle practices. The findings are really striking to us" (Nelson, 2000).

Epidemiologist Louise Brinton of the National Cancer Institute's Division of Cancer Epidemiology and Genetics notes the exceptionality of the foresight of the researchers starting this study years ago and appraising numerous risk factors. She states that over time the study has been adapted to continue to address new topics and continues to provide valuable outcomes and opportunities (Nelson, 2000). Harvard epidemiologist Graham Colditz (2016), Principal Investigator in the ongoing NHS, authored a study evaluating the impact of the previous 40 years of studies – NHS, NHS II, and NHS3 – from 1976 through 2016. Combined, this work has "demonstrated the public health impact and potential for prevention by summarizing evidence on risk factors. Approximately

90% of type 2 diabetes cases may be prevented by diet and lifestyle modifications alone," while approximately 80% of CHD is preventable with a healthy diet, 30 minutes of moderate physical activity most days of the week, moderation in alcohol (½–1 drink/day), and avoiding smoking. Additional findings are numerous and direct in their correlation. Breast cancer risk is linked to alcohol even at low levels of consumption. Teenage red meat consumption increases risk, while high fiber and fruit among adolescents decrease risk. For neurologic function and diseases, higher levels of cognitive functioning are related to higher intake of nuts, antioxidants, and following the plant-rich Mediterranean eating pattern. With regard to nutrition alone, the NHS studies have confirmed that the greatest risk factor for type 2 diabetes is excess adipose tissue, while weight across the life-span and obesity strongly associate with heart disease, numerous cancers, multiple sclerosis, kidney stones, and eye and skin conditions (Colditz, 2016).

The vast sum of epidemiological evidence from NHS and NHS2, combined with the Health Professionals' Follow-Up Study, convincingly demonstrates that a healthy diet, regular physical activity, moderation in alcohol, avoiding prolonged sitting and smoking, and maintaining a healthy weight can and would prevent most type 2 diabetes (Korat, et al., 2014)

2.2.4.2 Adventist Health Studies

As of this writing, there have been five Adventist Health Studies, based out of Loma Linda, CA; starting in 1958, these studies have looked at connections between lifestyle, particularly diet, and various diseases among members of the Seventh-Day Adventist church. This Christian community fosters healthy lifestyle behaviors, including abstaining from tobacco and alcohol and eating a vegetarian diet. These similarities across the population lower the likelihood of the confounding factors commonly found in other study cohorts (Loma Linda University Health, n.d.). Numerous papers continue to emerge from the ongoing Adventist Health Studies.

A study by Miles et al. (2019) notes that the impact of this dietary pattern is not only the absence of dietary elements from meat and/or dairy but also, importantly, the favorable effects of higher consumption of plant foods, with the associated increased levels of fiber, phytochemicals, and other beneficial compounds, that result in improved outcomes. According to the study, vegetarian diets are correlated with lower rates of diabetes, metabolic syndrome, colon cancer, and other cancers and manifest in improved waist circumference, blood pressure, blood sugar, serum fatty acid profiles, and triglycerides. Specific plant compounds and health correlations include serum carotenoids, and urine flavonoids perform anti-inflammatory and antioxidant roles, "neutralizing free radicals and protecting against cell damage and chronic diseases" (Miles et al., 2019). Isoflavones from soy and lignans from a wide variety of plant foods are protective against cancer, cardiovascular disease, and other chronic conditions (Miles et al., 2019).

Azemati et al. (2017) examined types of protein in relation to insulin resistance, which is a significant predictor of type 2 diabetes and an independent risk factor for heart disease, and found a direct correlation for animal protein increasing the risk of type 2 diabetes. Notably, vegetarian diets reduced the risk of diabetes, with the incidence lowest among vegans versus vegetarians and nonvegetarians (Azemati et al., 2017).

This association was also noted in an analysis by Le and Sabate (2014) demonstrating that vegetarian eating patterns are protective for cardiovascular disease, cardiometabolic risk factors, some cancers, and total mortality. The authors also found vegan eating patterns provide a further reduction in risk against type 2 diabetes, obesity, hypertension, and death from cardiovascular disease (Le & Sabate, 2014). Protein-based factor analysis by Tharrey et al. (2018) showed that elevated levels of protein from meat increased risk of CVD mortality, while consumption of protein from nuts and seeds is protective.

It has been demonstrated that, on average, it takes ten years for research to impact clinical practice (Morris, Wooding & Grant, 2011). Nurses are called on to disseminate nutrition research and engage patients and colleagues with this life-saving information. An annotated list of additional key studies that highlight the many benefits of a plant-based dietary pattern across disease states for prevention and treatment are provided in the supplement section of the chapter.

2.2.5 COVID-19 AND OPTIMAL NUTRITION

At the time of this writing, it is anticipated that the SARS-CoV-2 novel coronavirus and emerging variants will continue to put many people at risk for developing the acute respiratory tract infection COVID-19 (Fontanet et al., 2021), which was declared a pandemic by the WHO on March 11, 2020. Underlying medical conditions, including hypertension, type 2 diabetes, cardiovascular disease, and obesity, have been shown to increase the risk of severe outcomes from COVID-19. Public health recommendations have focused on vaccinations, personal protective equipment, social distancing, and handwashing, but have so far largely missed an opportunity to concurrently or prophylactically prescribe diet and lifestyle to treat underlying conditions and potentially mitigate COVID-19's impact.

Nutritional factors have been shown to benefit innate and adaptive immunity to viral diseases (Calder et al., 2020). A 2021 study looked at the dietary patterns of at-risk physicians and nurses with high rates of exposure in six countries, including the United States, and concluded that individuals who reported following a plant-based diet and plant-based or pescatarian diets that were higher in vegetables, legumes, and nuts and lower in poultry, red, and processed meats had 73% (OR 0.27, 95% CI 0.10 to 0.81) and 59% (OR 0.41, 95% CI 0.17 to 0.99) lower odds of moderate to severe COVID-19, respectively (Kim et al., 2021). These research findings are significant because this research is the first of its kind to report correlation between diet pattern quality and COVID-19 severity.

2.2.6 DIET PATTERNS – HOW ARE THEY DIFFERENT?

Extensive scientific evidence supports the use of a WFPB dietary pattern for the prevention and treatment of diet-related chronic diseases. Mediterranean (Becerra-Tomás et al., 2019) and vegetarian (Parker and Vadiveloo, 2019) diets are similar to WFPB, and when they most closely mimic WFPB, their health benefits increase (Clarys et al., 2014).

Dietary patterns centered around plants, which are nutrient-dense and rich in antioxidants, also reduce or eliminate exposure to dietary toxins such as saturated fat and cholesterol oxidation products. WFPB is the only dietary pattern proven to reverse heart disease (Ornish et al., 1990), the leading cause of death in the U.S. (Kochanek et al., 2019). On the other end of the dietary spectrum are animal-based diets, which may be classified as low-carbohydrate dietary patterns.

While there are definitely benefits to reducing carbohydrates from refined flour and sugar, there is harm in excluding or limiting carbohydrates found in fruits, vegetables, and whole grains. A meta-analysis of low-carb diets found mortality increased by 32% (Seidelmann et al., 2018). This is due to the bulk of the calories in these diets being from meat. Boxes 2.2 and 2.3 describe different diets. Nurses will want to be conversant in these dietary patterns and, in addition, will benefit personally and professionally from becoming familiar with the science, in order to utilize it, act as role models for it, and translate the science into patient-friendly education.

BOX 2.2   PLANT-PREDOMINANT (PLANT BASED) DIETARY PATTERNS

Whole Food Plant-Based (WFPB): Typically defined in the literature as a diet that emphasizes whole, plant-based, unrefined, unprocessed foods and limits/excludes meat, dairy, and eggs (Tuso et al. 2013).

   Mediterranean: Whole grains, fruits, vegetables, seeds, olive oil, beans, nuts, legumes, fish/seafood, poultry, eggs, dairy (cheese/yogurts), minimal other meats and sweets, and moderate wine (Clegg & Hill Gallant, 2019). Mediterranean diets that are the most health-promoting emphasize plants.

Blue Zones: Vegetables, fruits, grains, and legumes make up as much as 95% of the diet of five places around the world with the longest-living (100 years), healthiest populations (Buettner & Skemp).

DASH diet: This includes whole grains, vegetables, fruits, low fat/non-fat dairy, lean meats, poultry and fish, nuts/seeds/dry beans, fats/oils, and sweets (Clegg & Hill Gallant, 2019). Developed to treat hypertension.

Other dietary patterns include:

- **Vegetarian:** No animal products except for dairy products and eggs.
- **Vegan:** No animal products. Usually for ethical reasons (for the animals and environment) but not necessarily a healthy dietary pattern (for example, Oreos are vegan but not a healthy food).
- **Raw food, vegan diet:** Has the same exclusions as veganism as well as the exclusion of all foods cooked at temperatures greater than 118°F.
- **Lacto-vegetarian:** Excludes eggs, meat, seafood, and poultry and includes milk products.
- **Ovo-vegetarian:** Excludes meat, seafood, poultry, and dairy products and includes eggs.
- **Lacto-ovo vegetarian:** Excludes meat, seafood, and poultry and includes eggs and dairy products.

BOX 2.3   ANIMAL-BASED DIETS

A **paleo** dietary pattern (Katz and Meller, 2014) includes high intake of red/white meat, eggs, nuts, seeds, green vegetables, limited starchy vegetables, and moderate fruit, fats, and oils. Excludes legumes, grains, and dairy. Caloric breakdown: 50% fat, 30% protein, and 20% carbohydrate. Short-term gains from excluding fast foods, fried foods, processed meat, refined grain, refined sugar, concentrated fats and oils, high-fat dairy products, and alcohol. High meat diet results in high consumption of agrochemicals, endotoxins, environmental contaminants, heme iron, which is linked to insulin resistance, products of oxidation, saturated fat, and cholesterol and may up-regulate cancer-promoting genes.

A **keto** dietary pattern (Crosby et al., 2021) includes high amounts of red and white meat/poultry/fish/eggs, very high concentrated fats/oils/cheese, and very limited vegetables and fruits. Fat makes up 75% or more of calories, and up to 20% calories come from protein and 5% calories from carbohydrates. Excluded are: legumes, grains, and starchy vegetables. Reduces seizure frequency in some individuals and short-term reduction in blood sugar and weight. Found to lower bone mineral density, raise LDL-C, increase risk of having a child born with neural tube defect, and increase risk of cardiovascular disease and arrhythmias, diabetes, cancer, CKD, and Alzheimer's disease.

2.2.7   DIETARY RECOMMENDATIONS – A MATTER OF DEGREE AND DENSITY

A whole food plant-based dietary pattern is effective because it optimizes nutrient-dense foods while limiting or avoiding problematic foods. While there are benefits to every degree of improvement in dietary choices, i.e. whole-fruit topped oatmeal in place of a McDonalds' McMuffin for breakfast in the morning, the adage "all things in moderation" turns out to be poor nutrition advice.

As Michael Greger likes to say, "moderate changes in diet can leave one with moderate blindness, moderate kidney failure, and moderate amputations" (Greger, 2016). Just as medications are given in specific doses, the degree of diet change when optimally dosed is most effective. As demonstrated in previously noted NHS and Adventist Health Studies, a more intensive degree of dietary change (e.g. WFPB pattern) will be more effective than moderate changes. This is described in detail in the ACLM position paper "Type 2 Diabetes: Remission and Lifestyle Medicine" (Kelly, Karlsen, and Steinke, 2020).

The Executive Summary of the updated Dietary Guidelines for Americans 2020–2025 states that

> the scientific connection between food and health has been well documented for many decades, with substantial and increasingly robust evidence showing that a healthy lifestyle – including following a healthy dietary pattern-can help people achieve and maintain good health and reduce the risk of chronic diseases throughout all stages of the lifespan ... the core elements of a healthy dietary pattern are remarkably consistent across the lifespan and across health outcomes.
>
> (p. vii)

Importantly, the latest edition reflects a shift in three areas based on the evolved science: 1) today over 50% of adults have one or more chronic diseases linked to poor diet; therefore, the guidelines are based on the premise that nearly every American can benefit from moving to healthier dietary patterns; 2) there is new appreciation for the fact that people eat foods and not distinct nutrients, so guidance is based on following healthy dietary patterns as a whole; and 3) with a recognition of nutrition and healthy eating across the entire life of a person, the guidelines speak to this, beginning for the first time with guidance for infants and toddlers (Dietary Guidelines, 2020–2025).

The DGA four fundamental recommendations can be summarized as 1) follow a healthy dietary pattern across the lifespan; 2) consume nutrient-dense foods and beverage customized per culture, taste, and budget; 3) focus on nutrient-dense foods and beverages within calorie needs and balance; and 4) limit those items that are higher in added saturated fat, sodium, and sugar, and limit alcohol (DGA, 2020–2025). The DGA describes optimizing to a high degree a dietary pattern that is high in nutrient density and staying within healthy calorie limits.

How is nutrient density defined? Nutrient density, according to the DGA 2020–2025, refers to food products high in "vitamins, minerals, and other health-promoting components" with minimum added saturated fat, sodium, and sugar. Of importance is the fact that adequately and accurately defining the terms nutrient dense and nutrient density to reflect the science and to be usable by the public is a topic of interest and concern. Nutrient-dense, according to the National Cancer Institute (cancer.gov) is "food that is high in nutrients but relatively low in calories. Nutrient-dense foods contain vitamins, minerals, complex carbohydrates, lean protein, and healthy fats." This is discussed in more detail in Chapter 20 of this volume.

The European Food Information Council (EUFIC) recommends scoring foods for nutrient density based on the amount of specific nutrients per calorie or serving, otherwise known as nutrient profiling. The non-profit is focused on generating evidence-based recommendations that can empower and inform the dietary choices of the citizens of Europe (EUFIC, 2021).

Drewnowski et al. (2019) proposes a hybrid nutrient density scoring system that factors in one of the nutrient-rich food (NRF) models, which scores foods based on three nutrients to limit (saturated fat, sugar, sodium) per 100 kcal along, then factors in considerations for DG- recommended food groups such as those specifically called out in the guidelines, including whole grains, whole fruits, nuts, and green leafy vegetables. This creates a more useful and guideline-based hybrid according to the study and the illustrations provided. For example, in a comparison of white rice and brown rice, based on NRF alone, the two versions have close scores of 5 and 3, but when placed in the hybrid model, which accounts for food categories and patterns encouraged in the DGA, such as whole grains, the brown rice comes out at 38 while the white rice remains a 3 (Drewnowski et al., 2019).

There are challenges and opportunities to the "nutrient density approach to healthy eating"; Nicklas et al. (2014) note that although nutrient-dense foods are "widely recommended," an agreed-upon definition has not yet been developed, and there is much to be done in both defining and applying the term nutrient density. The paper highlights the potential of this as a tool for the public to use of, to make it easier and clearer for the public to make healthier food choices (Nicklas et al., 2014).

Energy density and nutrient density are two different concepts that are often used when discussing food quality. Energy density is also commonly referred to as calorie density, which is defined as the calories per gram of food and beverage in the diet. While following an energy density approach to food quality, it is very possible to easily consume high calorie-density food like alcohol and fatty foods. Nutrient density is defined as nutrients per unit. Nutrient density conceptualizes the food energy provided, ensuring that food nutrient and energy needs are met. The SAD is noted to be energy-rich and nutrient poor. The 2020 dietary guidelines suggest focusing on a nutrient-dense diet. There is conflicting literature on these definitions and parameters; nevertheless, a naturally nutrient-rich NNR score has been developed to address the mean percentage daily values (DVs) for 14 nutrients based on a 2000 kcal diet (Drewnowski, 2005). The current food and nutrition labeling guidelines and policies have yet to use NNR scores. Overall, it is clear that approximately 15% of Americans meet the healthy index criteria for a healthy diet. Additionally, over 20 million Americans live in food deserts where there is limited access to whole, plant-based nutritious food.

Micronutrients such as vitamins and minerals, along with many other phytochemicals, are needed in adequate amounts in order to achieve health. Joel Fuhrman developed the following formula to show how health is related to nutrient density of consumed food (Fuhrman, 2017):

H= N/C (Health = Nutrients/Calories)

The Aggregate Nutrient Density Index (ANDI) was developed by Fuhrman (2017) to rank nutrient density among common foods, based on how many nutrients each delivers to the body for each calorie consumed. The highest ranking, with a score of 1000, are cruciferous leafy greens such as kale, collard greens, mustard greens, and watercress. Some of the lowest rankings include items such as low-fat plain yogurt (28), chicken breast (24), beef (21), feta cheese (20), olive oil (10), white bread (9), and cola (1). Eating foods that are listed towards the top of the ANDI provides the most nutrient-dense calories. Eating a variety of these top-scorers provides micronutrient diversity, another consideration for achieving and sustaining good health (Fuhrman, 2017).

2.3 THE ESSENTIALS AND COMPETENCY-BASED EDUCATION

The foundations of the practice of lifestyle medicine for nurses at all educational levels align seamlessly with The Essentials (2021), grounded in competency-based education. According to The Essentials (AACN, 2021, p. 4), "competency-based education encourages conscious connections between knowledge and action", and the 10 Domains of Competency provide the education required for a nurse to be competent and prepared for practicing now and in the future. Importantly, competence is described as "progressive," developing across time, and reflective of both "internal and external factors and experiences of the student" (p. 15). The sub-competency levels correlate with the educational levels of nurses, and likewise there are corresponding levels and means for translation and implementation of lifestyle medicine principles in nursing practice, appropriately based upon a nurse's education and scope of practice. The Domains of Competence provide a nursing practice framework (AACN, 2021) and, likewise, a structure for interpreting and integrating the principles of lifestyle medicine at all levels of nursing education and practice.

Domain 1: Knowledge for Nursing Practice

- This Domain of Competence integrates, translates, and applies nursing knowledge and "unique ways of knowing" to that of other disciplines. We need look no further than the founder of modern nursing, Florence Nightingale, and her Environmental Theory, to appreciate the breadth of application and synergy between nursing and the tenets of lifestyle medicine.
- Nightingale's Environmental Theory calls for nurses to place the individual in the "best possible conditions for nature to restore or to preserve health" (Hegge, 2013).
- According to the ACLM, core competencies include "helping individuals and families adopt and sustain healthy behaviors that affect health and quality of life" (ACLM, n.d.).

Domain 2: Person-Centered Care

- This Domain of Competence relates to "person-centered care," centering on the individual in all of their contexts and noting that person-centered care is by its very nature, "holistic, individualized, just, respectful, compassionate, coordinated, evidence-based, and developmentally appropriate" (AACN, 2021).
- Lifestyle medicine is, in its very definition, "person-centered care." It is "the evidence-based practice of helping individuals and families adopt and sustain healthy behaviors that affect health and quality of life" (ACLM, n.d.).
- The person-centered LM competencies include that of assessment, specifically, to "assess the social, psychological and biological predispositions of patients' behaviors and the resulting health outcomes" and "patient and family readiness, willingness, and ability to make health behavior changes" (ACLM, n.d.).

Domain 3: Population Health

- This Domain of Competence speaks to population health across the healthcare system and emphasizes the vital role of leveraging partnerships, both traditional and non-traditional, in order to achieve more equitable health outcomes, particularly in disadvantaged communities (AACN, 2021).
- Here, too, Vodovotz et al. (2020) speaks to the worldview of lifestyle medicine and echoes the principles of Domain 3. The authors call out the "need to move beyond framing individual lifestyle behaviors as only personal 'choices' toward using an integrated model of socio-ecological influences on health, within which clinical application of lifestyle medicine is a foundational best practice component." The authors point to the fact that each patient, and every family, resides in and is impacted by overlapping environments, including air and water, housing and employment, education and community, and so human health and that of the broader environment are inextricably interrelated (Vodovotz et al., 2020).

Domain 4: Scholarship for Nursing Discipline

- This Domain of Competence speaks to the "generation, synthesis, translation, application, and dissemination of nursing knowledge to improve health and transform health care" (AACN, 2021).
- Lifestyle medicine competencies parallel Domain 4 and call for assisting patients in their lifestyle and health behavior self-management through utilization of practice guidelines that are nationally recognized (ACLM, n.d.).
- Echoing the intent of Domain 4, Benigas (2020) notes that at least 80% of all healthcare costs are related to treating ill health and disease caused by poor and often uninformed

choices in daily life, whether dietary or otherwise. Therefore, treatment must evolve and transform toward a lifestyle-based model that pinpoints and addresses these fundamental root causes. The author notes in parallel that patients likewise have the right to be fully informed of their options to utilize lifestyle medicine options to prevent, treat, and often reverse their disease (Benigas, 2020).

- The authors of Vodovotz et al. (2020) critique a absence in application of the science to improve human health, in a review of the recent U.S. National Institutes of Health (NIH) Prevention Research Portfolio, which indicates there are fundamentally no federal research projects dedicated to the study of lifestyle as an intervention for the treatment of the root causes of these chronic diseases, despite the overwhelming evidence for this being the number one cause of major chronic conditions in Americans (Vodovotz et al., 2020).

Domain 5: Quality and Safety

- This Domain of Competence highlights the core value to "enhance quality and minimize risk of harm through both system effectiveness and individual performance" (AACN, 2021).
- If, as the science clearly shows, the major causes of morbidity and mortality are lifestyle-related factors, particularly diet related, and if the treatment and interventions do not match the evidence, then there appears to be risk of harm, particularly in the data discussed thus far, in relation to the major causes of disease and death being lifestyle related. According to Kris-Etherton et al. (2015, p. 83), "most health care professionals are not adequately trained to address diet and nutrition-related issues with their patients, thus missing important opportunities to ameliorate chronic diseases and improve outcomes." This article appears not in the *American Journal of Lifestyle Medicine* but rather as an Annual Meeting Symposium Summary in the journal *Advances in Nutrition* (2015). It is actually very good news that an a priori in quality and safety for nurse domain competencies is the update, practice, and dissemination of the fundamentals of healthy dietary patterns for the prevention, treatment, and often reversal of conditions, where the prescription for the APRN and the health promotion guidance for BSN is education on food and lifestyle factors and resources for treating root causes of disease for patients and for the nurse herself (Kris-Etherton et al., 2015).

Domain 6: Interprofessional Partnerships

- This Domain of Competence speaks to the importance of collaboration across all spheres in order to "optimize care, enhance the healthcare experience, and strengthen outcomes" (AACN, 2021).
- The Lifestyle Medicine Competency of Management Skills could not be clearer in echoing the importance of relationships and collaboration. It is worth quoting here, to "establish effective relationships with patients and families to effect and sustain behavioral change using evidence-based counseling methods and tools and follow up," to "collaborate with patients and their families to develop evidence-based, achievable, specific, written action plans such as lifestyle prescriptions," and to "help patients manage and sustain healthy lifestyle practices, and refer patients to other health care professionals as needed for lifestyle-related conditions" (ACLM, n.d.).
- The LM Competence in Use of Office Equipment and Community Support additionally calls for LM professionals to leverage many tools, including to "have the ability to practice in an interdisciplinary team of health care providers and support a team approach" and to "use appropriate community referral resources that support the implementation of healthy lifestyles" (ACLM, n.d.).

Domain 7: Systems-Based Practice

- This Domain of Competence addresses the complexity of healthcare systems and its intersection with the need to proactively and successfully coordinate optimal care to a diverse group of patients.
- Vodovotz et al. (2020) once more describe the lifestyle medicine corollary to a nursing Domain of Competence, noting the complexity of diverse populations and factors affecting patient health and observing that in order to provide optimal care, all lifestyle and environmental factors are key to providing optimal care. It is worth quoting that "declining life expectancy and increasing all-cause mortality in the United States have been associated with unhealthy behaviors, socio-ecological factors, and preventable disease" (Vodovotz et al., para. 1).

Domain 8: Informatics and Healthcare Technologies

- This Domain of Competence acknowledges that "information and communication technologies and informatics processes are used to provide care, gather data, form information to drive decision making, and support professionals as they expand knowledge and wisdom for practice" (AACN, 2021, p. 11). Technology can be harnessed for the good of our patients.
- Here, too, lifestyle medicine competencies parallel that of the nursing Essentials. This is spelled out in the Competency Use of Office and Community Support, which calls on lifestyle medicine professionals to "develop and apply office systems and practices to support lifestyle medical care including decision support technology" and to "measure processes and outcomes to improve quality of lifestyle interventions in individuals and groups of patients" (ACLM, n.d.).
- In fact, lifestyle medicine is innovating and advocating not only for EMRs that collect and measure lifestyle-related data points and interventions but also for patient education and empowerment.
- According to the Health Information National Trends Survey, nearly half of adults went online first to obtain information on cancer versus approximately one in ten who contacted their physician first. Today, the evidence points to the value of digital health technology for educating patients and aiding in the development of skills and behaviors necessary for healthy lifestyle practices to treat chronic disease (Kuwabara et al., 2019).
- Lianov et al. (2019) describes an "explosion of digital health services and products" that can be an adjunct for health professionals to provide to patients but also it is particularly noteworthy that these tools can serve to bridge some social disparities in health. Article examples included mindfulness exercises and walks in nature and in addition, a myriad of free podcasts, videos, and even education on healthy eating.
- Additionally, Nowson et al. (2020) note the power, growing acceptance by health professionals and patients, and the opportunity imbued in leveraging telehealth for educational classes in cooking and nutrition and other lifestyle health education and care modalities,

Domain 9: Professionalism

- This Domain of Competence calls for the "formation and cultivation of a sustainable professional nursing identity" reflective of nursing's characteristics and values.
- A lifestyle medicine professional's identity, like a nurse's identity, calls for leadership to begin. In LM, this means first developing and manifesting a health-promoting lifestyle

and then serving as a role model and promoter in both practice and in the community (ACLM, n.d.).

Domain 10: Personal, Professional, and Leadership Development

- This Domain of Competence calls for "participation in activities and self-reflection that foster personal health, resilience, and well-being, lifelong learning, and support the acquisition of nursing expertise and assertion of leadership" (AACN, 2021, p. 11).
- In a study on health promotion and well-being, Matranga et al. (2020) found that, as a result of the research and practice of lifestyle medicine, there have been dynamic shifts in what is considered health, with a movement toward the concept of well-being. The researchers found a positive correlation between healthy lifestyles and feelings of well-being. The recommendations, like those of the Essentials Domain 10, call for individual cultivation of practices to support health, self-awareness, and growth.

2.4 NUTRITION AND THE NURSING PROCESS

The nursing process is a core commonality among the many different specialties of nursing. The five parts include assessment, diagnosis, planning, implementation, and evaluation. The process is essential to nursing practice in order to deliver holistic care to the patient and provide the best outcomes. Ackley et al. (2017, p. 10) explain that "typically, nursing care does not involve 'curing' the medical condition causing the symptom" and that usually the interventions focus on symptom management. However, in light of the evidence provided throughout this textbook, reversal of certain medical conditions is within the scope of nursing and should be considered throughout the nursing process.

2.4.1 ASSESSMENT

Nursing assessment is the foundation on which appropriate nursing diagnoses, planning, and interventions are based (Ackley et al., 2017). Assessment includes the collection of subjective and objective data across all dimensional characteristics of the patient: Biophysical, psychological, sociocultural, spiritual, and environmental. (Ackley et al., 2017). When considering lifestyle changes, it is important for the nurse to assess readiness to change. Determining the reason that the patient wants to make the change, the "why," is a useful finding that can help keep the patient on course to reaching her or his goals. The nurse needs to assess from a holistic, patient-centered approach, keeping in mind all of the factors about this individual: location, family, preferences, economic status, resources available, support system, health status, motivational factors, etc., considering existing support and potential barriers. If the patient states a willingness to make changes, then the nurse should work with that patient/family/care team to help make an appropriate goal and provide interventions that will set the patient up to help achieve the goal.

A short nutrition assessment is appropriate in some settings, and a more detailed nutrition assessment is warranted in others. A basic assessment should ask about frequency and quantity of intake of whole and minimally processed plant foods, including vegetables, fruits, whole grains, legumes, and nuts/seeds, as well as intake of animal products, highly processed foods, and added oils.

One of the simplest methods is to ask the question, "what do you eat and drink in a typical day, from the time you wake up until you go to sleep?" This approach will elicit useful information about the number of meals and snacks and the types of foods and beverages the patient likes to eat. Good follow-up questions would be, "how often do you eat out?" and "what do you order?" Questions are asked in a non-judgmental way.

BOX 2.4   EXAMPLES OF NUTRITION ASSESSMENT TOOLS

- 24-Hour Recall – see www.nutritools.org/tools
- Food Diary – see www.cdc.gov/diabetes/prevention/pdf/t2/Handouts-Food_Log.pdf or www.cdc.gov/healthyweight/pdf/food_diary_cdc.pdf
- Food Frequency Questionnaire – https://epi.grants.cancer.gov/dhq3/
- 5-Page Nutrition Assessment from ACLM and Loma Linda University Health (PDF available to members of ACLM at www.lifestylemedicine.org)
- Food Insecurity Screening Toolkit – https://hungerandhealth.feedingamerica.org/resource/food-insecurity-screening-toolkit/

It is estimated that 1 in 9 people in the United States struggle with hunger (Coleman-Jenson et al. 2019). Nurses have a unique opportunity to develop trusting relationships and assess for food insecurity. An assessment tool is linked in Box 2.4. An assessment may reveal a complicated nutrition history or comorbidities requiring special diets, such as eating disorders or thyroid disease. Nurses should seek out and refer patients to registered dietitian nutritionists with expertise in plant-based nutrition.

2.4.2   NURSING DIAGNOSIS

The nurse uses clinical reasoning to identify and prioritize nursing diagnoses – the human responses to actual or potential health problems (Ackley et al. 2017). The North American Nursing Diagnosis Association – International (NANDA-I) sets the standardized nursing diagnostic terminology "to ensure patient safety through evidence-based care, thereby improving the health care of all people" (NANDA International, 2021, para. 4). Diagnoses may be problem focused, a risk, health promoting, a syndrome, or a possibility. Nursing diagnosis can be independently treated by the nurse (Ackley et al., 2017). In Box 2.5, we consider some sample NANDA diagnoses related to human responses to actual or potential problems connected to nutrition.

BOX 2.5   SAMPLE NANDA NUTRITION AND LIFESTYLE DIAGNOSIS

Problem Focused:
- Altered nutrition: Less than body requirements
- Altered nutrition: More than body requirements
- Constipation related to low-fiber diet as evidenced by high intake of animal products and refined grains

Risk Diagnosis:
- At risk for breast cancer related to family history, diet history
- At risk for ovarian cancer
- At risk for colon cancer
- At risk for prostate cancer
- At risk for dementia
- At risk for depression
- At risk for anxiety
- At risk for increase all-cause mortality related to unhealthy dietary pattern

Health Promotion:
- Readiness for enhanced nutrition as evidenced by patient's verbalization of desire to enhance nutrition
- Metabolic syndrome
- Possible knowledge deficiency

Collaborative nursing diagnoses are patient problems that the nurse and other disciplines jointly monitor, plan, and implement patient care (Estes, 2013). NANDA- approved nursing diagnoses that are also medical diagnoses include Constipation, Anxiety, Urinary retention, Nausea, Diarrhea and Bowel Incontinence (Ackley et al., 2017). Based on the evidence supporting nutrition interventions, the following are examples of medical diagnoses could be included as nursing diagnosis:

- Dysbiosis
- Cardiovascular disease
- Type 2 diabetes
- Impaired kidney function (chronic kidney disease).

Considering the body of evidence that exists for the nutrition interventions, its role within the scope of practices of nurses and the public need for this information, additional diagnoses that specify WFPB nutrition should be proposed for NAND-I consideration.

2.4.3 PLANNING

Priorities are set based on Maslow's hierarchy of needs (Ackley et al., 2017). As basic needs are met, patients are able to work towards meeting, for example, esteem needs, such as independence or mastery that would come from nutrition knowledge and application that frees them from management of a chronic disease.

The nurse collaborates with the patient/family and caregiving team to identify the goal that they want to achieve and when would be a realistic time to reach the goal. SMART (Specific, Measurable, Attainable, Realistic, and Timed) goals are used to assist patients to create and achieve behavior change goals (Ackley et al., 2017). A SMART goal related to nutrition would be to "replace breakfast of bacon and eggs with a breakfast of oatmeal, fruit, and nuts five or more days a week." Nurses can assist patients in developing a goal and creating a plan for accountability.

2.4.4 IMPLEMENTATION

The nursing process calls for evidence-based nursing (EBN) (Ackley et al., 2017). Nutrition recommendations supported by peer-reviewed published research and practice guidelines have been presented throughout this chapter and may be used to develop nursing interventions that are appropriate for the patient and will help reach identified goals. Below are some examples of nursing interventions and their rationales.

For the patient with a nursing diagnosis that addresses food intake for a diet-related chronic disease, such as type 2 diabetes, hypertension, kidney disease, or a condition such as obesity or constipation:

- Complete a nutrition assessment to get a baseline on the amount of nutrition coming from whole plant foods and to determine how much fiber the patient is consuming. (Rationale: Fiber helps regulate hormone levels, cholesterol levels, improves bowel regularity.)

- Provide WFPB meals/snacks. (Rationale: WFPB nutrition provides a nutrient dense diet that has been proven to prevent/treat/ reverse…)
- Discourage the consumption of all animal products (meat, eggs, dairy). (Rationale: Animal products contain cholesterol, saturated fat, excess calories, etc.)
- Consult with a dietitian who is knowledgeable about WFPB dietary patterns. (Rationale: Interdisciplinary collaboration can help the patient achieve goals.)
- Educate the patient about eating WFPB. (Rationale: Knowledge is required for behavior change.)
- Provide WFPB resources such as websites, documentaries, or local cooking classes. (Rationale: Print/video/live resources support initiation and maintenance of behavior changes.)
- Provide community resources for patients that live in food desert areas. (Rationale: Access to health-promoting foods is required for improved nutrition status.)

This evidence needs to be incorporated into the new additions of nursing diagnosis handbooks that include the NANDA-approved nursing diagnosis.

2.4.5 EVALUATION

Evaluation is an important part of the nursing process but is especially critical to care plans involving nutrition and behavior change. Follow-up to interventions is planned to determine if goals were met. Interventions and goals may be revised with patients using coaching skills and positive psychology discussed in Chapter 30 and Chapter 6.

2.4.6 CASE SAMPLE – THE NURSING PROCESS WITH NUTRITION

Example of WFPB interventions incorporated in with NANDA-I Nursing Diagnosis:

Assessment data:

This is a 72-year-old male who is active (walks 2 miles 4 times a week) who presents for a routine physical exam. He complains of mild occasional swelling in both ankles and fatigue over the week. This client is a retired science teacher who lives with his spouse. She is in good health and is with him at the visit.

Vitals: BP – 140/64, HR – 72, RR – 18, Temp 98.9, SaO2 – 99%
Medications: Metoprolol 100 mg daily, Omeprazole 20 mg daily
History: Hypertension, GERD
Lab results: GFR of 46 mL/min, creatinine of 1.50 mg/dL, BUN of 25 (indicating chronic kidney disease)

The client and his spouse are surprised by the diagnosis of CKD. Client states he "does not want his kidneys to fail" and wants to know what he can do. Spouse states that she is willing to do whatever it takes to help her husband improve his health.

Nutrition assessment indicates that the patient eats animal protein and drinks 1% dairy milk at each meal; only eats 2 servings of vegetables a day; 1 serving of fruit; 2 servings of refined grains; and no serving of legumes. States he likes beans and ate a lot as a kid. Eats most meals at home. Client also drinks 3 (12 ounce) cans of cola a day and only 8 ounces of water a day. His wife usually does the cooking of the meals and the grocery shopping.

Nursing Diagnoses:

1. Impaired urinary elimination related to decreased renal function as evidenced by glomerular filtration rate (GFR) of 46 mL/min, creatinine of 1.50 mg/dL, and blood urea nitrogen (BUN) of 25, edema, decreased urine output.

Outcome 1: Client will demonstrate improved kidney function by 8 weeks (insert date) by labs of:
- GFR above 60 mL/min
- Creatinine below 1.35 mg/dL
- BUN below 22
- No edema

Outcome 2: Client will increase intake of whole plant foods by 8 weeks (insert date) by:
- Eating 5 servings of vegetables, 3 servings of fruits, and 3 or more servings of whole grains on 5 or more days/week.
- Replacing animal protein with plant protein, such as bean-based soups, stews, casseroles, and salads.
- Eliminating highly processed foods.
- Drinking only water and aiming for 4 or more 8 oz glasses during the daytime.

Interventions:

1. Complete a nutrition assessment to get a baseline on the amount of nutrition coming from whole plant foods.
2. Educate the client and spouse about WFPB eating pattern.
3. Educate the client and spouse about the benefits of WFPB, specifically kidney function benefits and blood pressure benefits.
4. Provide WFPB resources to client and spouse (refer to list below).
5. Provide documentaries about WFPB and disease prevention/reversal.
6. Provide WFPB meals/snacks examples such as pamphlets/magazines that have recipes.
7. Encourage clients and spouses to join WFPB online groups or in person local groups for support.
8. Refer to lifestyle medicine provider or WFPB dietitian.
9. Provide information on cooking/nutrition classes (Food for Life classes).
10. Educate the client on monitoring blood pressure.

Evaluation:

Outcome 1: Client met the goal of having improved kidney function as evidenced by GFR at 81 mL/min, a creatinine at 1.30 mg/dL, and BUN of 15. He has normal urinary elimination and no edema.

Outcome 2: Client met the goal of increasing his intake of whole plant foods and has stated that his GERD and level of energy have greatly improved. He now walks 2 miles every day. His blood pressure has decreased to 124/62 and he has been tapered off of his Metoprolol by his provider.

2.5 CONCLUSION

Nurses have many aspects of the holistic care that they provide to their patients. One of the most important components of care is also one of the most challenging – nutrition. This is due to the changing of professional requirements over time, non-science-based misinformation and a lack of holistic knowledge. Nurses should continue to advocate for our patients and play a key role in treating the body as a whole system, not just as individual diseases. And, as a whole system, when one disease condition begins to improve, others do as well because the body does not selectively heal.

There is a general lack of evidence-based nutrition education for nurses at all levels as well as for healthcare providers in general. Nurses are the largest healthcare professional group in the United

States. And where there is a lack in education, there is opportunity to grow and improve. Nutrition is fundamental in patient care for prevention, arrest, and possible reversal of chronic disease conditions such as cardiovascular disease, stroke, renal disease, certain types of cancers, obesity, and diabetes, to name a few. According to the CDC, 60% of Americans are living with at least one of the afore-mentioned chronic conditions, and these are leading causes of mortality and morbidity in the United States (Centers for Disease Control and Prevention, 2021). Some health experts agree that we are not living longer, but in fact dying longer. Chronic disease can lead to slow and progressive deteri-orating health with unnecessary suffering for patients and their families and loved ones. Fortunately, when armed with evidence-based nutrition founded upon the preponderance of scientific research, nurses can educate and advocate for themselves and their patients for improved long-term health outcomes, improved longevity, quality of life, and healthy years. Nutrition is so fundamental that it should be a vital sign along with blood pressure, respiration rate, heart rate, oxygen saturation, and temperature. A whole food, plant-based pattern is the only dietary pattern that has been shown to reverse cardiovascular disease. Not only is this dietary pattern arguably the healthiest, but it is also the kindest on the environment. Nurses should perform a nutrition assessment and incorporate evidence-based nutrition into all aspects of care.

Passion for nutrition in healthcare has led some nurses to establish employee wellness programs at their institutions, start campaigns to change hospital food, incorporate cooking demonstrations into group medical visits, teach cooking classes at food pantries, host nutrition CE programs, lead grocery store tours in their communities, address social disparities by teaching budget cooking at churches and food banks, testify before the U.S. Dietary Guidelines Advisory Committee on the need for nutrition advice that is based on scientific evidence and not industry promotion, and more.

Nutrition expertise offers professional and personal benefits. We have found the study and imple-mentation of nutrition to be rewarding and fun – the path to nutrition enlightenment often includes digging into published research, questioning nutrition dogma and nutrition fads, trying new foods, learning new cooking skills, seeking out farmer's markets, and sharing great meals with like-minded co-workers and/or with colleagues at nursing and multidisciplinary conferences. Box 2.6 is a personal vignette highlighting the importance of nutrition for self-care.

BOX 2.6   PERSONAL VIGNETTE #2: NUTRITION FOR A NURSE

I've been an RN, BSN, for almost 44 years. By the time I was 20 years into my career, I had become what so many of my patients were – obese, diabetic, hypertensive, and hyperlipid-emic. I spent the next 20 years managing my chronic diseases as conventional medical wisdom taught – count carbs, take medications as prescribed, try to be active. I kept my A1c at 6.5 or less. I yoyo dieted to stay as slim as I could – which ranged from 27 to 36 BMI. My choles-terol was usually over 200 and my triglycerides ranged 195 to 335. In 2016, I discovered a new diet that required weighing and measuring every morsel I ate. I managed to get down to 25 BMI and was off most medications. But I did not want to weigh everything I ate for the rest of my life. In January 2017, I read Dr Esselstyn's book – *Prevent and Reverse Heart Disease*. It was jaw-dropping information!! Many of his patients also had diabetes, and in reversing their heart disease, they reversed their diabetes, too. The magic? A whole foods, plant-based lifestyle. I made the switch on January 24, 2017. Five years later, I am not, and have not been, on any medications in all those years. I stay at a BMI of 24 or less. My A1c is usually 5.5. My labs usually report in this kind of range – A1C 5.5, glucose 63, HDL 56, LDL 85, Chol 162, triglycerides 98. No medications, no weighing and measuring what I eat! Just wonderful foods that are so satisfying and delicious!

I love the health and vitality I have at age 65. I feel better than I did 30 and 40 years ago. I have energy to exercise daily. I LOVE the foods I eat. My husband transitioned to WFPB with me. I'm sure he's the healthiest trucker on the road. I work in an office doing phone assessments. So, my sphere of influence is the nurses I work with. Recently, a nurse new to our office asked me about my prominently displayed plant-based pin. He had just gotten a rather sad report on his health from his PCP. I helped guide him and his wife to WFPB eating. They jumped right in and began moving toward plant-based eating. Three months, later his doctor was shocked at the turnaround in his lab results and his weight loss. He told him to keep up the great work. I have become a licensed Food for Life instructor and plan to work with this PCP in assisting other patients to improve their health rather than just managing their diseases.

My best advice? First, do this for yourself!! Second, YOU can impact the patients and co-workers in your sphere of influence. WFPB eating is evidence based with decades of strong research. Use your influence to help people stay well or regain their health. You can leave a legacy of changing the life trajectory of the people you are around. Grab the opportunity and make a difference in yourself and your world!!

Debbie Keele, RN, BSN

REFERENCES

Ackley, B. J., Ladwig, G. B., & Makic, M. B., (2017). *Nursing diagnosis handbook: An evidence-based guide to planning care.* (11th ed.). Elsevier.

American Association of Colleges of Nursing (AACN). (2021, April 6). *The Essentials: Core Competencies for Professional Nursing Education.* American Association of Colleges of Nursing: The Voice of Academic Nursing. www.aacnnursing.org/AACN-Essentials

American College of Lifestyle Medicine (ACLM). (n.d.). Core Competencies. www.lifestylemedicine.org/ACLM/About/Core_Competencies/ACLM/About/What_is_Lifestyle_Medicine_/Core_Competencies.aspx?hkey=949ce5f3-757f-4b12-b658-6170fa510390

American College of Lifestyle Medicine (ACLM). (n.d.). Lifestyle Medicine Tools and Resources. https://lifestylemedicine.org/ACLM/Resources/Tools_Resources/ACLM/Tools_and_Resources/Tools_and_Resources.aspx?hkey=8282b986-4ca1-4912-a1a9-b8e18e7b76c5

American Nurses Association. (2015). Code of Ethics for Nurses With Interpretive Statements. ANA.

Azemati, B., Rajaram, S., Jaceldo-Siegl, K., Sabate, J., Shavlik, D., Fraser, G. E., & Haddad, E. H. (2017). Animal-protein intake is associated with insulin resistance in Adventist Health Study 2 (AHS-2) calibration substudy participants: A cross-sectional analysis. *Current developments in nutrition, 1*(4), e000299.

Becerra-Tomás, N., Blanco Mejía, S., Viguiliouk, E., Khan, T., Kendall, C., Kahleova, H., Rahelić, D., Sievenpiper, J. L., & Salas-Salvadó, J. (2020). Mediterranean diet, cardiovascular disease and mortality in diabetes: A systematic review and meta-analysis of prospective cohort studies and randomized clinical trials. *Critical reviews in food science and nutrition, 60*(7), 1207–1227. https://doi.org/10.1080/10408398.2019.1565281

Benigas S. (2019). American college of lifestyle medicine: Vision, tenacity, transformation. *American journal of lifestyle medicine, 14*(1), 57–60. https://doi.org/10.1177/1559827619881094

Buettner, D., & Skemp, S. (2016). Blue sones: Lessons from the world's longest lived. *American journal of lifestyle medicine, 10*(5), 318–321. https://doi.org/10.1177/1559827616637066

Calder, P. C., Carr, A. C., Gombart, A. F., & Eggersdorfer, M. (2020). Optimal nutritional status for a well-functioning immune system is an important factor to protect against viral infections. *Nutrients, 12*(4), 1181. https://doi.org/10.3390/nu12041181

Campbell, T. Colin. (2013). *Whole: Rethinking the Science of Nutrition.* BenBella Books, Kindle edition.

Centers for Disease Control and Prevention. (2021). National Center for Chronic Disease Prevention and Health Promotion. www.cdc.gov/chronicdisease/index.htm

Clarys, P., Deliens, T., Huybrechts, I., Deriemaeker, P., Vanaelst, B., De Keyzer, W., Hebbelinck, M., & Mullie, P. (2014). Comparison of nutritional quality of the vegan, vegetarian, semi-vegetarian, pesco-vegetarian and omnivorous diet. *Nutrients, 6*(3), 1318–1332. https://doi.org/10.3390/nu6031318

Clegg, D. J., & Hill Gallant, K. M. (2019). Plant-based diets in CKD. *Clinical journal of the American Society of Nephrology*, *14*(1), 141–143. https://doi.org/10.2215/CJN.08960718

Colditz, G. A., Philpott, S. E., & Hankinson, S. E. (2016). The impact of the Nurses' Health Study on population health: Prevention, translation, and control. *American journal of public health*, *106*(9), 1540–1545. https://doi.org/10.2105/AJPH.2016.303343

Coleman-Jensen, A., Rabbitt, M. P., Gregory, C. A., & Singh, A. (2019). Household Food Security in the United States in 2018, ERR-270. U.S. Department of Agriculture, Economic Research Service. www.ers.usda.gov/webdocs/publications/94849/err-270.pdf?v=963.1

Crosby, L., Davis, B., Joshi, S., Jardine, M., Paul, J., Neola, M., & Barnard, N. D. (2021). Ketogenic diets and chronic disease: Weighing the benefits against the risks. *Frontiers in nutrition*, *403*. https://doi.org/10.3389/fnut.2021.702802

DiMaria-Ghalili, R. A., Mirtallo, J. M., Tobin, B. W., Hark, L., Van Horn, L., & Palmer, C. A. (2014). Challenges and opportunities for nutrition education and training in the health care professions: Intraprofessional and interprofessional call to action. *The American journal of clinical nutrition*, *99*(5), 1184S–1193S.

Drewnowski, A. (2005). Concept of a nutritious food: Toward a nutrient density score. *The American journal of clinical nutrition*, *82*(4), 721–732. https://academic.oup.com/ajcn/article/82/4/721/4607427

Drewnowski, A., Dwyer, J., King, J. C., & Weaver, C. M. (2019). A proposed nutrient density score that includes food groups and nutrients to better align with dietary guidance. *Nutrition Reviews*, *77*(6), 404–416.

Englert, D. M., Crocker, K. S., & Stotts, N. A. (1986). Nutrition education in schools of nursing in the United States. Part 1. The evolution of nutrition education in schools of nursing. *Journal of parenteral and enteral nutrition*, *10*(5), 522–527.

Estes, M. E. Z. (2013). *Health assessment and physical examination*. Cengage Learning.

EUFIC. (2021). *What Is Nutrient Density?* EUFIC. www.eufic.org/en/understanding-science/article/what-is-nutrient-density

Fontanet, A., Autran, B., Lina, B., Kieny, M. P., Karim, S., & Sridhar, D. (2021). SARS-CoV-2 variants and ending the COVID-19 pandemic. *Lancet (London, England)*, *397*(10278), 952–954. https://doi.org/10.1016/S0140-6736(21)00370-6

Ford, E. S., Bergmann, M. M., Kröger, J., Schienkiewitz, A., Weikert, C., & Boeing, H. (2009). Healthy living is the best revenge: Findings from the European prospective investigation into cancer and nutrition – Potsdam study. *Archives of internal medicine*, *169*(15), 1355–1362.

Fuhrman, J. (2017). ANDI food scores: Rating the nutrient density of foods. www.drfuhrman.com/blog/128/andi-food-scores-rating-the-nutrient-density-of-foods

Furman, D., Campisi, J., Verdin, E., Carrera-Bastos, P., Targ, S., Franceschi, C., … & Slavich, G. M. (2019). Chronic inflammation in the etiology of disease across the life span. *Nature medicine*, *25*(12), 1822–1832.

Greger, M. (2016). Diabetes reversal: Is it the calories or the food? [Video]. NutritionFacts.org. https://nutritionfacts.org/video/diabetes-reversal-is-it-the-calories-or-the-food

Hassenplug, L. W. (1960). Nursing education in universities. *Nursing outlook*, *8*, 92–95.

Hegge, M. (2013). Nightingale's Environmental Theory. *Nursing science quarterly*, *26*(3), 211–219. https://doi.org/10.1177/0894318413489255

Herdman, T. H. et al. (2021). NANDA international nursing diagnoses: Definitions and classification. (12th ed.). Thieme.

Huth, P. J., Fulgoni, V. L., Keast, D. R., Park, K., & Auestad, N. (2013). Major food sources of calories, added sugars, and saturated fat and their contribution to essential nutrient intakes in the US diet: Data from the national health and nutrition examination survey (2003–2006). *Nutrition Journal*, *12*(1), 1–10. https://doi.org/10.1186/1475-2891-12-116

Katz, D. L., & Meller, S. (2014). Can we say what diet is best for health? *Annual review of public health*, 35, 83–103.

Kelly, J., Karlsen, M., & Steinke, G. (2020). Type 2 diabetes remission and lifestyle medicine: A position statement from the American College of Lifestyle Medicine. *American Journal of Lifestyle Medicine*, *14*(4), 406–419. https://doi.org/10.1177/1559827620930962

Kim, H., Rebholz, C. M., Hegde, S., LaFiura, C., Raghavan, M., Lloyd, J. F., Cheng, S., & Seidelmann, S. B. (2021). Plant-based diets, pescatarian diets and COVID-19 severity: A population-based case–control study in six countries. *BMJ Nutrition, Prevention & Health*, *4*(1). https://doi.org/10.1136/bmjnph-2021-000272

Kochanek, K. D., Xu, J. Q., & Arias, E. (2019). Mortality in the United States, 2019. NCHS Data Brief, no 395. Hyattsville, MD: National Center for Health Statistics. 2020. www.cdc.gov/nchs/data/databriefs/db395-H.pdf

Korat, A. V. A., Willett, W. C., & Hu, F. B. (2014). Diet, lifestyle, and genetic risk factors for type 2 diabetes: A review from the Nurses' Health Study, Nurses' Health Study 2, and Health Professionals' Follow-up Study. *Current nutrition reports*, *3*(4), 345–354.

Kris-Etherton, P. M., Akabas, S. R., Douglas, P., Kohlmeier, M., Laur, C., Lenders, C. M., … & Saltzman, E. (2015). Nutrition competencies in health professionals' education and training: A new paradigm. *Advances in nutrition*, *6*(1), 83–87.

Kuwabara, A., Su, S., & Krauss, J. (2020). Utilizing digital health technologies for patient education in lifestyle medicine. *American journal of lifestyle medicine*, *14*(2), 137–142. https://doi.org/10.1177/1559827619892547

Kyu, H. H., Abate, D., Abate, K. H., Abay, S. M., Abbafati, C., Abbasi, N., Abbastabar, H., Abd-Allah, F., Abdela, J., Abdelalim, A., Abdollahpour, I., Abdulkader, R. S., Abebe, M., Abebe, Z., Abil, O. Z., Aboyans, V., Abrham, A. R., Abu-Raddad, L. J., Abu-Rmeileh, N. M. E. … & Murray, C. J. L. (2018). Global, regional, and national disability-adjusted life-years (DALYs) for 359 diseases and injuries and healthy life expectancy (HALE) for 195 countries and territories, 1990–2017: A systematic analysis for the Global Burden of Disease Study 2017. *The Lancet*, *392*(10159), 1859–1922. https://doi.org/10.1016/S0140-6736(18)32335-3

Le, L. T., & Sabaté, J. (2014). Beyond meatless, the health effects of vegan diets: Findings from the Adventist cohorts. *Nutrients*, *6*(6), 2131–2147.

Leitch, M.A. (1956). Educational standards for student nurses in the dietary department. *Journal of the American Dietetic Association*, *32*(4), 337–340.

Lianov, L. S., Fredrickson, B. L., Barron, C., Krishnaswami, J., & Wallace, A. (2019). Positive psychology in lifestyle medicine and health care: Strategies for implementation. *American journal of lifestyle medicine*, 13(5), 480–486. https://doi.org/10.1177/1559827619838992

Lichtenstein, A. H., Appel, L. J., Vadiveloo, M., Hu, F. B., Kris-Etherton, P. M., Rebholz, C. M., … & American Heart Association Council on Lifestyle and Cardiometabolic Health; Council on Arteriosclerosis, Thrombosis and Vascular Biology; Council on Cardiovascular Radiology and Intervention; Council on Clinical Cardiology; and Stroke Council. (2021). 2021 dietary guidance to improve cardiovascular health: A scientific statement from the American Heart Association. *Circulation*, *144*(23), e472–e487.

Liu, J., Rehm, C. D., Onopa, J., & Mozaffarian, D. (2020). Trends in diet quality among youth in the United States, 1999–2016. *JAMA*, *323*(12), 1161–1174. http://doi.org/10.1001/jama.2020.0878

Liu, J., Ren, Z. H., Qiang, H., Wu, J., Shen, M., Zhang, L., & Lyu, J. (2020). Trends in the incidence of diabetes mellitus: results from the Global Burden of Disease Study 2017 and implications for diabetes mellitus prevention. *BMC public health*, *20*(1), 1–12.

Logan, A. C., Prescott, S. L., & Katz, D. L. (2019). Golden age of medicine 2.0: Lifestyle medicine and planetary health prioritized. *Journal of lifestyle medicine*, *9*(2), 75.

Loma Linda University Health. (n.d.) Adventist Health Study. https://adventisthealthstudy.org/

Loprinzi, P. D., Branscum, A., Hanks, J., & Smit, E. (2016). Healthy lifestyle characteristics and their joint association with cardiovascular disease biomarkers in US adults. *Mayo Clinic Proceedings*, *91*(4), 432–442. https://doi.org/10.1016/j.mayocp.2016.01.009

Matranga, D., Restivo, V., Maniscalco, L., Bono, F., Pizzo, G., Lanza, G., … & Miceli, S. (2020). Lifestyle medicine and psychological well-being toward health promotion: A cross-sectional study on Palermo (Southern Italy) undergraduates. *International journal of environmental research and public health*, *17*(15), 5444.

Miles, F. L., Lloren, J. I. C., Haddad, E., Jaceldo-Siegl, K., Knutsen, S., Sabate, J., & Fraser, G. E. (2019). Plasma, urine, and adipose tissue biomarkers of dietary intake differ between vegetarian and non-vegetarian diet groups in the Adventist Health Study-2. *The journal of nutrition*, *149*(4), 667–675.

Morris, Z. S., Wooding, S., & Grant, J. (2011). The answer is 17 years, what is the question: Understanding time lags in translational research. *Journal of the Royal Society of Medicine*, *104*(12), 510–520.

Murphy SL, Kochanek KD, Xu JQ, Arias E. (2021). Mortality in the United States, 2020. NCHS Data Brief, no 427. Hyattsville, MD: National Center for Health Statistics. https://dx.doi.org/10.15620/cdc:112079

Murray, C. J. L. & The US Burden of Disease Collaborators (2018). The state of US health, 1990–2016: Burden of diseases, injuries, and risk factors among US states. *JAMA, 319*(14), 1444–1472. https//dx.doi.org/10.1001/jama.2018.0158

National Council of State Boards of Nursing. (2019). NCLEX examination statistics.

National Cancer Institute. *NCI Dictionary of Cancer Terms*. National Cancer Institute. (n.d.). www.cancer.gov/publications/dictionaries/cancer-terms/def/nutrient-dense-food

Nelson, N. J. (2000). Nurses' health study: Nurses helping science and themselves. *Journal of the National Cancer Institute, 92*(8), 597–599.

Nicklas, T. A., Drewnowski, A., & O'Neil, C. E. (2014). The nutrient density approach to healthy eating: Challenges and opportunities. *Public health nutrition, 17*(12), 2626–2636.

Nightingale, F. (1992). *Notes on nursing: What it is, and what it is not*. Lippincott Williams & Wilkins.

Nowson, C. (2020). Opportunities for innovation in nutrition education for health professionals. *BMJ nutrition, prevention & health, 3*(2), 126.

Nurses' Health Study (NHS). (n.d.). https://nurseshealthstudy.org/

Ornish, D., & Multicenter Lifestyle Demonstration Project Research Group. (1998). Avoiding revascularization with lifestyle changes: The Multicenter Lifestyle Demonstration Project. *The American journal of cardiology, 82*(10), 72–76.

Parker, H. W., & Vadiveloo, M. K. (2019). Diet quality of vegetarian diets compared with nonvegetarian diets: a systematic review. *Nutrition reviews, 77*(3), 144–160. https://doi.org/10.1093/nutrit/nuy067

Rippe, J. M. (Ed.). (2019). *Lifestyle Medicine*. CRC Press.

Schneider, E. C., Shah, A., Doty, M. M., Tikkanen, R., Fields, K., & Williams II, R. D. (2014). *Mirror, Mirror 2021: Reflecting Poorly*. The Commonwealth Fund.

Schulze, M. B., Martínez-González, M. A., Fung, T. T., Lichtenstein, A. H., & Forouhi, N. G. (2018). Food based dietary patterns and chronic disease prevention. *BMJ, 361*, k2396. https://doi.org/10.1136/bmj.k2396

Seidelmann, S. B., Claggett, B., Cheng, S., Henglin, M., Shah, A., Steffen, L. M., ... & Solomon, S. D. (2018). Dietary carbohydrate intake and mortality: A prospective cohort study and meta-analysis. *The Lancet Public Health, 3*(9), e419–e428. https://doi.org/10.1016/S2468-2667(18)30135-X

Shah, R., & Davis, B. (2020). *Nourish: The definitive plant-based nutrition guide for families*. Health Communications, Inc.

Slawson, D. L., Fitzgerald, N., & Morgan, K. T. (2013). Position of the Academy of Nutrition and Dietetics: The role of nutrition in health promotion and chronic disease prevention. *Journal of the Academy of Nutrition and Dietetics, 113*(7), 972–979.

Tharrey, M., Mariotti, F., Mashchak, A., Barbillon, P., Delattre, M., & Fraser, G. E. (2018). Patterns of plant and animal protein intake are strongly associated with cardiovascular mortality: The Adventist Health Study-2 cohort. *International journal of epidemiology, 47*(5), 1603–1612.

Tuso, P. J., Ismail, M. H., Ha, B. P., & Bartolotto, C. (2013). Nutritional update for physicians: Plant-based diets. *The permanente journal, 17*(2), 61.

U.S. Department of Health and Human Services and U.S. Department of Agriculture. (2020). *2020–2025 Dietary Guidelines for Americans*. 9th Edition. www.dietaryguidelines.gov/sites/default/files/2020-12/Dietary_Guidelines_for_Americans_2020-2025.pdf

U.S. Department of Health and Human Services and U.S. Department of Agriculture. (2015). *2015–2020 Dietary Guidelines for Americans*. 8th Edition. https://health.gov/our-work/food-nutrition/previous-dietary-guidelines/2015

Vodovotz, Y., Barnard, N., Hu, F. B., Jakicic, J., Lianov, L., Loveland, D., ... & Parkinson, M. D. (2020). Prioritized research for the prevention, treatment, and reversal of chronic disease: recommendations from the lifestyle medicine research summit. *Frontiers in Medicine, 7*, 959.

Vos, T., Abajobir, A. A., Abate, K. H., Abbafati, C., Abbas, K. M., Abd-Allah, F., ... & Criqui, M. H. (2017). Global, regional, and national incidence, prevalence, and years lived with disability for 328 diseases and injuries for 195 countries, 1990–2016: A systematic analysis for the Global Burden of Disease Study 2016. *The Lancet, 390*(10100), 1211–1259.

3 Structured Exercise, Lifestyle Physical Activity, and Cardiorespiratory Fitness in the Prevention and Treatment of Chronic Diseases

Barry A. Franklin[1] and Thomas F. O'Connell[2]

[1]Preventive Cardiology and Cardiac Rehabilitation

Beaumont Hospital

Royal Oak, Michigan, USA

Internal Medicine

Oakland University William Beaumont School of Medicine

Rochester, Michigan, USA

[2]Department of Cardiovascular Medicine

Beaumont Hospital

Royal Oak, Michigan, USA

CONTENTS

DOI: 10.1201/9781003178330-4

KEY POINTS

- Regular physical activity (PA), structured exercise training, and higher cardiorespiratory fitness (CRF) delay the development of atherosclerotic cardiovascular disease (CVD) and reduce the incidence of coronary heart disease (CHD) events.
- There is an inverse relationship between regular exercise, moderate-to-vigorous PA, and the incidence of type 2 diabetes mellitus (DM2) in men and women.
- The gradual progression of exercise intensities from moderate-to-vigorous to high intensity training regimens (in selected individuals) may result in even greater cardioprotective benefits.
- Increased levels of PA and/or CRF before hospitalization for acute coronary syndromes may confer more favorable short-term outcomes, potentially via exercise preconditioning.
- Moderate-to-vigorous PA, which corresponds to any activity ≥3 METs, has been consistently shown to reduce the health risks associated with chronic diseases and the likelihood of developing them.
- Walking is the most accessible and easily regulated exercise that can enhance health and CRF.
- In an era of escalating health care expenditures, structured exercise regimens, increased lifestyle PA, or both provide independent, additive, and complementary benefits for achieving improved health outcomes.

3.1   INTRODUCTION

Substantial epidemiologic, clinical, and basic science evidence suggests that regular physical activity (PA), structured exercise training, and higher cardiorespiratory fitness (CRF) delay the development of atherosclerotic cardiovascular disease (CVD) and reduce the incidence of coronary heart disease (CHD) events. PA is defined as bodily movement resulting from the contraction of skeletal muscle that increases energy expenditure above the resting level, that is, 1 metabolic equivalent (1 MET = 3.5 mL O_2/kg/min). Structured exercise training, which is considered a subcategory of PA, is defined as any planned intervention to improve or maintain CRF, health, athletic performance, or combinations thereof. Aerobic capacity (VO_2max) or CRF, commonly expressed as mL O_2/kg/min or multiples of the resting O_2 consumption (METs), can be directly measured during cardiopulmonary exercise testing or estimated from the attained workload (Franklin et al., 2020).

In an early meta-analysis of 43 studies of the relation between PA and CHD incidence, the relative risk of CHD in relation to physical inactivity ranged from 1.5 to 2.4, with a median value of 1.9 (Powell et al., 1987). Moreover, the relative risk of a sedentary lifestyle appeared to be similar in magnitude to that associated with other major CHD risk factors. Another systematic review and meta-analysis of 33 PA studies, including 883,372 participants, reported pooled risk reductions of 35% and 33% for CVD and all-cause mortality, respectively (Nocon et al., 2008). More recently, researchers analyzed data from two major ongoing cohort studies, the Nurses' Health Study (n = 78,865) and the Health Professionals Follow-Up Study (n = 44,354) to estimate the impact of lifestyle on life expectancy in the U.S. population (Li et al., 2018). Five low-risk lifestyle factors were considered: not smoking; body mass index 18.5 to 24.9 kg/m^2; *≥ 30 min/day of moderate-to-vigorous PA*; moderate alcohol consumption; and a healthy diet score. Up to 34 years of follow-up, adherence to all five lifestyle-related factors significantly increased life expectancy at age 50 years for both men and women, 12.2 and 14.0 years, respectively. The most physically active cohorts of men and women demonstrated 7– to 8–year gains in life expectancy!

This chapter reviews the impact of structured exercise/PA interventions in individuals with and without CHD, with specific reference to the cardiovascular benefits of regular moderate-to-vigorous PA and improved CRF, underlying mechanisms, related health outcomes (e.g., chronic disease, health care costs, hospitalization for acute coronary syndrome, short-term surgical results), exercise prescription, contemporary PA recommendations, value of progressing exercise training intensities, and complementary exercise interventions. Additional topics include exercise preparticipation screening, extreme exercise and cardiovascular health, using technology to promote PA, and strategies to enhance exercise compliance.

3.2 EFFECTS OF PHYSICAL ACTIVITY AND FITNESS ON CHRONIC DISEASES

Large epidemiologic studies have reported an inverse relationship between regular exercise, moderate-to-vigorous PA, and the incidence of type 2 diabetes mellitus (DM2) in men and women (Hu et al., 1999; Manson et al., 1992). These observations have been substantiated in interventional studies. The Finnish Diabetes Prevention Study found that participants with impaired fasting glucose who were counseled to engage in aerobic exercise, follow a specific diet, and reduce body weight by ≥5% had significantly better results on glucose tolerance testing after 3.2 years (mean duration) as compared with a control group (Tuomilehto et al., 2001). Similarly, the Diabetes Prevention Program Research Group Study evaluated participants with impaired fasting glucose who were randomized to placebo, metformin 850 mg twice daily, or lifestyle modification. Participants in the lifestyle modification group were advised to follow a specific diet and to exercise ≥150 minutes of week. The lifestyle intervention group had a 58% lower incidence of DM2 compared to placebo while the metformin group had a 31% lower incidence (Knowler et al., 2002). More recently, these investigations have been extended to evaluate the prognostic significance of CRF, specifically peak oxygen uptake (VO$_2$ peak). Jae et al. (2016) found that Korean men without DM2, CVD, or hypertension (HTN) were at 1.8 times greater risk of developing DM2 at 5-year follow-up (median) if they were unfit based on median values of age-specific VO$_2$ peak.

Multiple studies have confirmed an inverse relationship between PA, CRF, and the future development of HTN (Huai et al., 2013). A study of pre-hypertensive, male veterans assessed the incidence of HTN after 9.2 years stratified by CRF, expressed as peak METs. Compared to veterans who achieved >10 METs, the risk of future HTN was 36% higher in veterans achieving 8.6 to 10 METs, 66% higher in those achieving 6.6 to 8.5 METs, and 72% higher for those achieving ≤6.5 METs (Faselis et al., 2012). This demonstrates that not only is there an inverse relationship between CRF and incident HTN, but that the risk of developing HTN decreases in a graded manner according to exercise capacity.

HTN and DM2 are major risk factors for chronic kidney disease (CKD). However, exercise and improved CRF have been independently associated with a lower incidence of CKD. A study of male veterans found that the adjusted risk of developing CKD was 22% lower for each 1-MET increase in exercise capacity over 7.9 year follow up (median) (Kokkinos et al., 2015). These findings have also been extended to patients with diabetes (Nylen et al., 2015).

Finally, the impact of chronic exercise and improved CRF on incident atrial fibrillation (AF) and heart failure (HF) are also relevant. The relationship between exercise and AF is controversial. Multiple studies suggest a higher incidence of AF in vigorous exercisers, including elite endurance athletes, who participate in strenuous, long-term exercise (Aizer et al., 2009). However, other studies have reported an inverse relationship between CRF and the incidence of AF. One investigation found that the risk of AF was 21% lower for every 1-MET increase in exercise capacity (Qureshi et al., 2015). There have been multiple studies demonstrating benefits of exercise on future HF diagnoses and hospital admissions. One large cohort study showed that each 1-MET increase was associated with an 18% to 20% lower risk of HF hospitalization (Pandey et al., 2015). Among male veterans, each 1-MET increase in exercise capacity was associated with a 19% reduction in the incidence of HF (Myers et al., 2017). In aggregate, these data overwhelmingly support structured exercise, moderate-to-vigorous lifestyle PA, and improved CRF as preventive strategies for the most prevalent chronic diseases.

3.3 CARDIOPROTECTIVE EFFECTS OF CHRONIC AEROBIC EXERCISE: POTENTIAL UNDERLYING MECHANISMS

Regular moderate-to-vigorous PA has been shown to promote salutary anti-atherosclerotic, antithrombotic, anti-ischemic, and antiarrhythmic adaptations and is associated with beneficial physiological effects (Figure 3.1) (Boden et al., 2014). Specific anti-ischemic effects include reducing myocardial oxygen demand by lowering the rate-pressure product at rest and during any given submaximal workload, as well as increasing the period of diastole, during which coronary perfusion predominates. Improved coronary blood flow and endothelial function have also been

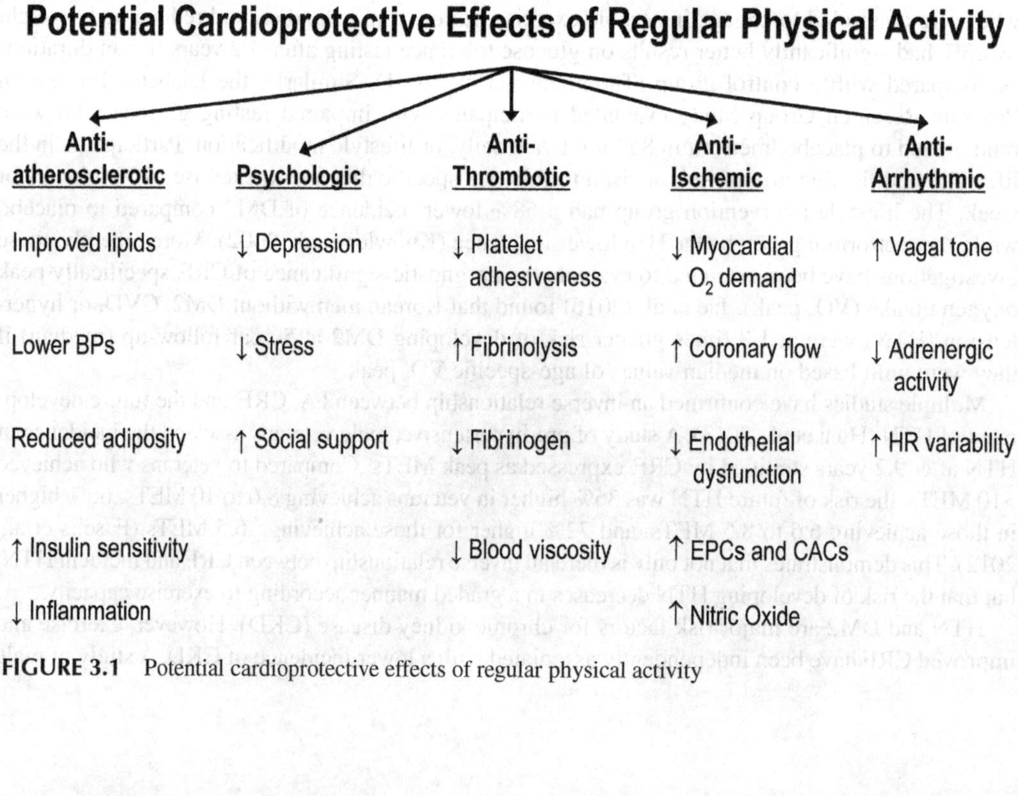

Potential Cardioprotective Effects of Regular Physical Activity

Anti-atherosclerotic	Psychologic	Anti-Thrombotic	Anti-Ischemic	Anti-Arrhythmic
Improved lipids	↓ Depression	↓ Platelet adhesiveness	↓ Myocardial O₂ demand	↑ Vagal tone
Lower BPs	↓ Stress	↑ Fibrinolysis	↑ Coronary flow	↓ Adrenergic activity
Reduced adiposity	↑ Social support	↓ Fibrinogen	↓ Endothelial dysfunction	↑ HR variability
↑ Insulin sensitivity		↓ Blood viscosity	↑ EPCs and CACs	
↓ Inflammation			↑ Nitric Oxide	

FIGURE 3.1 Potential cardioprotective effects of regular physical activity

TABLE 3.1

Multiple mechanisms by which vigorous-intensity exercise training may be more effective than moderate-intensity exercise at reducing cardiovascular risk[*]

↑	Parasympathetic tone
↑	Period of diastole and NO vasodilator function
↓	Shear stress on endothelial walls
↑	Artery compliance
↓	Plaque rupture
↓	Adverse ventricular remodeling
↓	Incident AF and/or HF
↓	Endothelial dysfunction and myocardial ischemia
↓	Arrhythmias
↑	Heart rate variability
↓	Sympathetic outflow
↓	Inflammation

NO = nitric oxide; AF = atrial fibrillation; HF = heart failure; ↑ = increased; ↓ = decreased.

[*] Adapted from Franklin, B. A., Kaminsky, L. A., & Kokkinos, P. (2018). Quantitating the dose of physical activity in secondary prevention: relation of exercise intensity to survival. *Mayo Clinic proceedings*, *93*(9), 1158–1163.

reported following exercise training (Niebauer & Cooke, 1996). Moreover, Green et al. (2008) proposed a cardioprotective "vascular conditioning" effect, including enhanced nitric oxide vasodilator function, improved vascular reactivity, altered vascular structure, or combinations thereof. Decreased vulnerability to threatening ventricular arrhythmias has also been postulated to reflect training-induced adaptations in autonomic control (i.e., attenuate sympathetic drive and increased vagal tone) (Wilson et al., 2016).

3.3.1 VIGOROUS VERSUS MODERATE INTENSITY PHYSICAL ACTIVITY

The gradual progression of exercise intensities, from moderate to vigorous to high intensity training regimens (in selected individuals), may result in even greater cardioprotective benefits. The mortality reduction associated with a 5-minute run approximates a 15-minute walk, and a 25-minute run is comparable with a 105-minute walk (Wen et al., 2011). Furthermore, at equivalent levels of total energy expenditure, vigorous exercise seems to be more effective than moderate-intensity exercise in reducing cardiovascular risk (Swain & Franklin, 2006). Vigorous exercise intensities are also more effective than moderate intensities at increasing CRF (Swain & Franklin, 2002). This has additional prognostic significance, since higher levels of CRF have been repeatedly shown to confer a lower risk of cardiovascular and all-cause mortality (Franklin, 2002). Specific mechanisms associated with the incremental and additive cardioprotective benefits of vigorous intensity exercise training are shown in Table 3.1 (Franklin, Kaminsky, et al., 2018).

3.4 IMPACT OF PHYSICAL ACTIVITY AND CARDIORESPIRATORY FITNESS ON HEALTH OUTCOMES

This section reviews the impact of PA and/or CRF on varied health outcomes, including the comparative benefits on the relative risks of CHD and CVD, cardiovascular and all-cause mortality, health care costs, hospitalization for acute coronary syndromes, and short-term elective surgical outcomes.

3.4.1 CRF AND PA AS SEPARATE RISK FACTORS: COMPARATIVE BENEFITS

Regular PA and improved CRF, expressed as METs, are reported to be cardioprotective. However, a meta-analysis concluded that these variables had significantly different relationships to CVD (Williams, 2001).[27] There was a 64% decline in the risk of heart disease from the least to the most fit, with a precipitous drop in risk comparing the lowest (0) to the next lowest fitness category (i.e., 25th percentile), but only a 30% decline from the least to the most physically active (Figure 3.2). It was concluded that being unfit warrants consideration as an independent risk factor, and that a low level of CRF increases the risk of CVD to a greater extent than merely being physically inactive.

3.4.2 CRF AND CARDIOVASCULAR AND ALL-CAUSE MORTALITY

In a seminal report, Blair et al. (1989) found an inverse relation between peak METs and cardio-vascular and all-cause mortality in a large cohort of healthy middle-aged subjects (n = 13,344), but suggested an "asymptote of gain" beyond which further improvements in CRF conferred no additional survival benefit. This asymptote was estimated to be ~9 and 10 METs for women and men, respectively, approximate cut points that have been substantiated by others (Gulati et al., 2003; Kodama et al., 2009; Kokkinos & Myers, 2010). Similarly, in a large cohort of asymptomatic women (n = 5721), Gulati et al. (2003) reported that after adjusting for age and Framingham Risk Score, CRF was a strong independent predictor of all-cause mortality. Over an 8-year follow-up, for each 1-MET increase in exercise capacity, there was a 17% reduction in mortality. On the other hand, in both studies – Blair et al. (1989) and Gulati et al. (2003) – an exercise capacity <5 METs identified population subsets with the highest mortality.

In another study of 20,590 U.S. veterans, the incidence of major cardiovascular events was 17% lower for every 1-MET increase in CRF. When compared with the least fit patients, the risk of car-diovascular events was ~70% lower for patients in the highest fitness category (Kokkinos et al., 2017). Others have reported that, irrespective of the risk factor profile, high-fit men and women have ~50% the 30-year CVD mortality as their low-fit counterparts (Wickramasinghe et al., 2014). Moreover, follow-up reports in the Cooper Clinic Longitudinal study have shown that, regardless of the coronary artery calcium score, higher levels of PA or CRF appear to confer a lower risk for all-cause and cardiovascular mortality (DeFina et al., 2019; Radford et al., 2018).

Collectively, these data suggest that in apparently healthy men and women, individuals with comorbid conditions (e.g., overweight/obesity, HTN, DM2), an elevated coronary calcium score,

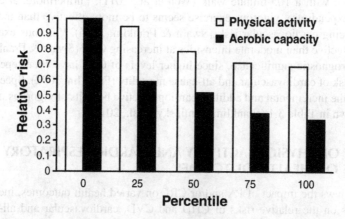

FIGURE 3.2 The risks of coronary heart disease and cardiovascular disease decrease linearly in association with increasing percentiles of physical activity

and those with suspected or known CHD, a low-level of CRF is an independent risk factor for all-cause and cardiovascular mortality. Low-fit subjects were ~2–3 times more likely to die during the follow-up as compared with their more fit counterparts. Among men and women with and without CHD, each 1 MET increase in exercise capacity is associated with an ~15% reduction in cardiovascular mortality (Boden et al., 2013; Kodama et al., 2009), which compares favorably with the survival benefit conferred by low-dose aspirin, statins, β-blockers, and angiotensin-converting enzyme inhibitors after acute myocardial infarction. In fact, a report demonstrated that CRF more accurately predicted 5-year mortality than left ventricular ejection fraction in patients with ST-segment elevation myocardial infarction treated with percutaneous coronary intervention (Dutcher et al., 2007).

3.4.3   CRF AND HEALTH CARE COSTS

Over the past 20 years, increasing data regarding the relations between CRF, habitual PA, and health care costs have become available. Most of the previously published cost-effectiveness data were derived from reviews and analytical models, rather than via a direct evaluation of the effect of measured exercise capacity on health care costs. A recent report linked lower intensities of peak daily energy expenditure, estimated from ambulatory electrocardiographic (ECG) monitoring, with increased health care utilization (George et al., 2017).

To examine the relationship between CRF, expressed as METs, and 1-year total health care costs in the year following the treadmill test, Weiss et al. (2004) studied 881 consecutive patients (mean age = 59 years; 95% men) who were referred for diagnostic treadmill testing. A relatively high proportion of patients had ≥1 coronary risk factors, whereas a notably smaller proportion had a history of documented CVD. In unadjusted analysis, inpatient and outpatient health care costs were incrementally lower by an average of 5.4% per MET increase ($P < 0.001$) (Figure 3.3). The biggest drop in health care costs went from an exercise capacity of <5 to 5.0 to 6.9 METs. Multivariable analysis further demonstrated that the peak METs achieved during exercise testing proved to be the most significant predictor of subsequent health care costs.

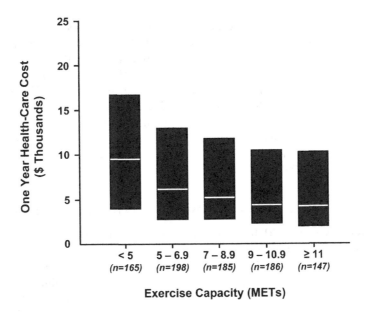

FIGURE 3.3   Relationship between exercise capacity, expressed as METs, and 1-year total health care costs in the year following the treadmill test

https://doi.org/10.1378/chest.126.2.608

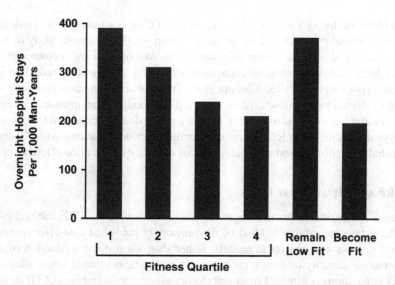

FIGURE 3.4 Inverse relationship between overnight hospital stays (per 1000 person-years) and increasing levels of fitness, after adjustment for potential confounding variables

Similarly, researchers at the Cooper Clinic/Institute conducted a prospective study of 6679 men (mean ± SD age = 44.8 ± 9.1 years; 97% white) to examine the relationship between CRF, estimated from treadmill test duration, and health care costs (i.e., incidence of physician office visits and overnight hospital stays) during the 1-year period before each of the two preventive medicine exams (Mitchell et al., 2004). A subset (n = 2974) also was evaluated to assess whether improvements in fitness were associated with reduced health care expenditures. Men in the top fitness quartile as well as those who became fit demonstrated health care utilization trends that amounted to a 53% reduction in direct health care costs (Figure 3.4).

More recently, Myers et al. (2018), using the Veterans Exercise Testing database, reported that each 1-MET higher level of CRF was associated with $1592 (USD) annual reduction in health care costs/person, corresponding to a 5.6% lower cost per MET. To clarify the impact of both CRF and body habitus on health care costs, de Silva and associates (2019) evaluated male veterans (n = 9789) over a 7-year period (de Silva et al., 2019). Each 1-MET higher level of CRF was associated with annual cost savings per person (USD) of $1346, $1823, and $2745 for normal-weight, overweight, and obese subjects, respectively. These findings and other reports suggest that increased levels of CRF as well as structured or leisure-time exercise interventions reduce the likelihood of using health care services and their associated costs (Ackermann et al., 2003; Franklin et al., 2020; Martin et al., 2006; Vestergaard et al., 2006).

3.4.4 Impact of Preadmission PA on Hospitalization for Acute Coronary Syndromes

Increased levels of PA and/or CRF before hospitalization for acute coronary syndromes may confer more favorable short-term outcomes, potentially via exercise preconditioning (Thijssen et al., 2018). A widely cited investigation of 2172 patients hospitalized for acute coronary syndromes (mean ± SD age = 65.5 ± 13 years; 76% men) evaluated the effect of pre-hospital admission PA status on in-hospital and 1-month post-discharge CVD health outcomes (Pitsavos et al., 2008). After adjusting for potential confounders, the most physically active cohort demonstrated 0.56-fold lower odds of in-hospital mortality and 0.80-fold lower odds of recurrent CVD events within the first 30 days of hospital discharge.

3.4.5 EXERCISE PRECONDITIONING: A CARDIOPROTECTIVE PHENOTYPE

Beyond the long-term adaptive benefits of vascular and architectural remodeling in those who adopt a physically active lifestyle, exercise preconditioning provides *immediate* cardioprotective benefits and improved clinical outcomes following acute cardiac events (Quindry & Franklin, 2021). These protective effects are widely underappreciated, occur after just one to three brief bouts (e.g., 20–30 min) of moderate intensity exercise, and persist for several days to more than a week after the last exercise session. Researchers believe the phenomenon may be due to transiently altered biochemical pathways or enhanced cardiac electrical stability. Interestingly, while moderate intensity exercise provides robust protection against acute myocardial infarction and threatening ventricular arrhythmias, higher intensity exercise does not bolster the magnitude of protection (Quindry & Franklin, 2021).

3.4.6 IMPACT OF PA AND CRF ON SURGICAL OUTCOMES

Recent studies suggest that in addition to being a strong predictor of cardiovascular and all-cause mortality in both asymptomatic and clinically referred populations, CRF could be especially helpful in the preoperative risk assessment of patients undergoing coronary artery bypass grafting (Figure 3.5) (Smith et al., 2013), abdominal aortic aneurysm repair, bariatric surgery (McCullough et al., 2006), and other surgical interventions (Kaminsky et al., 2013; Ross et al., 2016). Complications after surgery have been linked to reduced preoperative levels of PA or CRF (Figure 3.6) (Hoogeboom et al., 2014). It has been suggested that patients with higher levels of CRF are simply better able to cope with the aerobic and myocardial demands created by the trauma of major surgery. Reduced aerobic fitness may also be associated with greater numbers and greater severity of unhealthy comorbid conditions that individually or collectively could increase mortality. Another proposed explanation is that a low CRF identifies a subset of patients who are more difficult to operate on, requiring longer

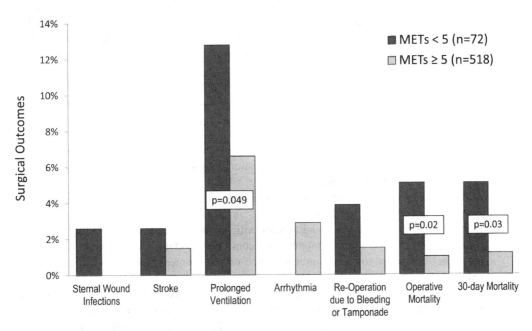

FIGURE 3.5 Short-term outcomes after coronary artery bypass grafting in patients with reduced presurgical cardiorespiratory fitness (<5 METs)

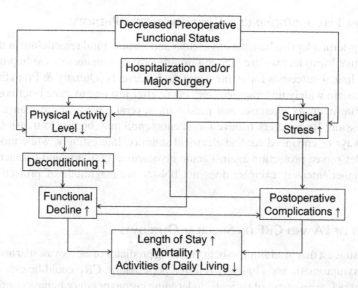

FIGURE 3.6 Possible impact of decreased preoperative physical activity or cardiorespiratory fitness on hospitalized patients undergoing emergent or elective surgery with specific reference to short-term outcomes

operative and intubation times, or those characterized by a high-risk, pro-inflammatory state that could be related to the development of heightened postoperative complications (Ross et al., 2016).

3.5 EXERCISE PREPARTICIPATION AND SCREENING PROCEDURES

Screening selected middle-aged and older individuals before participating in structured exercise and/or recreational PA and younger individuals prior to engaging in sports training and competitive activities remains controversial. In 2015, the American College of Sports Medicine (ACSM) published revised recommendations for exercise pre-participation screening (Riebe et al., 2015). The new algorithm focused on four major modulators of exercise-related acute cardiovascular events: (1) the individual's current level of PA; (2) known cardiovascular, metabolic, or renal disease (CMRD); (3) the presence of signs or symptoms suggestive of CVD; and (4) the desired or anticipated exercise intensity (Table 3.2) (Franklin et al., 2020). The new recommendations can be succinctly summarized by the following four points:

- Physically active asymptomatic individuals without known CMRD may continue their usual moderate or vigorous exercise and progress gradually as tolerated, according to contemporary ACSM guidelines (Riebe et al., 2017). Those who develop signs or symptoms of CMRD should immediately discontinue exercise and seek medical evaluation and clearance before resuming exercise of any intensity.
- Physically active asymptomatic individuals with known CMRD who have been medically evaluated within the previous 12 months may continue a moderate-intensity exercise program unless they develop signs or symptoms, which require immediate cessation of exercise and medical reassessment.
- Physically inactive individuals without known CMRD may begin light to moderate intensity exercise without medical clearance and, provided they remain asymptomatic, progress gradually in intensity as recommended by current ACSM guidelines (Riebe et al., 2017).
- Physically inactive individuals with known CMRD or signs/symptoms that are suggestive of these diseases should seek medical clearance before starting an exercise program, regardless of the intensity.

TABLE 3.2
Potential risk modulators of exercise-related acute cardiovascular events

Risk Modulator Category

Individual's Current Level of Activity
"Active" defined as performing planned, structured moderate-to-vigorous intensity PA ≥30 min at least
3 d·wk⁻¹, defined as 40% to 59% or ≥60% functional capacity, respectively

Presence of Signs and Symptoms Suggestive of CVD
Pain or discomfort at rest or with physical exertion in the chest, neck, jaw, arms, or other areas that may result
from myocardial ischemia
Unusual shortness of breath
Lightheadedness
Ankle swelling
Awareness of a rapid or irregular heart beat
Burning or cramping sensations in the lower extremities when walking short distances

Known CVD, Metabolic, or Renal Disease
Diabetes (type 1 and type 2 diabetes mellitus)
Renal disease
CVD including angina pectoris, previous myocardial infarction, coronary revascularization, heart surgery,
pacemaker, valve disease, heart failure, structural heart disease, or combinations thereof

Desired Exercise Intensity
Light: an intensity that evokes slight increases in heart rate and breathing (2 to 2.9 METs) or <40% FC
Moderate: an intensity that evokes noticeable increases in heart rate and breathing (3 to 5.9 METs) or 40%
to 59% FC
Vigorous: an intensity that evokes substantial increases in heart rate and breathing (≥6 METs) or ≥60% FC

PA = physical activity; CVD = cardiovascular disease; FC = functional capacity; and METs = metabolic equivalents
(1 MET = 3.5 mL O_2/kg/min). Copyright, American Heart Association.

Adapted from Franklin, B. A., Thompson, P. D., Al-Zaiti, S. S., Albert, C. M., Hivert, M.-F., Levine, B. D., Lobelo, F.,
Madan, K., Sharrief, A. Z., & Eijsvogels, T. M. (2020). Exercise-related acute cardiovascular events and potential deleterious
adaptations following long-term exercise training: placing the risks into perspective – an update: a scientific statement from
the American Heart Association. *Circulation, 141*(13), e705–e736.

3.5.1 Screening Exercise Testing

The exercise preparticipation health screening process should provide prudent assessment while
minimizing barriers to adopting a structured exercise regimen, increased lifestyle PA, or both (Riebe
et al., 2015). Unwarranted referral to health care providers for exercise screening may lead to a
high rate of false-positive exercise test responses in some populations, additional unnecessary non-
invasive/invasive follow-up studies, and financial and other burdens on the patient/client and health
care system (Franklin, 2014). The U.S. Preventive Services Task Force advised against routine
screening with resting or exercise ECGs in low-risk asymptomatic adults to prevent cardiovascular
events (Curry et al., 2018). Moreover, the Task Force review of randomized controlled trials of exercise ECG screening found no additional improvement in health outcomes, despite the inclusion of
higher-risk populations with diabetes mellitus (Jonas et al., 2018). Exercise testing may be helpful
for assessing cardiovascular disorders in selected patient subsets, including high-risk middle-aged
and older individuals who wish to pursue high-intensity endurance sports, individuals with atypical
chest pain, multiple risk factors, an elevated coronary artery calcium score, or a family history of
premature CHD, or those whom the clinician suspects may be ignoring symptoms or not giving an
accurate history (Franklin et al., 2020).

3.6   EXERCISE PRESCRIPTION/PROGRAMMING

Structured exercise training sessions should include a preliminary aerobic warm-up (~10 minutes), a continuous or accumulated aerobic conditioning phase (≥30 minutes), and a cool-down (5 to 10 minutes). The warm-up facilitates the transition from rest to the aerobic conditioning phase, reducing the potential for abnormal signs/symptoms (e.g., ischemic ST-segment depression, ventricular arrhythmias) that can occur with the onset of sudden strenuous exertion (Barnard et al., 1973). The ideal warm-up for any endurance activity is calisthenics followed by the training activity but at a lower intensity. A cool-down enhances venous return during recovery, decreasing the likelihood of hypotension and related manifestations, promotes more rapid removal of lactic acid than stationary recovery, and ameliorates the potential deleterious effects of the post-exercise rise in plasma catecholamines (Dimsdale et al., 1984).

3.6.1   EXERCISE MODALITIES/TRAINING INTENSITIES

The most effective exercises for the endurance or conditioning phase include walking, graded walking, jogging, running, stationary cycle ergometry, combined arm-leg ergometry, outdoor cycling, swimming, rope skipping, and rowing. Complementary PA recommendations include resistance training (Grafe et al., 2018; Jurca et al., 2005; McCartney et al., 1993; Williams et al., 2007) and increased lifestyle activity (Andersen et al., 1999; Dunn et al., 1999), both of which provide independent and additive benefits to an aerobic exercise regimen. To improve aerobic capacity or CRF, the "minimum" or threshold intensity for training is ~40–50% of the VO_2max, which corresponds to ~60–70% of the highest heart rate achieved during maximal or peak exercise testing. For patients who have not undergone recent exercise testing, we recommend the standing resting heart rate plus 20 to 30 beats/minute for the initial exercise intensity, using signs/symptoms and perceived exertion as additional intensity modulators (Franklin & Zhu, 2021). Over time, the exercise intensity should be gradually increased to 50–80% of aerobic capacity, which approximates 70–85% of the highest heart rate attained during exercise testing.

The widely used Borg rating of perceived exertion (RPE) scale provides an adjunctive methodology to regulate exercise intensity (Table 3.3) (Borg, 1982). Exercise rated as 12–15 (6–20 category scale), between "somewhat hard" and "hard," is generally considered appropriate. However, during the first 4–6 weeks of training, ratings of 11–13, corresponding to "fairly light" to "somewhat hard," are strongly recommended (Franklin & Zhu, 2021).

3.6.2   ENERGY EXPENDITURE OF PHYSICAL ACTIVITY: METs

The intensity of PA is objectively expressed as METs, where 1 MET (3.5 mL O_2/kg/min) corresponds to the resting metabolic rate. An increase in oxygen consumption or energy expenditure occurs as exercise intensity increases. Accordingly, PA may be quantified by using multiples of the resting energy expenditure; for example, 2 METs represents two times the resting oxygen consumption (Varghese et al., 2016).

To facilitate exercise prescription, a compendium of physical activities has been developed to quantify energy expenditures based on the ratio of estimated or measured work metabolic rate to a standard resting metabolic rate (Ainsworth et al., 2011). This involves recommending activities that are sufficiently below the MET capacity achieved during exercise testing. Walking at a leisurely pace uses about 2 to 3 METs, whereas faster walking speeds (e.g., 3.5 to 4.5 miles per hour [mph]) may approximate 4 to 5 METs. Singles tennis requires about 6 to 7 METs. In contrast, jogging and running typically require 8 to 10 or more METs, respectively (Franklin, Brinks, et al., 2018). Examples of light, moderate, and vigorous activities are shown in Table 3.4 (Ainsworth et al., 2011).

TABLE 3.3
Rating of perceived exertion

Category Scale

6	
7	Very Very Light
8	
9	Very Light
10	
11	Fairly Light
12	
13	Somewhat Hard
14	
15	Hard
16	
17	Very Hard
18	
19	Very, Very Hard
20	

Adapted from Borg, G. A. (1982). Psychophysical bases of perceived exertion. *Medicine and science in sports and exercise*, *14*, 377–381. https://doi.org/10.1249/00005768-198205000-00012

TABLE 3.4
Energy cost (METs) of common occupational and leisure-time activities

Light (<3.0 METs)	Moderate (3–<6 METs)	Vigorous (≥6 METs)
Cycling (stationary, light intensity)	Cycling (as transportation)	Cycling (race)
Fishing	Mowing lawn	Moving furniture
Golf	Swimming (moderate)	Swimming (fast)
Sweeping	Table tennis	Tennis
Walking slowly or strolling	Walking briskly or jogging	Walking briskly uphill

METs = metabolic equivalents

Adapted from Ainsworth, B. E., Haskell, W. L., Herrmann, S. D., Meckes, N., Bassett, D. R., Tudor-Locke, C., Greer, J. L., Vezina, J., Whitt-Glover, M. C., & Leon, A. S. (2011). 2011 Compendium of Physical Activities: a second update of codes and MET values. *Medicine and science in sports and exercise*, *43*(8), 1575–1581.

3.6.3   Energy Expenditure of Physical Activity: Heart Rate Index Equation

Wicks et al. (2011) reported a simple method for the prediction of oxygen uptake (METs) during PA in patients with and without CHD, including those taking β-blockers, using the heart rate index equation (Table 3.5).

3.6.4   Energy Expenditure of Treadmill Walking

The oxygen cost of horizontal and grade walking increases linearly and predictably for moderate paces; that is, between 50 and 100 m/min, and exponentially thereafter (Franklin et al. 2000).

TABLE 3.5
Changes in heart rate to estimate energy expenditure (METs) during daily activities*

The energy cost of any activity, expressed as METs, can be estimated from the resting and exercise heart rates using the equation:

METs = (6 × Heart Rate Index) − 5

where the Heart Rate Index equals the activity heart rate divided by the resting heart rate.

Example #1:

A tennis player's resting heart rate of 60 beats per minute (bpm) is increased to 120 bpm during a tennis match. His MET level is estimated as follows: 120 bpm/60 bpm = 2.0 Heart Rate Index which is multiplied by 6, yielding 12, from which we subtract 5, yielding an estimated 7 METs.

$$(120/60 \times 6) - 5 = (2 \times 6) - 5 = 7 \text{ METs}$$

Example #2:

A recreational walker with a resting heart rate of 70 bpm walks at 105 bpm. Her estimated MET level is....

$$(105/70 \times 6) - 5 = (1.5 \times 6) - 5 = 4 \text{ METs}$$

*Adapted from Wicks, J. R., Oldridge, N. B., Nielsen, L. K., & Vickers, C. E. (2011). HR index – a simple method for the prediction of oxygen uptake. *Medicine and science in sports and exercise*, 43(10), 2005–2012.

Consequently, oxygen consumption, expressed as mL/kg/min, can be estimated with a reasonable degree of accuracy for walking speeds within this range. Table 3.6 lists the approximate energy requirements in METs for varied walking speeds (1.7–3.75 mph) and percent grades (0–20%) (Franklin et al., 2000).

3.6.5 THE RULE OF 2 AND 3 MPH

Because most elderly, unfit, overweight/obese, or cardiac patients prefer to walk at more moderate paces, it should be recognized that walking on level ground at 2 and 3 mph speeds approximates 2 and 3 METs, respectively. Moreover, at a 2-mph walking speed, each 3.5% increase in treadmill grade adds ~1 MET to the gross energy expenditure. If a patient desires to walk at a 2-mph pace but requires a 4 MET workload for training, he/she would be advised to add 7% grade to this speed. For patients who can negotiate the faster walking speed (3 mph), recognize that each 2.5% increase in treadmill grade adds an additional MET to the gross energy cost. Accordingly, a workload of 3 mph, 5% grade, would approximate 5 METs. Using this practical rule can be helpful in counseling their patients regarding appropriate walking speeds and grades for training without the need for consulting tables or nomograms (Franklin & Gordon, 2009).

3.6.6 HOW MUCH EXERCISE IS ENOUGH?

Contemporary exercise guidelines or recommendations, the importance of progressing training intensities (METs) over time, and the concept of MET-minutes/week will also be briefly discussed relative to the recommended exercise dosage.

3.6.7 CONTEMPORARY PHYSICAL ACTIVITY RECOMMENDATIONS

Moderate-to-vigorous PA, which corresponds to any activity ≥3 METs, has been consistently shown to reduce the health risks associated with chronic diseases and the likelihood of developing them (Haskell et al., 2007).[76] To promote and maintain health, moderate-intensity PA (40–59% aerobic capacity or 3.0–5.9 METs) for a minimum of 30 minutes for five days each week, or vigorous

TABLE 3.6
Approximate energy requirements in METs for horizontal and graded walking*

Walking speed (mph)

Grade (%)	1.7	2.0	2.5	3.0	3.4	3.75
0	2.3	2.5	2.9	3.3	3.6	3.9
2.5	2.9	3.2	3.8	4.3	4.8	5.2
5.0	3.5	3.9	4.6	5.4	5.9	6.5
7.5	4.1	4.6	5.5	6.4	7.1	7.8
10.0	4.6	5.3	6.3	7.4	8.3	9.1
12.5	5.2	6.0	7.2	8.5	9.5	10.4
15.0	5.8	6.6	8.1	9.5	10.6	11.7
17.5	6.4	7.3	8.9	10.5	11.8	12.9
20.0	7.0	8.0	9.8	11.6	13.0	14.2

*Adapted from Franklin, B. A., Whaley, M. H., Howley, E. T., & Balady, G. J. (2000). *ACSM's Guidelines for Exercise Testing and Prescription*. Philadelphia: Lippincott Williams & Wilkins.

intensity PA (≥60% aerobic capacity or ≥6.0 METs) for a minimum of 20 minutes for three days each week, or combinations thereof, is recommended (Haskell et al., 2007). Although traditional recommendations suggest that accumulated moderate-to-vigorous intensity exercise bouts should last ≥10 minutes to achieve the 30-minute daily minimum, recent studies suggest that even shorter periods of exercise, accrued over time, can evoke cardiovascular and health benefits (Fan et al., 2013; Glazer et al., 2013).

3.6.8 Progression of Exercise Training Intensities for Optimal Benefits

Most middle-aged and older people, with and without CHD, initiate exercise programs at ~2 to 3 METs, corresponding to level walking at ~2 to 3 mph. Far too often, however, these individuals fail to increase the intensity of their exercise over time as their level of CRF improves (Squires et al., 2018). This failure prevents them from achieving the maximal possible reduction in their risk of CVD.

Numerous studies now suggest that a "good" level of CRF, determined by progressive exercise testing to fatigue, is a far better predictor of survival or longevity than merely being physically active. Because CRF can be influenced by age, sex, regular PA, and chronic disease, it is important to establish goal exercise training intensities, expressed as METs, which are likely to confer "good" CRF levels that are associated with long-term survival (Franklin et al., 2020).

Figure 3.7 shows age- and sex-adjusted "good" levels of CRF for men and women, based on the FRIEND database (Kaminsky et al., 2015), and the recommended training intensity (60–80% VO_2 reserve [VO_2R], expressed as METs) to achieve these fitness levels. Regression equations signify 70% VO_2R. Depending on their age, men should ideally be training between 5.0 and 10.5 METs and women between 3.7 and 7.6 METs. For example, using the FRIEND database, "good" CRF for a 65-year-old man approximates ≥8.7 METs. Accordingly, a training intensity of 5.6–7.2 METs, ~6.4 METs (70% VO_2R), achieved over time (3–12 months) should enable this patient to attain "good" fitness during subsequent exercise testing.

3.6.9 Understanding the Concept of MET-Minutes per Week

This metric enables clinicians and patients to translate the guideline-driven minimum recommendation (500 MET-minutes per week) into achievable goals by quantifying incremental or accumulated

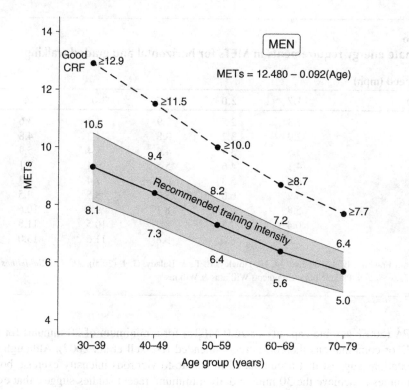

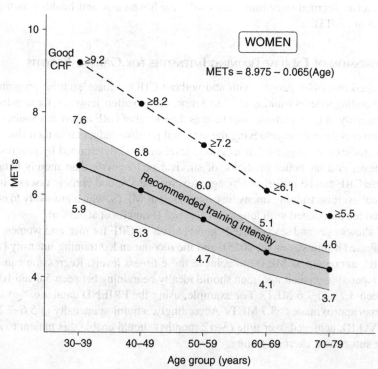

FIGURE 3.7 Age- and sex-adjusted "good" levels of cardiorespiratory fitness (CRF) for men and women and the recommended training intensity (60–80% VO_2R, expressed as METs) to achieve these fitness levels

https://doi.org/10.1093/eurjpc/zwaa094 with permission.

exercise in a simple formula: METs per activity × number of minutes/session × days/week = MET-minutes per week. For example, 60 minutes of walking at a 3-mph pace (3.5 METs), three days/week = 630 MET-min per week. Alternatively, 30 minutes of singles tennis (7 METs), three days/week = 630 MET-min per week. Or, for the distance runner, 20 minutes of running at a 6-mph pace (10 METs), three days/week = 600 MET-min per week. Because the ACSM recommends ≥500 to 1,000 MET-minutes per week (Garber et al., 2011), beyond usual activities, all three of these exercise programs would meet their criteria for an effective exercise dosage.

3.7 WALKING: THE UNDERVALUED PRESCRIPTION

Walking is the most accessible and easily regulated exercise that can enhance health and CRF. Moreover, inherent neuromuscular limitations to the speed of walking (and therefore, the rate of energy expenditure) establish it as the most appropriate activity to help prevent and treat chronic disease. Even at the slowest speeds (e.g., <2 mph), walking involves an aerobic requirement of ≥2 metabolic equivalents (METs) (Franklin et al., 1983).[83]

Advantages of a conventional walking program include a low drop-out rate, an easily tolerable work intensity, and fewer musculoskeletal and orthopedic problems of the legs, knees, and feet than jogging or running. It is also a "companionable" activity that requires no special equipment other than a pair of well-fitted athletic shoes. Variations of conventional walking programs, including walking with a backpack (Shoenfeld et al., 1980), swimming pool walking (Evans et al., 1978), dog walking (Bauman et al., 2001), and golf course walking (Parkkari et al., 2000), have also been shown to improve health and CRF and facilitate cardiovascular risk reduction.

3.7.1 WALKING DISTANCE AND SPEED AS PROGNOSTIC INDICATORS

Numerous studies and pooled analyses, in persons with and without CHD, have shown that weekly walking distance and walking speed are powerful predictors of mortality in middle-aged and older adults (Beatty et al., 2012; Cesari et al., 2005; Hakim et al., 1998; Kavanagh et al., 2008; Lo et al., 2015; Newman et al., 2006; Stanaway et al., 2011; Studenski et al., 2011; Yazdanyar et al., 2014). Hakim et al. (1998) studied the relation between distance walked per day and subsequent all-cause mortality in 707 nonsmoking retired men 61 to 81 years of age. Over a 12-year follow-up, there were 208 deaths. The mortality rate among those men who walked <1 mile/day was nearly twice that among those who walked >2 miles/day. Investigators concluded that regular distance walking is associated with a lower overall mortality rate in older, physically capable men.

Data from the Concord Health and Ageing in Men Project, a cohort study of 1705 healthy men ≥70 years living in several inner city suburbs in Sydney, Australia, were used to clarify the walking pace that may be associated with a heightened mortality (Stanaway et al., 2011). At baseline, walking speed was carefully measured at the usual pace, documenting the fastest time from two trials. A natural walking speed of ≤0.89 m/s (~2 mph) was most predictive of early mortality, while older men who walked at speeds greater than this were less likely to die during the 6-year follow-up. Moreover, no men who initially walked at speeds of ≥1.34 m/s (~3 mph) were among the 266 deaths reported (Stanaway et al., 2011). Interestingly, the walking speed associated with the highest mortality was similar to the gait speed (0.80 m/s), signifying the median life expectancy in a pooled analysis of nine cohort studies using individual data from diverse populations (n = 34,485 community-dwelling older adults, ≥65 years; 59.6% women) with baseline gait speed data. The pooled hazard ratio per each 0.1 m/s faster gait speed was 0.88 (Studenski et al., 2011).

In outpatients with stable CHD, the 6-minute walk test has been shown to provide independent and additive information beyond traditional risk factors and a prognostic significance over an 8-year follow-up, similar to CRF (peak METs) for predicting HF, myocardial infarction, and death (Beatty et al., 2012). In adults ≥65 years with HF, impairment in gait speed (<0.8 vs. ≥0.8 m/s), measured within one year before the diagnosis of incident HF, was independently associated with mortality (hazard ratio, 1.37), after adjusting for potential confounders (Lo et al., 2015). Collectively, these data suggest that greater daily walking distances and/or faster walking speeds are associated with increased survival. Nevertheless, additional clinical trials are needed before we can confidently state that favorably modifying either of these variables will improve outcomes in the elderly population.

3.8 BENEFITS AND RISKS OF HIGH-INTENSITY INTERVAL TRAINING

Cardiovascular exercise is one of the most effective lifestyle therapies in the prevention and treatment of coronary artery disease (CAD) (Quindry & Franklin, 2018). Typical cardiac rehabilitation exercise protocols incorporate moderate-intensity continuous training (MICT) where participants exercise at 50–75% of their peak or maximal attained heart rate (HRmax). Recently, there has been a heightened interest in high-intensity interval training (HIIT), which alternates high-intensity 30 to 240 second exercise bouts with periods of more moderate activity or passive recovery. An intensity of 85 to 100% HRmax is generally targeted during the most strenuous HIIT intervals (Gayda et al., 2016). In healthy individuals, HIIT has been shown to elicit similar improvements in body composition and aerobic capacity as compared with MICT but in an abbreviated training duration (Ross et al., 2016). HIIT has also been reported to increase post-exercise oxygen consumption, which has the potential to augment weight loss (Gibala et al., 2012). Despite some potential advantages of HIIT, questions remain regarding its safety and efficacy as compared with MICT in patients with CAD.

Patients with CAD are at a transiently increased risk of acute cardiac events during high intensity exercise. In one study, coronary patients participating in moderate or high intensity exercise experienced one acute cardiac event per 58,607 training hours; however, those exercising at high intensity were ~6 times more likely to experience an event (Rognmo et al., 2012). Contemporary risk stratification guidelines classify patients as low, moderate, or high risk based on signs or symptoms of residual myocardial ischemia, exercise capacity, ejection fraction, threatening ventricular arrhythmias, and other characteristics in the medical history (Thompson et al., 2007). To date, there have been 11 randomized controlled trials comparing HIIT to MICT in low to moderate risk patient subsets. Although there were no exercise-related cardiac events attributed to HIIT in any of these trials, HIIT has not been studied in high-risk populations (Quindry et al., 2019).

Head-to-head trials of HIIT and MICT in patients with CAD have yielded comparative data. The most studied HIIT protocol in CAD populations is a 12-week workout regimen where patients exercise in intervals of 4 × 4 minutes, achieving 85 to 95% of the peak attained heart rate during exercise testing with 3-minute interspersed bouts of active recovery. HIIT generally outperformed MICT when assessing VO_2 max, submaximal exercise performance, and cardiac performance. However, HIIT elicited comparable outcomes relative to MICT when assessing body weight, body composition, resting heart rate, resting blood pressure, exercise blood pressure, blood glucose, and blood lipids. Also, most studies comparing HIIT to MICT did not include a sedentary control group. Long-term comparisons of these exercise regimens in coronary patients are less clear. Moholdt et al. (2009) found greater improvements in aerobic capacity with HIIT as compared to MICT in patients six months after coronary artery bypass grafting. Conversely, Pattyn and colleagues found no difference in the benefits between HIIT and MICT in a multisite, randomized controlled trial in patients with CAD after 12 months (Pattyn et al., 2016).

When recommending a specific exercise regimen, it is also important to consider adherence as well as the characteristics of the patient population. Although there is a low drop-out rate in both HIIT and MICT cardiac rehabilitation programs, self-reported adherence to home-based HIIT is lower than MICT (Moholdt et al., 2012; Pattyn et al., 2016). Others have substantiated the fact that high intensity exercise regimens are less likely to retain participants (Haskell et al., 2007). This finding may be exaggerated in previously sedentary patients with CAD, many of whom comprise the populations participating in exercise-based cardiac rehabilitation. In summary, clinicians should consider patient characteristics, adherence, safety, and medical supervision when recommending HIIT to their patients and recognize that the potential advantages may be outweighed by decreased compliance and/or increased risks.

3.9 EXTREME EXERCISE AND CARDIOVASCULAR HEALTH: CHANGING PARADIGMS AND PERCEPTIONS

Reports documenting the favorable risk factor profiles and superb cardiac performance of long-distance runners, the limited use of anti-diabetic, antihypertensive, and cholesterol-lowering medications among endurance athletes, and the recent finding that regular aerobic exercise prevents cellular senescence in humans, have led an increasing number of middle-aged and older adults to adopt the notion that "more exercise is better" (Franklin & Billecke, 2012).

Clearly, 35 minutes of regular vigorous PA enhances CRF and health, but performing 3-hour bouts of strenuous PA does not multiply the health benefits. In fact, the added survival benefits of vigorous PA (i.e., running) appear to plateau beyond 35 minutes per day (Wen et al., 2011). Moreover, recent studies suggest that potentially adverse cardiovascular maladaptations may occur following high-volume and/or high-intensity long-term aerobic exercise training, which may attenuate the health benefits of a physically active lifestyle. Accelerated coronary artery calcification, exercise-induced cardiac biomarker release (e.g., cardiac troponin I and B-type natriuretic peptide), myocardial fibrosis, transient myocardial dysfunction, AF, plaque rupture and acute coronary thrombosis, and even sudden cardiac death have been reported (Eijsvogels et al., 2018; Franklin et al., 2020; O'Keefe et al., 2014).

If the current mantra "exercise is medicine" is embraced, there are indications and contraindications, and underdosing and overdosing are possible. The increased cardiovascular risks of vigorous to near-maximal exercise, especially over short (unaccustomed) bursts or extended durations, should be weighed against the benefits. Thus, extreme exercise may have a U-shaped or reverse J-shaped dose-response curve with a plateau in benefit or even adverse effects in individuals with a diseased or susceptible heart (e.g., hypertrophic cardiomyopathy) (Eijsvogels et al., 2018; Franklin et al., 2020). As an increasing proportion of the population are investing an unprecedented number of hours in intense endurance training and competition, the need for clinicians to clarify the associated risk–benefit ratio of this practice is apparent (Franklin & Billecke, 2012).

3.10 STRATEGIES TO ENHANCE EXERCISE ADOPTION AND ADHERENCE

The likelihood that patients will or will not engage in a particular lifestyle behavior is governed by a myriad of socioeconomic, attitudinal, and cultural factors, including their expectations of the benefits, costs, and consequences of that behavior. Lack of or a suboptimal social support system, social isolation, financial difficulties, declaring that they are too busy, and underlying psychosocial factors (e.g., depression, denial, chronic life stress) are often cited as common barriers to achieving successful lifestyle behavior changes (Franklin & Vanhecke, 2008; Spring et al., 2013; Williams et al., 2003). Strategizing with the patient to identify realistic options to overcome these barriers, real or perceived, is integral to changing unhealthy behaviors (Spring et al., 2013). In our experience, these discussions should be complemented by counseling strategies to overcome inertia with downscaled goals (Franklin et al., 2020).

3.10.1 Overcoming Inertia With Downscaled Goals

For many patients, setting initial goals and taking action for lifestyle modification (e.g., structured exercise program, increased lifestyle PA) may be unrealistic and overwhelming, especially if contemporary guidelines are embraced. Although inertia is a major barrier to making permanent lifestyle changes, it is also one of the easiest obstacles to overcome. We simply need to get patients to *act*. Any action they take, no matter how trivial, may help to gain momentum. For example, rather than counseling the habitually sedentary patient to exercise for ≥30 minutes/day on most days of the week, as contemporary guidelines suggest, our approach would be to recommend 10-minute moderate intensity exercise bouts (e.g., brisk walking), three times per week, over the initial month of physical conditioning (Franklin & Vanhecke, 2008). By making it easier to overcome inertia, this approach gets patients moving in the right direction, many of whom subsequently find themselves not only meeting but also exceeding these goals.

3.10.2 RECOMMENDATIONS TO ENHANCE EXERCISE ADHERENCE

Although many patients can be motivated to participate in an exercise program, especially if downscaled goals are initially adopted, maintaining the commitment can be challenging. Unfortunately, psychosocial variables or family/work-related responsibilities often outweigh the positive variables contributing to sustained interest and enthusiasm, leading to a decline in exercise adherence and program effectiveness. Several research-based counseling and motivational strategies may enhance patient interest and facilitate initiation of and compliance with a structured exercise program (Table 3.7). Additionally, we can improve exercise compliance by referring our patients to quality physical conditioning programs that employ certified, enthusiastic exercise professionals.

3.11 USING TECHNOLOGY TO PROMOTE PHYSICAL ACTIVITY

Digital tools such as social media, mobile games on smart phones and tablets, varied apps that promote PA, and activity trackers may assist in reducing barriers to structured exercise by helping patients with planning, increasing access to health-fitness programs, and providing daily goal reminders (Chaddha et al., 2017). Self-monitoring techniques, devices (e.g. pedometers, accelerometers, personalized activity intelligence (Nes et al., 2017), heart rate monitors), or apps can be helpful in this regard. Counseling and reinforcement can be handled over the phone, in Zoom chats, or via the Internet. Active-play video gaming can also be used to promote healthy weight and

---

TABLE 3.7
Strategies to enhance exercise compliance

Assess exercise habits and counsel patients to be physically active
Evaluate the patient's "Readiness to Change" and target interventions accordingly
Establish short-term, attainable goals; evaluate progress at subsequent office visits
Clarify the "whys" and "hows" of exercise
Minimize injury with a moderate exercise prescription; emphasize gradual progression
Advocate exercising with others (i.e., social support)
Avoid overemphasis of regimented calisthenics
Consider gender differences in activity programming
Provide positive reinforcement through periodic testing and feedback of results (fitness, fatness, blood
     pressure, cholesterol and glucose levels)
Recruit spouse support of the exercise program
Use progress charts or a computerized data system to record individual exercise achievements
Encourage patients to use certified, enthusiastic exercise professionals
Stress participation in activities that are enjoyable
Include an optional recreational game to the conditioning program format
Listen to music or watch television while exercising

regular PA in children and adolescents, middle-aged and older adults, and patients with chronic disease (Lieberman et al., 2011). One report, in healthy adults, noted that the aerobic requirements for Wii Sports and Wii Fit Plus game activities approximated 1.3 to 5.6 METs, which correspond to the energy expenditure associated with very slow (<1 mph) to extremely fast walking (~4.0 mph) (Miyachi et al., 2010). Others have suggested that using active-play video gaming, which can be readily accessible, highly competitive, and reinforcing (i.e., winning against an opponent), may serve as a gateway to structured exercise regimens. In aggregate, these data suggest that using technology, a contributor to the physical inactivity epidemic, can also be part of the solution (Chaddha et al., 2017).

3.12 CONCLUSION

Regular moderate-to-vigorous intensity exercise has been described as "a miracle drug that can benefit every part of the body and substantially extend lifespan" (Wen & Wu, 2012). The authors suggested that the cardiovascular and systemic health benefits of regular exercise are underestimated by many clinicians, who often fail to emphasize the salutary impact of regular PA and/or improved CRF, as well as the harms of physical inactivity, even though they routinely counsel patients about other modifiable cardiovascular risk factors, such as cigarette smoking, elevated cholesterol levels, obesity, diabetes, and hypertension.

In an era of escalating health care expenditures, structured exercise regimens, increased lifestyle PA, or both provide independent, additive, and complementary benefits for achieving improved health outcomes. If the salutary impact of regular exercise is to be applied and optimized, the prescription at present remains woefully underfilled for too many patients with and without CVD. Thus, the medical community should embrace this clinically proven, readily accessible, and cost-effective strategy as a *first-line therapy* to prevent and treat the skyrocketing prevalence of chronic diseases.

REFERENCES

Ackermann, R. T., Cheadle, A., Sandhu, N., Madsen, L., Wagner, E. H., & LoGerfo, J. P. (2003). Community exercise program use and changes in healthcare costs for older adults. *American journal of preventive medicine*, 25(3), 232–237.

Ainsworth, B. E., Haskell, W. L., Herrmann, S. D., Meckes, N., Bassett, D. R., Tudor-Locke, C., Greer, J. L., Vezina, J., Whitt-Glover, M. C., & Leon, A. S. (2011). 2011 Compendium of Physical Activities: a second update of codes and MET values. *Medicine and science in sports and exercise*, 43(8), 1575–1581.

Aizer, A., Gaziano, J. M., Cook, N. R., Manson, J. E., Buring, J. E., & Albert, C. M. (2009). Relation of vigorous exercise to risk of atrial fibrillation. *The American journal of cardiology*, 103(11), 1572–1577.

Andersen, R. E., Wadden, T. A., Bartlett, S. J., Zemel, B., Verde, T. J., & Franckowiak, S. C. (1999). Effects of lifestyle activity vs structured aerobic exercise in obese women: a randomized trial. *Jama*, 281(4), 335–340.

Barnard, R. J., Macalpin, R., Kattus, A. A., & Buckberg, G. D. (1973). Ischemic response to sudden strenuous exercise in healthy men. *Circulation*, 48(5), 936–942.

Bauman, A. E., Russell, S. J., Furber, S. E., & Dobson, A. J. (2001). The epidemiology of dog walking: an unmet need for human and canine health. *The medical journal of Australia*, 175(11–12), 632–634.

Beatty, A. L., Schiller, N. B., & Whooley, M. A. (2012). Six-minute walk test as a prognostic tool in stable coronary heart disease: data from the heart and soul study. *Archives of Internal Medicine*, 172(14), 1096–1102.

Blair, S. N., Kohl, H. W., Paffenbarger, R. S., Clark, D. G., Cooper, K. H., & Gibbons, L. W. (1989). Physical fitness and all-cause mortality: a prospective study of healthy men and women. *Jama*, 262(17), 2395–2401.

Boden, W. E., Franklin, B., Berra, K., Haskell, W. L., Calfas, K. J., Zimmerman, F. H., & Wenger, N. K. (2014). Exercise as a therapeutic intervention in patients with stable ischemic heart disease: an underfilled prescription. *The American journal of medicine*, 127(10), 905–911.

Boden, W. E., Franklin, B. A., & Wenger, N. K. (2013). Physical activity and structured exercise for patients with stable ischemic heart disease. *Jama*, *309*(2), 143–144.

Borg, G. A. (1982). Psychophysical bases of perceived exertion. *Medicine and science in sports and exercise*, *14*, 377–381. https://doi.org/10.1249/00005768-198205000-00012

Cesari, M., Kritchevsky, S. B., Penninx, B. W., Nicklas, B. J., Simonsick, E. M., Newman, A. B., Tylavsky, F. A., Brach, J. S., Satterfield, S., & Bauer, D. C. (2005). Prognostic value of usual gait speed in well-functioning older people – results from the Health, Aging and Body Composition Study. *Journal of the American Geriatrics Society*, *53*(10), 1675–1680.

Chaddha, A., Jackson, E. A., Richardson, C. R., & Franklin, B. A. (2017). Technology to help promote physical activity. *American journal of cardiology*, *119*(1), 149–152.

Curry, S. J., Krist, A. H., Owens, D. K., Barry, M. J., Caughey, A. B., Davidson, K. W., Doubeni, C. A., Epling, J. W., Kemper, A. R., & Kubik, M. (2018). Screening for cardiovascular disease risk with electrocardiography: US Preventive Services Task Force recommendation statement. *Jama*, *319*(22), 2308–2314.

de Silva, C. G. d. S., Kokkinos, P., Doom, R., Loganathan, D., Fonda, H., Chan, K., de Araújo, C. G. S., & Myers, J. (2019). Association between cardiorespiratory fitness, obesity, and health care costs: the Veterans Exercise Testing Study. *International journal of obesity*, *43*(11), 2225–2232.

DeFina, L. F., Radford, N. B., Barlow, C. E., Willis, B. L., Leonard, D., Haskell, W. L., Farrell, S. W., Pavlovic, A., Abel, K., & Berry, J. D. (2019). Association of all-cause and cardiovascular mortality with high levels of physical activity and concurrent coronary artery calcification. *JAMA cardiology*, *4*(2), 174–181.

Dimsdale, J. E., Hartley, L. H., Guiney, T., Ruskin, J. N., & Greenblatt, D. (1984). Postexercise peril: plasma catecholamines and exercise. *Jama*, *251*(5), 630–632.

Dunn, A. L., Marcus, B. H., Kampert, J. B., Garcia, M. E., Kohl III, H. W., & Blair, S. N. (1999). Comparison of lifestyle and structured interventions to increase physical activity and cardiorespiratory fitness: a randomized trial. *Jama*, *281*(4), 327–334.

Dutcher, J. R., Kahn, J., Grines, C., & Franklin, B. (2007). Comparison of left ventricular ejection fraction and exercise capacity as predictors of two-and five-year mortality following acute myocardial infarction. *The American journal of cardiology*, *99*(4), 436–441.

Eijsvogels, T. M., Thompson, P. D., & Franklin, B. A. (2018). The "extreme exercise hypothesis": recent findings and cardiovascular health implications. *Current treatment options in cardiovascular medicine*, *20*(10), 1–11.

Evans, B. W., Cureton, K. J., & Purvis, J. W. (1978). Metabolic and circulatory responses to walking and jogging in water. *Research Quarterly. American Alliance for Health, Physical Education and Recreation*, *49*(4), 442–449.

Fan, J. X., Brown, B. B., Hanson, H., Kowaleski-Jones, L., Smith, K. R., & Zick, C. D. (2013). Moderate to vigorous physical activity and weight outcomes: does every minute count? *American journal of health promotion*, *28*(1), 41–49.

Faselis, C., Doumas, M., Kokkinos, J. P., Panagiotakos, D., Kheirbek, R., Sheriff, H. M., Hare, K., Papademetriou, V., Fletcher, R., & Kokkinos, P. (2012). Exercise capacity and progression from prehypertension to hypertension. *Hypertension*, *60*(2), 333–338.

Franklin, B., Pamatmat, A., Johnson, S., Scherf, J., Mitchell, M., & Rubenfire, M. (1983). Metabolic cost of extremely slow walking in cardiac patients: implications for exercise testing and training. *Archives of physical medicine and rehabilitation*, *64*(11), 564–565.

Franklin, B. A. (2002). Survival of the fittest: evidence for high-risk and cardioprotective fitness levels. *Current sports medicine reports*, *1*(5), 257–259.

Franklin, B. A. (2014). Preventing exercise-related cardiovascular events: is a medical examination more urgent for physical activity or inactivity? *Circulation*, *129*(10), 1081–1084.

Franklin, B. A., Arena, R., Kaminsky, L. A., Peterman, J. E., Kokkinos, P., & Myers, J. (2020). Maximizing the cardioprotective benefits of exercise with age-, sex-, and fitness-adjusted target intensities for training. *European journal of preventive cardiology*. https://doi.org/10.1093/eurjpc/zwaa094

Franklin, B. A., & Billecke, S. (2012). Putting the benefits and risks of aerobic exercise in perspective. *Current sports medicine reports*, *11*(4), 201–208.

Franklin, B. A., Brinks, J., Berra, K., Lavie, C. J., Gordon, N. F., & Sperling, L. S. (2018). Using metabolic equivalents in clinical practice. *The American journal of cardiology*, *121*(3), 382–387.

Franklin, B. A., Brubaker, P. H., Harber, M. P., Lavie, C. J., Myers, J., & Kaminsky, L. A. (2020). The journal of cardiopulmonary rehabilitation and prevention at 40 years and its role in promoting lifestyle medicine for prevention of cardiovascular diseases: part 1. *Journal of cardiopulmonary rehabilitation and prevention*, *40*(3), 131–137.

Franklin, B. A., Kaminsky, L. A., & Kokkinos, P. (2018). Quantitating the dose of physical activity in secondary prevention: relation of exercise intensity to survival. *Mayo Clinic proceedings*, *93*(9), 1158–1163.

Franklin, B. A., Myers, J., & Kokkinos, P. (2020). Importance of lifestyle modification on cardiovascular risk reduction: counseling strategies to maximize patient outcomes. *Journal of cardiopulmonary rehabilitation and prevention*, *40*(3), 138–143.

Franklin, B. A., Thompson, P. D., Al-Zaiti, S. S., Albert, C. M., Hivert, M.-F., Levine, B. D., Lobelo, F., Madan, K., Sharrief, A. Z., & Eijsvogels, T. M. (2020). Exercise-related acute cardiovascular events and potential deleterious adaptations following long-term exercise training: placing the risks into perspective – an update: a scientific statement from the American Heart Association. *Circulation*, *141*(13), e705–e736.

Franklin, B. A., & Gordon, N. F. (2009). *Contemporary Diagnosis and Management in Cardiovascular Exercise*. Newton (PA): Handbooks in Health Care Company.

Franklin, B. A., & Vanhecke, T. E. (2008). Counseling patients to make cardioprotective lifestyle changes: strategies for success. *Preventive cardiology*, *11*(1), 50–55.

Franklin, B. A., Whaley, M. H., Howley, E. T., & Balady, G. J. (2000). *ACSM's Guidelines for Exercise Testing and Prescription*. Philadelphia: Lippincott Williams & Wilkins.

Franklin, B.A., & Zhu, W. (2021). *Home-Based Cardiac Rehabilitation: Helping Patients Help Themselves*. Monterey (CA): Healthy Learning.

Garber, C. E., Blissmer, B., Deschenes, M. R., Franklin, B. A., Lamonte, M. J., Lee, I.-M., Nieman, D. C., & Swain, D. P. (2011). American College of Sports Medicine position stand: quantity and quality of exercise for developing and maintaining cardiorespiratory, musculoskeletal, and neuromotor fitness in apparently healthy adults: guidance for prescribing exercise. *Medicine and science in sports and exercise*, *43*(7), 1334–1359.

Gayda, M., Ribeiro, P. A., Juneau, M., & Nigam, A. (2016). Comparison of different forms of exercise training in patients with cardiac disease: where does high-intensity interval training fit? *Canadian journal of cardiology*, *32*(4), 485–494.

George, J., Abdulla, R. K., Yeow, R., Aggarwal, A., Boura, J., Wegner, J., & Franklin, B. A. (2017). Daily energy expenditure and its relation to health care costs in patients undergoing ambulatory electrocardiographic monitoring. *American journal of cardiology*, *119*(4), 658–663.

Gibala, M. J., Little, J. P., MacDonald, M. J., & Hawley, J. A. (2012). Physiological adaptations to low-volume, high-intensity interval training in health and disease. *The journal of physiology*, *590*(5), 1077–1084.

Glazer, N. L., Lyass, A., Esliger, D. W., Blease, S. J., Freedson, P. S., Massaro, J. M., Murabito, J. M., & Vasan, R. S. (2013). Sustained and shorter bouts of physical activity are related to cardiovascular health. *Medicine and science in sports and exercise*, *45*(1), 109.

Grafe, K., Bendick, P., Burr, M., Boura, J., & Franklin, B. A. (2018). Effects of resistance training on vascular and hemodynamic responses in patients with coronary artery disease. *Research quarterly for exercise and sport*, *89*(4), 457–464.

Green, D. J., O'Driscoll, G., Joyner, M. J., & Cable, N. T. (2008). Exercise and cardiovascular risk reduction: time to update the rationale for exercise? *Journal of applied physiology*, *105*(2), 766–768.

Gulati, M., Pandey, D. K., Arnsdorf, M. F., Lauderdale, D. S., Thisted, R. A., Wicklund, R. H., Al-Hani, A. J., & Black, H. R. (2003). Exercise capacity and the risk of death in women: the St James Women Take Heart Project. *Circulation*, *108*(13), 1554–1559.

Hakim, A. A., Petrovitch, H., Burchfiel, C. M., Ross, G. W., Rodriguez, B. L., White, L. R., Yano, K., Curb, J. D., & Abbott, R. D. (1998). Effects of walking on mortality among nonsmoking retired men. *New England journal of medicine*, *338*(2), 94–99.

Haskell, W. L., Lee, I.-M., Pate, R. R., Powell, K. E., Blair, S. N., Franklin, B. A., Macera, C. A., Heath, G. W., Thompson, P. D., & Bauman, A. (2007). Physical activity and public health: updated recommendation for adults from the American College of Sports Medicine and the American Heart Association. *Circulation*, *116*(9), 1081.

Hoogeboom, T. J., Dronkers, J. J., Hulzebos, E. H., & van Meeteren, N. L. (2014). Merits of exercise therapy before and after major surgery. *Current opinion in anaesthesiology*, *27*(2), 161.

Hu, F. B., Sigal, R. J., Rich-Edwards, J. W., Colditz, G. A., Solomon, C. G., Willett, W. C., Speizer, F. E., & Manson, J. E. (1999). Walking compared with vigorous physical activity and risk of type 2 diabetes in women: a prospective study. *Jama*, *282*(15), 1433–1439.

Huai, P., Xun, H., Reilly, K. H., Wang, Y., Ma, W., & Xi, B. (2013). Physical activity and risk of hypertension: a meta-analysis of prospective cohort studies. *Hypertension*, *62*(6), 1021–1026.

Jae, S. Y., Franklin, B. A., Choo, J., Yoon, E. S., Choi, Y.-H., & Park, W. H. (2016). Fitness, body habitus, and the risk of incident type 2 diabetes mellitus in Korean men. *The American journal of cardiology*, *117*(4), 585–589.

Jonas, D. E., Reddy, S., Middleton, J. C., Barclay, C., Green, J., Baker, C., & Asher, G. N. (2018). Screening for cardiovascular disease risk with resting or exercise electrocardiography: evidence report and systematic review for the US Preventive Services Task Force. *Jama*, *319*(22), 2315–2328.

Jurca, R., Lamonte, M. J., Barlow, C. E., Kampert, J. B., Church, T. S., & Blair, S. N. (2005). Association of muscular strength with incidence of metabolic syndrome in men. *Medicine and science in sports and exercise*, *37*(11), 1849.

Kaminsky, L. A., Arena, R., Beckie, T. M., Brubaker, P. H., Church, T. S., Forman, D. E., Franklin, B. A., Gulati, M., Lavie, C. J., & Myers, J. (2013). The importance of cardiorespiratory fitness in the United States: the need for a national registry: a policy statement from the American Heart Association. *Circulation*, *127*(5), 652–662.

Kaminsky, L. A., Arena, R., & Myers, J. (2015). Reference standards for cardiorespiratory fitness measured with cardiopulmonary exercise testing: data from the Fitness Registry and the Importance of Exercise National Database. *Mayo Clinic proceedings*, *90*(11), 1515–1523.

Kavanagh, T., Hamm, L. F., Beyene, J., Mertens, D. J., Kennedy, J., Campbell, R., Fallah, S., & Shephard, R. J. (2008). Usefulness of improvement in walking distance versus peak oxygen uptake in predicting prognosis after myocardial infarction and/or coronary artery bypass grafting in men. *The American journal of cardiology*, *101*(10), 1423–1427.

Knowler, W. C., Barrett-Connor, E., Fowler, S. E., Hamman, R. F., Lachin, J. M., Walker, E. A., & Nathan, D. M. (2002). Reduction in the incidence of type 2 diabetes with lifestyle intervention or metformin. *New England journal of medicine*, *346*(6), 393–403. https://doi.org/10.1056/NEJMoa012512

Kodama, S., Saito, K., Tanaka, S., Maki, M., Yachi, Y., Asumi, M., Sugawara, A., Totsuka, K., Shimano, H., & Ohashi, Y. (2009). Cardiorespiratory fitness as a quantitative predictor of all-cause mortality and cardiovascular events in healthy men and women: a meta-analysis. *Jama*, *301*(19), 2024–2035.

Kokkinos, P., Faselis, C., Myers, J., Sui, X., Zhang, J., Tsimploulis, A., Chawla, L., & Palant, C. (2015). Exercise capacity and risk of chronic kidney disease in US veterans: a cohort study. *Mayo Clinic proceedings*, *90*(4), 461–468.

Kokkinos, P., & Myers, J. (2010). Exercise and physical activity: clinical outcomes and applications. *Circulation*, *122*(16), 1637–1648.

Kokkinos, P. F., Faselis, C., Myers, J., Narayan, P., Sui, X., Zhang, J., Lavie, C. J., Moore, H., Karasik, P., & Fletcher, R. (2017). Cardiorespiratory fitness and incidence of major adverse cardiovascular events in US veterans: a cohort study. *Mayo Clinic proceedings*, *92*(1), 39–48.

Li, Y., Pan, A., Wang, D. D., Liu, X., Dhana, K., Franco, O. H., Kaptoge, S., Di Angelantonio, E., Stampfer, M., & Willett, W. C. (2018). Impact of healthy lifestyle factors on life expectancies in the US population. *Circulation*, *138*(4), 345–355.

Lieberman, D. A., Chamberlin, B., Medina Jr, E., Franklin, B. A., Sanner, B. M., & Vafiadis, D. K. (2011). The power of play: Innovations in Getting Active Summit 2011: a science panel proceedings report from the American Heart Association. *Circulation*, *123*(21), 2507–2516.

Lo, A. X., Donnelly, J. P., McGwin Jr, G., Bittner, V., Ahmed, A., & Brown, C. J. (2015). Impact of gait speed and instrumental activities of daily living on all-cause mortality in adults ≥65 years with heart failure. *The American journal of cardiology*, *115*(6), 797–801.

Manson, J. E., Nathan, D. M., Krolewski, A. S., Stampfer, M. J., Willett, W. C., & Hennekens, C. H. (1992). A prospective study of exercise and incidence of diabetes among US male physicians. *Jama*, *268*(1), 63–67.

Martin, M. Y., Powell, M. P., Peel, C., Zhu, S., & Allman, R. (2006). Leisure-time physical activity and health-care utilization in older adults. *Journal of aging and physical activity*, *14*(4), 392–410.

McCartney, N., McKelvie, R., Martin, J., Sale, D., & MacDougall, J. (1993). Weight-training-induced attenuation of the circulatory response of older males to weight lifting. *Journal of applied physiology*, *74*(3), 1056–1060.

McCullough, P. A., Gallagher, M. J., Dejong, A. T., Sandberg, K. R., Trivax, J. E., Alexander, D., Kasturi, G., Jafri, S. M., Krause, K. R., & Chengelis, D. L. (2006). Cardiorespiratory fitness and short-term complications after bariatric surgery. *Chest*, *130*(2), 517–525.

Mitchell, T. L., Gibbons, L. W., Devers, S. M., & Earnest, C. P. (2004). Effects of cardiorespiratory fitness on healthcare utilization. *Medicine and science in sports and exercise*, *36*(12), 2088–2092.

Miyachi, M., Yamamoto, K., Ohkawara, K., & Tanaka, S. (2010). METs in adults while playing active video games: a metabolic chamber study. *Medicine and science in sports and exercise*, *42*(6), 1149–1153.

Moholdt, T., Bekken Vold, M., Grimsmo, J., Slørdahl, S. A., & Wisløff, U. (2012). Home-based aerobic interval training improves peak oxygen uptake equal to residential cardiac rehabilitation: a randomized, controlled trial. *PloS one*, *7*(7), e41199.

Moholdt, T. T., Amundsen, B. H., Rustad, L. A., Wahba, A., Løvø, K. T., Gullikstad, L. R., Bye, A., Skogvoll, E., Wisløff, U., & Slørdahl, S. A. (2009). Aerobic interval training versus continuous moderate exercise after coronary artery bypass surgery: a randomized study of cardiovascular effects and quality of life. *American heart journal*, *158*(6), 1031–1037.

Myers, J., Doom, R., King, R., Fonda, H., Chan, K., Kokkinos, P., & Rehkopf, D. H. (2018). Association between cardiorespiratory fitness and health care costs: the veterans exercise testing study. *Mayo Clinic proceedings*, *93*(1), 48–55.

Myers, J., Kokkinos, P., Chan, K., Dandekar, E., Yilmaz, B., Nagare, A., Faselis, C., & Soofi, M. (2017). Cardiorespiratory fitness and reclassification of risk for incidence of heart failure: the Veterans Exercise Testing Study. *Circulation: heart failure*, *10*(6), e003780.

Nes, B. M., Gutvik, C. R., Lavie, C. J., Nauman, J., & Wisløff, U. (2017). Personalized activity intelligence (PAI) for prevention of cardiovascular disease and promotion of physical activity. *The American journal of medicine*, *130*(3), 328–336.

Newman, A. B., Simonsick, E. M., Naydeck, B. L., Boudreau, R. M., Kritchevsky, S. B., Nevitt, M. C., Pahor, M., Satterfield, S., Brach, J. S., & Studenski, S. A. (2006). Association of long-distance corridor walk performance with mortality, cardiovascular disease, mobility limitation, and disability. *Jama*, *295*(17), 2018–2026.

Niebauer, J., & Cooke, J. P. (1996). Cardiovascular effects of exercise: role of endothelial shear stress. *Journal of the American College of Cardiology*, *28*(7), 1652–1660.

Nocon, M., Hiemann, T., Müller-Riemenschneider, F., Thalau, F., Roll, S., & Willich, S. N. (2008). Association of physical activity with all-cause and cardiovascular mortality: a systematic review and meta-analysis. *European journal of preventive cardiology*, *15*(3), 239–246.

Nylen, E. S., Gandhi, S. M., Kheirbek, R., & Kokkinos, P. (2015). Enhanced fitness and renal function in type 2 diabetes. *Diabetic medicine*, *32*(10), 1342–1345.

O'Keefe, J. H., Franklin, B., & Lavie, C. J. (2014). Exercising for health and longevity vs peak performance: different regimens for different goals. *Mayo Clinic proceedings*, *89*(9), 1171–1175.

Pandey, A., Patel, M., Gao, A., Willis, B. L., Das, S. R., Leonard, D., Drazner, M. H., de Lemos, J. A., DeFina, L., & Berry, J. D. (2015). Changes in mid-life fitness predicts heart failure risk at a later age independent of interval development of cardiac and noncardiac risk factors: the Cooper Center Longitudinal Study. *American heart journal*, *169*(2), 290–297. e291.

Parkkari, J., Natri, A., Kannus, P., Mänttäri, A., Laukkanen, R., Haapasalo, H., Nenonen, A., Pasanen, M., Oja, P., & Vuori, I. (2000). A controlled trial of the health benefits of regular walking on a golf course. *The American journal of medicine*, *109*(2), 102–108.

Pattyn, N., Vanhees, L., Cornelissen, V. A., Coeckelberghs, E., De Maeyer, C., Goetschalckx, K., Possemiers, N., Wuyts, K., Van Craenenbroeck, E. M., & Beckers, P. J. (2016). The long-term effects of a randomized trial comparing aerobic interval versus continuous training in coronary artery disease patients: 1-year data from the SAINTEX-CAD study. *European journal of preventive cardiology*, *23*(11), 1154–1164.

Pitsavos, C., Kavouras, S. A., Panagiotakos, D. B., Arapi, S., Anastasiou, C. A., Zombolos, S., Stravopodis, P., Mantas, Y., Kogias, Y., & Antonoulas, A. (2008). Physical activity status and acute coronary syndromes survival: the GREECS (Greek Study of Acute Coronary Syndromes) study. *Journal of the American College of Cardiology*, *51*(21), 2034–2039.

Powell, K. E., Thompson, P. D., Caspersen, C. J., & Kendrick, J. S. (1987). Physical activity and the incidence of coronary heart disease. *Annual review of public health*, *8*(1), 253–287.

Quindry, J. C., & Franklin, B. A. (2018). Cardioprotective exercise and pharmacologic interventions as complementary antidotes to cardiovascular disease. *Exercise and sport sciences reviews*, *46*(1), 5–17.

Quindry, J. C., & Franklin, B. A. (2021). Exercise preconditioning as a cardioprotective phenotype. *The American journal of cardiology*.

Quindry, J. C., Franklin, B. A., Chapman, M., Humphrey, R., & Mathis, S. (2019). Benefits and risks of high-intensity interval training in patients with coronary artery disease. *The American journal of cardiology*, *123*(8), 1370–1377.

Qureshi, W. T., Alirhayim, Z., Blaha, M. J., Juraschek, S. P., Keteyian, S. J., Brawner, C. A., & Al-Mallah, M. H. (2015). Cardiorespiratory fitness and risk of incident atrial fibrillation: results from the Henry Ford Exercise Testing (FIT) Project. *Circulation*, *131*(21), 1827–1834.

Radford, N. B., DeFina, L. F., Leonard, D., Barlow, C. E., Willis, B. L., Gibbons, L. W., Gilchrist, S. C., Khera, A., & Levine, B. D. (2018). Cardiorespiratory fitness, coronary artery calcium, and cardiovascular disease events in a cohort of generally healthy middle-age men: results from the Cooper Center Longitudinal Study. *Circulation*, *137*(18), 1888–1895.

Riebe, D., Franklin, B. A., Thompson, P. D., Garber, C. E., Whitfield, G. P., Magal, M., & Pescatello, L. S. (2015). Updating ACSM's recommendations for exercise preparticipation health screening. *Medicine & Science in Sports & Exercise*, *47*(11), 2473–2479. https://doi.org/10.1249/MSS.0000000000000664

Riebe, D., Ehrman, J. K., Liguori, G., Magal, M. (2017). *ACSM's Guidelines for Exercise Testing and Prescription* (10th ed.). Philadelphia, PA: Lippincott Williams & Williams.

Rognmo, Ø., Moholdt, T., Bakken, H., Hole, T., Mølstad, P., Myhr, N. E., Grimsmo, J., & Wisløff, U. (2012). Cardiovascular risk of high-versus moderate-intensity aerobic exercise in coronary heart disease patients. *Circulation*, *126*(12), 1436–1440.

Ross, L. M., Porter, R. R., & Durstine, J. L. (2016). High-intensity interval training (HIIT) for patients with chronic diseases. *Journal of sport and health science*, *5*(2), 139–144.

Ross, R., Blair, S. N., Arena, R., Church, T. S., Després, J.-P., Franklin, B. A., Haskell, W. L., Kaminsky, L. A., Levine, B. D., & Lavie, C. J. (2016). Importance of assessing cardiorespiratory fitness in clinical practice: a case for fitness as a clinical vital sign: a scientific statement from the American Heart Association. *Circulation*, *134*(24), e653–e699.

Shoenfeld, Y., Keren, G., Shimoni, T., Birnfeld, C., & Sohar, E. (1980). Walking: a method for rapid improvement of physical fitness. *Jama*, *243*(20), 2062–2063.

Smith, J. L., Verrill, T. A., Boura, J. A., Sakwa, M. P., Shannon, F. L., & Franklin, B. A. (2013). Effect of cardiorespiratory fitness on short-term morbidity and mortality after coronary artery bypass grafting. *The American journal of cardiology*, *112*(8), 1104–1109.

Spring, B., Ockene, J. K., Gidding, S. S., Mozaffarian, D., Moore, S., Rosal, M. C., Brown, M. D., Vafiadis, D. K., Cohen, D. L., & Burke, L. E. (2013). Better population health through behavior change in adults: a call to action. *Circulation*, *128*(19), 2169–2176.

Squires, R. W., Kaminsky, L. A., Porcari, J. P., Ruff, J. E., Savage, P. D., & Williams, M. A. (2018). Progression of exercise training in early outpatient cardiac rehabilitation. *Journal of cardiopulmonary rehabilitation and prevention*, *38*(3), 139–146.

Stanaway, F. F., Gnjidic, D., Blyth, F. M., Couteur, D. G. L., Naganathan, V., Waite, L., Seibel, M. J., Handelsman, D. J., Sambrook, P. N., & Cumming, R. G. (2011). How fast does the Grim Reaper walk? Receiver operating characteristics curve analysis in healthy men aged 70 and over. *British medical journal*, *343*, d7679. https://doi.org/10.1136/bmj.d7679

Studenski, S., Perera, S., Patel, K., Rosano, C., Faulkner, K., Inzitari, M., Brach, J., Chandler, J., Cawthon, P., & Connor, E. B. (2011). Gait speed and survival in older adults. *Jama*, *305*(1), 50–58.

Swain, D. P., & Franklin, B. A. (2002). VO2 reserve and the minimal intensity for improving cardiorespiratory fitness. *Medicine and science in sports and exercise*, *34*(1), 152–157.

Swain, D. P., & Franklin, B. A. (2006). Comparison of cardioprotective benefits of vigorous versus moderate intensity aerobic exercise. *The American journal of cardiology*, *97*(1), 141–147.

Thijssen, D. H., Redington, A., George, K. P., Hopman, M. T., & Jones, H. (2018). Association of exercise preconditioning with immediate cardioprotection: a review. *JAMA cardiology*, *3*(2), 169–176.

Thompson, P. D., Franklin, B. A., Balady, G. J., Blair, S. N., Corrado, D., Estes, N. A. M., Fulton, J. E., Gordon, N. F., Haskell, W. L., Link, M. S., Maron, B. J., Mittleman, M. A., Pelliccia, A., Wenger, N. K., Willich, S. N., & Costa, F. (2007). Exercise and Acute Cardiovascular Events. *Circulation*, *115*(17), 2358–2368. https://doi.org/10.1161/CIRCULATIONAHA.107.181485

Tuomilehto, J., Lindström, J., Eriksson, J. G., Valle, T. T., Hämäläinen, H., Ilanne-Parikka, P., Keinänen-Kiukaanniemi, S., Laakso, M., Louheranta, A., & Rastas, M. (2001). Prevention of type 2 diabetes mellitus by changes in lifestyle among subjects with impaired glucose tolerance. *New England journal of medicine, 344*(18), 1343–1350.

Varghese, T., Schultz, W. M., McCue, A. A., Lambert, C. T., Sandesara, P. B., Eapen, D. J., Gordon, N. F., Franklin, B. A., & Sperling, L. S. (2016). Physical activity in the prevention of coronary heart disease: implications for the clinician. *Heart, 102*(12), 904–909.

Vestergaard, S., Andersen, C. K., Korsholm, L., & Puggaard, L. (2006). Exercise intervention of 65+-year-old men and women: functional ability and health care costs. *Aging clinical and experimental research, 18*(3), 227–234.

Weiss, J. P., Froelicher, V. F., Myers, J. N., & Heidenreich, P. A. (2004). Health-care costs and exercise capacity. *Chest, 126*(2), 608–613. https://doi.org/10.1378/chest.126.2.608

Wen, C. P., Wai, J. P. M., Tsai, M. K., Yang, Y. C., Cheng, T. Y. D., Lee, M.-C., Chan, H. T., Tsao, C. K., Tsai, S. P., & Wu, X. (2011). Minimum amount of physical activity for reduced mortality and extended life expectancy: a prospective cohort study. *The lancet, 378*(9798), 1244–1253.

Wen, C. P., & Wu, X. (2012). Stressing harms of physical inactivity to promote exercise. *The lancet, 380*(9838), 192–193.

Wickramasinghe, C. D., Ayers, C. R., Das, S., De Lemos, J. A., Willis, B. L., & Berry, J. D. (2014). Prediction of 30-year risk for cardiovascular mortality by fitness and risk factor levels: the Cooper Center Longitudinal Study. *Circulation: cardiovascular quality and outcomes, 7*(4), 597–602.

Wicks, J. R., Oldridge, N. B., Nielsen, L. K., & Vickers, C. E. (2011). HR index--a simple method for the prediction of oxygen uptake. *Medicine and science in sports and exercise, 43*(10), 2005–2012.

Williams, M. A., Haskell, W. L., Ades, P. A., Amsterdam, E. A., Bittner, V., Franklin, B. A., Gulanick, M., Laing, S. T., & Stewart, K. J. (2007). Resistance exercise in individuals with and without cardiovascular disease: 2007 update: a scientific statement from the American Heart Association Council on Clinical Cardiology and Council on Nutrition, Physical Activity, and Metabolism. *Circulation, 116*(5), 572–584.

Williams, P. T. (2001). Physical fitness and activity as separate heart disease risk factors: a meta-analysis. *Medicine and science in sports and exercise, 33*(5), 754.

Williams, R. B., Barefoot, J. C., & Schneiderman, N. (2003). Psychosocial risk factors for cardiovascular disease: more than one culprit at work. *Jama, 290*(16), 2190–2192.

Wilson, M. G., Ellison, G. M., & Cable, N. T. (2016). Basic science behind the cardiovascular benefits of exercise. *British journal of sports medicine, 50*(2), 93–99.

Yazdanyar, A., Aziz, M. M., Enright, P. L., Edmundowicz, D., Boudreau, R., Sutton-Tyrell, K., Kuller, L., & Newman, A. B. (2014). Association between 6-minute walk test and all-cause mortality, coronary heart disease–specific mortality, and incident coronary heart disease. *Journal of aging and health, 26*(4), 583–599.

4 Sleep Science

Glenn S. Brassington[1] and Glenn T. Brassington[1]
[1]Department of Psychology
Sonoma State University, Rohnert Park, CA, USA

CONTENTS

KEY POINTS

- Sufficient quality sleep is associated with reduced mortality and disease prevention.
- Sleep duration, deep sleep, and REM sleep decrease from birth to age 40.
- Older adults, women, and members of ethnic/racial minority groups have greater difficulty achieving sufficient health sleep.
- Sleep is determined by the interaction of sleep drive, circadian rhythm, physiological arousal, cognitive arousal, and the sleep environment.
- By implementing sleep management principles and guidelines, nurses can prevent disease, improve treatment outcomes, and improve the quality of life of their patients.

A good laugh and a long sleep are the two best cures.

                                      – An Irish proverb

DOI: 10.1201/9781003178330-5

4.1 INTRODUCTION

Imagine that a patient arrives at a medical clinic unable to focus her attention. She is disoriented and having problems with her memory, feeling fatigued and depressed, and her lab results are worrisome. Now, imagine how you would feel if you could offer this patient a treatment that works in 1–14 days, is free of medication side effects, requires no physical therapy, no access to transportation, no fees, and is already something the patient is doing. In this chapter, you will learn about such a treatment—it is called sleep.

Over millions of years, modern humans have evolved to require sleeping for an average of one-third of their lives, or approximately 25–30 years. Recently, researchers have measured neural activity in zebrafish that are analogous to humans (i.e., slow-wave and rapid-eye-movement sleep). These observations indicate that human sleep has been maintained as an essential evolutionary adaptation for the past 450 million years (Leung et al., 2019). The preservation of this behavior suggests that sleep has played an important role in the evolution and survival of the human species. Unfortunately, more than one-third of American and Canadian adults are not getting enough sleep (i.e., less than the 7 hours per night recommended by public health authorities) to promote health and prevent disease (Chaput, Wong, et al., 2017; Liu et al., 2016). Insufficient sleep results in a significant amount of preventable disease and suffering around the world (Chattu et al., 2018). Hence, it is essential that nurses have the necessary knowledge to promote healthy sleep in their patients.

In this chapter, we will discuss five main topics: (1) what is sleep, (2) how is sleep measured, (3) healthy sleep across the lifespan, (4) sleep in the prevention and treatment of disease, and (5) sleep management principles and guidelines. It is expected that after reading this chapter, nurses will have the knowledge and resources to improve the sleep of their patients and, in so doing, their effectiveness in prevention and treating mental and physical diseases. This chapter will focus on the use of lifestyle factors in promoting healthy sleep. For information about the diagnosis and treatment of sleep disorders requiring non-lifestyle medical treatment, please see review by Bukhari and colleagues (2021).

4.2 WHAT IS SLEEP?

Sleep has been defined in behavioral terms as a "reversible behavioral state of perceptual disengagement from and unresponsiveness to the environment" (Carskadon & Dement, 2017). During sleep, we are to a great degree cut off from sensory information from the environment, but unlike a coma, we can easily be awakened. At the same time as we are cut off from the environment, our organism is undergoing a great deal of activity and change compared to that observed in waking hours. In contrast to sleep, fatigue is a type of tiredness that does not improve with sleep and a lightened workload. Two distinct types of sleep have been defined by researchers: non-rapid eye movement (NREM) and rapid eye movement (REM) sleep. Beginning in the 1960s, sleep was defined as consisting of five stages (Carskadon & Dement, 2017; Rechtschaffen & Kales, 1968): four NREM stages and one REM stage. However, in 2007, the *American Academy of Sleep Medicine (AASM)* reduced the number of stages to four, by combining NREM stages 3 and 4 and creating a new manual for scoring sleep (Berry et al., 2015). We will be using the AASM defined stages in this chapter.

As we sleep, we move through three stages of NREM sleep (i.e., N1, N2, N3) and one stage of REM sleep (i.e., R). Sleep cycles are approximately 60 minutes in length from birth to age 5 and approximately 90 minutes thereafter. Characteristic changes in brain activity, eye movement, body temperature, and muscle tension define each stage of sleep. N1 sleep is considered light sleep and lasts only a few minutes after the onset of sleep. In this stage, brain and muscle activity begin to slow and occasional muscle twitching can be observed. N2 sleep is also considered light sleep where brain activity continues to decrease as indicated by the appearance of high-voltage slow waves beginning to appear on the electroencephalograph (EEG). These changes in brain activity are accompanied by steady decreases in respiration rate, heart rate, and body temperature. N3 sleep is considered very deep sleep in which breathing becomes rhythmic, muscle activity is limited, and the majority of brain activity consists of slow delta waves (i.e., high voltage, slow wave) on the EEG. N3 sleep is often referred to as slow-wave sleep (SWS), deep sleep, or delta wave sleep. As brain activity decreases and sleep deepens, greater external stimulus is needed to awaken one from sleep. The final stage of each sleep cycle is referred to as R sleep. R sleep is characterized by rapid eye movement, muscle atonia, and EEG desynchronization (i.e., low voltage sawtooth brain waves that resemble wakefulness), increased heart rate, and rapid shallow breathing. The high levels of brain activity during R sleep resemble the brain activity seen during waking life and has led to it being referred to as paradoxical sleep.

4.3 HOW IS SLEEP MEASURED?

A variety of assessments have been created to describe the changes that occur during sleep. The most commonly used measures that constitute the operational definitions of sleep include: polysomnography, mobile devices, Multiple Sleep Onset Latency Test, questionnaires, and sleep diaries. Each of these methods of quantifying sleep is described below.

4.3.1 POLYSOMNOGRAPHY

Polysomnography is a set of physiological recordings taken during sleep. The primary parameters assessed during sleep are as follows: (1) EEG records electrical activity on the scalp associated with neurons in the brain, (2) electrooculography (EOG) records eye movement, (3) electromyography (EMG) records skeletal muscle activity, (4) pneumotachometry records respiratory airflow, and (5) pulse oximetry records the percentage of oxygen in the blood. EEG, EOG, and EMG are used to quantify the stages of sleep, while pneumotachometry and pulse oximetry are used to diagnose disordered breathing.

4.3.2 MOBILE DEVICES

Although polysomnography is considered the "gold standard" in assessing sleep, newer technologies being developed that are less expensive, do not tend to disrupt sleep, and capture daytime functioning. One such device is often referred to as an actigraph or actimeter. Typically, the actigraph is placed on the wrist and records movement with an accelerometer that is then analyzed by a microprocessor to determine how much time the user was awake or asleep (Stone & Ancoli-Israel, 2017). Actigraphy has been shown to be a valid measure of total sleep time and nighttime awakening (Sadeh, 2011; Smith et al., 2018). More recently, commercial bed sensors have been developed to assess sleep by monitoring body movement, breathing, and cardiac activities. These micro-bend fiber optic sensors are placed under the mattress and feed data to a mobile device for analysis (Tal et al., 2017). Many emerging technologies (e.g., wireless EEG, smartwatches/fitness trackers, mobile phone sensing, ultrasound sensors, and WiFi/radio-signal approaches) hold promise for monitoring sleep in the general population (Perez-Pozuelo et al., 2020). Nevertheless, while the reliability and validity of some commercial devices are good for quantifying total sleep time and nighttime awakening, little evidence supports their ability to accurately assess sleep quality and all of the four stages of sleep (Stone et al., 2020). Hence, it is important to use caution when interpreting data about the quality of a patient's sleep when it is derived from existing commercial technologies. Imtiaz conducted a review of 90 studies examining 13 sensing modalities and concluded that EEG is the only sensing modality that is capable of identifying all of the stages of sleep (Imtiaz, 2021).

4.3.3 Multiple Sleep Latency Test

To assess how much physiological drive a person has to sleep, patients are given 4–6 opportunities to take naps during the day and record the amount of time it takes them to fall asleep (Carskadon et al., 1986). Sleep latency in normal adults is from 10 to 20 minutes with pathological sleepiness as a mean sleep latency of 5–6 minutes. This shorter latency to sleep onset suggests that the participant is experiencing a very strong drive to sleep during the day and indicates insufficient quality nighttime sleep (Carskadon & Dement, 2017).

4.3.4 Questionnaires

Self-report questionnaires assess patients' subjective experience of the quantity and quality of their sleep and provide normative data upon which each patient can be compared. The following are three brief measures that can be used to assess sleep and daytime dysfunction in clinical and research settings.

4.3.4.1 The Pittsburgh Sleep Quality Index (PSQI)

The PSQI is the most widely used self-report measure of sleep quality and daytime functioning (Buysse et al., 1989). Participants answer a series of questions about their sleep over the previous month. The PSQI provides a global score of sleep quality and seven subscales: sleep quality, sleep latency, sleep duration, sleep efficiency, sleep disturbances, use of medication, and daytime dysfunction.

4.3.4.2 The Epworth Sleepiness Scale (ESS)

The ESS is a widely used measure of daytime sleepiness (Johns, 1991). On the ESS, participants rate from (0) slight to (3) high the likelihood that they would "doze" in a variety of situations, such as "sitting and reading," "sitting and talking to someone," and "in a car, while stopped for a few minutes in traffic." Daytime sleepiness is an indicator of whether a patient's sleep is of sufficient quality to sustain alertness during the day.

4.3.4.3 The Satisfaction, Alertness, Timing, Efficiency, and Duration (SATED) Questionnaire

The SATED is a reliable and valid measure of sleep health in the general public (Ravyts et al., 2021; Buysse, 2014). The questionnaire evaluates five dimensions of sleep health, including (1) satisfaction: "Are you satisfied with your sleep?"; (2) alertness: "Do you stay awake all day without dozing?"; (3) timing: "Are you asleep (or trying to sleep) between 2:00 a.m. and 4:00 a.m.?"; (4) efficiency: "Do you spend less than 30 minutes awake at night? This includes the time it takes to fall asleep and awakenings from sleep"; and (5) duration: "Do you sleep between 6 and 8 hours per day?" Patients are asked to respond on a 0–2-point scale: 0–Rarely/Never, 1–Sometimes, 2–Usually/Always, resulting in a 0 to 10-point scale. This measure can be administered in the clinical setting in a few minutes and used to encourage patients to discuss any concerns they have about their sleep and to promote healthy sleep.

4.3.5 Sleep Diaries

Although the above retrospective measures provide important information about a patient's recollection of her nighttime sleep and daytime sleepiness, prospective sleep diaries—also referred to as a sleep log or sleep journal—help overcome some of the biases caused by memories being incomplete and selective. A sleep diary is frequently completed for two weeks and requests participants provide information about their sleep (e.g., when you went to bed, how long it took to fall asleep,

Sleep Diary

Day of the Week							
Complete in the evening before bed							
Number of alcoholic beverages							
Time of last alcoholic beverage							
Number of caffeinated beverages							
Time of last caffeinated beverage							
Minutes of moderate exercise							
Time of last exercise							
Minutes of meditation/breathing exercises							
Did you do any activity in bed except sleep and sex?							
Name of stimulating medication (e.g., diet pills)							
Dose of stimulating medication							
Number of cigarettes smoked							
Time of last cigarette smoked							
Number of daytime naps							
Total minutes spent napping							
Name of sleep medication							
Dose of sleep medication							
Time you turned off lights and attempted to sleep							
Complete during the night							
Nighttime awakening #1 (time you woke up)							
Nighttime awakening #1 (minutes awake)							
Reason you awakened							
Nighttime awakening #2 (time you woke up)							
Nighttime awakening #2 (minutes awake)							
Reason you awakened							
Complete upon awakening in the morning							
Minutes you spent in bed NOT sleeping last night							
Time you woke up in the morning							
Time you got out of bed							
Minutes it took you to fall asleep last night							
How rested do you feel on a scale from (1=not at all rested to 10=very rested)?							
Was the room you slept in comfortable (yes or no)?							

FIGURE 4.1 Sleep Log

nighttime awakenings, etc.) and factors that might impair sleep (e.g., caffeine consumption, anxiety, and stressful activities engaged in before bed). Sleep diary data are used to help patients identify how much quality sleep they are getting and how cognitive, behavioral, and environmental factors may be affecting their sleep (see Figure 4.1).

4.4 HEALTHY SLEEP ACROSS THE LIFESPAN

Sleep patterns change across the lifespan in a variety of ways due to normal development associated with age, sex, race/ethnicity, and participation in health-promoting behaviors (e.g., nutrition, exercise, relaxation/meditation). Humans from in utero to end of life exhibit differences in all of the main dimensions of sleep: total sleep time, length of sleep cycles, number of nighttime awakenings, sleep efficiency, and time in each stage of sleep (i.e., N1, N2, N3, and R). Nevertheless, more data exists to describe the sleep of young and middle-aged adults compared to infants, children, and older adults. We will briefly describe some of the characteristics of sleep at each stage of development based on the most recent systematic reviews and meta-analyses (Galland et al., 2012; Iglowstein et al., 2003; Kocevska et al., 2021; Li et al., 2018; Ohayon et al., 2004; Olds et al., 2010).

The emergence of different sleep states begins in the womb. Fetuses spend approximately 95% of their time sleeping. At approximately 32 weeks of gestation, N1–N3 sleep (i.e., quiet sleep), R sleep (i.e., active sleep), and wakefulness can be observed with fetal ultrasound (Mirmiran et al., 2003). The most significant changes in sleep across the lifespan are seen in infants and young children. From birth to 1 year, baby's sleep cycles are approximately 50–60 minutes in length and awakenings occur frequently during the day and night, especially in the first 10–12 weeks of life, but become increasingly nocturnal thereafter (Galland et al., 2012). Between ages 1 and 5, children continue to take naps but tend to discontinue them as they enter pre-school. Sleep duration is approximately 12.8 hours in infants, 11.9 hours in toddler/preschool, and 9.2 hours in children. Overall, total sleep time, time in bed, and sleep efficiency decrease from birth to age 12.

As a child moves through childhood and adolescence, total sleep time, N3 sleep (i.e., slow wave, deep sleep) and R sleep latency (i.e., the time from sleep onset to the first epoch of R sleep) all decrease while N2 (i.e., light sleep) increases. By age 5, REM sleep has decreased to 20–25% of total sleep and will stay at this proportion of sleep throughout adulthood. Other dimensions of sleep appear not to change during this stage of development (Ohayon et al., 2004). Total sleep time for children 6–13 years old has been reported to be 10.6 (+/– 1.0) hours and 7.7 (+/– 1.1) hours for adolescents 14–17 years old (Kocevska et al., 2021), based on a meta-analytic review of 1.1 million people.

As one moves through adulthood, total sleep time continues to decrease, stabilizing at about age 40. Average sleep time is 7.5 (+/– 1.1) hours at age 18–25, 7.2 (+/– 1.1) hours at age 26–40, 7.0 (+/– 1.1) hours at age 41–65, and also 7.0 (+/– 1.1) hours over 65 years (Kocevska et al., 2021). N3 and R sleep also decrease but stabilize by age 50–60. Patients also have more trouble falling asleep, maintaining sleep, and waking too early in the morning as they age. Small but significant sex differences were reported with women having less total sleep time, greater sleep latency, less N3, and less REM sleep during adulthood. These data are consistent with other studies indicating that women experience slightly poorer sleep as they age compared to men. However, it is important to note that women's sleep remains understudied (Mallampalli & Carter, 2014).

Women experience sleep differently than men (Pengo et al., 2018). Unlike in previous reviews on sleep across the lifespan, Pengo and Colleagues address sex differences in sleep during the major developmental stages of a woman's life: childhood, adolescence/puberty, reproductive years, pregnancy, perimenopause, and aging. What follows is a brief summary of the findings from their review. There are currently no reported sex differences in neonates, infants, and younger children (Galland et al., 2012; Liu et al., 2005). However, sex differences in sleep have been reported with the first menstrual cycle as sexual hormones (i.e., estradiol and progesterone) begin to affect the duration and quality of sleep. Menstrual hormonal changes are associated with increased EEG activity associated with memory consolidation in NREM sleep in the postovulatory luteal phase of the menstrual cycle.

During pregnancy, significant anatomical and physiological changes (e.g., gastroesophageal reflux, musculoskeletal discomfort, uterine contractions, and nocturia) can reduce sleep duration and increase sleep fragmentation. Pregnant women in their third trimester sleep approximately 30 minutes less than their non-pregnant peers and are more likely to sleep too short (<6 hrs) or too long (>9 hrs) per night. A meta-analysis of 11,000 participants cited by Pengo and Colleagues concluded that 46% of women experienced poor sleep during pregnancy and that sleep worsens from the second to third trimester (Sedov et al., 2018). It is estimated that <40–60% of women in perimenopause or post-menopause sleep less and experience poorer sleep quality

TABLE 4.1
Summary of recommended sleep duration across the lifespan

Developmental stage	Recommended hrs of sleep
Newborns (0–3 months)	14–17
Infants (4–11 months)	12–15
Toddler (1–2 years)	11–14
Preschool (3–5 years)	10–13
School-age (6–13 years)	9–11
Teenagers (14–17 years)	8–10
Young adult (18–25 years)	7–9
Adult (26–64 years)	7–9
Older adult (65+ years)	7–8

Hirshkowitz, M., Whiton, K., Albert, S. M., Alessi, C., Bruni, O., DonCarlos, L., Hazen, N., Herman, J., Adams Hillard, P. J., Katz, E. S., Kheirandish-Gozal, L., Neubauer, D. N., O'Donnell, A. E., Ohayon, M., Peever, J., Rawding, R., Sachdeva, R. C., Setters, B., Vitiello, M. V., & Ware, J. C. (2015). National Sleep Foundation's updated sleep duration recommendations: Final report. *Sleep Health*, *1*(4), 233–243. https://dx.doi.org/10.1016/j.sleh.2015.10.004

than pre-menopause. There are several potential mechanisms by which sleep may be affected in perimenopause and beyond, including vasomotor symptoms (i.e., hot flashes and night sweats), hormonal changes, age-related changes, depression, and sleep disordered breathing (Pengo et al., 2018). Very little is known about the sleep architecture (i.e., stages of sleep) of women in the peri-menopausal and postmenopausal stages of development. A great deal of future research needs to be conducted to clearly describe changes in sleep duration, sleep quality, and sleep architecture across the lifespan in women.

Over the past five years, research has begun to assess the sleep of people of non-European descent. Johnson and Colleagues (2019) reviewed all studies that assessed the sleep of the main categories of racial/ethnic minority groups defined by the United States Office of Management and Budget: American Indian/Alaskan Native, Asian, African American/Black, Hispanic/Latino, and Native Hawaiian/Pacific Islander. They reported that the majority of studies were not published until the early 2000s. They concluded that compared to people of European descent, Asian, African American, Non-Hispanic/Latino, Native Hawaiian, and Pacific Islander groups had shorter sleep duration and poorer sleep quality. In terms of daytime sleepiness, Asian people reported less daytime sleepiness, Blacks reported more daytime sleepiness, and there were mixed results for Hispanic/Latino people. Overall, sleep complaints were greater in people of Asian descent and lower in Hispanic/Latino descent. Several reviews support the notion that sleep health and sleep problems are not equal across racial/ethnic groups, are associated with health disparities, and require further study (Egan et al., 2017; Grandner et al., 2016; Johnson et al., 2019).

The American Academy of Sleep Medicine (AASM), the Sleep Research Society (SRS), and the National Sleep Foundation (NSF) created separate expert panels to review research to determine recommended sleep for healthy people across the lifespan. The AASM and SRS in their joint statement recommended that adults aged 18 to 60 years sleep 7–9 hours per night for optimal health. Although these organizations were not able to reach significant agreement to make a firm recommendation for sleeping 6–7 hours or >9 hours, the median vote by the panel was that these ranges of sleep are insufficient to promote health (Watson et al., 2015). The NSF provided recommendations (see Table 4.1) for age intervals from newborns to older adults, with the need for sleep decreasing from birth to adulthood and stabilizing thereafter (Hirshkowitz et al., 2015).

4.5   SLEEP IN THE PREVENTION AND TREATMENT OF DISEASE

The duration and quality of sleep affects all of the major organ systems and physiological processes in the human body. Insufficient sleep has been linked to increased mortality and many of the leading causes of death around the world (Cappuccio et al., 2010; Chattu et al., 2018). Numerous studies have demonstrated that insufficient sleep is related to all-cause mortality, metabolic syndrome, diabetes/impaired glucose metabolism, obesity, cancer, hypertension, coronary heart disease, accidents, impaired neurobehavioral performance, injuries, and mental health in young children (Chaput, Gray, et al., 2017), school-aged children (Chaput et al., 2016), and adults (Buysse, 2014; He et al., 2020). The strongest cumulative evidence for the deleterious effect of short sleep (<6 hours per night) on health outcomes comes from a meta-analysis of 5,172,710 participants from 153 studies (Itani et al., 2017). Short sleep was significantly associated with increased mortality, diabetes mellitus, hypertension, cardiovascular disease, coronary heart disease, and obesity. In another meta-analysis of the same data, Jike et al., 2018 reported that sleeping more than 9 hours per night was associated with the same mortality and disease risk and the addition of stroke. These meta-analyses indicate that there is an optimal range for sleep (i.e., 7–9 hours in adults) that reduces mortality and risk for disease.

Although there was not sufficient data in Itani and colleagues' meta-analysis to assess depression, sleep disturbances and short sleep have been identified as risk factors for depression elsewhere (Kalmbach et al., 2017; Li et al., 2016). Further support for the role of sleep as a causal factor for mental health problems comes from a study of 3755 participants who received digital cognitive behavioral therapy for insomnia (Freeman et al., 2017), in which insomnia mediated changes in paranoia and hallucinations. Finally, sleep problems have been shown to be a risk factor for falls in older adults (Brassington et al., 2000; Stone et al., 2014).

Although the majority of studies have identified the importance of sleep duration in mortality and disease risk, fewer studies have examined the role of sleep timing and sleep consistency (Chaput et al., 2020). Sleep timing refers to the time of day that sleep occurs, and sleep consistency refers to the day-to-day variability in bedtime/wake-up times and sleep duration. Chaput and Colleagues (2020) reviewed 41 studies and concluded that later sleep timing, less consistency in sleep, and social jet lag were associated with poor health outcomes in adults aged 18–64 years. The healthiest sleep patterns were reported to be: (1) earlier sleep timing, (2) regularity in sleep patterns with consistent bedtimes and wake-up times, and (3) catch-up sleep on the weekends. These data indicate that it is necessary but not sufficient to get the recommended hours of quality sleep to promote health; patients must also be encouraged to develop a regular sleep schedule.

Some mediators have been identified to explain the mechanism by which insufficient sleep causes disease. These variables include inflammatory markers (e.g., IL-beta, TNF-alpha, IL-6, and CRP), autonomic activation (i.e., sympathetic output), vascular indices (e.g., endothelial function, cell adhesion molecules), lifestyle, and health status (Hall et al., 2015; Mullington et al., 2010). Although more research is needed to fully explain the pathways by which sleep affects risk for disease, it does appear reasonable to suggest that insufficient sleep induces a stress response in the body, causing damage to cells and arteries that predispose one to disease as well as reducing health-promoting behaviors such as exercise and good nutrition (Irwin, 2019).

4.6   SLEEP MANAGEMENT PRINCIPLES AND GUIDELINES

Two main approaches to promoting health in clinical and non-clinical settings are sleep hygiene education (SHE) and cognitive behavior therapy for insomnia (CBT-I). SHE includes a set of behavioral and environmental recommendations designed to promote healthy sleep. Patients are usually given a list of behaviors to engage in and avoid. Although there are many versions of SHE, the most common areas discussed with patients are caffeine, alcohol, tobacco, exercise, stress, noise, sleep consistency, and daytime napping (Irish et al., 2015). Providers of SHE do not need specific education about sleep to administer this intervention. CBT-I is an approach to treating insomnia that seeks to modify dysfunctional cognitions and behaviors that interfere with sleep. An important dimension of CBT-I, not generally present in SHE, is educating patients about the biological and psychological processes that facilitate healthy sleep (Taylor et al., 2019). CBT-I requires a strong understanding of how to assess sleep problems and apply the principles and strategies with patients over 4–6 sessions. Research indicates that SHE improves sleep in adults without sleep problems (Murawski et al., 2018). However, in clinical settings, CBT-I achieves superior results to SHE whether delivered online or in person (Luik et al., 2017; van Straten et al., 2018). The sleep management principles discussed below are drawn from both interventions.

In working with patients to improve their sleep, it is important to explain first the biological and psychological processes that determine sleep quality. Following this explanation, patients should be encouraged to modify cognitive, behavioral, and environmental variables to improve their sleep provided in the guidelines. It is important to assess how each guideline is functioning to facilitate sleep in a particular patient. Guidelines are derived from biological and psychological principles, but they are not absolutes. For example, one of the sleep management guidelines is to "avoid taking naps during the day." This guideline is based on the principle that daytime naps reduce physiological drive to sleep and thus may delay sleep onset. However, it is possible that a patient could take a short nap in the early afternoon to improve work performance and not delay sleep onset provided the drive to sleep was not significantly reduced.

Sleep and wakefulness are under homeostatic and circadian alerting control. Homeostatic control refers to the phenomenon that the longer we are awake or not experiencing specific sleep stages, the greater the drive to make up for the lost sleep or sleep stage. This is referred to as "sleep drive." Circadian control of the sleep–wake rhythm consists of biochemical, physiological, and behavioral processes that encourage wakefulness and is referred to as the "circadian alerting rhythm." When these two regulatory mechanisms are working in synchrony, patients are able to enter into sleep at regular times each evening, experience deeper stages of sleep (i.e., N3 sleep), and remain asleep until it is time to awake and arise from bed feeling rested. Unfortunately, these two main regulators of sleep can be disrupted by behaviors that increase alertness and wakefulness when sleep is desired. Working with patients to improve their sleep should begin with a brief description of the physiological and psychological factors that cause the initiation and maintenance of sleep and wakefulness: (1) sleep drive, (2) circadian alerting rhythm, (3) physiological arousal, (4) cognitive arousal, and (5) sleep environment, followed by the behaviors that affect these factors. We present each sleep management principle and its associated guidelines below.

4.6.1 SLEEP DRIVE

The drive to sleep is often referred to as a person's sleep debt. This debt is built up by being awake and is paid back by sleeping. It is not possible to have zero sleep drive, because as soon as one does one will wake up and begin accruing sleep debt. The key understanding here is that it is not intention to sleep that promotes sleep but rather the body's drive to sleep that has been built up during wakefulness. Trying to sleep can actually be counterproductive as it generally increases arousal and inhibits sleep.

Further, falling asleep is not the major problem reported by most people, as many people are routinely experiencing sleep debt due to curtailing sleep to engage in other priorities. The more common problem is nighttime awakenings and not entering into the deeper stages of restful sleep. Nighttime awakenings often occur as the sleep debt is paid back during the night and the sleep drive diminished. This lack of sleep drive may make it possible for internal (e.g., worries) or external factors (noises) to wake the patient.

Recommendations related to sleep drive are as follows:

- **Do not go to bed until you feel sleepy.** If a patient has not accrued sufficient sleep drive, they will not be able to fall asleep, even if they are relaxed, comfortable, and in a safe sleep environment. A common problem is for a patient to go to bed several hours earlier than is customary for her the night before an important activity (e.g., an examination, meeting, etc.) scheduled for the following morning. This often leads to a patient lying in bed and worrying about not being able to sleep and the negative effects this will have on her performance the following day. Remind patients that morning wake time determines that night's sleep time by increasing the drive to sleep throughout the day.
- **Do not take daytime or evening naps.** Daytime naps reduce sleep drive and may lead to delays in sleep onset and nighttime awakenings. The exception to this recommendation is if daytime naps of less than one hour reduce daytime sleepiness and improve performance but do *not* reduce sleep drive to a point that it makes it impossible for a patient to fall asleep or remain asleep during the night.

4.6.2 Circadian Alerting Rhythm

The circadian rhythm or body clock coordinates the timing of all biological processes. Some physiological processes need to be turned on at certain times of the day and night and others need to be turned off. For example, the digestive system needs to be less active in the night so that one can sleep, while body temperature needs to be lowered during the night to help one enter into deeper stages of sleep. It has been posited by many sleep researchers that the circadian alerting rhythm works in opposition to the sleep drive in order to help us stay awake during the day and consolidate sleep at night. The circadian alerting exerts its effect by creating biological changes that keep us alert and then withdraws these changes in order to let the sleep drive take its effect. For example, melatonin release after dark causes the circadian clock to withdraw its alerting influence.

It is now believed that our sleep–wake circadian rhythm is 10–15 minutes longer than 24 hours, requiring us to reset our internal clock each day. The daily pattern of action of the circadian alerting rhythm is to begin to alert the organism at about 9 a.m. and to increase alertness slowly until 9 p.m. with the greatest alerting effect occurring between 6 a.m. and 9 p.m. The circadian alerting rhythm decreases its action slowly and almost completely withdrawn between 3 a.m. and 6 a.m. Figure 4.2 depicts this process, known as the Opponent Process Model (Edgar, 1993). The "afternoon dip"

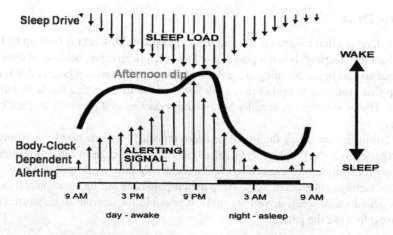

FIGURE 4.2   Opponent Process Model of sleep

(i.e., between 1 and 3 p.m.) in energy is associated with the withdrawal of circadian alerting and increasing sleep drive.

Recommendations related to circadian alerting rhythm are as follows:

- **Expose the body to as much sunlight as possible early in the day and as little sunlight and artificial light (e.g., light bulbs, digital screens light) in the evening as possible.** Light inhibits the production of melatonin and signals the body that it needs to remain alert.
- **Get up and go to bed at approximately the same time (within one hour) every day.** Maintaining a consistent schedule will help the circadian alerting facilitate alertness during the day and withdraw its effects in the evening. It is not uncommon for patients to go to sleep after midnight in the later days of the week only to find that they are not able to fall asleep when they try to sleep before midnight in the earlier days of the week. Moving the sleep and wake schedule is equivalent to creating a physiological state similar to that associated with jet lag every week.
- **Avoid consuming excess fluids prior to sleeping and avoid eating and all other activities (e.g., smoking, using electronic devices) during the night.** Urination and digestion are shut down by the circadian clock to promote sleep. Eating and engaging in other activities in the night can lead to hormonal changes related to hunger and arousal that can cause future nighttime awakenings.
- **Eat on a consistent schedule during the day and early evening. Do not skip meals. Include healthy foods in one's diet such as fruits, vegetables, and legumes.** Circadian alerting is associated with eating. Circadian alerting is less likely to withdraw its effects when patients eat late into the evening and during the night. Also, healthy eating is associated with overall better physiological functioning responsible for circadian alerting activities.
- **Do not exercise within four hours of bedtime.** Exercise raises core body temperature promoting alertness. However, core body temperature tends to decrease within four hours of exercise.

4.6.3 Physiological Arousal

Sleep requires quiescence of the arousal system. Muscle tension needs to be reduced to a minimum, respiration needs to slow, and the body needs to feel comfortable to encourage sleep. Conversely, physiological arousal (e.g., muscle tensions, pain, stress hormones) prohibits sleep. Commonly referred to as the fight-or-flight syndrome, physiological arousal is associated with alertness and a physiological state of preparing for action. In the case of a real threat, the least adaptive thing to do is sleep. A person who is attacked while deeply sleeping is unlikely to survive. Hence, arousal is associated with fragmented and shallow sleep because an aroused organism is not able to let go of external monitoring for fear that they will be unable to defend themselves.

Recommendations related to physiological arousal are as follows:

- **Do not eat or drink anything containing caffeine after 4 p.m., or within six hours of bedtime.** Identify all of the foods (e.g., chocolate and ice cream), drinks (e.g., decaffeinated coffee, tea, beer, and flavored waters), and medications (e.g., some over-the-counter cold, headache, and pain relief medications) that contain caffeine. Some patients are more sensitive to the tiredness-blocking effects of caffeine and need to completely eliminate consumption in order to facilitate sleep. Encourage patients not to consume nicotine. Patients who have developed tolerance to these substances may need to slowly reduce their consumption before experiencing improved sleep as withdrawal symptoms can also inhibit sleep.
- **Engage in pleasant, stress-reducing activities and nurturing supportive relationships.** Pleasant activities (e.g., reading a book, speaking with a friend, and gazing at the stars) can

significantly relax the body and buffer the effects of external stressors that often lead to sleep-inhibiting hyper-arousal (e.g., muscle tension, elevated blood pressures).

- **Practice relaxation training exercises (e.g., diaphragmatic breathing, autogenic relaxation, progressive muscle relaxation, Tai Chi, and meditation) during the day and in the evening before sleeping.** Patients should try to reduce their response to daytime and evening stressors as much as possible using these techniques. It may take some patients weeks to months to develop a strong consistent relaxation response using these techniques, while other patients may experience relaxation on their first attempt. It is important to communicate to patients that control over the relaxation response is possible for everyone and increases over time. A physically relaxed or "rest and digest" state is an important factor involved in initiating sleep. Reduced muscle tension indicates to patients that they do not have to use energy to accomplish a task or meet a challenge but rather can let go of daily activities and enter into repose.

- **Do not drink alcohol two hours before bedtime.** Alcohol may cause a patient to fall asleep quickly but it alters sleep architecture (i.e., reduces R sleep) during the night and is associated with nighttime awakenings.

4.6.4 Cognitive Arousal

Attention to and processing the external and internal world needs to diminish for sleep to occur. One of the biggest barriers to this process of withdrawing from ourselves and the world is excessive thoughts about problems in one's life. Thinking about losses, fears, or injustices interferes with sleep by increasing cognitive activity, effort, vigilance, or arousal. This type of problem solving and preparation for future action is incompatible with the type of diffuse attention required to enter into sleep. For many busy people, as soon as their bodies begin to relax, their minds begin to ruminate about a flood of problems to be solved, which only serves to heighten their alertness. For other people, being in bed is one of the only times in the day that they feel is "their own time," and they resist the urge to sleep so they can enjoy some time of solitude. Another type of cognition that can interfere with sleep arises when patients worry that they will not be able to fall asleep and get the rest they need to perform well the next day.

Recommendations related to cognitive arousal are as follows:

- **Do not try to initiate sleep.** Trying to sleep is incompatible with the withdrawal of attention and effort required to enter into sleep. Patients should tell themselves to "let sleep happen" and console themselves with the notion that they will eventually sleep, especially as their sleep drive increases. This letting go of effort often leads to sleep.

- **Avoid working on unpleasant or frustrating tasks just prior to bedtime.** Patients should be encouraged to identify activities that increase their mental activity and limit their participation in these activities as long before bed as possible.

- **Use the last hour prior to bedtime to engage in activities that are enjoyable and relaxing (e.g., taking a warm shower, drinking herb tea).** Patients should be encouraged to create evening routines that shift cognitive processing away from problem solving to enjoying pleasant activities in the moments before going to bed. Patients should try to engage in less cognitively demanding activities before going to bed.

- **Schedule a brief time (e.g., 5–10 minutes) to write about worries and things one needs to do the following day and let them go before bed.** The idea is to let the worries flow out onto the page with the understanding that they have been captured, will not be lost in the night, and will be readily available to pursue upon awakening. This can also be done during the night if it helps foster sleep. This activity provides a time to identify things that cannot be changed while sleeping but that the patient wants to make sure are not forgotten upon awakening. Patients often have difficulty initiating and maintaining sleep because they are afraid that they will forget to do something important when they awaken.

- **Imagine one's thoughts slowly becoming quieter.** A helpful exercise to help patients quiet their mind is called "landing the helicopters." In bed, before sleeping, patients imagine that their thoughts are like the blades of a helicopter and that they hear the blades turn less and less quickly until they stop. For some patients, this pre-sleep routine helps them reduce ruminating, let go of the demands of the day, and transition to sleep.

4.6.5 SLEEP ENVIRONMENT

The sleep environment can have a positive or negative effect on sleep. It is important for patients to learn to associate their bed and bedroom with sleep. If the environment in which a patient sleeps is dark, quiet, relaxing, comfortable, and perceived as safe, she will have a better chance of maintaining sufficient restful restorative sleep. Conversely, if light, sound, and temperature change significantly during the night, sleep will likely be interrupted, shorter in duration, less deep, and less restorative. Sleep is an inherently unsafe behavior for every species of animal, as defense against predators is not possible during sleep. Hence, it is adaptive to have shallow fragmented sleep in an environment that is perceived as unsafe (e.g., high-crime neighborhoods and war zones) and awaken rapidly when changes in the environment suggest danger. Unfortunately for modern humans, this alerting response, which has helped us survive, does not tend to distinguish between environmental changes that indicated true danger (i.e., imminent attack) and changes due to modern technology (e.g., traffic noise and light bulbs).

Recommendations related to sleep environment are as follows:

- **If you go to bed and remain awake for longer than 20 minutes, get out of bed and do something not cognitively, emotionally, or physically stimulating (e.g., sit in a chair facing a wall). Do not return to bed until you feel sleepy. If you return to bed, but again cannot fall asleep for longer than 20 minutes, repeat the instructions.** This behavior will lead to fewer nighttime awakenings and reduce the time it takes to fall back to sleep when one does awaken. Patients need to associate their bed with sleeping. They need to understand that lying in bed and not sleeping is not the same type of rest afforded by sleep and that this behavior will increase awake time at night. Spending more time in bed not sleeping creates a stronger association between the bed and wakefulness, making it increasingly more difficult to initiate sleep and fall asleep after a nighttime awakening.
- **Do not engage in any activity other than sleep (and sex) in bed.** The patient's bed should serve as a cue for sleep (i.e., associate the bed with sleep). Patients should be encouraged not to use electronic devices, watch TV, read, listen to the radio, or do any activity other than sleep and sex in bed.
- **Make the sleep environment conducive to sleep.** Patients should darken the room as much as possible in the night (e.g., use blackout blinds or an eye mask). They should arrange for a comfortable temperature and minimal levels of sound. It is important to avoid using a radio, stereo, television, or electronic device to help one sleep. Patients should make the bedroom feel as safe and secure as possible. They should consider closing and locking windows/doors and using an alarm system. These devices can "off-load" the responsibility for monitoring the environment to an external device, letting the patient enter into and maintain deep sleep throughout the night.

4.7 CONCLUSION

One-third of a human's life is spent sleeping. During sleep, the human brain and body undergo a myriad of changes, cycling through NREM and REM sleep approximately every 60–90 minutes throughout the night. Sufficient quality sleep (i.e., 7–9 hours per night in adulthood) is essential to promoting health, preventing disease, and reducing mortality. The human and monetary cost of insufficient sleep around the world is staggering, with approximately one-third of the world not getting the recommended amount of sleep. Insufficient sleep is associated with risk factors (e.g., inflammatory markers, autonomic activation, vascular abnormalities, lifestyle, and health status) for major diseases (e.g., cardiovascular disease, cancer, and diabetes) affecting the world. Nurses should educate patients about the physiological and psychological factors that facilitate sleep and wakefulness: (1) sleep debt, (2) circadian rhythm alerting, (3) physiological arousal, (4) cognitive arousal, and (5) the sleep environment. After patients understand the interrelationship among these principles, behavioral sleep management guidelines (e.g., go to bed when one is sleepy, maintain a consistent sleep/wakeup schedule, relaxation training, practice "landing the helicopters," get out of bed when not sleeping) should be tailored to facilitate each patient's sleep. Nurses are uniquely positioned to promote health and improve medical care by educating patients about how to get a good night's sleep.

REFERENCES

Berry, R. B., Brooks, R., Gamaldo, C. E., Harding, S. M., Lloyd, R. M., Marcus, C. L., & Vaughn, B. V. (2015). *The AASM Manual for the Scoring of Sleep and Associated Events: Rules, Terminology and Technical Specifications, Version 2.2.* American Academy of Sleep Medicine. www.aasmnet.org

Brassington, G. S., King, A. C., & Bliwise, D. L. (2000). Sleep problems as a risk factor for falls in a sample of community-dwelling adults aged 64–99 years. *Journal of the American Geriatrics Society, 48*(10), 1234–1240. https://doi.org/10.1111/j.1532-5415.2000.tb02596.x

Bukari, M. A. A., Alghtani, M. A. M., Aljohani, Z. S., Qasem, A. A. A., & Alhazmi, I. H. M. (2021). Diagnosis and treatment of sleep disorders: A brief review. *International Journal of Medicine in Developing Countries, 5*(1), 364–369. https://doi.org/10.24911/IJMDC.51-1604917632

Buysse, D. J. (2014). Sleep health: Can we define it? Does it matter? *Sleep, 37*(1), 9–17. https://doi.org/10.5665/sleep.3298

Cappuccio, F. P., D'Elia, L., Strazzullo, P., & Miller, M. A. (2010). Sleep duration and all-cause mortality: A systematic review and meta-analysis of prospective studies. *Sleep: Journal of Sleep and Sleep Disorders Research, 33*(5), 585–592. http://dx.doi.org/10.1093/sleep/33.5.585

Carskadon, M. A., & Dement, W. C. (2017). Normal human sleep: An overview. In M. Kryger, T. Roth, & W. C. Dement (Eds.), *Principles and Practice of Sleep Medicine (Sixth Edition)* (pp. 15–24. e13). Elsevier. https://doi.org/10.1016/B978-0-323-24288-2.00002-7

Carskadon, M. A., Dement, W. C., Mitler, M. M., Roth, T., Westbrook, P. R., & Keenan, S. (1986). Guidelines for the multiple sleep latency test (MSLT): A standard measure of sleepiness. *Sleep: Journal of Sleep Research & Sleep Medicine, 9*(4), 519–524. http://dx.doi.org/10.1093/sleep/9.4.519

Chaput, J. P., Dutil, C., Featherstone, R., Ross, R., Giangregorio, L., Saunders, T. J., Janssen, I., Poitras, V. J., Kho, M. E., Ross-White, A., Zankar, S., & Carrier, J. (2020). Sleep timing, sleep consistency, and health in adults: A systematic review. *Applied Physiology, Nutrition, and Metabolism, 45*(10 (Suppl. 2)), S232–S247. https://doi.org/10.1139/apnm-2020-0032

Chaput, J. P., Gray, C. E., Poitras, V. J., Carson, V., Gruber, R., Birken, C. S., MacLean, J. E., Aubert, S., Sampson, M., & Tremblay, M. S. (2017). Systematic review of the relationships between sleep duration and health indicators in the early years (0–4 years). *BMC Public Health, 17*(Suppl 5), 855. https://doi.org/10.1186/s12889-017-4850-2

Chaput, J. P., Gray, C. E., Poitras, V. J., Carson, V., Gruber, R., Olds, T., Weiss, S. K., Connor Gorber, S., Kho, M. E., Sampson, M., Belanger, K., Eryuzlu, S., Callender, L., & Tremblay, M. S. (2016). Systematic review of the relationships between sleep duration and health indicators in school-aged children and youth. *Applied Physiology, Nutrition, & Metabolism = Physiologie Appliquee, Nutrition et Metabolisme, 41*(6 Suppl 3), S266–282. https://doi.org/10.1139/apnm-2015-0627

Chaput, J. P., Wong, S. L., & Michaud, I. (2017). Duration and quality of sleep among Canadians aged 18 to 79. *Health Reports, 28*(9), 28–33. http://ovidsp.ovid.com/ovidweb.cgi?T=JS&PAGE=reference&D=med14&NEWS=N&AN=28930365

Chattu, V. K., Manzar, M. D., Kumary, S., Burman, D., Spence, D. W., & Pandi-Perumal, S. R. (2018). The global problem of insufficient sleep and its serious public health implications. *Healthcare*, 7(1), 20. https://dx.doi.org/10.3390/healthcare7010001

Edgar, D. M. D., W.C.; Fuller, C.A. (1993). Effect of SCN lesions on sleep in squirrel monkeys: Evidence for opponent processes in sleep–wake regulation. *The Journal of Neuroscience*, 13(3), 1065–1079.

Egan, K. J., Knutson, K. L., Pereira, A. C., & von Schantz, M. (2017). The role of race and ethnicity in sleep, circadian rhythms and cardiovascular health. *Sleep Medicine Reviews*, 33, 70–78. http://dx.doi.org/10.1016/j.smrv.2016.05.004

Freeman, D., Sheaves, B., Goodwin, G. M., Yu, L.-M., Nickless, A., Harrison, P. J., Emsley, R., Luik, A. I., Foster, R. G., Wadekar, V., Hinds, C., Gumley, A., Jones, R., Lightman, S., Jones, S., Bentall, R., Kinderman, P., Rowse, G., Brugha, T., … Espie, C. A. (2017). The effects of improving sleep on mental health (OASIS): A randomised controlled trial with mediation analysis. *The Lancet Psychiatry*, 4(10), 749–758. http://dx.doi.org/10.1016/S2215-0366%2817%2930328-0

Galland, B. C., Taylor, B. J., Elder, D. E., & Herbison, P. (2012). Normal sleep patterns in infants and children: A systematic review of observational studies. *Sleep Medicine Reviews*, 16(3), 213–222. http://dx.doi.org/10.1016/j.smrv.2011.06.001

Grandner, M. A., Williams, N. J., Knutson, K. L., Roberts, D., & Jean-Louis, G. (2016). Sleep disparity, race/ethnicity, and socioeconomic position. *Sleep Medicine*, 18, 7–18. http://dx.doi.org/10.1016/j.sleep.2015.01.020

Hall, M. H., Smagula, S. F., Boudreau, R. M., Ayonayon, H. N., Goldman, S. E., Harris, T. B., Naydeck, B. L., Rubin, S. M., Samuelsson, L., Satterfield, S., Stone, K. L., Visser, M., & Newman, A. B. (2015). Association between sleep duration and mortality is mediated by markers of inflammation and health in older adults: The Health, Aging and Body Composition Study. *Sleep: Journal of Sleep and Sleep Disorders Research*, 38(2), 189–195. http://dx.doi.org/10.5665/sleep.4394

He, M., Deng, X., Zhu, Y., Huan, L., & Niu, W. (2020). The relationship between sleep duration and all-cause mortality in the older people: An updated and dose-response meta-analysis. *BMC Public Health*, 20(1), 1179. https://dx.doi.org/10.1186/s12889-020-09275-3

Hirshkowitz, M., Whiton, K., Albert, S. M., Alessi, C., Bruni, O., DonCarlos, L., Hazen, N., Herman, J., Adams Hillard, P. J., Katz, E. S., Kheirandish-Gozal, L., Neubauer, D. N., O'Donnell, A. E., Ohayon, M., Peever, J., Rawding, R., Sachdeva, R. C., Setters, B., Vitiello, M. V., & Ware, J. C. (2015). National Sleep Foundation's updated sleep duration recommendations: Final report. *Sleep Health*, 1(4), 233–243. https://dx.doi.org/10.1016/j.sleh.2015.10.004

Iglowstein, I., Jenni, O. G., Molinari, L., & Largo, R. H. (2003). Sleep duration from infancy to adolescence: Reference values and generational trends. *Pediatrics*, 111(2), 302–307. https://doi.org/10.1542/peds.111.2.302

Imtiaz, S. A. (2021). A systematic review of sensing technologies for wearable sleep staging. *Sensors*, 21(5), 24. https://dx.doi.org/10.3390/s21051562

Irish, L. A., Kline, C. E., Gunn, H. E., Buysse, D. J., & Hall, M. H. (2015). The role of sleep hygiene in promoting public health: A review of empirical evidence. *Sleep Medicine Reviews*, 22, 23–36. http://dx.doi.org/10.1016/j.smrv.2014.10.001

Irwin, M. R. (2019). Sleep and inflammation: Partners in sickness and in health. *Nature Reviews. Immunology*, 19(11), 702–715. https://dx.doi.org/10.1038/s41577-019-0190-z

Itani, O., Jike, M., Watanabe, N., & Kaneita, Y. (2017). Short sleep duration and health outcomes: A systematic review, meta-analysis, and meta-regression. *Sleep Medicine*, 32, 246–256. https://doi.org/10.1016/j.sleep.2016.08.006

Jike, M., Itani, O., Watanabe, N., Buysse, D. J., & Kaneita, Y. (2018). Long sleep duration and health outcomes: A systematic review, meta-analysis and meta-regression. *Sleep Medicine Reviews*, 39, 25–36. http://dx.doi.org/10.1016/j.smrv.2017.06.011

Johnson, D. A., Jackson, C. L., Williams, N. J., & Alcantara, C. (2019). Are sleep patterns influenced by race/ethnicity—a marker of relative advantage or disadvantage? Evidence to date. *Nature & Science of Sleep*, 11, 79–95. https://doi.org/10.2147/NSS.S169312

Kalmbach, D. A., Arnedt, J., Song, P. X., Guille, C., & Sen, S. (2017). Sleep disturbance and short sleep as risk factors for depression and perceived medical errors in first-year residents. *Sleep: Journal of Sleep and Sleep Disorders Research*, 40(3), 1–8. http://dx.doi.org/10.1093/sleep/zsw073

Kocevska, D., Lysen, T. S., Dotinga, A., Koopman-Verhoeff, M. E., Luijk, M., Antypa, N., Biermasz, N. R., Blokstra, A., Brug, J., Burk, W. J., Comijs, H. C., Corpeleijn, E., Dashti, H. S., de Bruin, E. J., de Graaf, R., Derks, I. P. M., Dewald-Kaufmann, J. F., Elders, P. J. M., Gemke, R., ... Tiemeier, H. (2021). Sleep characteristics across the lifespan in 1.1 million people from the Netherlands, United Kingdom and United States: A systematic review and meta-analysis. *Nature Human Behaviour, 5*(1), 113–122. https://dx.doi.org/10.1038/s41562-020-00965-x

Leung, L. C., Wang, G. X., Madelaine, R., Skariah, G., Kawakami, K., Deisseroth, K., Urban, A. E., & Mourrain, P. (2019). Neural signatures of sleep in zebrafish. *Nature, 571*(7764), 198–204. https://doi.org/10.1038/s41586-019-1336-7

Li, J., Vitiello, M. V., & Gooneratne, N. S. (2018). Sleep in normal aging. *Sleep Medicine Clinics, 13*(1), 1–11. http://dx.doi.org/10.1016/j.jsmc.2017.09.001

Li, L., Wu, C., Gan, Y., Qu, X., & Lu, Z. (2016). Insomnia and the risk of depression: A meta-analysis of prospective cohort studies. *BMC Psychiatry, 375*, 16. http://dx.doi.org/10.1186/s12888-016-1075-3

Liu, X., Liu, L., Owens, J. A., & Kaplan, D. L. (2005). Sleep patterns and sleep problems among school-children in the United States and China. *Pediatrics, 115*(1 Suppl), 241–249. https://doi.org/10.1542/peds.2004-0815F

Liu, Y., Wheaton, A. G., Chapman, D. P., Cunningham, T. J., Lu, H., & Croft, J. B. (2016). Prevalence of healthy sleep duration among adults—United States, 2014. *MMWR Morbidity and Mortality Weekly Report, 65*(6), 137–141. https://doi.org/10.15585/mmwr.mm6506a1

Luik, A. I., Kyle, S. D., & Espie, C. A. (2017). Digital cognitive behavioral therapy (dCBT) for insomnia: A state-of-the-science review. *Current Sleep Medicine Reports, 3*(2), 48–56. https://dx.doi.org/10.1007/s40675-017-0065-4

Mallampalli, M. P., & Carter, C. L. (2014). Exploring sex and gender differences in sleep health: A society for women's health research report. *Journal of Women's Health, 23*(7), 553–562. https://doi.org/10.1089/jwh.2014.4816

Mirmiran, M., Maas, Y. G., & Ariagno, R. L. (2003). Development of fetal and neonatal sleep and circadian rhythms. *Sleep Medicine Reviews, 7*(4), 321–334. https://doi.org/10.1053/smrv.2002.0243

Mullington, J. M., Simpson, N. S., Meier-Ewert, H. K., & Haack, M. (2010). Sleep loss and inflammation. *Best Practice & Research Clinical Endocrinology & Metabolism, 24*(5), 775–784. https://dx.doi.org/10.1016/j.beem.2010.08.014

Murawski, B., Wade, L., Plotnikoff, R. C., Lubans, D. R., & Duncan, M. J. (2018). A systematic review and meta-analysis of cognitive and behavioral interventions to improve sleep health in adults without sleep disorders. *Sleep Medicine Reviews, 40*, 160–169. http://dx.doi.org/10.1016/j.smrv.2017.12.003

Ohayon, M. M., Carskadon, M. A., Guilleminault, C., & Vitiello, M. V. (2004). Meta-analysis of quantitative sleep parameters from childhood to old age in healthy individuals: Developing normative sleep values across the human lifespan. *Sleep: Journal of Sleep and Sleep Disorders Research, 27*(7), 1255–1273. http://dx.doi.org/10.1093/sleep/27.7.1255

Olds, T., Blunden, S., Petkov, J., & Forchino, F. (2010). The relationships between sex, age, geography and time in bed in adolescents: A meta-analysis of data from 23 countries. *Sleep Medicine Reviews, 14*(6), 371–378. http://dx.doi.org/10.1016/j.smrv.2009.12.002

Pengo, M. F., Won, C. H., & Bourjeily, G. (2018). Sleep in women across the life span. *Chest, 154*(1), 196–206. https://dx.doi.org/10.1016/j.chest.2018.04.005

Perez-Pozuelo, I., Zhai, B., Palotti, J., Mall, R., Aupetit, M., Garcia-Gomez, J. M., Taheri, S., Guan, Y., & Fernandez-Luque, L. (2020). The future of sleep health: A data-driven revolution in sleep science and medicine. *NPJ Digital Medicine, 3*, 42. https://doi.org/10.1038/s41746-020-0244-4

Ravyts, S. G., Dzierzewski, J. M., Perez, E., Donovan, E. K., & Dautovich, N. D. (2021). Sleep health as measured by RU SATED: A psychometric evaluation. *Behavioral Sleep Medicine, 19*(1), 48–56. https://doi.org/10.1080/15402002.2019.1701474

Rechtschaffen, A., & Kales, A. (Eds.). (1968). *A Manual of Standardized Terminology, Techniques, and Scoring System for Sleep Stages of Human Subjects*. Brain Information Service/Brain Research Institute. https://doi.org/10.1001/archpsyc.1969.01740140118016

Sadeh, A. (2011). The role and validity of actigraphy in sleep medicine: An update. *Sleep Medicine Reviews, 15*(4), 259–267. http://dx.doi.org/10.1016/j.smrv.2010.10.001

Sedov, I. D., Cameron, E. E., Madigan, S., & Tomfohr-Madsen, L. M. (2018). Sleep quality during pregnancy: A meta-analysis. *Sleep Medicine Reviews, 38*, 168–176. http://dx.doi.org/10.1016/j.smrv.2017.06.005

Smith, M. T., McCrae, C. S., Cheung, J., Martin, J. L., Harrod, C. G., Heald, J. L., & Carden, K. A. (2018). Use of actigraphy for the evaluation of sleep disorders and circadian rhythm sleep-wake disorders: An American Academy of Sleep Medicine systematic review, meta-analysis, and GRADE assessment. *Journal of Clinical Sleep Medicine*, *14*(7), 1209–1230. https://dx.doi.org/10.5664/jcsm.7228

Stone, J. D., Rentz, L. E., Forsey, J., Ramadan, J., Markwald, R. R., Finomore, V. S., Galster, S. M., Rezai, A., & Hagen, J. A. (2020). Evaluations of commercial sleep technologies for objective monitoring during routine sleeping conditions. *Nature & Science of Sleep*, *12*, 821–842. https://dx.doi.org/10.2147/NSS.S270705

Stone, K. L., & Ancoli-Israel, S. (2017). Chapter 171—Actigraphy. In M. Kryger, T. Roth, & W. C. Dement (Eds.), *Principles and Practice of Sleep Medicine (Sixth Edition)* (pp. 1671–1678.e1674). Elsevier. https://doi.org/10.1016/B978-0-323-24288-2.00171-9

Stone, K. L., Blackwell, T. L., Ancoli-Israel, S., Cauley, J. A., Redline, S., Marshall, L. M., Ensrud, K. E., & Osteoporotic Fractures in Men Study Group. (2014). Sleep disturbances and risk of falls in older community-dwelling men: The outcomes of sleep disorders in Older Men (MrOS Sleep) Study. *Journal of the American Geriatrics Society*, *62*(2), 299–305. https://doi.org/10.1111/jgs.12649

Tal, A., Shinar, Z., Shaki, D., Codish, S., & Goldbart, A. (2017). Validation of contact-free sleep monitoring device with comparison to polysomnography. *Journal of Clinical Sleep Medicine*, *13*(3), 517–522. https://dx.doi.org/10.5664/jcsm.6514

Taylor, D. J., Peterson, A. L., Goodie, J. L., Grieser, E., Hryshko-Mullen, A. S., Rowan, A., Wilkerson, A., Pruiksma, K. E., Dietch, J. R., Hall-Clark, B., & Fina, B. (2019). *Cognitive-behavioral therapy for insomnia in the military: Therapist guide*. University of Arizona Insomnia and Sleep Health Research Laboratory. http://insomnia.arizona.edu/CBTI-M

van Straten, A., van der Zweerde, T., Kleiboer, A., Cuijpers, P., Morin, C. M., & Lancee, J. (2018). Cognitive and behavioral therapies in the treatment of insomnia: A meta-analysis. *Sleep Medicine Reviews*, *38*, 3–16. http://dx.doi.org/10.1016/j.smrv.2017.02.001

Watson, N. F., Badr, M., Belenky, G., Bliwise, D. L., Buxton, O. M., Buysse, D., Dinges, D. F., Gangwisch, J., Grandner, M. A., Kushida, C., Malhotra, R. K., Martin, J. L., Patel, S. R., Quan, S. F., Tasali, E., Twery, M., Croft, J. B., Maher, E., Barrett, J. A., … Heald, J. L. (2015). Joint consensus statement of the American Academy of Sleep Medicine and Sleep Research Society on the recommended amount of sleep for a healthy adult: Methodology and discussion. *Sleep: Journal of Sleep and Sleep Disorders Research*, *38*(8), 1161–1183. http://dx.doi.org/10.5665/sleep.4886

5 Emotional Wellness and Stress Resilience

Elizabeth R. Click[1] and Alyssa Vela[2]
[1]FPB School of Nursing
Case Western Reserve University, Cleveland, USA
[2]Cardiac Behavioral Medicine
Bluhm Cardiovascular Institute of Northwestern, Chicago, USA
Northwestern University Feinberg School of Medicine, Chicago, USA

CONTENTS

DOI: 10.1201/9781003178330-6

KEY POINTS

- Emotional wellness and stress resilience are critical for overall health and well-being.
- Evidence-based skills and strategies exist to enhance emotional wellness and stress resilience.
- Nurses are able to implement best practices in a variety of settings to foster stress resilience and to enhance emotional wellness with patients of any age.

5.1 INTRODUCTION

Emotional wellness focuses on effectively handling life stressors during times of change and challenge, as well as during times of peace and calm. Being aware of emotions, understanding them, and accepting emotions experienced are hallmarks of emotional wellness. Within the comprehensive scope of wellness, the emotional dimension is critical for overall health. Indeed, the rise in reports of threats to emotional wellness for all ages emphasizes the importance of emotions and stress resilience for overall quality of life. Figure 5.1 portrays the interconnected nature of these concepts.

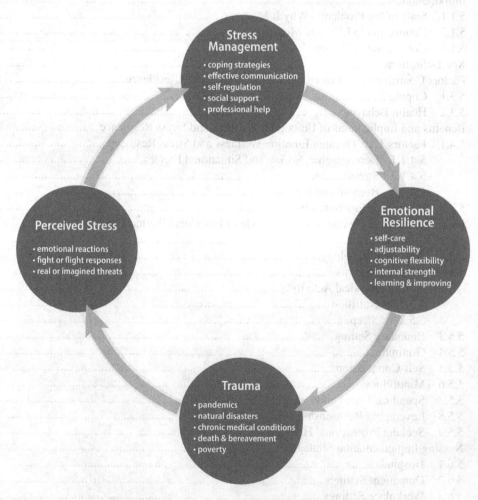

FIGURE 5.1   Interconnectedness of emotional wellness and stress resilience

5.1.1 State of the Problem – Why It Matters

Human beings are complex, with our bodies, minds, and spirits working together in intricate ways. When considering life experiences and health across the lifespan, a variety of dimensions are critical to examine. While physical health is typically identified as important to address first, emotional and mental health are equally as impactful. As more is understood about the detailed interconnections between the physical body and mind, the significance of emotional wellness has been elevated. Recent healthcare reports further highlight the value of emotional wellness and stress resilience. Increasing numbers of people experience acute and chronic emotional and mental health issues that affect overall health (Figueroa et al., 2020). More mental health claims have been incurred by patients with conditions that are expensive to treat (Davenport et al., 2020). Suicide is the tenth leading cause of death in the United States and is the second leading cause of death for ages 10 through 34 (Hedegaard et al., 2020). Given the synergistic effects of physical, emotional, and mental wellness, emotional wellness and stress resilience must be well understood and embraced by nurses so that they can experience full emotional well-being and benefit their patients.

5.1.2 Connection to Lifestyle Medicine

Chronic stress is pervasive within daily life, negatively influences health, and increases chronic illness in the U.S. More than three-quarters of visits to healthcare providers are related to high levels of daily stress (Avey et al., 2003); however, stress management counseling is not prevalent during primary care visits and is the least likely aspect of lifestyle to be addressed (Nerurkar et al., 2013). This connection between stress and ill health is so significant that stress management has been identified as one of six pillars of lifestyle medicine practice (Rippe, 2018). Research indicates that practice of stress management techniques makes a significant difference in ameliorating the negative effects of stress. Lifestyle medicine is a critical driver for moving our sick care system into a true healthcare system, and stress resilience is critical for emotional wellness and overall well-being.

5.1.3 Connection to Nursing Education and Practice

Nursing education has emphasized the importance of health promotion in contributing to health across the lifespan for decades. One of the foremost theorists, Nola Pender, PhD, conceptualized the importance of health promotion to nursing practice in 1982; seven editions have since been published (Pender, Murdaugh & Parsons, 2014). Nevertheless, there has been less emphasis placed on prevention within nursing education than on acute and chronic health conditions. Thus, there is opportunity to view health from a holistic perspective by emphasizing wellness. This book provides the opportunity to delve into critical wellness elements and understand the impact of lifestyle factors on overall health.

5.2 KEY DEFINITIONS

Like many psychosocial constructs, there are many definitions of wellness and related terms. As defined by the World Health Organization (WHO), *wellness* is more than the absence of disease or suffering; it is a dynamic state of being that includes physical, mental, and social domains (Misselbrook, 2014). Further definitions of wellness emphasize an active process that consists of a culmination of health behavior decisions (Misselbrook, 2014). The active term wellness differs from *well-being*, which is often defined as a momentary state of health. The American Psychological Association's (2021a) definition of well-being is a state characterized by contentment, happiness, good quality of life, a good outlook, good mental and physical health, and little distress. *Emotional wellness* means to be able to cope with the stressors of life and to adapt when faced with difficulties.

Emotional wellness can be identified by supportive relationships, the ability to experience and express a broad range of emotions, and a healthy concept of oneself (Stewart-Brown, 1998). It is also important to note that these terms are not associated with only the experience of constant positive emotions. When emotions and/or state of being is predominantly negative, individuals may experience a decline in quality of life (QOL).

One factor that has the most impact on well-being and wellness is stress. *Stress* is defined as a response to internal and/or external stimuli that results in a physiological and/or psychological response. The physiological stress response impacts most organ systems and often shows up with physical symptoms such as sweating, heart palpitations, dry mouth, shortness of breath, and fidgeting. Those symptoms are often accompanied by a negative emotional and/or affective response (Cohen et al., 2007; Selye, 1993). Severe stress can result in especially profound physiological symptoms, which are understood as *general adaptation syndrome* (*GAS*). GAS occurs in stages: 1) alarm, which is characterized by shock and associated with a decrease in muscle tone, temperature, and blood pressure, as well as countershock, during which the sympathetic nervous system is aroused; 2) resistance, also known as adaptation, during which stabilization occurs but at heightened physiological levels (i.e. high blood pressure which can result in hypertension); and 3) exhaustion, which is the breakdown of the coping and adaptation that occurs in response to the severe stressor. Exhaustion is often characterized by poor sleep, difficulty concentrating, restlessness, mood changes, and irritability (Selye, 1993).

Stressors themselves vary greatly in not only intensity but also duration. Stress occurs in three forms: acute stress, episodic stress, and chronic stress. *Acute stress* is a physiological and/or psychological response to a brief and episodic event that is perceived as stressful. The acute stress response is often likened to the fight-or-flight response of the sympathetic nervous system and, like the stressor, is acute and terminates after a brief, distinct period of time. For many people, receiving a shot with the experience of the needle and brief pain associated, is an example of an acute stressor (Selye, 1993). *Episodic stress* refers to the culmination of many acute stressors that interfere with life and result in increasing levels of distress. For individuals experiencing episodic stress, what may seem minor acute stressors, such as running late, or being stuck in traffic, trigger a cascade effect in which more situations are perceived as stressors, with resulting physiological and psychological effects. *Chronic stress* occurs in response to a prolonged external or internal stressor and results in chronic physical and/or psychological responses. The stressor itself does not need to remain present, as the stress response can be triggered by only recall of the stressor (Wheaton, 1997). Examples of chronic stress include: a work environment that is perceived as bad and stressful, and living through the COVID-19 pandemic. Individuals can experience the effects of chronic stress related to negative early childhood events, trauma history, and lifetime experiences of discrimination (Wheaton, 1997). While often related to chronic stress, burnout is a distinct term.

Work-related stress and exposure to trauma can build over time and spill into other aspects of life and functional status, in the form of burnout (Beck, 2011; Delgado, Upton, Ranse, Furness, & Foster, 2017). While burnout is not a diagnosable condition in the United States, it has been recognized as an important construct and is listed as a condition in the ICD-10 (Merlo & Rippe, 2020). *Burnout* is defined as a state of total mental, physical, and/or emotional exhaustion, often in the context of chronic stress (American Psychological Association, 2021b). The term burnout is typically applied to professional exhaustion, and much of the research has been conducted among individuals in caregiving professions, such as nursing. Burnout is associated with a decrease in motivation, changes in performance, and negative perception of self. Research suggests that burnout tends to build over time, and with greater burnout, employees tend to experience greater perceived work stress. Thus, stress and burnout are mutually reinforcing (de Oliveira et al., 2019). Of note, *caregiver stress* and *caregiver fatigue* are distinct from burnout, as they refer to the stress and multidimensional fatigue when caring for a family member or loved one (i.e. a parent with dementia), rather than professional

TABLE 5.1
Key emotional wellness definitions

Term	Definition
Wellness	Dynamic ongoing process that includes physical, mental, and social domains and is more than absence of disease.
Well-being	A momentary state of health characterized by contentment, happiness, good quality of life, a good outlook, good mental and physical health, and little distress.
Emotional wellness	To be able to cope with the stressors of life and to adapt when faced with difficulties, have healthy relationships, healthy self-concept, and be able to experience a range of emotions.
Stress	A response to internal and/or external stimuli that results in a physiological and/or psychological response. Symptoms include sweating, heart palpitations, dry mouth, and negative emotions.
Acute stress	Physiological and/or psychological response to a brief and episodic event that is perceived as stressful.
Episodic stress	The culmination of many acute stressors that start to interfere with life and result in increasing levels of distress
Chronic stress	Response to a prolonged external or internal stressor, that may not always be present, and results in chronic physical and/or psychological responses.
Burnout	A state of total mental, physical, and/or emotional exhaustion, often in the context of chronic stress. Typically specific to work/professional life.
Caregiver stress/fatigue	The stress and multidimensional fatigue when someone provides for a family member or loved one, outside of professional responsibilities.
Resilience	Process and outcome of adapting to difficult experiences by adjusting to internal and external demands with psychological and behavioral flexibility.

caregiving (McDaniel & Allen, 2012). One of the most potent influencing factors on stress, trauma, and burnout is resilience.

Fortunately, the majority of people are at least moderately resilient and able to prevent and/or recover from significant stress and/or burnout (Zhuang-Shuang & Hasson, 2020). *Resilience* is defined as both the process and the outcome of adapting to difficult experiences by adjusting to internal and external demands with psychological and behavioral flexibility (Aburn et al., 2010). Research has indicated that resilience is influenced by one's outlook and view of the world, access to quality social support, and sufficient coping strategies. These foundational concepts outlined in this section will be discussed further throughout the chapter. See Table 5.1.

5.3   FACTORS CONTRIBUTING TO EMOTIONAL WELLNESS AND STRESS RESILIENCE

Key factors that influence emotional wellness and stress resilience include coping skills and health behaviors. Ability to adapt and cope with stressors and job demands, and having realistic expectations, has been associated with resilience and has positive implications for work and daily life. Resilience can be learned through skill building and practice (Brennan, 2016). Resilience occurs within context, meaning that the individual factors that prime an individual for resilience when faced with a stressful situation are influenced by the larger sociocultural context (Fletcher & Sarkar, 2013). For example, social support in the context of stressful experiences or trauma bolsters resilience. However, since the onset of the COVID-19 pandemic, coping and resilience have been negatively impacted by individual and systemic stressors for all providers, inadequate resources, and mood changes that made it challenging to cope to buffer the effects of stress (Huang et al., 2020). Thus, coping skills and health behaviors, such as diet and physical activity, are critical for emotional wellness and stress resilience.

5.3.1 Coping

One of the key factors in the development and maintenance of resilience is sufficient quantity and quality of coping skills and the ability to employ them as needed. Coping skills are behavioral or cognitive strategies that allow an individual to adapt to situations (American Psychological Association, 2021c). They are critical to maintaining emotional wellness and preventing issues related to stress and require intentional effort. Coping skills are typically utilized to minimize the psychological harm a situation may cause (Carroll, 2013). Coping is often divided into two types: problem-focused (also called solution-focused) and emotion-focused. Problem-focused coping strategies emphasize addressing or resolving the sources of stress and include strategies such as information seeking and removing oneself from the stressful environment or situation. Rather than resolving the stressor, emotion-focused coping focuses on addressing the emotions related to a stressor and includes strategies such as relaxation techniques and positive self-talk (Carroll, 2013). Research has also suggested differences in perception and experience of stress, both within and outside of the workplace. Individual differences in coping skills appear to vary based on age, gender, and job type (Nekoranec & Kmosena, 2015). Factors that influence workplace stress include: working conditions, such as hours, deadlines, and pressure to perform; work relationships; organizational culture; and professional development. Individual perceptions of stress also vary based on personality, professional identity, and available coping skills (Nekoranec & Kmosena, 2015).

Coping, and factors that influence coping, have an important influence on nursing students and nurses in the field. Research suggests there are many factors that influence coping skills for nurses, including age, level of experience, and environment, including the setting in which one works (Laal & Aliramaie, 2010). A 2017 review identified moderate to high levels of stress among nursing students, with stress related to workload, negative interactions with instructors, and patient care. Nursing students tend to use problem-focused coping strategies to address such stressors, for example developing new strategies to solve problems. From an emotion-focused perspective, finding meaning in situations and challenges was also an important coping skill for nursing students (Labrague et al., 2017). Following graduation, nurses experience workplace stress, regardless of role.

Coping is also relevant to nurses who are in practice. Workplace experiences of nurse managers indicate they experience moderate levels of stress related to insufficient resources, financial responsibilities, and overall workload. Having the power to make decisions and/or have control over situations was a key predictor of workplace stress for nurse managers. Coping skills were related to reliance on interpersonal relationships with team members, including members of the administration (Labrague et al., 2018). Overall, the type and utility of coping strategies is dependent upon personality, outlook, and workplace or educational environmental factors. Coping strategies also overlap with good health behaviors (i.e. exercise) to allow for effective coping, while poor health behaviors (i.e. smoking) can result in further stress and barriers to coping.

5.3.2 Health Behaviors

Good health behaviors, which includes nutritious diet, sufficient physical activity, good quality and quantity of sleep, managing stress, and limiting substance use, all influence emotional wellness. As the field of lifestyle medicine develops, there is further evidence for the role of health behaviors and lifestyle in psychological well-being and quality of life (Morton, 2018). Health behaviors have been associated with the prevention of poor mental health and a fostering of good emotional well-being, independent of or as an adjunct to traditional forms of therapy and psychopharmacology for mental health conditions (Morton, 2018). For example, engaging in physical activity, such as taking a brief walk to reduce stress and improve mood, is a well-established and effective strategy (Penedo & Dahn, 2005). Poor health behaviors, such as turning to sugar or alcohol to cope with stress, are forms of unhealthy coping that often result in further stress and negative outcomes (Bremner et al., 2020).

5.4 BENEFITS AND IMPLICATIONS OF EMOTIONAL WELLNESS AND STRESS RESILIENCE

There are numerous benefits associated with emotional wellness, including psychological and physical benefits like enhanced productivity and resilience. The factors and implications are discussed within this section.

5.4.1 FACTORS THAT THREATEN EMOTION WELLNESS AND STRESS RESILIENCE

The factors that threaten emotional wellness and stress resilience include demographic, social, and situational factors as well as experiences of stress, burnout, and fatigue.

5.4.1.1 Demographic, Social, and Situational Factors

Research has identified a variety of factors that may affect emotional wellness. Demographic factors, such as gender, age, race, and marital status, impact emotional health. Social and situational factors, such as low socioeconomic status, social connections, and living conditions, may also serve as threats to emotional wellness. A significant body of published literature focuses on each of these factor sets.

When examining demographic factors impacted by stress, a lifespan approach is generally taken. Stress impacts children, adolescents, and young, middle, and older adults in different ways. Children and adolescents may experience stress in relation to self-esteem, gender, personality, social support, family makeup, health, and past experiences with stress (Pender et al., 2014). Young and middle-aged adults often deal with stressors related to career pursuits, relationships, child-bearing, and child-rearing. During older adulthood, some stressors experienced during youth may diminish, while others may be amplified. For example, managing sadness and loss often becomes more significant as people age. Changing health status and physical capability may also impact the effect of stress for older adults.

Maslow's Hierarchy of Needs is also relevant to this discussion given the connection between basic life resources as precursors to developing strong psychological and emotional wellness (Mathes, 1981). When basic biological and physiological needs (e.g. eating, cleansing, water, sleep, etc.) are not met in a person's life, those deficiencies may impact the ability and motivation of that person to grow and develop in other more advanced stages (e.g. safety, self-esteem, belonging, cognitive, and self-actualization). This means that those individuals lacking fundamental daily life resources may be predisposed to experiencing greater threats to emotional wellness, and possibly less stress resilience, than those who have those basic life needs fulfilled. Maslow's Hierarchy of Needs serves as a strong example of the importance of basic, psychological, and self-fulfillment needs in achieving holistic well-being.

Lack of access to resources, or low socioeconomic status, places individuals at increased risk for mental health issues (Kivimaki et al., 2020). From that economic perspective, socioeconomic status begins a cascade over time connecting emotional wellness and physical health. Stated differently, not having enough financial resources may threaten emotional wellness and stress resilience, which then may lead to additional problems such as substance abuse and various physical health issues.

Another social factor that impacts emotional wellness and stress resilience is social determinants of health. This concept refers to the conditions and environments in which people live, work, play, and age and impact health, functioning, and quality of life outcomes (Office of Disease Prevention and Health Promotion [ODHP], n.d.). In the past few years, increased awareness of the powerful impact of social determinants of health has also highlighted the unique needs of those who may experience implicit bias and systemic racism in their daily life experience. Implicit bias is defined as automatically evoked mental associations about social groups based on inequalities and stereotypes in the environment (Payne & Hannay, 2021). Implicit bias may serve as an indicator of the level of systemic racism in an environment. Systemic racism refers to structures within society that systematically disadvantage marginalized groups (Payne & Hannay, 2021). The recent rise in awareness of discrimination and racism in society has led to more published literature that describes the impact of those experiences on stress resilience and emotional wellness (Williams, 2018). Understanding these factors is critical as they also serve as threats to emotional wellness and stress resilience.

A lifespan perspective is also relevant to this discussion of social factors. For example, adverse childhood events (ACEs) may impact individuals in a variety of ways as they age. ACEs are defined as stressful or traumatic events that occur in a child's life prior to 18 years of age (Gilgoff, Singh, Koita, Gentile & Marques, 2020). Research has identified numerous sequelae connecting ACEs with a variety of negative health and behavioral outcomes. Understanding an individual's full life experience is critical to learning more about their emotional wellness and stress resilience.

Finally, situational factors, such as social connections and living circumstances, also affect emotional wellness and stress resilience. Social relationships have short and long-term effects with the impacts experienced throughout the lifespan (Umberson & Montez, 2011). Social isolation has a negative impact on mental health and led to new threats to emotional wellness during the COVID-19 pandemic (Sher, 2020). Each person experiences circumstances differently, so fully understanding an individual's perspective, and all factors associated with their life, is necessary in order to implement appropriate treatment. The complex interplay between these factors makes it difficult to generalize outcomes and experiences for all people, so more investigation is necessary (Ungar & Theron, 2020).

5.4.1.2 Stress

When individuals experience stress repeatedly, significant negative issues can develop that have a comprehensive effect. Not only do acute (e.g., increased heart rate, blood pressure, respiratory rate, etc.) and chronic health conditions (e.g. high blood pressure, heart disease, chest pain, diabetes, headaches, gastrointestinal issues, insomnia, etc.) develop, they may worsen over time as a result of continued stress (Suvarna et al., 2020). Mental health conditions impacted by stress include increased incidence of anxiety and depression, worrying, forgetfulness, and inability to focus. The effects of stress on emotional wellness are evidenced by agitation, frustration, moodiness, loneliness, low self-esteem, and feeling overwhelmed. No aspect of individual wellness is spared when high stress levels exist in daily life (Guidi et al., 2021). Behavioral issues, such as changes in appetite and eating patterns, increased substance use, procrastination, avoidance, and nervous fidgeting may also develop following stressful events. While stress is part of everyday life, experiencing chronic stress may lead to a variety of long-term health consequences. Learning how to manage stress effectively is critical for overall well-being.

5.4.1.3 Burnout and Fatigue

Caregiving professions, such as nursing, are prone to experiencing burnout (Zhang et al., 2018). As with stress, burnout has a comprehensive effect on health and leads to physical, mental, and emotional issues. Physical issues experienced in association with burnout may include: fatigue, headache, pain, hypercholesterolemia, type 2 diabetes, cardiovascular and gastrointestinal issues, severe injury, and mortality before 45 years of age. Mental and emotional consequences related to burnout may include: depression, insomnia, use of psychotropic medications, and hospitalization for mental health disorders. Occupational issues, such as job dissatisfaction, absenteeism, and presenteeism, may develop in relation to burnout (Salvagioni et al., 2017). Comprehensive approaches are needed that address work environment, job demands, and individual coping strategies to minimize the experience and detrimental effects of burnout. The effects of experiencing stress and burnout can lead to fatigue and emotional exhaustion for nurses. When increased work demands, limited job control, and low levels of job support are present in a work environment, individuals may be predisposed to experiencing emotional exhaustion and burnout (Aronsson et al., 2017) and could benefit from structural and psychological empowerment within the workplace (Zhang, Ye & Li, 2018).

5.4.2 BENEFITS OF EMOTIONAL WELLNESS

There are also a number of psychological and physical benefits associated with emotional wellness, including enhanced productivity and psychological resilience. While these are not the only benefits of emotional wellness, they are the focus of the current chapter. Absenteeism, presenteeism, and the economic burdens associated with mental health issues are significant (Goetzel et al., 2004). Understanding the impact of mental health conditions on productivity highlights the importance of emotional wellness as a work force imperative. Evidence of this association can be seen in the HERO Scorecard® study, which found a relationship between higher HERO scores and better company performance on the Standard & Poor's (S&P) 500 Index (Grossmeier et al., 2016).

Resilience is not only a benefit of well-being but also a supportive resource in maintaining emotional wellness. Learning how to build resilience is a critical strategy to achieving overall well-being. Practicing the use of attending and attuning, to move from negativity to positivity, helps achieve resilience over time (Graham, 2019). "Attending" to emotions involves focusing on the present experience – what an individual is feeling at that time, without judgment. Once aware of present feelings, you can move on to "attuning." During this stage, you are working towards a "felt sense" of various emotions experienced in the moment. Taking time to identify emotions is important; then a response can be chosen. Opportunities for learning and growth are possible through this ongoing practice. Developing emotional awareness builds the base for future experience of emotions (GGSC, 2021).

5.5 EVIDENCE AND BEST-PRACTICES FOR A LIFESTYLE OF EMOTIONAL WELLNESS AND STRESS RESILIENCE

Developing emotional awareness and using internal and external resources (e.g., positivity orientation, talking with supportive friends and colleagues, utilizing evidence-based practices to work through issues, etc.) to attain balance helps resilience build over time. The brain is trained to be aware of, and to focus on, those feelings that enhance emotional wellness and resilience. By tuning into positive emotions frequently each day, inner resilience reserves can be strengthened.

5.5.1 POSITIVE PSYCHOLOGY

Much of the research on practices to support a lifestyle of emotional wellness have a foundation in positive psychology. Positive psychology was developed by psychologist Martin Seligman, PhD, and is defined as "the science of subjective experience, positive individual traits, and positive institutions promises to improve quality of life and prevent the pathologies that arrive when life is barren and meaningless" (Seligman & Csikszentmihalyi, 2014). A meta-analysis of randomized controlled trials (RCT) testing positive psychology interventions found that across self-help, individual, and group therapy modalities, positive psychology interventions were associated with enhanced well-being and, in some cases, reduction of depressive symptoms (Bolier et al., 2013). The science of positive psychology has been important in laying groundwork for clinical interventions that foster pleasure, engagement, and meaning in life, all factors that are critical to emotional well-being (Duckworth et al., 2005).

5.5.2 HEALTH BEHAVIORS

Healthy behaviors, including attention to physical activity, healthy eating, and restful sleep, are explained next.

5.5.2.1 Physical Activity

Emotional resilience is enhanced through physical activity (Gil-Beltran et al., 2020); both occasional and regular activity facilitate emotional well-being (Bernstein & McNally, 2018). Physiological benefits are due to the increase in endorphins, serotonin, and dopamine that develop in response to physical activity practice. Those neurotransmitters are responsible for emotional regulation and stress reduction (Gil-Beltran et al., 2020). The bidirectional relationship between physical activity and stress was investigated by Schultchen et al. (2019). The literature also highlights the benefits of physical activity in decreasing psychological ill-health (i.e. depression, stress, negative affect, and psychological distress) and how physical activity increases psychological well-being (i.e. self-image, satisfaction with life and happiness, and psychological well-being) among adolescents and adults (Rector et al., 2019, Rodriguez-Ayllon et al., 2019, Meyer et al., 2020).

5.5.2.2 Nutrition

Nutrition, a core aspect of lifestyle, is critical to overall health. While this knowledge has been well established for decades, the effect of nutrition on emotional wellness is still being explored. Understanding of the mind–body connection has developed as research focused on the microbiome has grown. The microbiome is a complex ecosystem of microbes in and around the human body, with the majority of microbes living in the gut. The microbiome facilitates digestion, regulates immunity, aids in synthesis of some vitamins, fosters growth and development, and stimulates neurons to send signals to the brain via the vagus nerve (Bull & Plummer, 2014; Galland, 2014). Studies have identified the modulating effect of the gastrointestinal microbiome on behavior through the neuroendocrine and immune systems (Sylvia & Demas, 2018), a complex, scientific relationship. Similarly, positive effects on well-being were found by Mujcic and Oswald (2016) following fruit and vegetable consumption. Yet, inconsistent findings within other studies highlight the need for more research to better understand the intricate relationship between food and emotional wellness (Schultchen et al., 2019).

5.5.2.3 Sleep

An insidious connection exists between sleep, non-restorative sleep, and stress, as well as restorative sleep and emotional wellness. Stress, in the form of anxiety, worry, frustration and resentment, are closely aligned with insomnia and may account for up to 50% of those cases (WELCOA, 2016). When people do not sleep well, they may experience irritability, anxiety, and depression. The effects of this cycle – poor sleep, stress, and decreased emotional wellness – impact brain resilience (Parrino & Vaudano, 2018). For those engaged in shift work, sleep issues have a deleterious effect on physical and mental health (Torquati et al., 2019). Following best practice guidelines for better sleep may diminish the negative effects of sleep on the stress experience and help maintain emotional health.

5.5.3 BOUNDARY SETTING

Understanding and applying one's limits with respect to time as well as physical and emotional energy is critical for maintaining emotional wellness and preventing fatigue and burnout. Boundary setting is applicable to personal and professional situations. Boundary setting acknowledges the finite resources each person has and can allow for select use of such resources (Mellner et al., 2014). Emotional boundary setting is relevant to the patient-facing work done by nurses. Research acknowledges the emotional toll of nursing, and that individual and contextual factors play an important role in protecting nurses from emotional and psychological exhaustion (Kinman & Leggetter, 2016). For professional boundaries with patients and coworkers, professional boundary-setting appears to play an important role. A study on the well-being of nurses who provided at-home care to older adults specifically noted the importance of boundary setting for job satisfaction and well-being (McGarry, 2010).

5.5.4 Gratitude

Cultivating gratitude is a powerful way to strengthen emotions and positively affect daily well-being. Engaging in deliberate activities to foster gratitude may produce profound benefits from this relatively simple shift in perspective. When focus is on value and finding meaning, a "positive begets positive" mindset has the capacity to expand over time. Simple acts of gratitude can improve mental health for healthcare clinicians (Chen et al., 2015). While the benefits can be significant, some research has questioned outcomes associated with gratitude (Dickens, 2017) and the impact of gratitude on overall health (Boggiss et al., 2020).

5.5.5 Self-Compassion

When we are kind and compassionate towards ourselves, hormones such as endorphins and oxytocin are released, which enhances our sense of well-being and deactivates the flight-or-fight response. Research indicates that self-compassionate people are better able to deal with traumatic life events (Germer & Neff, 2015). Happiness, life satisfaction, motivation, improved relationships, better physical health, and less anxiety and depression are additional outcomes associated with self-compassion practices (Neff & Germer, 2019; Neff, 2011). Practicing self-compassion is suggested for nurses due to the positive effects on well-being (Benzo et al., 2017) and the contribution of that practice to emotional wellness.

5.5.6 Mindfulness

During mindfulness practice, one chooses to focus on the present moment and to accept "what is" without judgment. Present awareness and intentional mindfulness practice are an excellent way to build mindful attention and resilience (Graham, 2019). Mindfulness-based stress reduction (MBSR) has been studied extensively for over 30 years (Zinn, 2021). That practice enhances emotional wellness and leads to positive physical health effects, such as improved glycemic control in diabetics (Kian et al., 2018), improved blood pressure (Park & Han, 2017), decreased experience of chronic pain (Hilton et al., 2017; Majeed, Ali & Sudak, 2018), and fewer headaches (Probyn et al., 2017; Seng et al., 2019), anxiety, and depression (Gonzalez-Valeri et al., 2019). While all can benefit, MBSR is an especially effective strategy for improving nurses' mental health (Guillamie et al., 2017).

5.5.7 Spending Time Outdoors

Self-perceived nature deprivation is associated with diminished well-being, while spending time in nature fosters individual well-being, even in times of emotional distress (Tomasso et al., 2021). The use of nature-based prescriptions fosters social connection as well as mental and physical well-being for vulnerable populations (Leavell et al., 2019). Evidence has grown over the last decade regarding the positive health effects associated with spending time in nature. This evolution in knowledge has been influenced by the increased amount of time many people spend indoors while at work, home, and school.

5.5.8 Leveraging Relationships

Healthy interpersonal relations play an important role in well-being and resilience. Personal and professional relationships contribute to emotional wellness, burnout mitigation, and job satisfaction for nurses. High-quality social support through interpersonal relationships has been associated with better mental health and emotional well-being (Harandi et al., 2017). High-quality team coordination, as well as psychological safety or feeling emotionally comfortable with professional team members, has been associated with better mental health and less emotional strain, as well as better patient and medical-center outcomes (Welp & Manser, 2016). Seeking out life-enhancing personal and professional relationships, and leveraging those relationships to bolster emotional well-being, is important and effective.

5.5.9 Seeking Professional Help

While not often discussed, many individuals in helping professions, such as nursing, require professional mental health treatment and support. Rates of mental health conditions have been on the rise globally, with one in five American adults meeting criteria for a mental disorder (Mental Health America, 2019; National Institute of Mental Health, 2021). Despite high rates of depression, anxiety, trauma, and suicide among medical professionals, stigma related to mental health and treatment seeking is arguably more pervasive (Melnyk, 2020). Further, mental health stigma has been associated with gaps in treatment seeking (Sickel et al., 2014). Recent data indicates that in 2019 less than 50% of people with a mental health condition sought treatment (National Institute of Mental Health, 2021). Given rates of mental health symptoms and illness, and the stressful nature of the work, nurses are encouraged to attend to their own mental health as well as to support and encourage colleagues to do so.

5.6 NURSING IMPLEMENTATION STRATEGIES

Nurses can benefit from emotional wellness and stress resilience practices within a wide variety of settings. The American Nurses Association (ANA) and the American Nurses Foundation (ANF) developed the Well-Being Initiative (ANA, 2021), which offers free resources to foster nurses' mental health and well-being. Emotional wellness and stress resilience are critical for productivity, personal and professional quality of life, and overall wellness.

5.6.1 Hospitals

The hospital environment may be quite stressful for patients given the sounds, activities, and people present. Lifestyle behaviors, such as diet, sleep, activity, and socialization are all impacted by hospitalization. Dealing with those situations may be moderately to significantly stressful. Strategies to alleviate hospital-associated stressors might include listening to the patient describe their current experiences; coaching patients through relaxation exercises to dissipate stress; facilitating communication between patients and family members so that the emotional well-being of all can be encouraged; and identifying additional stress management strategies that the patient finds beneficial. Increasing numbers of hospitals now offer workplace wellness programs. Programs address physical activity, nutrition, and tobacco cessation among employees (Mulder et al., 2020). Stress management should also be a critical focus as research has identified beneficial effects of resiliency techniques for nurses (Grabbe et al., 2020).

5.6.2 OUTPATIENT SETTINGS

Interventions designed to enhance stress resilience and emotional wellness can also be practiced within outpatient settings. Nurses address wellness when working in pediatric clinics with children and families. Emotional support may be needed for parents and children when diseases are newly diagnosed, when children are fearful of healthcare visits, and to enhance stress resilience for children, middle-aged, and older teens experiencing stress in relation to daily life and school issues. Care, compassion and emotional support are helpful for adults experiencing health issues, such as cancer (Leao et al., 2021) and life stress.

5.6.3 WORKPLACE SETTINGS

Nurses that work in occupational health or worksite wellness positions offer educational workshops to minimize negative effects of stress. Integration of emotional wellness programs within the work setting has grown, with the majority of worksites offering wellness programs within the U.S. (Mattke et al., 2013). Those efforts generally prioritize stress management education and skills practice so that employees foster their own stress resilience over time. Inclusion of physical activity programming is also a key component of comprehensive worksite wellness programs targeting stress reduction (Click, 2017). Regular practice of healthy lifestyle behaviors facilitates wellness and builds coping reserves that foster engagement and productivity at work (Gil-Beltran et al., 2020). The need for nurse stress resilience is clear given the job demands associated within the nurses' work environments (Yu et al., 2019).

5.7 CONCLUSION

This chapter discussed an overview of the importance of emotional wellness and stress resilience for nurses. Given the professional demands of nursing, coupled with personal stressors, nurses are prone to ill effects of stress, fatigue, distress, and burnout. The COVID-19 pandemic further highlighted the physical and mental health implications of stress, trauma, and burnout, and how nurses in particular are affected. Fortunately, the negative implications of stress can be mitigated, and emotional wellness and resilience can be fostered through healthy lifestyle factors, including diet, physical activity, sleep, and healthy interpersonal relationships. There are myriad evidence-based practices, from mindfulness, to gratitude practices, to seeking professional help that can further support nurses' goals to improve and/or maintain good quality of life by effectively managing stress and attending to emotional wellness. Such strategies are relevant to the nursing profession, regardless of workplace or setting, and are also applicable to life outside of work. While the effects of stress can be vastly harmful, there is abundant research to support that people are generally resilient, that resilience can be learned, and that emotional wellness can be cultivated through engagement in key lifestyle behaviors.

REFERENCES

Aburn, G., Gott, M., and Hoare, K. (2016). What is resilience? An integrative review of the empirical literature. *Journal of Advanced Nursing*, 72(5), 980–1000.

American Nurses Association. (2021, January 23). *The well-being initiative*. ANA. www.nursingworld.org/practice-policy/work-environment/health-safety/disaster-preparedness/coronavirus/what-you-need-to-know/the-well-being-initiative/

Aronsson, G., Theorell, T., Grape, T., Hammarstrom, A., Hogstedt, C., Marteinsdottir, I., Skoog, I., Traskman-Bendz, L. and Hall, C. (2017). A systematic review including meta-analysis of work environment and burnout symptoms. *BMC Public Health*, 17(1), 264. https://doi.org/10.1186/s12889-017-4153-7

American Psychological Association. (2021a). APA Dictionary: Well-Being. https://dictionary.apa.org/well-being

American Psychological Association. (2021b). APA Dictionary: Burnout. https://dictionary.apa.org/burnout

American Psychological Association. (2021c). APA Dictionary: Coping Strategy. https://dictionary.apa.org/coping-strategy

Avey, H., Matheny, K. B., Robbins, A., and Jacobson, T. A. (2003). Health care providers' training, perceptions, and practices regarding stress and health outcomes. *Journal of the National Medical Association*, *95*(9), 833, 836–845.

Beck, C. T. (2011). Secondary traumatic stress in nurses: A systematic review. *Archives of Psychiatric Nursing*, *25*(1), 1–10.

Benzo, R. P., Kirsch, J. L., and Nelson, C. (2017). Compassion, mindfulness, and the happiness of healthcare workers. *Explore*, *13*(3), 201–206. https://doi.org/10.1016/j.explore.2017.02.001

Bernstein, E. E., and McNally, R. J. (2018). Exercise as a buffer against difficulties with emotion regulation: A pathway to emotional well-being. *Behaviour Research and Therapy*, *109*, 29–36. https://doi.org/10.1016.j.brat.2018.07.010

Boggiss, A. L., Consedine, N. S., Brenton-Peters, J. M., Hofman, P. L. and Serlachius, A. S. (2020). A systematic review of gratitude interventions: Effects on physical health and health behaviors. *Journal of Psychosomatic Research*, *135*, 1–10. https://doi.org/10.1016/j.brat.2018.07.010

Bolier, L., Haverman, M., Westerhof, G. J., Riper, H., Smit, F., and Bohlmeijer, E. (2013). Positive psychology interventions: A meta-analysis of randomized controlled studies. *BMC Public Health*, *13*(1), 119. https://doi.org/10.1186/1471-2458-13-119

Bremner, J. D., Moazzami, K., Wittbrodt, M. T., Nye, J. A., Lima, B. B., Gillespie, C. F., … Vaccarino, V. (2020). Diet, stress and mental health. *Nutrients*, *12*(8), 2428. https://doi.org/10.3390/nu12082428

Brennan, I. R. (2016). When is violence not a crime? Factors associated with victims' labelling of violence as a crime. *International Review of Victimology*, *22*(1), 3–23. https://doi.org/10.1177/0269758015610849

Bull, M. J., and Plummer, N. T. (2014). Part 1: The human gut microbiome in health and disease. *Integrative Medicine: A Clinician's Journal*, *13*(6), 17–22.

Carroll, L. (2013). Problem-focused coping. In M. D. Gellman and J. R. Turner (Eds.), *Encyclopedia of behavioral medicine* (pp. 1540–1541). Springer. https://doi.org/10.1007/978-1-4419-1005-9_1171

Chen, S. T., Tsui, P. K., and Lam, J. H. M. (2015). Improving mental health in health care practitioners: Randomized control trial of a gratitude intervention. *Journal of Consulting and Clinical Psychology*, *83*(1), 177–183. https://doi.org/10.1037/a0037895

Cohen, S., Janicki-Deverts, D., and Miller, G. E. (2007). Psychological stress and disease. *JAMA*, *298*(14), 1685–1687.

Click, E. R. (2017). Creating a culture of health – one university's experience. *Health Matrix: Journal of Law-Medicine*, *27*, 417–434.

Davenport, S., Gray, T. J., and Melek, S. (2020, February 15). *How do individuals with behavioral health conditions contribute to physical and total healthcare spending?* Milliman Research Report. www.milliman.com/-/media/milliman/pdfs/articles/milliman-high-cost-patient-study-2020.ashx

de Oliveira, S. M., de Alcantara Sousa, L. V., Gadelha, M. d. S. V., and do Nascimento, V. B. (2019). Prevention actions of burnout syndrome in nurses: An integrating literature review. *Clinical Practice and Epidemiology in Mental Health: CP & EMH*, *15*, 64.

Delgado, C., Upton, D., Ranse, K., Furness, T., and Foster, K. (2017). Nurses' resilience and the emotional labour of nursing work: An integrative review of empirical literature. *International Journal of Nursing Studies*, *70*, 71–88.

Dickens, L. R. (2017). Using gratitude to promote positive change: A series of meta-analyses investigating the effectiveness of gratitude interventions. *Basic and Applied Social Psychology*, *39*(4), 193–208. https://doi.org/10.1080/01973533.2017.1323638

Duckworth, A. L., Tracy, A. S., and Seligman, M. E. P. (2005). Positive psychology in clinical practice. *Annual Review of Clinical Psychology*, *1*(1), 629–651. https://doi.org/10.1146/annurev.clinpsy.1.102803.144154

Figueroa, J. F., Phelan, J., and Orav, J. (2020). Association of mental health disorders with healthcare spending in the Medicare population. *JAMA Network Open*, *3*(3), e201210. https://doi.org/10.1001/jamanetworkopen.2020.1210

Fletcher, D., and Sarkar, M. (2013). Psychological resilience: A review and critique of definitions, concepts, and theory. *European Psychologist*, *18*(1), 12–23. https://doi.org/10.1027/1016-9040/a000124

Galland, L. (2014). The gut microbiome and the brain. *Journal of Medicinal Food*, *17*(12), 1261–1272. https://doi.org/10.1089/jmf.2014.7000

Germer, C. K., and Neff, K. D. (2015). Cultivating self-compassion in trauma survivors. In V. M. Follette, J. Briere, D. Rozelle, J. W. Hopper, and D. I. Rome (Eds.), *Mindfulness-oriented interventions for trauma: Integrating contemplative practices* (pp. 43–58). The Guilford Press.

Gil-Beltran, E., Meneghal, I., Llorens, S., and Salanova, M. (2020). Get vigorous with physical exercise and improve your well-being at work! *International Journal of Environmental Research and Public Health*, *17*(17), 6384.

Gilgoff, R., Singh, L., Koita, K., Gentile, B., and Marques, S.S. (2020). Adverse childhood experiences, outcomes, and interventions. *Pediatric Clinics of North America*, *67*(2), 259–273. https://doi.org/10.1016/j.pcl.2019.12.001

Goetzel, R. Z., Long, S. R., Ozminkowski, R. J., Hawkins, K., Wang, S., & Lynch, W. (2004). Health, absence, disability, and presenteeism cost estimates of certain physical and mental health conditions affecting US employers. *Journal of Occupational and Environmental Medicine*, *46*(4), 398–412.

Gonzalez-Valeri, G., Zurita-Ortega, F., Ubago-Jimenez, J. L., and Puertas-Molero, P. (2019). Use of meditation and cognitive behavioral therapies for the treatment of stress, depression and anxiety in students. A systematic review and meta-analysis. *International Journal of Environmental Research and Public Health*, *16*(22), 4394. https://doi.org/10.3390/ijerph16224393

Grabbe, L., Higgins, M. K., Baird, M., Craven, P. A. and Fratello, S. S. (2020). The Community Resilience Model® to promote nurse well-being. *Nursing Outlook*, *68*(3), 324–336. https://doi.org/10.1016/j.outlook.2019.11.002

Graham, L. (2019). *Train your brain to build resilience*. Mindful. www.mindful.org/train-your-brain-to-build-resilience/

Greater Good Science Center (GGSC). (2021, January 27). GGSC. https://ggsc.berkeley.edu/who_we_serve/educators/online_courses_for_educators?utm_source=Greater+Good+Science+Center&utm_campaign=fc190365cf-ED_NEWSLETTER_JANUARY_2021&utm_medium=email&utm_term=0_5ae73e326e-fc190365cf-50922771

Grossmeier, J., Fabius, R., Flynn, J. P., Noeldner, S. P., Fabius, D., Goetzel, R. Z., and Anderson, D. F. (2016). Linking workplace health promotion best practices and organizational financial performance: Tracking market performance of companies with highest scores on the HERO scorecard. *JOEM*, *58*(1), 16–23.

Guidi, J., Lucente, M., Sonino, N., and Fava, G. A. (2021). Allostatic load and its impact on health: A systematic review. *Psychotherapy and Psychosomatics*, *90*, 11–27. https://doi.org/10.1159/000510696

Guillamie, L., Boiral, O., and Champagne, J. (2017). A mixed-methods systematic review of the effects of mindfulness on nurses. *Journal of Advanced Nursing*, *73*(5), 1017–1034. https://doi.org/10.1111/jan.13176

Harandi, T. F., Taghinasab, M. M., and Nayeri, T. D. (2017). The correlation of social support with mental health: A meta-analysis. *Electronic Physician*, *9*(9), 5212.

Hedegaard, J., Curtin, S. C., and Warner, M. (2020). Increase in suicide mortality in the United States, 1999–2018. *NCHS Data Brief*, *362*, 1–8.

Hilton, L., Hempel, S., Ewing, B. A., Apaydin, E., Xenakis, L., Newberry, S., Colaiaco, B., Ruelaz Maher, A., Hanman, R. M., Sorbero, M. E., and Maglione, M. A. (2017). Mindfulness meditation for chronic pain: Systematic review and meta-analysis. *Annals of Behavioral Medicine*, *51*, 199–213. https://doi.org/10.1007/s12160-016-9844-2

Huang, L., Wang, Y., Liu, J., Ye, P., Cheng, B., Xu, H., ... Ning, G. (2020). Factors associated with resilience among medical staff in radiology departments during the outbreak of 2019 novel coronavirus disease (COVID-19): A cross-sectional study. *Medical Science Monitor*, *26*. https://doi.org/10.12659/msm.925669

Kian, A. A., Vahdani, B., Noorbala, A. A., Nejatisafa, A., Arbabi, M., Zenoozian, S., and Nakhjavani, M. (2018). The impact of mindfulness-based stress reduction on emotional wellbeing and glycemic control of patients with type 2 diabetes mellitus. *Journal of Diabetes Research*, 1–6. https://doi.org/10.1155/2018/1986820

Kinman, G., and Leggetter, S. (2016). Emotional labour and wellbeing: What protects nurses? *Healthcare*, *4*(4), 89. https://doi.org/10.3390/healthcare4040089

Kivimaki, M., Batty, G. D., Pentti, J., Shipley, M. J., Sipilo, P. N., Nyberg, S. T., Suominen, S. B., Oksanen, T., Stenholm, S., Virtanen, M., Marmot, M. G., Singh-Manoux, A., Brunner, E. J., Lindbohm, J. V., Ferrie,

J. A., and Vahtera, J. (2020). Association between socioeconomic status and the development of mental and physical health conditions in adulthood: A multi-cohort study. *The Lancet*, *5*, e140–e149.

Laal, M., and Aliramaie, N. (2010). Nursing and coping with stress. *International Journal of Collaborative Research on Internal Medicine & Public Health*, *2*(5), 0–0.

Labrague, L. J., McEnroe-Petitte, D. M., Gloe, D., Thomas, L., Papathanasiou, I. V., and Tsaras, K. (2017). A literature review on stress and coping strategies in nursing students. *Journal of Mental Health*, *26*(5), 471–480.

Labrague, L. J., McEnroe-Petitte, D. M., Leocadio, M. C., Van Bogaert, P., and Cummings, G. G. (2018). Stress and ways of coping among nurse managers: An integrative review. *Journal of Clinical Nursing*, *27*(7–8), 1346–1359.

Leao, D. C., Pereira, E. R., Silva, R. M., Garca-Caro, M. P., Cruz-Quintana, F., and Rocha, R. C. (2021). Spiritual and emotional experience with a diagnosis of breast cancer: A scoping review. *Cancer Nursing*, *Publish Ahead of Print*. https://doi.org/10.1097/NCC.0000000000000936

Leavell, M. A., Leiferman, J. A., Gascon, M., Braddick, F., Gonzalez, J. C., and Litt, J. S. (2019). Nature-based social prescribing in urban settings to improve social connectedness and mental well-being: A review. *Current Environmental Health Reports*, *6*, 297–308.

Mathes, E. W. (1981). Maslow's hierarchy of needs as a guide for living. *Journal of Humanistic Psychology*, *21*(4), 69–72.

Mattke, S., Schnyer, C., and Van Busum, K. R. (2013). A review of the U.S. workplace wellness market. *Rand Health Quarterly*, *3*, 7.

Majeed, M. H., Ali, A. A., and Sudak, D. M. (2018). Mindfulness-based interventions for chronic pain: Evidence and applications. *Asian Journal of Psychiatry*, *32*, 79–83. https://doi.org/10.1016/ajp.2017.11.025

McDaniel, K. R., and Allen, D. G. (2012). Working and care-giving: The impact on caregiver stress, family–work conflict, and burnout. *Journal of Life Care Planning*, *10*(4), 21–32.

McGarry, J. (2010). Relationships between nurses and older people within the home: Exploring the boundaries of care. *International Journal of Older People Nursing*, *5*(4), 265–273. https://doi.org/10.1111/j.1748-3743.2009.00192.x

Mellner, C., Aronsson, G., and Kecklund, G. (2014). Boundary management preferences, boundary control, and work-life balance among full-time employed professionals in knowledge-intensive, flexible work. *Nordic Journal of Working Life Studies*, *4*(4), 7–23.

Melnyk, B. M. (2020). Burnout, depression and suicide in nurses/clinicians and learners: An urgent call for action to enhance professional well-being and healthcare safety. *Worldviews on Evidence-Based Nursing*, *17*(1), 2–5.

Mental Health America. (2019). *The state of mental health in America*. https://mhanational.org/sites/default/files/2019-09/2019%20MH%20in%20America%20Final.pdf

Merlo, G., and Rippe, J. (2020). Physician burnout: A lifestyle medicine perspective. *American Journal of Lifestyle Medicine*, *15*(2), 148–157. https://doi.org/10.1177/1559827620980420

Meyer, J., McDowell, C., Lansing, J., Brower, C., Smith, L., Tully, M., and Herring, M. (2020). Changes in physical activity and sedentary behavior in response to COVID-19 and their associations with mental health in 3052 US adults. *International Journal of Environmental Research and Public Health*, *17*(18), 6469. https://doi.org/10.3390/ijerph17186469

Misselbrook, D. (2014). W is for wellbeing and the WHO definition of health. *British Journal of General Practice*, *64*(628), 582–582. https://doi.org/10.3399/bjgp14x682381

Morton, D. P. (2018). Combining lifestyle medicine and positive psychology to improve mental health and emotional well-being. *American Journal of Lifestyle Medicine*, *12*(5), 370–374. https://doi.org/10.1177/1559827618766482

Mulder, L., Belay, B., Mukhtar, Q., Lang, J. E., Harris, D., and Onufrak, S. (2020). Prevalence of workplace health practices and policies in hospitals: Results from the workplace health in America study. *American Journal of Health Promotion*, *34*(8), 867–875. https://doi.org/10.1177/0890117120905232

Mujcic, R., and Oswald, A. J. (2016). Evolution of well-being and happiness after increases in consumption of fruits and vegetables. *American Journal of Public Health*, *106*(8), 1504–1510. https://doi.org/10.2105/AJPH.2016.303260

National Institute of Mental Health. (2021, January 3). Mental illness. www.nimh.nih.gov/health/statistics/mental-illness.shtml

Neff, K. (2011). *Self-compassion*. New York, NY: HarperCollins.

Neff, K., and Germer, C. (2019). *The transformative effects of mindful self-compassion*. Mindful: Healthy Mind, Healthy Life. www.mindful.org/the-transformative-effects-of-mindful-self-compassion

Nekoranec, J., and Kmosena, M. (2015). Stress in the workplace-sources, effects and coping strategies. *Review of the Air Force Academy*, *1*(28), 163–170.

Nerurkar, A., Bitton, A., Davis, R. B., Phillips, R. S., and Yeh, G. (2013). When physicians counsel about stress: Results of a national study. *JAMA Internal Medicine*, *173*(1), 76–77. https://doi.org/10.1001/2013.jamainternmed.480

Park, S., and Han, K.S. (2017). Blood pressure response to meditation and yoga: A systematic review and meta-analysis. *Journal of Alternative and Complementary Medicine*, *23*(9), 685–695. https://doi.org/10.1089/acm.2016.0234

Parrino, L., and Vaudano, A. E. (2018). The resilient brain and the guardians of sleep – New perspectives on old assumptions. *Sleep Medicine Reviews*, *39*, 98–107.

Payne, B. K., and Hannay, J. W. (2021). Implicit bias reflects systemic racism. *Trends in Cognitive Sciences*, *25*(11), 927–936. https://doi.org/10.1016/j.tics.2021.08.001

Pender, N., Murdaugh, C., and Parsons, M.A. (2014). *Health promotion in nursing practice*. Pearson.

Penedo, F. J., and Dahn, J. R. (2005). Exercise and well-being: A review of mental and physical health benefits associated with physical activity. *Current Opinion in Psychiatry*, *18*(2), 189–193.

Probyn, K., Bowers, J., Mistry, D., Caldwell, F., Underwood, M., Patel, S., Sandhu, H. K., Matharu, M., and Pincus, T. (2017). Non-pharmacological self-management for people living with migraine or tension-type headache: A systematic review including analysis of intervention components. *BMJ*, *7*(8), e016670. https://doi.org/10.1136/bmjopen-2017-016670

Rector, J. L., Christ, S. L., and Friedman, E. M. (2019). Well-being and long-term physical activity participation in midlife adults: A latent class analysis. *Annals of Behavioral Medicine*, *53*(1), 53–64. https://doi.org/10.1093/abm/kay016

Rippe, J.M. (2018). Lifestyle medicine: The health promoting power of daily habits and practices. *American Journal of Lifestyle Medicine*, *12*(6), 499–512. https://doi.org/10.1177/1559827618785554

Rodriguez-Ayllon, M. I., Cadenas-Sanchez, C., Estevez-Lopez, F., Munoz, N. E., Mora-Gonzalez, J., Migueles, J. H., Molina-Garcia, P., Henriksson, H., Mena-Molina, A., Martinez-Vizcaino, V., Catena, A., Log, M., Erickson, K. I., Lubans, D. R., Ortega, F. B., and Esteban-Cornejo, I. (2019). Role of physical activity and sedentary behavior in the mental health of preschoolers, children and adolescents: A systematic review and meta-analysis. *Sports Medicine*, *49*(9). https://doi.org/10.1007/s40279-019-01099-5

Salvagioni, J., Melanda, F. N., Mesas, A. E., Gonzalez, A. D., Gabani, F. L. and de Andrade, S. M. (2017). Physical, psychological and occupational consequences of job burnout: A systematic review of prospective studies. *PLoS One*, *12*(10), e0185781. https://doi.org/10.1371/journal.pone.0185781

Schultchen, D., Reichenberger, J., Mittle, T., Weh, T. R. M., Smyth, J. M., Blechert, J., and Pollatos, O. (2019). Bidirectional relationship of stress and affect with physical activity and healthy eating. *British Journal of Health Psychology*, *24*(2), 315–333. https://doi.org/10.1111/bjhp.12355

Seligman, M. E. P., and Csikszentmihalyi, M. (2014). Positive psychology: An introduction. In *Flow and the foundations of positive psychology* (pp. 279–298): Springer. https://doi.org/10.1007/978-94-017-9088-8_18

Selye, H. (1993). History of the stress concept. In L. Goldberger & S. Breznitz (Eds.), *Handbook of stress: Theoretical and clinical aspects* (pp. 7–17). Free Press.

Sickel, A. E., Seacat, J. D., and Nabors, N. A. (2014). Mental health stigma update: A review of consequences. *Advances in Mental Health*, *12*(3), 202–215.

Seng, E. K., Singer, A. B., Metts, C., Grinberg, A. S., Patel, Z. S., Marzouk, M., Rosenberg, L., Day, M., Minen, M. T., Lipton, R. B., and Buse, D. C. (2019). Does mindfulness-based cognitive therapy for migraine reduce migraine-related disability in people with episodic and chronic migraine? A phase 2b pilot randomized clinical trial. *Headache*, *59*(9), 1448–1467. https://doi.org/10.1111/head.13657

Sher, K. (2020). The impact of the COVID-19 pandemic on suicide rates. *QJM*, *113*(10), 707–712. https://doi.org/10.1093/qjmed/hcaa202

Stewart-Brown, S. (1998). Emotional wellbeing and its relation to health: Physical disease may well result from emotional distress. *BMJ*, *317*, 1608–1609. https://doi.org/10.1136/bmj.317.7173.1608

Suvarna, B., Suvarna, A., Phillips, R., Juster, R. P., McDermott, B., and Sarnyai, Z. (2020). Health risk behaviours and allostatic load: A systematic review. *Neuroscience and Biobehavioral Reviews*, *108*, 694–711. https://doi.org/10.1016/j.neubiorev.2019.12.020

Sylvia, K. E., and Demas, G. E. (2018). A gut reaction: Microbiome–brain–immune interactions modulate social and affective behaviors. *Hormones and Behavior*, *99*, 41–49.

Tomasso, L. P., Yin, J., Guillermo, J., Laurent, C., Chen, J. T., Catalano, P. J., and Spengler, J. D. (2021). The relationship between nature deprivation and individual wellbeing across urban gradients under COVID-19. *International Journal of Environmental Research and Public Health*, *18*(4), 1511. https://doi.org/10.3390/ijerph18041511

Torquati, L., Mielke, G. I., Brown, W. J., Burton, N. W., and Kolbe-Alexander, T. L. (2019). Shift work and poor mental health: A meta-analysis of longitudinal studies. *American Journal of Public Health*, *109*(11), e13–e20. https://doi.org/10.2105/AJPH.2019.305278

Umberson, D., and Montez, J. K. (2011). Social relationships and health: A flashpoint for health policy. *Journal of Health and Social Behavior*, *51*, s54–s66. https://doi.org/10.1177/0022146510383501

Ungar, M., and Theron, L. (2020). Resilience and mental health: How multisystemic processes contribute to positive outcomes. *The Lancet*, *7*, 441–448. https://doi.org/10.1177/0022146510383501

Wellness Councils of America (WELCOA). (2016). *A good night's sleep – Addressing insomnia, stress and digital toxicity*. Omaha, NE: WELCOA.

Welp, A., and Manser, T. (2016). Integrating teamwork, clinician occupational well-being and patient safety – development of a conceptual framework based on a systematic review. *BMC Health Services Research*, *16*(1), 1–44.

Wheaton, B. (1997). The nature of chronic stress. In *Coping with chronic stress* (pp. 43–73): Springer.

Williams, D. (2018). Stress and the mental health of populations of color: Advancing our understanding of race-related stressors. *Journal of Health and Social Behavior*, *59*(4), 466–485.

Yu, F., Raphael, D., Mackay, L., Smith, M., and King, A. (2019). Personal and work-related factors associated with nurse resilience: A systematic review. *International Journal of Nursing Studies*, *93*, 129–140. https://doi.org/10.1016/j.ijnurstu.2019.02.014

Zhang, Y., Han, W., Qin, W., Yin, H., Zhang, C., Kong, C., and Wang, Y. (2018). Extent of compassion satisfaction, compassion fatigue and burnout in nursing: A meta-analysis. *Journal of Nursing Management*, *26*(7), 810–819. https://doi.org/10.1111/jonm.12589

Zhang, S., Ye, H., and Li, Y. (2018). Correlates of structural empowerment, psychological empowerment and emotional exhaustion among registered nurses: A meta-analysis. *Applied Nursing Research*, *42*, 9–16. https://doi.org/10.1016/j.apnr.2018.04.006

Zhuang-Shaung, L., and Hasson, F. (2020). Resilience, stress, and psychological well-being in nursing students: A systematic review. *Nurse Education Today*, *90*.

Zinn, J. K. (2021). Mindfulness based stress reduction. Accessed on February 10, 2021 from https://mbsrtraining.com/jon-kabat-zinn/

6 Happiness and Social Connectivity

Alyssa Vela[1,2] and Lisa Kamsickas[2]
[1]Cardiac Behavioral Medicine
Bluhm Cardiovascular Institute of Northwestern, Chicago, USA
[2]Northwestern University Feinberg School of Medicine, Chicago, USA

CONTENTS

KEY POINTS

- Happiness and positive affect are important for quality of life and job satisfaction.
- Social connectivity and healthy interpersonal relationships are also crucial for quality of life.
- Positive psychology interventions and healthy lifestyle behaviors can bolster both happiness and social connectivity.

6.1 INTRODUCTION: HAPPINESS AND WHY IT MATTERS

While there are many definitions of happiness, happiness is an emotional state involving positive feelings. For example, happiness can be distinguished by feelings of joy, satisfaction, contentment, and fulfillment. Happiness can also refer to the present moment or, more broadly, to someone's overall feelings about his or her life at a given time (Oishi & Westgate, 2021; Lyubomirsky, 2007). Because happiness is a broad construct with many definitions, and often difficult to measure, well-being and affect are constructs that are well studied, as they impact subjective happiness. The personal and professional happiness of nurses is greatly impacted by their experiences of positive and negative affect and their social connectivity, both of which will be explored in this chapter. Table 6.1 defines happiness, as well as other key terms, that will be used throughout this chapter.

Nurses are critical to healthcare systems and structures in the United States, comprising the largest proportion of any healthcare workers. For years, there have been concerns about a nursing shortage in the United States, with recent data indicating that over 11 million more nurses will be needed within the next few years (Haddad et al., 2021). However, nurses generally experience low

DOI: 10.1201/9781003178330-7

TABLE 6.1
Key Happiness and Social Connectivity Terms and Definitions

Term	Definition
Happiness	Various positive or pleasant emotions, ranging from contentment to intense joy
Health behavior	An action that can improve health or decrease disease risk
Healthy relationship	A connection with another individual in which there is mutual respect, trust, compromise, and anger control
Positive affect	Pleasurable emotions or the extent to which someone subjectively experiences positive moods
Positive psychology	A field of psychology focused on human flourishing
Prosocial behavior	An action that helps others
Resilience	The ability to withstand adversity and recover quickly from difficulties
Social connectivity	Feeling close to others by belonging to a social relationship or network
Well-being	A state of overall contentment and fulfillment, including, but not limited to, mental health and outlook, physical health, and interpersonal relationships

job satisfaction and high rates of burnout. Resultantly, the nursing profession has high turnover rates, which further contribute to understaffing (Haddad et al., 2021). More specifically, factors such as schedule dissatisfaction, heavy workload, and unsatisfactory work–life balance have been associated with burnout among nurses, which has, in turn, been associated with intent to leave one's position (Flynn & Ironside, 2018). Given the personal and systemic implications of overwhelmingly negative emotions, burnout, and high turnover rates in the nursing profession, understanding the science related to happiness and social connectivity is crucial for nurses.

While much of the attention surrounding mental health, quality of life, and job satisfaction emphasizes factors, such as stress, that detract from happiness, there is also a rich body of science that focuses on the positive. While work as a nurse can be stressful, and challenges are inevitable, creating and maintaining a positive mood can increase motivation, enjoyment, and productivity in the workplace (Martin, 2005). Further, research suggests that one does not need to naturally gravitate towards or constantly feel happiness or positive emotions. Instead, positive psychology interventions can be utilized to foster positive affect, resilience, and more optimal functioning within and outside of work (Froman, 2010; Martin, 2005). Positive psychology and interventions that promote positive affect align with the premise of lifestyle medicine. For example, coupling lifestyle medicine and positive psychology, which emphasizes individual strengths, may effectively foster good mental health and well-being (Morton, 2018). Additionally, social connectivity and healthy interpersonal relationships, two topics positive psychologists study, are critical for boosting positive affect and overall quality of life.

6.2   KEY CONCEPTS AND THEORETICAL FRAMEWORKS

Various models of well-being have been proposed to understand the factors individuals need to flourish. Maslow's hierarchy of needs proposed that there are many factors that contribute to individuals' ability to thrive or function as their best selves (Maslow, 1971). These factors include having basic physiological needs met (e.g., breathing, food, water); experiencing safety and security, love and belonging, and self-esteem; and feeling like they have meaning, purpose, and fulfillment in their lives (Maslow, 1943). Abraham Maslow was one of the first psychologists to focus on human growth and overall well-being and was the first to coin the term *positive psychology* (Maslow, 1954).

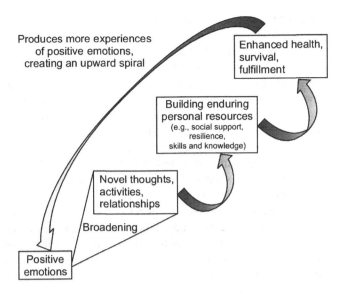

FIGURE 6.1   Potential Impact of Positive Emotions

(Reprinted from *Advances in Experimental Social Psychology*, 47, Barbara L. Fredrickson, Positive emotions broaden and build, 1–53, Copyright (2013) with permission from Elsevier.)

Positive psychology has since become a major area of scientific study and practice that focuses on humans' optimal functioning and has been defined as "the scientific study of what makes life worth living" (Seligman & Csikszentmihalyi, 2000, p. 5).

Despite Maslow's foundational work, the field of positive psychology was not established until almost the 20th century. Martin Seligman, one of the founders of positive psychology, encouraged researchers to study the positive aspects of life and wanted their experiments to be methodologically sound (Seligman, 2002). Seligman thus created the PERMA model, a theory of well-being that contains five elements needed to create a flourishing life: positive emotions, engagement, relationships, meaning, and accomplishments (Seligman, 2011). While there are many properties to each of these elements, some include that they individually contribute to well-being, are pursued for their own sakes and not merely to attain the other elements, and can be measured and defined independently from the other elements (Seligman, 2018).

Positive emotions can buffer against and counteract the damaging physical and mental effects of stress (Pressman et al., 2019). The protective effect of positive emotions also extends to the maladaptive behaviors that commonly occur in response to stress, such as feeling overwhelmed or engaging in unhealthy coping techniques (e.g., drinking alcohol). The broaden-and-build theory of positive emotions, created by Barbara Fredrickson, posits that this buffering happens because experiencing positive emotions broadens individuals' awareness and behavior (Fredrickson, 2013). As a result, positive affect prompts people to build social, intellectual, and physical resources and induces creativity and curiosity, cultivating an upward spiral of health, positive emotion, and life satisfaction (e.g., Cohn et al., 2009; Pressman et al., 2019). Concomitantly, experiencing chronic stress may reduce these resources and abilities (Folkman & Moskowitz, 2000). See Figure 6.1.

6.3   NEUROBIOLOGICAL DETERMINANTS OF POSITIVE AFFECT

The ongoing development of neuroimaging techniques over the past several decades has allowed for an emerging understanding of the neurological bases of emotion, including some of the specific neural circuits that contribute to the experience of negative and positive emotions. Presently, affect is thought to be a largely sub-neocortical process, meaning that subcortical areas of the brain are critical in the generation of emotion (Burgdorf & Panksepp, 2006). Emerging research highlights the role of the ventral striatum, a structure in the brain's forebrain that is involved in reward pathways. For example, one study found that the interaction between ventral striatum activity and recent life stressors, after controlling for psychosocial confounds (i.e., adverse childhood events), was associated with increased positive affect. For those with low ventral striatum reactivity, greater life stress was associated with less positive affect (Nikolova et al., 2012). Positive affect has also been associated with the ability to regulate and maintain physiological processes that keep internal conditions steady (e.g., body temperature; Burgdorf & Panksepp, 2006). Thus, while several brain structures are likely involved in the experience of positive emotions, research is beginning to pin-point the neurological processes involved in positive affect.

Beyond the neurological determinants, positive affect has been associated with several beneficial biological and cognitive outcomes. A 2005 study indicated an inverse relationship between positive affect and cortisol. The study also found that happiness was inversely related to systolic blood pressure. Further, happiness was associated with lower heart rate throughout the day and lesser fibrinogen stress response. The biological correlates assessed were stable at three-year follow-up (Steptoe & Wardle, 2005). Additionally, positive emotional states are understood to allow for an increase in self-control by inhibiting automatic or impulsive reactions, thus allowing for increased breadth of attention in visual and linguistic domains (Rowe et al., 2007). Thus, opportunities to foster positive affect are important to improve physical health outcomes, cognitive functioning, and general well-being.

6.4 PROSOCIAL BEHAVIOR

One such opportunity to foster positive affect is engaging in prosocial behaviors, or acts that help others (i.e., cooperating), as positive affect is influenced by interactions with others and social relationships. Prosocial behaviors, or acts that help others (i.e., helping, cooperating), and positive affect bidirectionally reinforce each other (Snippe et al., 2018). For example, engagement in an average of one to two acts of prosocial behavior may buffer against the negative implications of stress and support overall mental health, further bolstering the beneficial consequences of experiencing positive emotion (Raposa et al., 2016). Expressing gratitude may also influence prosocial behavior by contributing to feelings of value by encouraging a sense of connection with others (Grant & Gino, 2010). However, having fewer racial biases and being open-minded increases the likelihood of participating in prosocial behavior, further indicating the importance of identifying and addressing biases in healthcare (Stepanikova et al., 2011). Therefore, prosocial behavior can result in a multitude of personal and social benefits, such as fostering a sense of connection, promoting trust, and increasing positive emotion.

The nature of the nursing profession offers opportunities for prosocial behavior, such as helping a colleague move a patient from their bed to a chair, and highlights the role of rapport in relationships between nurses and their co-workers and patients. Prosocial behavior among nurses in the workplace can benefit individual and team relationships and mental health. For example, by helping another nurse with a patient, nurses can experience positive emotion, support their team, and provide strong patient care. A meta-analysis explored the effects of communal motivation, or motivation to care for the well-being of others, and found that communal motivation appears to result in improved well-being for both members of a relationship (Le et al., 2018). Further, prosocial behavior contributes to resilience, which is highly relevant to the experiences of nurses who are regularly exposed to difficult situations and trauma (Turner, 2014). Finally, acts that demonstrate caring and support aid in the development and maintenance of healthy long-term relationships, including friendship and romantic relationships (Rusbult & Agnew, 2010; Stavrova & Ehlebracht, 2015). Consequently, engaging in prosocial behavior can result in many benefits.

6.5 SOCIAL CONNECTIVITY: WHY IT MATTERS

Healthy and meaningful relationships are important during nurses' education, in the workplace, and outside of the workplace, as they have implications for mental health, affect, job satisfaction, and stress resilience. Thus, creating and maintaining healthy relationships are crucial to individuals' happiness and well-being (Saphire-Bernstein & Taylor, 2013). More specifically, social support has been shown to be a protective factor for physical and mental health outcomes, while it also supports nurses' ability to optimize their work lives by preventing burnout, reducing turnover, and supporting job satisfaction (Orgambídez-Ramos & de Almeida, 2017; Velando-Soriano et al., 2019).

6.5.1 Psychological Benefits of Social Connectivity and Positive Affect

While many studies about psychological benefits and healthy relationships are correlational, the abundance of literature revealing links between these constructs suggest they are bidirectional. In other words, having supportive relationships enhances subjective well-being, and perceiving one's own well-being as high results in stronger relationships (Diener & Tay, 2017; Lyubomirsky et al., 2005). Happiness enhances relationships by boosting individuals' levels of sociability and strengthening the quality of social interactions (Diener & Tay, 2017). Participants who reported greater levels of positive emotions throughout the day also reported more social connectedness, emotional and practical support, optimism and adaptive coping responses, and lower levels of depression (Steptoe et al., 2008a). These findings remained after controlling for age, gender, household income, paid employment, smoking status, and negative affect. Happy people find spending time with others more rewarding and have higher life satisfaction compared to less happy individuals (Diener & Tay, 2017). Further, partners in committed relationships produce less of the stress hormone cortisol and are less responsive to psychological stress (Maestripieri et al., 2010). Contrarily, relationship conflict and lower social support advance depression, emotional stress responses, and damaging health behaviors (Kiecolt-Glaser et al., 2010). Moreover, loneliness can make individuals more sensitive to social threats, impair executive functioning, cause worse sleep, and negatively affect mental and physical well-being (Cacioppo & Cacioppo, 2014). Therefore, healthy relationships are linked with numerous personal and social advantages and are thus crucial for well-being.

Happier individuals also report greater quantity and better quality of friendships and family relationships (Diener & Seligman, 2002). The hallmark 75-year longitudinal Harvard Study of Adult Development found that the quality of people's relationships predicted their happiness and well-being throughout their lives (Vaillant, 2012). Strong social connections help individuals cope with adversity, can sustain or prolong late-life cognitive and physical health, and are better predictors of happiness throughout life compared to social class, IQ, or genes (Feeney & Collins, 2015; Vaillant, 2012). Happy people are also generally more popular and likable (Boehm & Lyubomirsky, 2008). The described connection between happiness and relationships exists across cultures and sociocultural regions (Tay & Diener, 2011; Diener & Tay, 2017). Thus, creating and sustaining quality social relationships appears to be a crucial component to satisfaction and fulfillment in life.

6.5.2 Physical Health Benefits of Social Connectivity and Positive Affect

The vast benefits of social connections extend beyond the psychological and include physical health benefits. Some of the physical health benefits linked with social connectivity include stronger cognitive health, less vulnerability to progressive decline (Haslam et al., 2014), favorable physiological function, better sleep (Steptoe et al, 2008b), increased recovery and survival following surgery (Neuman & Werner, 2016), enhanced immune function (Martino et al., 2017), and less vulnerability to health challenges negatively affecting happiness (Waldinger & Schulz, 2010). The abundance of research consistently linking social connectivity and positive affect to decreased morbidity and mortality rates validates the reliability of this relationship (Diener & Chan, 2011). Indeed, a meta-analysis of 148 prospective studies revealed that participants' likelihood of survival increased by 50% for those who had stronger social ties (Holt-Lunstad et al., 2010). This association may be mediated by actual or perceived isolation, even after considering demographic factors and baseline health (Holt-Lunstad et al., 2015; Steptoe et al., 2013). Some other health outcomes linked with positive affect, which are likely tied with interpersonal interactions, include decreased rates and severity of heart disease (Boehm & Kubzansky, 2012; DuBois et al., 2015), fewer objective and subjective symptoms of illness (Doyle et al., 2006), resistance to flu and cold (Cohen et al., 2003), slower disease progression (Ironson & Hayward, 2008), and less pain (Strand et al., 2007). A study of over 1000 individuals with coronary heart disease found that positive affect was associated with better health behaviors, including sleep, physical activity, medication adherence, and not smoking cigarettes. Further, the authors found that increased positive affect was correlated with improved physical activity, sleep, and medication adherence over five-year follow-up (Sin et al., 2015). Therefore, social connectivity and positive affect are associated with multiple beneficial health consequences and health behaviors, which, in turn, lead to greater overall well-being and quality of life.

Various conceptual frameworks exist to try to understand the links between social relationships and health outcomes (Pietromonaco & Collins, 2017). As presented earlier, these correlations may be due to higher levels of positive affect or, as a result, protective psychosocial characteristics, felt support, or social control, among other potential mediators (Kok et al., 2013; Pressman et al., 2019; Steptoe et al., 2008a). Close family members or friends can also indirectly influence individuals' health by helping them monitor symptoms, adhere to medication regimens, attend medical appointments, and create and sustain challenging lifestyle decisions (Martire & Helgeson, 2017). In doing so, strong social connections can delay or prevent chronic conditions (Umberson & Karas Montez, 2010). Physiologically, supportive interactions can boost immune, endocrine, and cardiovascular functions and reduce allostatic load, which is when someone starts to feel weary and exhausted from chronic, cumulative stress (Umberson & Karas Montez, 2010). While research continues to be conducted regarding exactly how social relationships affect health outcomes and vice versa, there appears to be a network of ways these constructs are related and contribute to overall well-being.

6.6   SOCIAL RELATIONSHIPS WITHIN THE WORKPLACE

Organizational culture and relationships in the workplace play an important role in well-being. Nurses' professional relationships, particularly those with supervisors, impact their well-being, which in turn has implications for nursing staff turnover (Brunetto et al., 2013b). Another study found that almost half of intentions to leave hospital-based nursing positions were associated with poor well-being, a lack of teamwork, and a challenging relationship between nurses and their supervisors (Brunetto et al., 2013a). Thus, it is critical to attend to, foster, and support healthy relationships in the workplace to allow for nurses' well-being.

Modeling workplace relationships begins at the student–instructor and student–preceptor levels. A study of nursing students engaged in their clinical rotations found that the professional working relationship between a nursing student and their preceptor supported the preceptor's ability to well assess and promote knowledge. A strong professional relationship between a preceptor and a student also allows the preceptor to provide the student with an appropriate level of autonomy in the clinical setting (Haitana & Bland, 2011). At the level of nurse managers, one study found that interpersonal relationships were the strongest predictor of engagement in the workplace. Nurse managers can also further reinforce nurses' effort and willingness to help co-workers to improve workplace relationships (Clark et al., 2014). Interventions that offer mentorship, mutual respect, and promote autonomy and resilience have been found to foster workplace relationships and well-being (Latham et al., 2008). Thus, an environment and team that encourages healthy interpersonal relationships aids engagement and may impact communication, hiring, and retention of nursing staff (Warshawsky et al., 2012).

6.7   SOCIAL RELATIONSHIPS OUTSIDE OF THE WORKPLACE

Given the challenging nature of nursing work, it is important to understand how personal relationships benefit nurses' well-being and influence their quality of life. A study of over 1000 nurses found that social support was a significant predictor of quality of life, including physical, psychological, environmental, and social domains (Kowitlawkul et al., 2019). The benefits of healthy relationships in one's personal life are also understood to boost overall well-being and thus improve job satisfaction and engagement. As noted earlier, one of the most important findings of the hallmark 75-year longitudinal Harvard Study of Adult Development was that meaningful interpersonal relationships were the strongest predictor of good quality of life (Vaillant, 2002). Further, marital satisfaction was found to be protective of mental health, with older adults who reported happy marriages also noting less physical pain and mood lability (Vaillant, 2002). Thus, fostering and maintaining quality interpersonal relationships, particularly intimate relationships outside of the workplace, is critical to mental health and well-being. Nurses will likely benefit from leveraging their social support to bolster their ability to cope with work-related stressors.

6.8   FOSTERING PERSONAL WELL-BEING

Multiple health behaviors have been linked with increased positive affect and improved relationships. Good health behaviors, some of which will soon be described, have been associated with lesser anxiety, depression, and stress (Keniger et al., 2013; Mandelosi et al., 2018; Vyazovskiy, 2015). Exercise, for example, can create structural and functional alterations in the brain that can result in biological and psychological benefits, which positively affect cognition and well-being (Fernandes et al., 2017; Mandelosi et al., 2018). Along with numerous physical health benefits, physical activity increases confidence and emotional stability, among many other positive outcomes (Mandelosi et al., 2018). It can also treat unhealthy and addictive behaviors, which, in turn, can positively influence one's overall well-being and relationships (Giesen et al., 2015). Similarly, obtaining high caliber sleep is crucial to individuals' quality of life, as it helps with energy balance, emotional regulation, and restoration, as well as other imperative outcomes that influence psychological and physical health and relationships (Vyazovskiy, 2015). Conversely, sleep deprivation results in worse brain functioning, toxin buildup, and potential challenges in cognitive abilities, behavior, and judgment (Eugene & Masiak, 2015). Another health behavior with numerous beneficial outcomes is spending time in nature (Petersen et al., 2021). Some of the many advantages of exposure to nature include improved psychological well-being, increased cognitive ability and function, decreased mental fatigue, improved perceived health, social empowerment, improved social support, and increased spiritual well-being (Keniger et al., 2013). Finally, giving to others has been associated with less hostility and better physical functioning, among other positive outcomes. The beneficial consequences of helping others may be from replacing negative, self-centered emotions with positive emotions, such as compassion and care (Seppala et al., 2013). Though there are other benefits of these activities that were not listed, these are simple behaviors that can drastically improve one's quality of life.

There are also activities that can psychologically improve individuals' quality of life, well-being, and, thus, relationships. Each of the following activities is associated with reduced stress, depression, and anxiety (Coles et al., 2019; Goyal et al., 2014; Hunt et al., 2018; Jans-Beken et al., 2019; O'Day & Heimberg, 2021). First, meditation is a technique by which individuals train their attention and awareness to calm their minds and regulate their emotions. In the workplace, practicing meditation benefits individuals' mental health and social relationships, can lessen role conflicts, and can enhance organizational innovativeness and development (Cheng, 2016). Meditation has also been positively correlated with decreased pain symptoms, improved blood pressure, smoking cessation, improved cognitive function, decreased worry, and increased longevity (Fortney & Taylor, 2010). Another simple intervention to improve well-being is to smile. Facial feedback affects emotions, so smiling can amplify or weaken emotional experiences (Coles et al., 2019; Pressman et al., 2020). In turn, smiling can increase one's positive emotion and ease psychologically uncomfortable or painful situations (Coles et al., 2019; Folkman, 2008). Smiling also builds and enhances relationships, such as through increasing the perception of trustworthiness and prompting others to smile, too (Dimberg & Söderkvist, 2010; Johnston et al., 2010; Papa & Bonanno, 2008). Finally, practicing gratitude can improve life satisfaction, self-esteem, emotional well-being, and social well-being, among many other outcomes (Jans-Beken et al., 2019; Rash et al., 2011). These few activities can be quickly and easily completed, even while at work, and can have substantial benefits on one's mood.

Since the strain experienced by nurses is often high (Boamah & Laschinger, 2016), attending to relationships and engaging in activities that evoke positive affect outside of work is likely to foster increased job satisfaction, stress reduction, improved health, and decreased work overload (Chunta, 2020; Poulose & Sudarsan, 2017). Spending time with friends and family can improve individuals' well-being and, thus, their relationships (Hudson et al., 2020). Strong relationships can also prevent burnout in nurses (Kravits et al., 2010). However, time spent with others is generally decreasing, while time spent on social media is increasing (Twenge et al., 2019). Consequently, limiting social media use can decrease loneliness (Hunt et al., 2018). Numerous positive psychology interventions and activities exist to improve well-being (Carr et al., 2020), and some activities presented in this chapter can be implemented by nurses to benefit their well-being, increase their positive affect, and enhance their relationships.

6.9 CONCLUSION

Nurses are critical to healthcare; thus, the happiness and well-being of nurses is critical to healthcare. Attending to the implications of both positive and negative affect, as well as to the relationship between these two constructs, can allow nurses to effectively manage work-related stress, prevent burnout and staff turnover, and allow for optimal interpersonal relationships within and outside of the workplace (Johnston et al., 2013; Larsen et al., 2017). Further, positive psychology practices and interventions can be utilized to foster positive affect, which, in turn, enhance physical and psychological health and well-being. Positive affect boosts the quality of relationships, which are understood to be one of the most important factors for good quality of life (Diener & Chan, 2011; Diener & Seligman, 2002; Kiecolt-Glaser et al., 2002; Steptoe et al., 2010). Thus, nurses have an opportunity to specifically attend to and cultivate positive affect to support their own well-being and to have a positive impact on students, co-workers, patients, friends, and family.

REFERENCES

Boamah, S. A., & Laschinger, H. (2016). The influence of areas of work–life fit and work–life interference on burnout and turnover intentions among new graduate nurses. *Journal of Nursing Management, 24*(2), E164–E174. https://doi.org/10.1111/jonm.12318

Boehm, J. K., & Kubzansky, L. D. (2012). The heart's content: The association between positive psychological well-being and cardiovascular health. *Psychological Bulletin, 138*(4), 655–691. https://doi.org/10.1037/a0027448

Boehm, J. K., & Lyubomirsky, S. (2008). Does happiness promote career success? *Journal of Career Assessment, 16*(1), 101–116. https//doi.org/10.1177/1069072707308140

Brunetto, Y., Shriberg, A., Farr-Wharton, R., Shacklock, K., Newman, S., & Dienger, J. (2013a). The importance of supervisor–nurse relationships, teamwork, wellbeing, affective commitment and retention of North American nurses. *Journal of Nursing Management, 21*(6), 827–837. https://doi.org/10.1111/jonm.12111

Brunetto, Y., Xerri, M., Shriberg, A., Farr-Wharton, R., Shacklock, K., Newman, S., & Dienger, J. (2013b). The impact of workplace relationships on engagement, well-being, commitment and turnover for nurses in Australia and the USA. *Journal of Advanced Nursing, 69*(12), 2786–2799. https://doi.org/10.1111/jan.12165

Burgdorf, J., & Panksepp, J. (2006). The neurobiology of positive emotions. *Neuroscience & Biobehavioral Reviews*, *30*(2), 173–187. https://doi.org/10.1016/j.neubiorev.2005.06.001

Cacioppo, J. T., & Cacioppo, S. (2014). Social relationships and health: The toxic effects of perceived social isolation. *Social and Personality Psychology Compass*, *8*(2), 58–72. https://doi.org/10.1111/spc3.12087

Carr, A., Cullen, K., Keeney, C., Canning, C., Mooney, O., Chinseallaigh, E., & O'Dowd, A. (2020). Effectiveness of positive psychology interventions: A systematic review and meta-analysis. *The Journal of Positive Psychology*, 1–21. https://doi.org/10.1080/17439760.2020.1818807

Cheng, F. K. (2016). What does meditation contribute to workplace? An integrative review. *Journal of Psychological Issues in Organizational Culture*, *6*(4), 18–34. https://doi.org/10.1002/jpoc.21195

Chunta, K. S. (2020). New nurse leaders: Creating a work–life balance and finding joy in work. *Journal of Radiology Nursing*, *39*(2), 86–88. https://doi.org/10.1016/j.jradnu.2019.12.007

Clark, O. L., Zickar, M. J., & Jex, S. M. (2014). Role definition as a moderator of the relationship between safety climate and organizational citizenship behavior among hospital nurses. *Journal of Business and Psychology*, *29*(1), 101–110. https://doi.org/10.1007/s10869-013-9302-0

Cohen, S., Doyle, W. J., Turner, R. B., Alper, C. M., & Skoner, D. P. (2003). Emotional style and susceptibility to the common cold. *Psychosomatic Medicine*, *65*(4), 652–657. https://doi.org/10.1097/01.psy.0000077508.57784.da

Cohn, M. A., Fredrickson, B. L., Brown, S. L., Mikels, J. A., & Conway, A. M. (2009). Happiness unpacked: Positive emotions increase life satisfaction by building resilience. *Emotion*, *9*(3), 361–368. https://doi.org/10.1037/a0015952

Coles, N. A., Larsen, J. T., & Lench, H. C. (2019). A meta-analysis of the facial feedback literature: Effects of facial feedback on emotional experience are small and variable. *Psychological Bulletin*, *145*(6), 610–651. https://doi.org/10.1037/bul0000194

Diener, E., & Chan, M. Y. (2011). Happy people live longer: Subjective well-being contributes to health and longevity. *Applied Psychology: Health and Well-Being*, *3*(1), 1–43. https://doi.org/10.1111/j.1758-0854.2010.01045.x

Diener, E., & Seligman, M. E. P. (2002). Very happy people. *Psychological Science*, *13*(1), 81–84. https://doi.org/10.1111/1467-9280.00415

Diener, E. & Tay, L. (2017). A scientific review of the remarkable benefits of happiness for successful and healthy living. In *Happiness: Transforming the development landscape* (pp. 90–117). The Centre for Bhutan Studies and GNH.

Dimberg, U., & Söderkvist, S. (2011). The voluntary facial action technique: A method to test the facial feedback hypothesis. *Journal of Nonverbal Behavior*, *35*(1), 17–33. https://doi.org/10.1007/s10919-010-0098-6

Doyle, W. J., Gentile, D. A., & Cohen, S. (2006). Emotional style, nasal cytokines, and illness expression after experimental rhinovirus exposure. *Brain, Behavior, and Immunity*, *20*(2), 175–181. https://doi.org/10.1016/j.bbi.2005.05.005

DuBois, C. M., Lopez, O. V., Beale, E. E., Healy, B. C., Boehm, J. K., & Huffman, J. C. (2015). Relationships between positive psychological constructs and health outcomes in patients with cardiovascular disease: A systematic review. *International Journal of Cardiology*, *195*, 265–280. https://doi.org/10.1016/j.ijcard.2015.05.121

Eugene, A. R., & Masiak, J. (2015). The neuroprotective aspects of sleep. *MEDtube Science*, *3*(1), 35–40. www.ncbi.nlm.nih.gov/pmc/articles/PMC4651462/

Feeney, B. C., & Collins, N. L. (2015). A new look at social support: A theoretical perspective on thriving through relationships. *Personality and Social Psychology Review*, *19*(2), 113–147. https://doi.org/10.1177/1088868314544222

Fernandes, J., Arida, R. M., & Gomez-Pinilla, F. (2017). Physical exercise as an epigenetic modulator of brain plasticity and cognition. *Neuroscience & Biobehavioral Reviews*, *80*, 443–456. https://doi.org/10.1016/j.neubiorev.2017.06.012

Flynn, L., & Ironside, P. M. (2018). Burnout and its contributing factors among midlevel academic nurse leaders. *Journal of Nursing Education*, *57*(1), 28–34. https://doi.org/10.3928/01484834-20180102-06

Folkman, S. (2008). The case for positive emotions in the stress process. *Anxiety, Stress, and Coping*, *21*(1), 3–14. https://doi.org/10.1080/10615800701740457

Folkman, S., & Moskowitz, J. T. (2000). Positive affect and the other side of coping. *American Psychologist*, *55*(6), 647–654. https://doi.org/10.1037/0003-066X.55.6.647

Fortney, L., & Taylor, M. (2010). Meditation in medical practice: A review of the evidence and practice. *Primary Care: Clinics in Office Practice*, *37*(1), 81–90. https://doi.org/10.1016/j.pop.2009.09.004

Fredrickson, B. L. (2013). Chapter one – Positive emotions broaden and build. In P. Devine & A. Plant (Eds.), *Advances in experimental social psychology* (Vol. 47, pp. 1–53). Academic Press. https://doi.org/10.1016/B978-0-12-407236-7.00001-2

Froman, L. (2010). Positive psychology in the workplace. *Journal of Adult Development*, *17*(2), 59–69. https://doi.org/10.1007/s10804-009-9080-0

Giesen, E. S., Deimel, H., & Bloch, W. (2015). Clinical exercise interventions in alcohol use disorders: A systematic review. *Journal of Substance Abuse Treatment*, *52*, 1–9. https://doi.org/10.1016/j.jsat.2014.12.001

Goyal, M., Singh, S., Sibinga, E. M. S., Gould, N. F., Rowland-Seymour, A., Sharma, R., Berger, Z., Sleicher, D., Maron, D. D., Shihab, H. M., Ranasinghe, P. D., Linn, S., Saha, S., Bass, E. B., & Haythornthwaite, J. A. (2014). Meditation programs for psychological stress and well-being. *JAMA Internal Medicine*, *174*(3), 357–368. https://doi.org/10.1001/jamainternmed.2013.13018

Grant, A. M., & Gino, F. (2010). A little thanks goes a long way: Explaining why gratitude expressions motivate prosocial behavior. *Journal of Personality and Social Psychology*, *98*(6), 946–955. https://doi.org/10.1037/a0017935

Haddad, L. M., Annamaraju, P., & Toney-Butler, T. J. (2021). Nursing shortage. In *StatPearls*. StatPearls Publishing. www.ncbi.nlm.nih.gov/books/NBK493175/

Haitana, J., & Bland, M. (2011). Building relationships: The key to preceptoring nursing students. *Nursing Praxis in New Zealand*, *27*(1), 4–12.

Haslam, C., Cruwys, T., & Haslam, S. A. (2014). "The we's have it": Evidence for the distinctive benefits of group engagement in enhancing cognitive health in aging. *Social Science & Medicine*, *120*, 57–66. https://doi.org/10.1016/j.socscimed.2014.08.037

Holt-Lunstad, J., Smith, T. B., Baker, M., Harris, T., & Stephenson, D. (2015). Loneliness and social isolation as risk factors for mortality: A meta-analytic review. *Perspectives on Psychological Science: A Journal of the Association for Psychological Science*, *10*(2), 227–237. https://doi.org/10.1177/1745691614568352

Holt-Lunstad, J., Smith, T. B., & Layton, J. B. (2010). Social relationships and mortality risk: A meta-analytic review. *PLOS Medicine*, *7*(7), e1000316. https://doi.org/10.1371/journal.pmed.1000316

Hudson, N. W., Lucas, R. E., & Donnellan, M. B. (2020). Are we happier with others? An investigation of the links between spending time with others and subjective well-being. *Journal of Personality and Social Psychology*, *119*(3), 672–694. https://doi.org/10.1037/pspp0000290

Hunt, M. G., Marx, R., Lipson, C., & Young, J. (2018). No more FOMO: Limiting social media decreases loneliness and depression. *Journal of Social and Clinical Psychology*, *37*(10), 751–768. https://doi.org/10.1521/jscp.2018.37.10.751

Ironson, G., & Hayward, H. (2008). Do positive psychosocial factors predict disease progression in HIV-1? A review of the evidence. *Psychosomatic Medicine*, *70*(5), 546–554. https://doi.org/10.1097/PSY.0b013e318177216c

Jans-Beken, L., Jacobs, N., Janssens, M., Peeters, S., Reijnders, J., Lechner, L., & Lataster, J. (2019). Gratitude and health: An updated review. *The Journal of Positive Psychology*, *15*(6), 1–40. https://doi.org/10.1080/17439760.2019.1651888

Johnston, D. W., Jones, M. C., Charles, K., McCann, S. K., & McKee, L. (2013). Stress in nurses: Stress-related affect and its determinants examined over the nursing day. *Annals of Behavioral Medicine*, *45*(3), 348–356. https://doi.org/10.1007/s12160-012-9458-2

Johnston, L., Miles, L., & Macrae, C. N. (2010). Why are you smiling at me? Social functions of enjoyment and non-enjoyment smiles. *British Journal of Social Psychology*, *49*(1), 107–127. https://doi.org/10.1348/014466609X412476

Keniger, L. E., Gaston, K. J., Irvine, K. N., & Fuller, R. A. (2013). What are the benefits of interacting with nature? *International Journal of Environmental Research and Public Health*, *10*, 913–935. https://doi.org/10.3390/ijerph10030913

Kiecolt-Glaser, J. K., Gouin, J.-P., & Hantsoo, L. (2010). Close relationships, inflammation, and health. *Neuroscience and Biobehavioral Reviews*, *35*(1), 33–38. https://doi.org/10.1016/j.neubiorev.2009.09.003

Kiecolt-Glaser, J. K., McGuire, L., Robles, T. F., & Glaser, R. (2002). Emotions, morbidity, and mortality: New perspectives from psychoneuroimmunology. *Annual Review of Psychology*, *53*, 83–107. https://doi.org/10.1146/annurev.psych.53.100901.135217

Kok, B. E., Coffey, K. A., Cohn, M. A., Catalino, L. I., Vacharkulksemsuk, T., Algoe, S. B., Brantley, M., & Fredrickson, B. L. (2013). How positive emotions build physical health: Perceived positive social connections account for the upward spiral between positive emotions and vagal tone. *Psychological Science*, 24(7), 1123–1132. https://doi.org/10.1177/0956797612470827

Kowitlawkul, Y., Yap, S. F., Makabe, S., Chan, S., Takagai, J., Tam, W. W. S., & Nurumal, M. S. (2019). Investigating nurses' quality of life and work–life balance statuses in Singapore. *International Nursing Review*, 66(1), 61–69. https://doi.org/10.1111/inr.12457

Kravits, K., McAllister-Black, R., Grant, M., & Kirk, C. (2010). Self-care strategies for nurses: A psycho-educational intervention for stress reduction and the prevention of burnout. *Applied Nursing Research*, 23(3), 130–138. https://doi.org/10.1016/j.apnr.2008.08.002

Larsen, J. T., Hershfield, Hal. E., Stastny, B. J., & Hester, N. (2017). On the relationship between positive and negative affect: Their correlation and their co-occurrence. *Emotion*, 17(2), 323–336. https://doi.org/10.1037/emo0000231

Latham, C. L., Hogan, M., & Ringl, K. (2008). Nurses supporting nurses: Creating a mentoring program for staff nurses to improve the workforce environment. *Nursing Administration Quarterly*, 32(1), 27–39. https://doi.org/10.1097/01.NAQ.0000305945.23569.2b

Le, B. M., Impett, E. A., Lemay Jr., E. P., Muise, A., & Tskhay, K. O. (2018). Communal motivation and well-being in interpersonal relationships: An integrative review and meta-analysis. *Psychological Bulletin*, 144(1), 1–25. https://doi.org/10.1037/bul0000133

Lyubomirsky, S., King, L., & Diener, E. (2005). The benefits of frequent positive affect: Does happiness lead to success? *Psychological Bulletin*, 131(6), 803–855. https://doi.org/10.1037/0033-2909.131.6.803

Maestripieri, D., M. Baran, N., Sapienza, P., & Zingales, L. (2010). Between- and within-sex variation in hormonal responses to psychological stress in a large sample of college students. *Stress*, 13(5), 413–424. https:/doi.org/10.3109/10253891003681137

Mandolesi, L., Polverino, A., Montuori, S., Foti, F., Ferraioli, G., Sorrentino, P., & Sorrentino, G. (2018). Effects of physical exercise on cognitive functioning and wellbeing: Biological and psychological benefits. *Frontiers in Psychology*, 9, 509. https://doi.org/10.3389/fpsyg.2018.00509

Martin, A. J. (2005). The role of positive psychology in enhancing satisfaction, motivation, and productivity in the workplace. *Journal of Organizational Behavior Management*, 24(1–2), 113–133. https://doi.org/10.1300/J075v24n01_07

Martino, J., Pegg, J., & Frates, E.P. (2017). The connection prescription: Using the power of social interactions and the deep desire for connectedness to empower health and wellness. *American Journal of Lifestyle Medicine*, 11(6), 466–475. https://doi.org/10.1177/1559827615608788

Martire, L. M., & Helgeson, V. S. (2017). Close relationships and the management of chronic illness: Associations and interventions. *The American Psychologist*, 72(6), 601–612. https://doi.org/10.1037/amp0000066

Maslow, A. H. (1943). A theory of human motivation. *Psychological Review*, 50(4), 370–396. https://doi.org/10.1037/h0054346

Maslow, A. H. (1954). *Motivation and personality*. Harpers.

Maslow, A. H. (1971). *The farther reaches of human nature*. Arkana/Penguin Books.

Morton, D. P. (2018). Combining lifestyle medicine and positive psychology to improve mental health and emotional well-being. *American Journal of Lifestyle Medicine*, 12(5), 370–374. https://doi.org/10.1177/1559827618766482

Neuman, M. D., & Werner, R. M. (2016). Marital status and postoperative functional recovery. *JAMA Surgery*, 151(2), 194–196. https://doi.org/10.1001/jamasurg.2015.3240

Nikolova, Y. S., Bogdan, R., Brigidi, B. D., & Hariri, A. R. (2012). Ventral striatum reactivity to reward and recent life stress interact to predict positive affect. *Biological Psychiatry*, 72(2), 157–163. https://doi.org/10.1016/j.biopsych.2012.03.014

O'Day, E. B., & Heimberg, R. G. (2021). Social media use, social anxiety, and loneliness: A systematic review. *Computers in Human Behavior Reports*, 3, 100070. https://doi.org/10.1016/j.chbr.2021.100070

Oishi, S. & Westgate, E. C. (2021) A psychologically rich life: Beyond happiness and meaning. *Psychological Review*, 1–22. Aug. PMID: 34383524. DOI: 10.1037/rev0000317

Orgambídez-Ramos, A., & de Almeida, H. (2017). Work engagement, social support, and job satisfaction in Portuguese nursing staff: A winning combination. *Applied Nursing Research*, 36, 37–41. https://doi.org/10.1016/j.apnr.2017.05.012

Papa, A., & Bonanno, G. A. (2008). Smiling in the face of adversity: The interpersonal and intrapersonal functions of smiling. *Emotion, 8*(1), 1–12. https://doi.org/10.1037/1528-3542.8.1.1

Petersen, E., Bischoff, A., Liedtke, G., & Martin, A. J. (2021). How does being solo in nature affect well-being? Evidence from Norway, Germany and New Zealand. *International Journal of Environmental Research and Public Health, 18*(7897), 1–21. https://doi.org/10.3390/ijerph18157897

Pietromonaco, P. R., & Collins, N. L. (2017). Interpersonal mechanisms linking close relationships to health. *The American Psychologist, 72*(6), 531–542. https://doi.org/10.1037/amp0000129

Poulose, S., & Sudarsan, N. (2017). Assessing the influence of work-life balance dimensions among nurses in the healthcare sector. *Journal of Management Development, 36*(3), 427–437. https://doi.org/10.1108/JMD-12-2015-0188

Pressman, S. D., Jenkins, B. N., & Moskowitz, J. T. (2019). Positive affect and health: What do we know and where next should we go? *Annual Review of Psychology, 70*(1), 627–650. https://doi.org/10.1146/annu rev-psych-010418-102955

Pressman, S. D., Acevedo, A. M., Hammond, K. V., & Kraft-Feil, T. L. (2020). Smile (or grimace) through the pain? The effects of experimentally manipulated facial expressions on needle-injection responses. *Emotion, 21*(6), 1188–1203. https://doi.org/10.1037/emo0000913

Raposa, E. B., Laws, H. B., & Ansell, E. B. (2016). Prosocial behavior mitigates the negative effects of stress in everyday life. *Clinical Psychological Science, 4*(4), 691–698. https://doi.org/10.1177/216770261 5611073

Rash, J. A., Matsuba, M. K., & Prkachin, K. M. (2011). Gratitude and well-being: Who benefits the most from a gratitude intervention? *Applied Psychology: Health and Well-Being, 3*(3), 350–369. https://doi.org/10.1111/j.1758-0854.2011.01058.x

Rowe, G., Hirsh, J. B., & Anderson, A. K. (2007). Positive affect increases the breadth of attentional selection. *Proceedings of the National Academy of Sciences, 104*(1), 383–388. https://doi.org/10.1073/pnas.060 5198104

Rusbult, C. E., & Agnew, C. R. (2010). Prosocial motivation and behavior in close relationships. In M. Mikulincer & P. R. Shaver (Eds.), *Prosocial motives, emotions, and behavior: The better angels of our nature* (pp. 327–345). American Psychological Association. https://doi.org/10.1037/12061-017

Saphire-Bernstein, S., & Taylor, S. E. (2013). Close relationships and happiness. In I. Boniwell, S. A. David & A. C. Ayers (Eds.), *Oxford handbook of happiness* (pp. 821–833). Oxford University Press. https://doi.org/10.1093/oxfordhb/9780199557257.013.0060

Seligman, M. (2018). PERMA and the building blocks of well-being. *The Journal of Positive Psychology, 13*(4), 333–335. https://doi.org/10.1080/17439760.2018.1437466

Seligman, M. E. P. (2002). *Authentic happiness: Using the new positive psychology to realize your potential for lasting fulfillment.* Free Press.

Seligman, M. E. P. (2011). *Flourish: A visionary new understanding of happiness and well-being.* Free Press.

Seligman, M. E. P., & Csikszentmihalyi, M. (2000). Positive psychology: An introduction. *American Psychologist, 55*(1), 5–14. https://doi.org/10.1037/0003-066X.55.1.5

Seppala, Emma, Timothy Rossomando, & James R. Doty. (2013). Social connection and compassion: Important predictors of health and well-being. *Social Research: An International Quarterly, 80*(2), 411–430.

Sin, N. L., Moskowitz, J. T., & Whooley, M. A. (2015). Positive affect and health behaviors across five years in patients with coronary heart disease: The heart and soul study. *Psychosomatic Medicine, 77*(9), 1058–1066. https://doi.org/10.1097/PSY.0000000000000238

Snippe, E., Jeronimus, B. F., aan het Rot, M., Bos, E. H., de Jonge, P., & Wichers, M. (2018). The reciprocity of prosocial behavior and positive affect in daily life. *Journal of Personality, 86*(2), 139–146. https://doi.org/10.1111/jopy.12299

Stavrova, O., & Ehlebracht, D. (2015). A longitudinal analysis of romantic relationship formation: The effect of prosocial behavior. *Social Psychological and Personality Science, 6*(5), 521–527. https://doi.org/10.1177/1948550614568867

Stepanikova, I., Triplett, J., & Simpson, B. (2011). Implicit racial bias and prosocial behavior. *Social Science Research, 40*(4), 1186–1195. https://doi.org/10.1016/j.ssresearch.2011.02.004

Steptoe, A., O'Donnell, K., Marmot, M., & Wardle, J. (2010). Positive affect and psychosocial processes related to health. *British Journal of Psychology, 99*(2), 211–227. https://doi.org/10.1111/j.2044-8295.2008.tb00474.x

Steptoe, A., O'Donnell, K., Marmot, M., & Wardle, J. (2008a). Positive affect and psychosocial processes related to health. *British Journal of Psychology*, *99*(2), 211–227. https://doi.org/10.1111/j.2044-8295.2008.tb00474.x

Steptoe, A., O'Donnell, K., Marmot, M., & Wardle, J. (2008b). Positive affect, psychological well-being, and good sleep. *Journal of Psychosomatic Research*, *64*(4), 409–415. https://doi.org/10.1016/j.jpsycho res.2007.11.008

Steptoe, A., Shankar, A., Demakakos, P., & Wardle, J. (2013). Social isolation, loneliness, and all-cause mortality in older men and women. *Proceedings of the National Academy of Sciences*, *110*(15), 5797–5801. https://doi.org/10.1073/pnas.1219686110

Steptoe, A., & Wardle, J. (2005). Positive affect and biological function in everyday life. *Neurobiology of Aging*, *26*(1, Supplement), 108–112. https://doi.org/10.1016/j.neurobiolaging.2005.08.016

Strand, E. B., Kerns, R. D., Christie, A., Haavik-Nilsen, K., Klokkerud, M., & Finset, A. (2007). Higher levels of pain readiness to change and more positive affect reduce pain reports – A weekly assessment study on arthritis patients. *Pain*, *127*(3), 204–213. https://doi.org/10.1016/j.pain.2006.08.015

Tay, L., & Diener, E. (2011). Needs and subjective well-being around the world. *Journal of Personality and Social Psychology*, *101*(2), 354–365. https://doi.org/10.1037/a0023779

Turner, S. B. (2014). The resilient nurse: An emerging concept. *Nurse Leader*, *12*(6), 71–90. https://doi.org/10.1016/j.mnl.2014.03.013

Twenge, J. M., Spitzberg, B. H., & Campbell, W. K. (2019). Less in-person social interaction with peers among U.S. adolescents in the 21st century and links to loneliness. *Journal of Social and Personal Relationships*, *36*(6), 1892–1913. https://doi.org/10.1177/0265407519836170

Umberson, D., & Karas Montez, J. (2010). Social relationships and health: A flashpoint for health policy. *Journal of Health and Social Behavior*, *51*(1, Supplement), S54–S66. https://doi.org/10.1177/00221 46510383501

Vaillant, G. (2002). *Aging well: Surprising guideposts to a happier life*. Scribe Publications.

Vaillant, G. E. (2012). *Triumphs of experience*. Harvard University Press. www.jstor.org/stable/j.ctt2jbxs1

Velando-Soriano, A., Ortega-Campos, E., Gómez-Urquiza, J. L., Ramírez-Baena, L., De La Fuente, E. I., Cañadas-De La Fuente, G. A. (2019). Impact of social support in preventing burnout syndrome in nurses: A systematic review. *Japan Journal of Nursing Science*, *17*(1), e12269. https://doi.org/10.1111/jjns.12269

Vyazovskiy, V. V. (2015). Sleep, recovery, and metaregulation: Explaining the benefits of sleep. *Nature and Science of Sleep*, *7*, 171–184. https://doi.org/10.2147/NSS.S54036

Waldinger, R. J., & Schulz, M. S. (2010). What's love got to do with it?: Social functioning, perceived health, and daily happiness in married octogenarians. *Psychology and Aging*, *25*(2), 422–431. https://doi.org/10.1037/a0019087

Warshawsky, N. E., Havens, D. S., & Knafl, G. (2012). The influence of interpersonal relationships on nurse managers' work engagement and proactive work behavior. *The Journal of Nursing Administration*, *42*(9), 418–425. https://doi.org/10.1097/NNA.0b013e3182668129

7 Substance Use Risk Reduction

Michelle Knapp[1] and Donna McCabe[1]
[1]Rory Meyers College of Nursing
New York University
New York, New York, USA

CONTENTS

KEY POINTS

- Substance use occurs on a spectrum from abstinence to severe and disordered use.
- Chronic administration of a substance contributes to epigenetic changes that precipitate and exacerbate mental and medical illness.
- The etiology of substance use is complex, and comprehensive treatment is needed to address the multilayered biopsychosocial issues that hinder recovery from substance use problems.
- Motivational interviewing is an effective technique to help an individual move through stages of change toward abstinence.
- Harm reduction seeks to reduce risk associated with substance use and maybe useful for individuals as they work toward abstinence.
- Diet, exercise, group or individual therapies, and other nonpharmacologic modalities can be effective in addressing substance use and its multilayered etiologies.

DOI: 10.1201/9781003178330-8

7.1   INTRODUCTION

Substance use is pervasive in society and ubiquitous across cultures and populations. According to the 2021 World Drug Report, the United Nations found that about 275 million people used substances in the past year, while more than 36 million people had a substance use disorder (SUD) (United Nations, 2021). More than 19 million people over the age of 18 in the United States had a substance use disorder in 2019 (Substance Abuse and Mental Health Services Administration [SAMHSA], 2020).

Substance consumption rates are directly correlated with mortality and physical and mental health (Shield et al., 2017; Charlet & Heintz, 2017). Legal substances pose a great burden on society but are not necessarily less harmful. SAMHSA (2020) reports that alcohol continues to be the most used and misused substance among all age groups and races. Cannabis use has increased among all age groups, significantly for 12–17-year-olds. Cannabis use can be dangerous; in adolescents it is linked to a decline in IQ, risk for developing suicidal ideation, and risk for developing psychotic disorders in adulthood (Meier et al., 2012; Di Forti et al., 2019; McHugh et al., 2017). Since its legalization in several states, marijuana use has remained high across races and special populations in the United States. Use during pregnancy is dangerous, connected with a variety of sociodemographic factors that place these women at-risk, and has been shown to be associated with fetal growth restriction, stillbirth, preterm birth, and neonatal intensive care unit admission (Metz and Borgelt, 2018; Stickrath, 2019).

The opioid overdose epidemic of the 21st century is an example of implications for misuse of legal substances. Although this epidemic led to substantial policy changes and treatment gains with opioid agonist therapies, prescription opioids continue to be misused by almost 10 million people in the US (SAMHSA, 2020). Benzodiazepines are also legal, and misuse remains a problem (SAMHSA, 2020). These sedatives and hypnotics are commonly prescribed to treat anxiety and sleep problems, but due subsequent neurobiological changes in the body, overuse can worsen these conditions.

While cigarette use has decreased over the past several decades, nicotine vaping devices have introduced a new public health problem (SAMHSA, 2020). Since 2014, the e-cigarette has been the most frequently used addictive tobacco product by youth (Wang et al., 2018). Caffeine is another misused substance that is legal and readily available to individuals of all ages. Estimates are difficult to gather, but literature shows that globally about 10–13% of people are affected with problematic use, at higher rates in individuals with other SUDs (Sweeney et al., 2020).

Most people who have substance use problems do not receive treatment, partly due to treatment availability and partly because patients feel that they do not have a problem (SAMHSA, 2018). Individuals with substance use problems are overrepresented in emergency departments, hospital clinics, and primary care settings. Nurses in any setting are well positioned to address substance use problems with patients. The main goal of substance use treatment is to reduce or eliminate consumption to recommended limits. This requires a dynamic approach that targets multiple domains of a person's life beyond a pharmaceutical approach.

7.1.1   ETIOLOGIES OF SUBSTANCE USE DISORDERS

Substances are psychoactive chemicals that produce effects through intoxication. SUDs develop over time with repeated administration of the substance; this is commonly referred to as "addiction." Addiction is defined as a chronic, relapsing disorder characterized by compulsive substance seeking, continued use despite harmful consequences, and long-lasting changes in the brain. It is a complex brain disorder and a mental illness with multilayered etiologies that can vary across individuals (National Institute on Drug Abuse [NIDA], 2020).

7.1.1.1 Psychopathology: Self-Medication Hypothesis and Co-Occurring Disorders

In 1985, Edward John Khantzian, a psychiatrist, psychoanalyst, and professor of psychiatry at Harvard University, published his landmark article, "The Self-Medication Hypothesis of Addictive Disorders." Khantzian originated the self-medication hypothesis of substance use, identifying substance use as a symptom of a person trying to modify response to external stressors; the substance ameliorates distress rooted in psychological suffering (Khantzian, 1985). The hypothesis helps to explain why most individuals with a substance use disorder have a co-occurring mental health condition. In 2019, more than 9 million people in the United States had a primary mental illness with an SUD (SAMHSA, 2020). Substance use can precipitate or exacerbate mental health conditions. Some of the most common include anxiety, depression, bipolar disorder, trauma-related disorders, panic disorder, and personality disorders (American Psychiatric Association [APA], 2013). There is also a significant overlap of eating disorders with substance use, possibly related to the behavioral association and broad personality subtypes with emotional and behavioral dysregulation found among individuals with eating disorders (Thompson et al., 2008; Eskander et al., 2020). Trauma has a profound effect on risk for developing an SUD. The ACE (Adverse Childhood Experiences) landmark study in the 1990s showed that compounding adverse childhood events are strongly correlated with substance use problems in adulthood (Felletti et al., 1998). More recently, a secondary analysis of data from the National Longitudinal Study of Adolescent to Adult Health (N=11279) corroborated those results (Letendre & Reed., 2017).

7.1.1.2 Neurobiology of Substance Use Disorders

The addiction cycle is best explained with three core phases that are rooted in the mesocortical striatal pathway. These areas of the brain help to regulate motivation and behavior, thus the main stages of a developing and persisting substance use problem: binge/intoxication, negative reward, and preoccupation (Koob & Volkow, 2010; 2016). These phases contribute to the conditioning of the reward pathway in the brain (see Table 7.1). When a person without a substance use disorder binges and becomes intoxicated, the person is positively rewarded. Several neurochemicals (e.g., dopamine, serotonin, glutamate, gaba) are released, affecting the motivational neurocircuitry in the reward pathway area of the brain. When the substance is repeatedly introduced to the body, neuroadaptations occur. The brain develops a tolerance to the substance, requiring higher doses to achieve the same effect. With chronic administration and changes to this reward pathway, the person experiences dependence—meaning they depend on the substance to feel "normal"—or in homeostasis. The person then becomes preoccupied with obtaining the substance again to relieve this withdrawal-related dysphoria.

7.1.1.3 Genetics and Epigenetics

Large meta-analyses (MAs) have provided some understanding of the impact genetics have on the phenotypic traits of individuals who develop substance use problems, including genetic correlation with substance use and other mental illness (Walters et al., 2018; Lui et al., 2019; Polimanti et al., 2019). The relationship between genetics and behavior-related pathology is most richly explained through epigenetics. Epigenetics is the study of gene expression changes that occur without changing the sequence of the genes and is a science that helps us to better understand phenotypic trait expression (Allis & Jenuwein, 2016). As people engage in harmful behaviors, cellular toxicity induces modifications to DNA methylation and histones; healthy communication between cells is disrupted, leading to pathological conditions. While these changes occur in every area of the body, key areas of the reward pathway are heavily targeted with problematic substance use (Walker et al., 2018)

TABLE 7.1
The three stages of addiction: binge/intoxication, withdrawal, craving: neuroadaptation contributes to conditioned reinforcement

Stage	Associated Behaviors and Feelings	Major Neurotransmitters Implicated	Neurocircuitry
Positive reward	Incentive salience, intoxication/binging, rewarding rush, "incentive salience"	Dopamine	Basal ganglia, nucleus accumbens, VTA
Negative reward	Negative emotional state, withdrawal/dysphoria, anhedonia, irritability	Glutamate, gaba	Basal forebrain, extended amygdala, habenula
Preoccupation/anticipation	Substance-seeking, loss of control over substance consumption, irritability, anxiety	Glutamate	Prefrontal cortex, amygdala, hippocampus,

Koob, G. F., & Volkow, N. D. (2010). Neurocircuitry of addiction. *Neuropsychopharmacology: Official Publication of the American College of Neuropsychopharmacology*, *35*(1), 217–238. https://doi.org/10.1038/npp.2009.110

Koob, G. F., & Volkow, N. D. (2016). Neurobiology of addiction: A neurocircuitry analysis. *The Lancet Psychiatry*, *3*(8), 760–773. https://doi.org/10.1016/S2215-0366(16)00104-8

Volkow, N. D., Koob, G. F., & McLellan, A. T. (2016). Neurobiologic advances from the brain disease model of addiction. *The New England Journal of Medicine*, *374*(4), 363–371. https://doi.org/10.1056/NEJMra1511480

Nicotine has received substantial attention in epigenetic studies demonstrating the pervasive effect on readily available nicotine and the consequences to DNA (Joehanes et al., 2016). Importantly, epigenetic changes also contribute to the traits seen in other psychiatric and medical disorders (Blacker et al., 2019; Kuehner et al., 2019; Moosavi et al., 2016). Epigenetic damage related to smoking seems to be reversible with behavior change (McCartney et al., 2018). Lifestyle medicine treatments are partially behavioral and may have a profound impact on recovery from addiction and co-occurring conditions.

7.1.2 Classification

7.1.2.1 Spectrum of Use

Substance use occurs on a spectrum from abstinence to substance use disorder (see Figure 7.1).

Risky substance use is any pattern of use (quantity, frequency, duration) that increases an individual's risk of causing harm to self or others. SUDs are found on the far right of the spectrum, caused by repeated misuse. Core features of a substance use disorder include impaired control, social impairment, risky use, and craving (see Table 7.2) (NIDA, 2018). Substances are classified by their intoxication effects. *The Diagnostic and Statistical Manual of Mental Disorders* (5th ed.) (APA, 2013) outlines criteria for all substance use disorders (see Table 7.3). Most categories of substances include disorders, including intoxication, withdrawal, and substance use disorder (mild, moderate, or severe). Individuals also will commonly use more than one substance at a time. Importantly, many individuals with severe substance use problems diagnostically qualify for more than one chronic substance use syndrome at any given time (e.g. alcohol induced intoxication while having an alcohol use disorder).

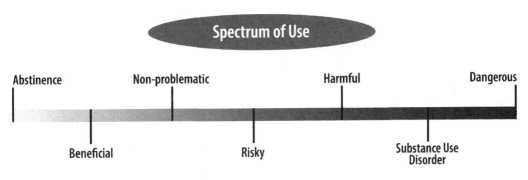

FIGURE 7.1 Spectrum of substance use

TABLE 7.2
Classification of substances with consequences of toxic exposure

Substance	Category	Consequences of Use
Alcohol	Depressant	Depression, anxiety, cardiac, increased sensitivity to pain, weakened immune function, sleep problems, hepatic and renal diseases
Opioids	Depressant	Opioid-induced hyperalgesia, low testosterone, low estrogen, GI problems, skin conditions, secondary infections
Cocaine, amphetamines	Stimulant	Dysphoria, nervousness, insomnia, stroke, GI problems, irregular heartbeat, elevated blood pressure, acute psychosis, chronic psychotic disorders, skin conditions, secondary infections, tooth and gum decay
Caffeine	Stimulant	Dysphoria, nervousness, insomnia, GI problems, irregular heartbeat, elevated blood pressure
Tobacco	Stimulant	Headaches, attentional problems, GI problems, cardiac illness, respiratory illness, tooth staining and decay
Cannabis, synthetic cannabis	Hallucinogen	Nervousness, paranoia, psychosis, adult-onset psychotic disorders, tooth staining and decay
Anabolic-androgenic steroids	Steroids	Depression, mood swings, frank paranoia, secondary infection, gynecomastia, enlarged prostate, elevated blood pressure, elevated glucose, decreased high-density lipoprotein

Levounis, P., Zerbo, E., & Aggarwal, R. (2016). *Pocket guide to addiction assessment and treatment.* American Psychiatric Publishing.

7.1.2.2 Recommended Limits

Currently, only alcohol and caffeine have recommended daily limits. Literature has identified benefits of moderate alcohol consumption on cardiac and metabolic conditions (Standridge et al., 2004). A recent meta-analysis found that moderate coffee consumption (2–4 cups/day) was associated with reduced mortality compared to no coffee consumption (Kim et al., 2019). The recommended daily limit for adults is no more than 4–5 standard cups (US Food and Drug Administration, n.d.).

Due to potential damage to the developing brain, alcohol is not recommended in the United States for consumption under the age of 21. The Centers for Disease Control ([CDC] 2021a) provides guidance on what constitutes a standard alcoholic drink (see Table 7.4). The maximum number of drinks per week for men ages 18–65 is 14 and women is 7. The CDC (2021b) also gives guidelines to identify binge consumption of alcohol (see Table 7.5).

TABLE 7.3
Criteria for substance use disorders

Physiological Changes:
- Tolerance to substance
- Withdrawal from substance

Note: if the substance is taken as prescribed, these criteria are not valid.

Loss of Control Over Use:
- Larger amounts and/or longer periods of substance use
- Feeling incapable of cutting back or controlling use of substance
- Increased time spent obtaining, using, or recovering the substance
- Craving the substance
- Compulsion to use the substance

Continued Use Despite Negative Consequences:
- Role failure or reduction of activities at work, home, school, other settings
- Social and relationship problems
- Reducing recreational activities
- Physical hazards
- Physiological harm

Severity:
- Mild: 1–3 criteria
- Moderate: 4–5 criteria
- Severe: 6 or more criteria

American Psychiatric Association. (2013). *Diagnostic and statistical manual of mental disorders (DSM-5)* (5th ed.).

TABLE 7.4
CDC standard alcohol drink

Standard Drink	Equivalent Beverage
A standard drink in the United States: Approximately 14.0 g (0.6 oz) of pure alcohol	12 oz beer (5% alcohol) 8 oz malt liquor (7% alcohol) 5 oz wine (12% alcohol) 1.5 oz or one shot of 80 proof (40% alcohol) distilled spirits or liquor (gin, rum, vodka, whiskey)

Centers for Disease Control and Prevention. (2021, May 11). *Standard drink.* Alcohol and Public Health: Frequently Asked Questions. www.cdc.gov/alcohol/fact-sheets/alcohol-use.htm

TABLE 7.5
CDC alcohol consumption definitions

Type of Alcohol Consumption	Definition
Heavy alcohol drinking	The quantity of alcohol consumed in one week by men or women: • Men: 15 or more drinks • Women: 8 or more drinks
Binge alcohol drinking	Pattern of drinking alcohol that corresponds to the number of alcoholic drinks consumed usually within a two-hour period (on a single occasion) by men and women • Men: 5 or more drinks • Women: 4 or more drinks

Centers for Disease Control and Prevention. (2021, May 11). *What is excessive drinking?* Alcohol and Public Health: Frequently Asked Questions. www.cdc.gov/alcohol/fact-sheets/alcohol-use.htm

7.2 LIFESTYLE-BASED THERAPIES TO TREAT SUBSTANCE USE DISORDERS

Research from the past 30 years suggests that addiction is a chronic illness. Given the complex etiologic persuasion, interventions must focus beyond stopping illicit use to address compounded biopsychosocial aspects of the illness. Lifestyle modification approaches should be culturally informed and patient-centered.

7.2.1 THEORETICAL APPROACH

Abstinence and harm reduction are two theoretical frameworks that guide the nurse to help individuals reduce or eliminate consumption of a substance. Both approaches include behaviorally focused interventions that benefit multiple domains of a person's life. A recent systematic review (SR) of 63 studies found lower prevalence of psychiatric episodes, decreased depression and anxiety, lower psychosocial stress levels, better social functioning, decreased medical morbidity, and socioeconomic benefit for substance use reduction or abstinence (Charlet & Heintz, 2017). Harm reduction also includes community-based interventions to decrease secondary risk associated with use (e.g., cellulitis related to injection, death secondary to overdose) (Carrico et al., 2014; Gilchrist et al., 2017).

The abstinence approach has historically driven policy and treatment. Per the clinical guidelines issued by the National Institute on Alcohol Abuse and Alcoholism ([NIAAA] 2005), abstinence is the safest course for most individuals with alcohol use disorders. The NIAAA (2005) recommends discussing individualized goals with patients and continued engagement if the person continues to use substances. Harm reduction helps to bridge the gap for many people who continue to use substances while working toward a goal of abstinence.

In 1960, E. Morton Jellinek (1960), a physiologist, alcoholism researcher, and founder of the Yale Center of Alcohol Studies, challenged the abstinence model (*The Disease Concept of Alcoholism*). He proposed that individuals labeled as alcoholics should be treated as physiologically sick people rather than moral failures. His harm reduction work focused on helping people to reduce the negative consequences of continued substance use. Under the harm reduction model, patients create short- and long-term goals that can change over time (see Table 7.6). The nurse uses motivational techniques to support the patient as they continuously realign their goals (Hawk et al., 2017). Harm reduction techniques to decrease substance use include:

- **Gradualism:** Making incremental changes tends to be more manageable for individuals (Hawk et al., 2017; Boucher et al., 2017). These changes occur over time and may ebb and flow.
- **Practicing refusal skills:** When a client's perceived self-efficacy is greater than the threat, the client often avoids the behavior (Choi et al., 2013). Part of practicing refusal skills is learning to replace harmful behavior with healthier behavior.
- **Redefining success:** The harm reduction philosophy inherently redefines success as it rejects the assumption that any return to use of a substance stops progress (Knapp & Kozikowski, 2020).

TABLE 7.6
Harm reduction goals

Goals	Example
Short term	To change the frequency of substance use
	To change the quantity of substance use
	To reduce the amount of money spent on the substance
Long term	To obtain employment
	To rebuild family relationships
	To begin a stable exercise and diet regimen

Early attempts at abstinence seem to fare well with overall outcomes of alcohol consumption. An analysis of the Combined Pharmacotherapies and Behavioral Interventions (COMBINE) clinical trial (N=954) found that early abstinence was significantly associated with fewer drinks per drinking day, number of drinking and heavy drinking days, longer time to first drinking, and first heavy drinking day. For a person trying to stop consuming alcohol, early consumption was significantly associated with continued consumption (Dunn et al., 2019).

Feasibility and outcomes of harm reduction techniques in alcohol use are mixed and may depend on the degree of consumption. Data analyses from Project MATCH (Matching Alcoholism Treatments to Client Heterogeneity) found that the likelihood of maintaining moderate drinking was lower in severely dependent patients (Witkiewitz, 2008). Nonetheless, a recent secondary analysis of the COMBINE study data (N = 1,383) examined heavy drinking patterns up to 16 months and found that two-thirds had a 64% reduction in drinking frequency and a 38% reduction in drinking intensity from pretreatment drinking levels (Witkiewitz et al., 2017).

While it is beyond the scope of this chapter to discuss medication therapies for substance use problems, it should be noted that there are FDA-approved medications to treat tobacco, alcohol, and opioid use disorders. These medications help to decrease or stop substance use and misuse and provide the individual time to engage in lifestyle modification. For example, smoking cessation is difficult for most and individuals could benefit from pharmacologic intervention. Sixty-eight percent of smokers in the United States want to stop, but most relapse within 24 hours of trying to quit, and 45% of individuals who are abstinent at six months experience subsequent relapse (Babb et al., 2017). More than 90% of people who smoke attempt to quit multiple times (Babb et al., 2017). Nicotine cessation has been shown to work best with nicotine replacement therapies or medications such as bupropion or varenicline (Anthenelli et al., 2016; Stapleton, et al., 2013).

Likewise, opioid use relapse is high for individuals with severe opioid use disorders without medications. Medications to treat opioid use disorder such as methadone and buprenorphine have been shown to have good success rates with moderate to severe opioid use disorder, although this may be dose dependent (Mattick et al., 2004; 2014). Extended-release naltrexone is an opioid antagonist shown to have good efficacy to stop illicit opioid use in individuals who are highly motivated (Lee et al., 2018). This medication also has also shown benefits in early treatment of alcohol use disorders (Ciraulo et al., 2008).

7.2.2 INTERVENTIONS

There is a vast amount of literature to support motivational interviewing (MI), which is a directive, patient-centered intervention that can be integrated into screening and brief intervention (Knapp & McCabe, 2019). Miller and Rollnick's (2013) stages of change and MI are founded in the work of DiClemente and Prochaska's (1998) Transtheoretical Change Model, which states that individuals make the decision to change over time, moving in and out of stages from precontemplation, contemplation, preparation, action, and maintenance (see Table 7.7 and Figure 7.2). Nurses use MI techniques to explore and resolve ambivalence such as developing discrepancy, eliciting change talk, and rolling with resistance to change. All conversations should use the OARS approach: open-ended questions, affirmations, reflections, and summarizing (Knapp & McCabe, 2019) (see Table 7.8). In a meta-analysis (MA) of 59 trials, MI corroborated results of prior reviews and was found to be significantly better than no intervention, and about the same with other types of psychotherapeutic intervention in the short/medium range follow-up (Smedslund et al., 2011). MI has also been found to be more effective than no intervention for adolescents and to have an impact on substance use among minority populations (Foxcraft et al., 2016; Hettema et al., 2005).

TABLE 7.7
Examples of Miller and Rollnick's (2013) stages of change based on the work of DiClemente and Prochaska (1998)

Stage of Change	Description
Pre-contemplation	The individual is largely unaware that their behavior is problematic and/or produces negative consequences.
Contemplation	The individual has changed behavior within about six months, recognizing that their behavior may be problematic, yet still might feel ambivalent about change.
Preparation	The individual is ready to take action within about the next 30 days and begin to prepare for change.
Action	The individual has recently changed their behavior and continue to modify behaviors.
Maintenance	The individual has sustained their behavior change for typically longer than about six months and is working to prevent relapse.

Miller, W. R., & Rollnick, S. (2013). *Motivational interviewing: Helping people change* (3rd ed.). Guilford Press.

DiClemente, C., & Prochaska, J. (1998). Toward a comprehensive, transtheoretical model of change. In W. R. Miller and N. Heather (Eds.), *Treating addictive behaviours* (2nd ed., pp. 3–24). Plenum Press.

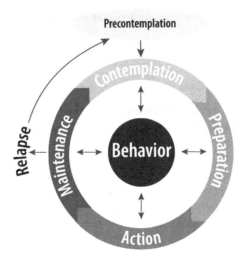

FIGURE 7.2   The stages of change

TABLE 7.8
OARS-style questions

Open-ended questions	What are you most worried about as a result of your use?
Affirmations	I see you've done a lot of work to cut back on your smoking.
Reflections	What I am hearing you say is that it is important to you that you stop drinking alcohol.
Summaries	Here's what we have discussed today. …Is there anything that I missed, or anything else you want to share?

TABLE 7.9

American Society of Addiction Medicine criteria for level of care and treatment are based on patient assessment and needs. Phases include: screening, assessment and diagnosis, and treatment

6 Dimensions of Patient-Centered Assessment	1. Acute intoxication and/or withdrawal potential 2. Biomedical conditions and complications 3. Emotional, behavioral, or cognitive conditions and complications 4. Readiness to change 5. Relapse, continued use, or continued problem potential 6. Recovery/living environment
Levels of Care (Guided by the 6 Dimensions)	1. Outpatient 2. Intensive Outpatient or partial hospitalization 3. Residential treatment 4. Medically managed intensive outpatient (Note: Dimensions 4-6 have No impact on determining this level)
2 Key Phases of Treatment	1. Detox & Stabilization: risks and safety, antagonist/agonist medications, symptomatic medications to treat withdrawal or intoxication stages 2. Rehabilitation and Maintenance Treatments: medications, psychotherapy, group therapy, stabilize psychiatric conditions

Rastegar, D., & Fingerhood, M. (2016). *The American Society of Addiction Medicine handbook of addiction medicine* (p. 370). Oxford University Press.

7.2.3 DETERMINING LEVEL OF CARE

One of the most challenging aspects of treatment is determining the level of care that is suitable for the patient—and receiving the necessary buy-in from the patient themself. There is also often resistance on the patient's side; family members are either supportive or unsupportive. Social challenges continue (e.g. lack of housing, problems with finances) that can severely disrupt the engagement process. Medical and psychiatric illness can complicate matters, and the care becomes increasingly complex in these cases. Levels of care are based on these factors and other patient-specific needs (see Table 7.9). Some individuals require an inpatient detoxification period due to risk of seizure (e.g. benzodiazepines, alcohol). During this time, the patient is provided a tapered medication regimen using medications that mimic the substance in order to safely discontinue the substance. Some patients will require substantial social support in an abstinent environment such as an inpatient rehabilitation (7 to 30 days) or even a long-term residential program (six months to one or more years). Outpatient treatment should continue indefinitely depending on the patient's needs and motivation to maintain abstinence.

7.2.4 SCREENING, BRIEF INTERVENTION, AND REFERRAL TO TREATMENT

SBIRT is a universal screening and prevention approach. It includes (S) screening, brief intervention (BI) including education, and referral to treatment (RT) when indicated. SBIRT can be used in any setting to determine if a person has problematic substance use (e.g., emergency room, primary care office, hospital clinic, homecare visit). Discussion of abstinence and harm reduction techniques can be integrated into screening and BI, even with a negative screen. For the positive screen, the nurse should also explore the patient's substance use and provide education and referral to treatment if necessary. Inpatient detoxification is recommended for individuals with risk of withdrawal seizures, certain chronic medical conditions (e.g., cirrhosis, renal failure), severe, persistent mental illness (e.g., schizophrenia, bipolar disorder), and moderate to high suicide risk. Detoxifications and longer-term rehabilitation programs provide individuals a controlled setting; this helps them to recondition their brains and removes them from certain conditioned cue cravings that prompted prior use of substances.

The United States Preventive Service Task Force (2020) recommends screening for unhealthy drug use in all adults over the age of 18 years (Krist et al., 2020). The American Academy of Pediatrics recommends screening for substance use in all primary care visits in children ages 12 to 17 years old (Levy et al., 2016). The NIDA screening tools can be used in adults 18 and over (see Resources 7.8). The NIDA Quick Screen alcohol question originates from Smith and colleagues (2009), and this single alcohol screener was 81.8% sensitive and 79.3% specific for identifying unhealthy alcohol use. The NIDA Quick Screen follows the NIDA recommended consumption limits. The NIDA Quick Screen for Other Substances was adapted from a single question screener by Smith and colleagues (2010), which was 100% sensitive and 73.5% specific for detection of a drug use disorder. A positive screen for illicit substance use, tobacco, or misuse of prescription drugs identifies risky use and necessitates exploration and referral for further intervention.

Brief interventions that follow screening should take into consideration where the patient lies on the continuum and if the patient wants to change the use. Questions are asked using nonjudgmental, open-ended questions. The brief intervention lasts from 5 to 30 minutes and helps the nurse to gauge readiness for change; it should be framed in a way that keeps the conversation open for further intervention (Knapp & McCabe, 2019).

Brief intervention has shown most efficacy for alcohol, opioids, and tobacco. Unfortunately, the literature is limited in that, if screening is not performed, then it cannot be included for evidence with SBIRT. To date, there are no randomized controlled trials (RCTs) that compare screening with BI to no screening with BI. BI has been found to be mostly effective for alcohol use, particularly on risky alcohol consumption (van Amsterdam & van den Brink, 2013; Chambers et al., 2016; Willenbring, 2014). A review of 32 controlled trials found that one session of brief intervention can make an effect on alcohol consumption (Bien et al., 1993). More recent literature supports that more than one session of BI is needed to decrease alcohol consumption (about three drinks per week) at one year with some contact with a primary care provider (Jonas et al., 2014). Brief intervention also has a small amount of literature to support its effectiveness for smoking cessation and opioid use problems. In 2015, an RCT of emergency room patients with harmful opioid use found that brief intervention with medication and a referral to a primary care provider reported decreased opioid use at one month (D'Onofrio et al., 2015). Another RCT was conducted in inner-city teaching hospital outpatient clinics with 3- and 6-months follow-up by blinded observers and found that brief intervention helped to significantly decrease heroin and cocaine use among women, people of color, and homeless in urgent care clinics (Bernstein et al., 2005). Likewise, brief intervention is found to be somewhat effective for tobacco users with or without smoking cessation pharmacotherapies (Patnode et al., 2015; Anthenelli et al., 2016).

7.2.5 INDIVIDUAL AND GROUP PSYCHOTHERAPIES

Psychotherapy helps patients to address both the substance use and other psychosocial problems that contribute to the addiction cycle. Group psychotherapy helps patients to strengthen social connectedness, while individual psychotherapy helps to increase one's awareness of their patterned behavior to make the necessary changes for enduring recovery—in all aspects of their lives. Patients should be referred for psychotherapy when they are willing to engage. It has been hypothesized that different types of psychotherapy work better during different stages of change, and that cognitive behavioral approaches can work across the span of the illness (Prochaska and DiClemente, 1992).

There is a vast amount of evidence to support cognitive behavioral therapy (CBT), which focuses on cognitive distortions and maladaptive behaviors that lead to continued, repetitive use. A recent MA of 30 RCTs found that CBT was more effective than no treatment or minimal treatment, and that it seems to have the most benefit for alcohol consumption earlier on in treatment (Magill et al., 2019). Magill and Ray (2009) had performed an earlier comprehensive MA of 53 controlled trials on adults using alcohol or illicit substances and found that 58% receiving CBT had better outcomes versus comparison treatment.

Psychodynamic therapy aligns with Khantizian's (1985; 2017; 2018) self-medication hypothesis and views substance use to deal with psychological distress as related to external stressors. Throughout the course of treatment, there is great focus on affective (emotional) regulation and development of self-esteem. The patient becomes more aware of the role that early childhood development had in their current substance use. Ultimately, the long-term goal is to help the patient's ego function by bolstering and developing healthy defense mechanisms to help them function better. While the literature for psychodynamic therapy in SUDs is limited, there is an emerging body of evidence for co-morbid conditions such as depression, anxiety, and personality pathology, particularly with longer-term treatment (Leichsenring et al., 2008; Taylor et al, 2012; Town et al., 2012). This supports the benefit of psychodynamic therapy for addressing the multilayered etiologies of substance use.

7.2.6 SELF-HELP GROUPS

Alcoholics Anonymous (AA) and other 12-step programs are abstinence-focused and founded on the original work of Bill Miller, guided by the *Big Book* (AA, 2002), first published in 1939. Self-help groups provide social support and connectedness that is often foregone with SUDs. AA meetings are free of charge and can be found anywhere in the world. There has been a substantial slate of observational and quasi-experimental studies over the years to support AA as a viable means to long-term recovery. A recent Cochrane Review of 27 studies (21 RCTs/quasi-RCTs, 5 non-randomized, and 1 purely economic study) (N=10,565) provides high quality evidence that manualized peer-led and professionally delivered treatments that facilitate AA involvement are more effective than other established treatments, such as CBT, for increasing abstinence for up to three years (Kelly et al., 2020).

There are other options for self-help that have emerged over the past few decades. These groups, like AA, are usually offered both in-person and online (e.g., Women for Sobriety (WFS), LifeRing Secular Recovery (LifeRing), and SMART Recovery; see Resources 7.8). There is an emerging literature base for these approaches, but it is still underdeveloped.

7.3 MINDFULNESS

Mindfulness practices are rooted in ancient traditions, intended to help the patient develop a focus on the present rather than worrying about the past or future. Many of the newer approaches to mindfulness integrate components of CBT and 12-step techniques. There have been several studies over the past several years that show its benefit in treating mental health conditions, including SUDs, across a variety of sub-groups. Witkiewitz and colleagues (2014) found women involved in the criminal justice system had significantly reduced substance use days and fewer legal and medical problems compared to the usual treatment program. The treatment program was designed to reduce relapse and was delivered in a residential setting. There is also evidence that mindfulness helps to reduce tobacco smoking for several months after the intervention (Brewer et al., 2011)

7.4 EXERCISE

Exercise in relation to treatment of addictions is an emerging field. Exercise has a host of implications for health, and the nurse should refer to the chapters specific to this topic for guidance on exercise recommendations. A MA of 22 RCTs found that exercise significantly increased abstinence rates among users of heroin, cocaine, alcohol, and nicotine (Wang et al., 2014). There were also significant reductions in anxiety and depression, and it helped to ease symptoms of withdrawal. This study supports several earlier studies across substances and populations. Importantly, most studies have been done in an inpatient setting, and there are often low adherence and high attrition rates after the individuals leave treatment; therefore, individuals might benefit from a structured exercise plan (Weinstock et al., 2017). The nurse should help the patient to integrate a lifestyle approach to exercise during the course of recovery.

7.5 DIET

Substance use impacts a person's nutrition in many ways. The basic physiological harm to the body can affect immune function via nutritional deficiencies and hormonal imbalances that impede healing. For example, chronic alcohol use leads to decreased thiamine and folic acid levels, while chronic exposure to alcohol, opioids, and other substances can alter testosterone and estrogen levels (see Table 7.3). A review of the literature by Jeynes and Gibson (2017) provides support for the essential role that a healthy diet plays in recovery. The nurse should approach this subject with guidance from the lifestyle medicine approach to nutrition.

7.6 ACUPUNCTURE

Acupuncture has been used to treat substance-related problems for more than three decades. While literature shows minimal effect in eliminating substance use, a 2016 RCT ($N=280$) found that acupuncture did correlate with lower anxiety and sleeping problems, even for those with psychiatric comorbidity (Ahlberg et al., 2016). Acupuncture has long been used to address pain and may be beneficial in that regard for substance users. Substances mask pain and sometimes cause hyperalgesia, intensifying pain when a person tries to reduce substance use (Yi et al., 2015). Acupuncture might also help to alleviate other symptoms associated with substance use. A small study done in Canada showed that offering voluntary, drop-in appointments for acupuncture ($N=2,755$ visits) helped to reduce withdrawal symptoms (hallucinations, stomach cramps, insomnia, nausea, sweating, heart palpitations) in the context of a community harm reduction model therapy for reduction of substance use (Janssen et al., 2005).

7.7 CONCLUSION

SUDs are chronic psychiatric conditions with complex etiologies and treatments. The nurse is in an ideal position to identify problematic substance use and intervene with patient-centered recommendations based on lifestyle modifications such as psychotherapy, self-help groups, diet, exercise, acupuncture, and mindfulness.

7.8 RESOURCES

7.8.1 SUBSTANCE USE SCREENING TOOLS

1. NIDA Quick Screen for Alcohol and Other Substances: https://archives.drugabuse.gov/ publications/resource-guide-screening-drug-use-in-general-medical-settings/nida-quick-screen
2. NIDA-Modified ASSIST: www.drugabuse.gov/sites/default/files/pdf/nmassist.pdf
3. CAGE Questionnaire: www.mdcalc.com/cage-questions-alcohol-use

7.8.2 SELF-HELP GROUPS

1. Alcoholics Anonymous: www.aa.org/
   Benefits include efficacy for sustained abstinence and reduction of substance consumption; free of charge; offered globally; strong social support network
2. SMART Recovery: www.smartrecovery.org/
   Benefits include social support, CBT/rational emotive behavior therapy style, ideal for individuals who want a very structured program

REFERENCES

Alcoholics anonymous big book (4th ed.). (2002). Alcoholics Anonymous World Services.

Ahlberg, R., Skårberg, K., Brus, O., & Kjellin, L. (2016). Auricular acupuncture for substance use: A randomized controlled trial of effects on anxiety, sleep, drug use and use of addiction treatment services. *Substance Abuse Treatment, Prevention, and Policy, 11*(1), 24. https://doi.org/10.1186/s13011-016-0068-z

Allis, C. D., & Jenuwein, T. (2016). The molecular hallmarks of epigenetic control. *Nature Reviews Genetics, 17*, 487–500. https://doi.org/10.1038/nrg.2016.59

American Psychiatric Association. (2013). *Diagnostic and statistical manual of mental disorders (DSM-5)* (5th ed.).

Anthenelli, R. M., Benowitz, N. L., West, R., St Aubin, L., McRae, T., Lawrence, D., Ascher, J., Russ, C., Krishen, A., & Evins, A. E. (2016). Neuropsychiatric safety and efficacy of varenicline, bupropion, and nicotine patch in smokers with and without psychiatric disorders (EAGLES): A double-blind, randomised, placebo-controlled clinical trial. *The Lancet, 387*(10037), 2507–2520. https://doi.org/10.1016/S0140-6736(16)30272-0

Babb, S., Malarcher, A., Schauer, G., Asman K., Jamal, G., Asman K., & Jamal, A. (2017). *Quitting smoking among adults — United States, 2000–2015* (Morbidity and Mortality Weekly Report, Vol. 65, No. 52). U.S. Department of Health & Human Services, Centers for Disease Control and Prevention. www.cdc.gov/mmwr/volumes/65/wr/mm6552a1.htm

Bernstein, J., Bernstein, E., Tassiopoulos, K., Heeren, T., Levenson, S., & Hingson, R. (2005). Brief motivational intervention at a clinic visit reduces cocaine and heroin use. *Drug and Alcohol Dependence, 77*(1), 49–59. https://doi.org/10.1016/j.drugalcdep.2004.07.006

Bien, T.H., Miller, W.R., & Tonigan, J.S. (1993). Brief interventions for alcohol problems: A review. *Addiction, 88*(3), 315–335.

Blacker, C. J., Frye, M. A., Morava, E., Kozicz, T., & Veldic, M. (2019). A review of epigenetics of PTSD in comorbid psychiatric conditions. *Genes, 10*(2), 140. https://doi.org/10.3390/genes10020140

Boucher, L. M., Marshall, Z., Martin, A., Larose-Hébert, K., Flynn, J. V., Lalonde, C., Pineau, D., Bigelow, J., Rose, T., Chase, R., Boyd, R., Tyndall, M., & Kendall, C. (2017). Expanding conceptualizations of harm reduction: Results from a qualitative community-based participatory research study with people who inject drugs. *Harm Reduction Journal, 14*(1), 18. https://doi.org/10.1186/s12954-017-0145-2

Brewer, J. A., Mallik, S., Babuscio, T. A., Nich, C., Johnson, H. E., Deleone, C. M., Minnix-Cotton, C. A., Byrne, S. A., Kober, H., Weinstein, A. J., Carroll, K. M., & Rounsaville, B. J. (2011). Mindfulness training for smoking cessation: Results from a randomized controlled trial. *Drug and Alcohol Dependence, 119*(1–2), 72–80. https://doi.org/10.1016/j.drugalcdep.2011.05.027

Carrico, A. W., Flentje, A., Gruber, V. A., Woods, W. J., Discepola, M. V., Dilworth, S. E., Neilands, T. B., Jain, J., & Siever, M. D. (2014). Community-based harm reduction substance abuse treatment with methamphetamine-using men who have sex with men. *Journal of Urban Health: Bulletin of the New York Academy of Medicine, 91*(3), 555–567. https://doi.org/10.1007/s11524-014-9870-y

Centers for Disease Control and Prevention. (May 11, 2021a). *Standard drink.* Alcohol and Public Health: Frequently Asked Questions. www.cdc.gov/alcohol/fact-sheets/alcohol-use.htm

Centers for Disease Control and Prevention. (May 11, 2021b). *What is excessive drinking?* Alcohol and Public Health: Frequently Asked Questions. www.cdc.gov/alcohol/fact-sheets/alcohol-use.htm

Chambers, J. E., Brooks, A. C., Medvin, R., Metzger, D. S., Lauby, J., Carpenedo, C. M., Favor, K. E., & Kirby, K. C. (2016). Examining multi-session brief intervention for substance use in primary care: Research methods of a randomized controlled trial. *Addiction Science & Clinical Practice, 11*(1), 8. https://doi.org/10.1186/s13722-016-0057-6

Charlet, K., & Heinz, A. (2017). Harm reduction—a systematic review on effects of alcohol reduction on physical and mental symptoms. *Addiction Biology*, *22*(5), 1119–1159. https://doi.org/10.1111/adb.12414

Choi, H. J., Krieger, J. L., & Hecht, M. L. (2013). Reconceptualizing efficacy in substance use prevention research: Refusal response efficacy and drug resistance self-efficacy in adolescent substance use. *Health Communication*, *28*(1), 40–52. https://doi.org/10.1080/10410236.2012.720245

Ciraulo, D. A., Dong, Q., Silverman, B. L., Gastfriend, D. R., & Pettinati, H. M. (2008). Early treatment response in alcohol dependence with extended-release naltrexone. *The Journal of Clinical Psychiatry*, *69*(2), 190–195. https://doi.org/10.4088/jcp.v69n0204

DiClemente C, Prochaska J. (1998). Toward a comprehensive, transtheoretical model of change. In W. R. Miller and N. Heather (Eds.), *Treating addictive behaviours* (2nd ed., pp. 3–24). Plenum Press.

Di Forti, M., Quattrone, D., Freeman, T. P., Tripoli, G., Gayer-Anderson, C., Quigley, H., Rodriguez, V., Jongsma, H. E., Ferraro, L., La Cascia, C., La Barbera, D., Tarricone, I., Berardi, D., Szöke, A., Arango, C., Tortelli, A., Velthorst, E., Bernardo, M., Del-Ben, C. M., Menezes, P. R., … EU-GEI WP2 Group (2019). The contribution of cannabis use to variation in the incidence of psychotic disorder across Europe (EU-GEI): A multicentre case-control study. *The Lancet Psychiatry*, *6*(5), 427–436. https://doi.org/10.1016/S2215-0366(19)30048-3

D'Onofrio, G., O'Connor, P. G., Pantalon, M. V., Chawarski, M. C., Busch, S. H., Owens, P. H., Bernstein, S. L., & Fiellin, D. A. (2015). Emergency department-initiated buprenorphine/naloxone treatment for opioid dependence: A randomized clinical trial. *JAMA*, *313*(16), 1636–1644. https://doi.org/10.1001/jama.2015.3474

Dunn, K. E., Harrison, J. A., Leoutsakos, J. M., Han, D., & Strain, E. C. (2017). Continuous abstinence during early alcohol treatment is significantly associated with positive treatment outcomes, independent of duration of abstinence. *Alcohol and Alcoholism*, *52*(1), 72–79. https://doi.org/10.1093/alcalc/agw059

Eskander, N., Chakrapani, S., & Ghani, M. R. (2020). The risk of substance use among adolescents and adults with eating disorders. *Cureus*, *12*(9), e10309. https://doi.org/10.7759/cureus.10309

Felitti, V. J., Anda, R. F., Nordenberg, D., Williamson, D. F., Spitz, A. M., Edwards, V., Koss, M. P., & Marks, J. S. (1998). Relationship of childhood abuse and household dysfunction to many of the leading causes of death in adults: The Adverse Childhood Experiences (ACE) Study. *American Journal of Preventive Medicine*, *14*(4), 245–258. https://doi.org/10.1016/s0749-3797(98)00017-8

Foxcroft, D. R., Coombes, L., Wood, S., Allen, D., Almeida Santimano, N. M., & Moreira, M. T. (2016). Motivational interviewing for the prevention of alcohol misuse in young adults. *The Cochrane Database of Systematic Reviews*, *7*(7), CD007025.

Gilchrist, G., Swan, D., Widyaratna, K., Marquez-Arrico, J. E., Hughes, E., Mdege, N. D., Martyn-St James, M., & Tirado-Munoz, J. (2017). A systematic review and meta-analysis of psychosocial interventions to reduce drug and sexual blood borne virus risk behaviours among people who inject drugs. *AIDS and Behavior*, *21*(7), 1791–1811. https://doi.org/10.1007/s10461-017-1755-0

Hawk, M., Coulter, R. W., Egan, J. E., Fisk, S., Friedman, M. R., Tula, M., & Kinsky, S. (2017). Harm reduction principles for healthcare settings. *Harm Reduction Journal*, *14*, 70. https://doi.org/10.1186/s12954-017-0196-4

Hettema, J., Steele, J., & Miller, W. R. (2005). Motivational interviewing. *Annual Review of Clinical Psychology*, *1*, 91–111. https://doi.org/10.1146/annurev.clinpsy.1.102803.143833

Janssen, P. A., Demorest, L. C., & Whynot, E. M. (2005). Acupuncture for substance abuse treatment in the Downtown Eastside of Vancouver. *Journal of Urban Health: Bulletin of the New York Academy of Medicine*, *82*(2), 285–295. https://doi.org/10.1093/jurban/jti054

Jellinek, E. M. (1960). *The disease concept of alcoholism*. Hillhouse Press.

Jeynes, K. D., & Gibson, E. L. (2017). The importance of nutrition in aiding recovery from substance use disorders: A review. *Drug and Alcohol Dependence*, *179*, 229–239. https://doi.org/10.1016/j.drugalcdep.2017.07.006

Joehanes, R., Just, A. C., Marioni, R. E., Pilling, L. C., Reynolds, L. M., Mandaviya, P. R., Guan, W., Xu, T., Elks, C. E., Aslibekyan, S., Moreno-Macias, H., Smith, J. A., Brody, J. A., Dhingra, R., Yousefi, P., Pankow, J. S., Kunze, S., Shah, S. H., McRae, A. F., Lohman, K., … London, S. J. (2016). Epigenetic signatures of cigarette smoking. *Circulation. Cardiovascular Genetics*, *9*(5), 436–447. https://doi.org/10.1161/CIRCGENETICS.116.001506

Jonas, D. E., Amick, H. R., Feltner, C., Bobashev, G., Thomas, K., Winners, R., Kim, M. M., Shanahan, E., Gass, E., Rowe, C. J., & Garbutt, J. (2014). *Pharmacotherapy for adults with alcohol-use disorders in outpatient settings: AHRQ comparative effectiveness review no. 134.* Agency for Healthcare Research and Quality. https://effectivehealthcare.ahrq.gov/products/alcohol-misuse-drug-therapy/policymaker

Kelly, J. F., Humphreys, K., & Ferri, M. (2020). Alcoholics Anonymous and other 12-step programs for alcohol use disorder. *The Cochrane Database of Systematic Reviews*, *3*(3), CD012880. https://doi.org/10.1002/14651858.CD012880.pub2

Khantzian, E. J. (1985). The self-medication hypothesis of addictive disorders: Focus on heroin and cocaine dependence. *American Journal of Psychiatry*, *142*(11), 1259–1264. https://doi.org/10.1176/ajp.142.11.1259

Khantzian, E. J. (2017, February 21). The theory of self-medication and addiction. *Psychiatric Times*, *34*(2). www.psychiatrictimes.com/addiction/ theory-self-medication-and-addiction

Khantzian, E. J. (2018). *Treating addiction: Beyond the pain.* Rowman & Littlefield.

Kim, Y., Je, Y., & Giovannucci, E. (2019). Coffee consumption and all-cause and cause-specific mortality: A meta-analysis by potential modifiers. *European Journal of Epidemiology*, *34*(8), 731–752. https://doi.org/10.1007/s10654-019-00524-3

Knapp, M., & Kozikowski, A. (2021). Harm reduction psychotherapy: A client with a substance use disorder. In C. Knight and K. Wheeler (Eds.), *Case study approach to psychotherapy for advanced practice psychiatric nurses*. Springer.

Knapp, M. M., & McCabe, D. E. (2019). Screening and interventions for substance use in primary care. *The Nurse Practitioner*, *44*(8), 48–55. https://doi.org/10.1097/01.NPR.0000574672.26862.24

Koob, G. F., & Volkow, N. D. (2010). Neurocircuitry of addiction. *Neuropsychopharmacology: Official Publication of the American College of Neuropsychopharmacology*, *35*(1), 217–238. https://doi.org/10.1038/npp.2009.110

Koob, G. F., & Volkow, N. D. (2016). Neurobiology of addiction: A neurocircuitry analysis. *The Lancet Psychiatry*, *3*(8), 760–773. https://doi.org/10.1016/S2215-0366(16)00104-8

Krist, A. H., Davidson, K. W., Mangione, C. M., Barry, M. J., Cabana, M., Caughey, A. B., … & US Preventive Services Task Force. (2020). Screening for unhealthy drug use: US Preventive Services Task Force recommendation statement. *Jama*, *323*(22), 2301–2309.

Kuehner, J. N., Bruggeman, E. C., Wen, Z., & Yao, B. (2019). Epigenetic regulations in neuropsychiatric disorders. *Frontiers in Genetics*, *10*, 268. https://doi.org/10.3389/fgene.2019.00268

Lee, J. D., Nunes, E. V., Jr., Novo, P., Bachrach, K., Bailey, G. L., Bhatt, S., Farkas, S., Fishman, M., Gauthier, P., Hodgkins, C. C., King, J., Lindblad, R., Liu, D., Matthews, A. G., May, J., Peavy, K. M., Ross, S., Salazar, D., Schkolnik, P., Shmueli-Blumberg, D., … Rotrosen, J. (2018). Comparative effectiveness of extended-release naltrexone versus buprenorphine-naloxone for opioid relapse prevention (X:BOT): A multicentre, open-label, randomised controlled trial. *The Lancet*, *391*(10118), 309–318. https://doi.org/10.1016/S0140-6736(17)32812-X

LeTendre, M. L., & Reed, M. B. (2017). The effect of adverse childhood experience on clinical diagnosis of a substance use disorder: Results of a nationally representative study. *Substance Use & Misuse*, *52*(6), 689–697. https://doi.org/10.1080/10826084.2016.1253746

Levounis, P., Zerbo, E., & Aggarwal, R. (2016). *Pocket guide to addiction assessment and treatment.* American Psychiatric Publishing.

Leichsenring, F., & Rabung, S. (2008). Effectiveness of long-term psychodynamic psychotherapy: A meta-analysis. *JAMA*, *300*(13), 1551–1565. https://doi.org/10.1001/jama.300.13.1551

Levy, S. J., Williams, J. F., Committee on Substance Use and Prevention, Ryan, S. A., Gonzalez, P. K., Patrick, S. W., Quigley, J., Siqueira, L., Smith, V. C., & Walker, L. R. (2016). Substance use screening, brief intervention, and referral to treatment. *Pediatrics*, *138*(1), e20161211. https://doi.org/10.1542/peds.2016-1211

Liu, M., Jiang, Y., Wedow, R., Li, Y., Brazel, D. M., Chen, F., Datta, G., Davila-Velderrain, J., McGuire, D., Tian, C., Zhan, X., 23andMe Research Team, HUNT All-In Psychiatry, Choquet, H., Docherty, A. R., Faul, J. D., Foerster, J. R., Fritsche, L. G., Gabrielsen, M. E., Gordon, S. D., … Vrieze, S. (2019). Association studies of up to 1.2 million individuals yield new insights into the genetic etiology of tobacco and alcohol use. *Nature Genetics*, *51*(2), 237–244. https://doi.org/10.1038/s41588-018-0307-5

Magill, M., & Ray, L. A. (2009). Cognitive-behavioral treatment with adult alcohol and illicit drug users: A meta-analysis of randomized controlled trials. *Journal of Studies on Alcohol and Drugs*, *70*(4), 516–527. https://doi.org/10.15288/jsad.2009.70.516

Magill, M., Ray, L., Kiluk, B., Hoadley, A., Bernstein, M., Tonigan, J. S., & Carroll, K. (2019). A meta-analysis of cognitive-behavioral therapy for alcohol or other drug use disorders: Treatment efficacy by contrast condition. *Journal of Consulting and Clinical Psychology*, *87*(12), 1093–1105. https://doi.org/10.1037/ccp0000447

Mattick, R. P., Kimber, J., Breen, C., & Davoli, M. (2004). Buprenorphine maintenance versus placebo or methadone maintenance for opioid dependence. *The Cochrane Database of Systematic Reviews*, (3), CD002207. https://doi.org/10.1002/14651858.CD002207.pub2

Mattick, R. P., Breen, C., Kimber, J., & Davoli, M. (2014). Buprenorphine maintenance versus placebo or methadone maintenance for opioid dependence. *The Cochrane Database of Systematic Reviews*, (2), CD002207. https://doi.org/10.1002/14651858.CD002207.pub4

McCartney, D. L., Stevenson, A. J., Hillary, R. F., Walker, R. M., Bermingham, M. L., Morris, S. W., Clarke, T. K., Campbell, A., Murray, A. D., Whalley, H. C., Porteous, D. J., Visscher, P. M., McIntosh, A. M., Evans, K. L., Deary, I. J., & Marioni, R. E. (2018). Epigenetic signatures of starting and stopping smoking. *EBioMedicine*, *37*, 214–220. https://doi.org/10.1016/j.ebiom.2018.10.051

McHugh, M. J., McGorry, P. D., Yung, A. R., Lin, A., Wood, S. J., Hartmann, J. A., & Nelson, B. (2017). Cannabis-induced attenuated psychotic symptoms: Implications for prognosis in young people at ultra-high risk for psychosis. *Psychological Medicine*, *47*(4), 616–626. https://doi-org/10.1017/S0033291716002671

Meier, M. H., Caspi, A., Ambler, A., Harrington, H., Houts, R., Keefe, R. S., McDonald, K., Ward, A., Poulton, R., & Moffitt, T. E. (2012). Persistent cannabis users show neuropsychological decline from childhood to midlife. *Proceedings of the National Academy of Sciences of the United States of America*, *109*(40), E2657–E2664. https://doi.org/10.1073/pnas.1206820109

Metz, T. D., & Borgelt, L. M. (2018). Marijuana use in pregnancy and while breastfeeding. *Obstetrics and Gynecology*, *132*(5), 1198–1210. https://doi.org/10.1097/AOG.0000000000002878

Miller, W. R., & Rollnick, S. (2013). *Motivational interviewing: Helping people change* (3rd ed.). Guilford Press.

Moosavi, A., & Motevalizadeh Ardekani, A. (2016). Role of epigenetics in biology and human diseases. *Iranian Biomedical Journal*, *20*(5), 246–258. https://doi.org/10.22045/ibj.2016.01

National Institute on Alcohol Abuse and Alcoholism. (2005). *Helping patients who drink too much: A clinician's guide*. US Department of Health and Human Services. https://pubs.niaaa.nih.gov/publications/practitioner/cliniciansguide2005/guide.pdf

National Institute on Drug Abuse. (2018, July). The science of drug use and addiction: The basics. www.drugabuse.gov/publications/media-guide/science-drug-use-addiction-basics

NIDA. (2020, July 13). Drug Misuse and Addiction. Retrieved on April 13, 2022, from https://nida.nih.gov/publications/drugs-brains-behavior-science-addiction/drug-misuse-addiction

Patnode, C. D., Henderson, J. T., Thompson, J. H., Senger, C. A., Fortmann, S. P., & Whitlock, E. P. (2015). Behavioral counseling and pharmacotherapy interventions for tobacco cessation in adults, including pregnant women: A review of reviews for the U.S. Preventive Services Task Force. *Annals of Internal Medicine*, *163*(8), 608–621. https://doi.org/10.7326/M15-0171

Polimanti, R., Peterson, R. E., Ong, J. S., MacGregor, S., Edwards, A. C., Clarke, T. K., Frank, J., Gerring, Z., Gillespie, N. A., Lind, P. A., Maes, H. H., Martin, N. G., Mbarek, H., Medland, S. E., Streit, F., Major Depressive Disorder Working Group of the Psychiatric Genomics Consortium, Agrawal, A., Edenberg, H. J., Kendler, K. S., Lewis, C. M., ... Derks, E. M. (2019). Evidence of causal effect of major depression on alcohol dependence: Findings from the psychiatric genomics consortium. *Psychological Medicine*, *49*(7), 1218–1226. https://doi.org/10.1017/S0033291719000667

Prochaska, J. O., DiClemente, C. C., & Norcross, J. C. (1992). In search of how people change: Applications to addictive behaviors. *The American Psychologist*, *47*(9), 1102–1114. https://doi.org/10.1037//0003-066x.47.9.1102

Rastegar, D., & Fingerhood, M. (2016). *The American Society of Addiction Medicine handbook of addiction medicine*. Oxford University Press.

Shield, K. D., Gmel, G., Gmel, G., Mäkelä, P., Probst, C., Room, R., & Rehm, J. (2017). Life-time risk of mortality due to different levels of alcohol consumption in seven European countries: Implications for low-risk drinking guidelines. *Addiction*, *112*(9), 1535–1544. https://doi.org/10.1111/add.13827

Smedslund, G., Berg, R. C., Hammerstrøm, K. T., Steiro, A., Leiknes, K. A., Dahl, H. M., & Karlsen, K. (2011). Motivational interviewing for substance abuse. *The Cochrane Database of Systematic Reviews*, (5), CD008063. https://doi.org/10.1002/14651858.CD008063.pub2

Smith, P. C., Schmidt, S. M., Allensworth-Davies, D., & Saitz, R. (2009). Primary care validation of a single-question alcohol screening test. *Journal of General Internal Medicine*, *24*(7), 783–788. https://doi.org/10.1007/s11606-009-0928-6

Smith, P. C., Schmidt, S. M., Allensworth-Davies, D., & Saitz, R. (2010). A single-question screening test for drug use in primary care. *Archives of Internal Medicine*, *170*(13), 1155–1160. https://doi.org/10.1001/archinternmed.2010.140

Standridge, J. B., Zylstra, R. G., & Adams, S. M. (2004). Alcohol consumption: An overview of benefits and risks. *Southern Medical Journal*, *97*(7), 664–672. https://pubmed.ncbi.nlm.nih.gov/15301124

Stapleton, J., West, R., Hajek, P., Wheeler, J., Vangeli, E., Abdi, Z., O'Gara, C., McRobbie, H., Humphrey, K., Ali, R., Strang, J., & Sutherland, G. (2013). Randomized trial of nicotine replacement therapy (NRT), bupropion and NRT plus bupropion for smoking cessation: Effectiveness in clinical practice. *Addiction*, *108*(12), 2193–2201. https://doi.org/10.1111/add.12304

Stickrath E. (2019). Marijuana use in pregnancy: An updated look at marijuana use and its impact on pregnancy. *Clinical Obstetrics and Gynecology*, *62*(1), 185–190. https://doi.org/10.1097/GRF.0000000000000415

Sweeney, M. M., Weaver, D. C., Vincent, K. B., Arria, A. M., & Griffiths, R. R. (2020). Prevalence and correlates of caffeine use disorder symptoms among a United States sample. *Journal of Caffeine and Adenosine Research*, *10*(1), 4–11. https://doi.org/10.1089/caff.2019.0020

Substance Abuse and Mental Health Services Administration. (2018). *Key substance use and mental health indicators in the United States: Results from the 2017 National Survey on Drug Use and Health*. Center for Behavioral Health Statistics and Quality, Substance Abuse and Mental Health Services Administration.

Substance Abuse and Mental Health Services Administration. (2020). *Key substance use and mental health indicators in the United States: Results from the 2019 National Survey on Drug Use and Health*. Center for Behavioral Health Statistics and Quality, Substance Abuse and Mental Health Services Administration. www.samhsa.gov/data/

Taylor, D., Carlyle, J. A., McPherson, S., Rost, F., Thomas, R., & Fonagy, P. (2012). Tavistock Adult Depression Study (TADS): A randomised controlled trial of psychoanalytic psychotherapy for treatment-resistant/treatment-refractory forms of depression. *BMC Psychiatry*, *12*, 60. https://doi.org/10.1186/1471-244X-12-60

Thompson-Brenner, H., Eddy, K. T., Franko, D. L., Dorer, D., Vashchenko, M., & Herzog, D. B. (2008). Personality pathology and substance abuse in eating disorders: a longitudinal study. *The International Journal of Eating Disorders*, *41*(3), 203–208. https://doi.org/10.1002/eat.20489

Town, J. M., Diener, M. J., Abbass, A., Leichsenring, F., Driessen, E., & Rabung, S. (2012). A meta-analysis of psychodynamic psychotherapy outcomes: Evaluating the effects of research-specific procedures. *Psychotherapy*, *49*(3), 276–290. https://doi.org/10.1037/a0029564

United Nations Office on Drugs and Crime. (2021, June 21). World Drug Report. www.unodc.org/unodc/en/data-and-analysis/wdr2021.html

US Food and Drug Administration. (n.d.) Spilling the beans: How much caffeine is too much? www.fda.gov/consumers/consumer-updates/spilling-beans-how-much-caffeine-too-much

van Amsterdam, J., & van den Brink, W. (2013). Reduced-risk drinking as a viable treatment goal in problematic alcohol use and alcohol dependence. *Journal of Psychopharmacology*, *27*(11), 987–997. https://doi.org/10.1177/0269881113495320

Volkow, N. D., Koob, G. F., & McLellan, A. T. (2016). Neurobiologic advances from the brain disease model of addiction. *The New England Journal of Medicine*, *374*(4), 363–371. https://doi.org/10.1056/NEJMra1511480

Walker, D. M., & Nestler, E. J. (2018). Neuroepigenetics and addiction. *Handbook of Clinical Neurology*, *148*, 747–765. https://doi.org/10.1016/B978-0-444-64076-5.00048-X

Walters, R. K., Polimanti, R., Johnson, E. C., McClintick, J. N., Adams, M. J., Adkins, A. E., Aliev, F., Bacanu, S. A., Batzler, A., Bertelsen, S., Biernacka, J. M., Bigdeli, T. B., Chen, L. S., Clarke, T. K., Chou, Y. L., Degenhardt, F., Docherty, A. R., Edwards, A. C., Fontanillas, P., Foo, J. C., … Agrawal, A. (2018). Transancestral GWAS of alcohol dependence reveals common genetic underpinnings with psychiatric disorders. *Nature Neuroscience*, *21*(12), 1656–1669. https://doi.org/10.1038/s41593-018-0275-1

Wang, D., Wang, Y., Wang, Y., Li, R., & Zhou, C. (2014). Impact of physical exercise on substance use disorders: A meta-analysis. *PloS One*, *9*(10), e110728. https://doi.org/10.1371/journal.pone.0110728

Wang, T.W., Gentzke, A., Sharapova, S., Cullen, K.A., Ambrose, B.K., & Jamal, A. (2018) *Tobacco product use among middle and high school students—United States, 2011–2017* (Morbidity and Mortality Weekly

Report, Vol. 67, No. 22). U.S. Department of Health and Human Services, Centers for Disease Control and Prevention. www.cdc.gov/mmwr/volumes/67/wr/mm6722a3.htm

Weinstock, J., Farney, M. R., Elrod, N. M., Henderson, C. E., & Weiss, E. P. (2017). Exercise as an adjunctive treatment for substance use disorders: Rationale and intervention description. *Journal of Substance Abuse Treatment, 72*, 40–47. https://doi.org/10.1016/j.jsat.2016.09.002

Willenbring, M. L. (2013). Gaps in clinical prevention and treatment for alcohol use disorders: Costs, consequences, and strategies. *Alcohol Research: Current Reviews, 35*(2), 238–243.

Witkiewitz K. (2008). Lapses following alcohol treatment: Modeling the falls from the wagon. *Journal of Studies on Alcohol and Drugs, 69*(4), 594–604. https://doi.org/10.15288/jsad.2008.69.594

Witkiewitz, K., Warner, K., Sully, B., Barricks, A., Stauffer, C., Thompson, B. L., & Luoma, J. B. (2014). Randomized trial comparing mindfulness-based relapse prevention with relapse prevention for women offenders at a residential addiction treatment center. *Substance Use & Misuse, 49*(5), 536–546. https://doi.org/10.3109/10826084.2013.856922

Witkiewitz, K., Wilson, A. D., Pearson, M. R., Hallgren, K. A., Falk, D. E., Litten, R. Z., Kranzler, H. R., Mann, K. F., Hasin, D. S., O'Malley, S. S., & Anton, R. F. (2017). Temporal stability of heavy drinking days and drinking reductions among heavy drinkers in the COMBINE study. *Alcoholism, Clinical and Experimental Research, 41*(5), 1054–1062. https://doi.org/10.1111/acer.13371

Yi, P., & Pryzbylkowski, P. (2015). Opioid induced hyperalgesia. *Pain Medicine, 16*(Suppl 1), S32–S36. https://doi.org/10.1111/pme.12914

8 Environmental Toxins

Mikki Meadows-Oliver
Rory Meyers College of Nursing
New York University
New York, New York, USA

CONTENTS

KEY POINTS

- Environmental toxins are ubiquitous in our environment. They affect the air we breathe, the water and food we ingest, and the places we live and play.
- Air pollution exposure is widespread, and air pollutants may be encountered in both the indoor and outdoor environments. Common air pollutants to which humans are exposed include environmental tobacco smoke, ground level ozone, and particulate matter.
- Common environmental toxins found in the built environment include bisphenol A (BPA), phthalates, lead, and radon. Radon is the second leading cause of lung cancer after cigarette smoking.
- Environmental toxins found in food and drink include arsenic, lead, mercury, and pesticides. Arsenic, lead, and mercury are naturally occurring elements in the Earth's crust. Pesticides (which include herbicides, insecticides, and fungicides) are man-made environmental toxins.
- In the United States, low-income communities and communities of color often face disproportionate burdens of exposure to environmental toxins both inside and outside of the home.
- In addition to individual lifestyle factors, conditions such as hypertension, obesity, and type 2 diabetes may be affected by exposures to endocrine disrupting chemicals and disparities in exposures to environmental toxins.
- Global commitment by governments worldwide is needed to reduce the use of environmental toxins in order to protect human health and the environment.

DOI: 10.1201/9781003178330-9

8.1 INTRODUCTION

Human health is influenced by the air we breathe, the water and food we ingest, and our built environment. The built environment encompasses man-made structures that provide spaces where people live, work, go to school, or take part in recreational activities (Environmental Protection Agency [EPA], 2020). Toxins and toxicants are present in each of these environments. Toxins are poisonous substances produced by animals, plants, or microorganisms such as bacteria. An example of a toxin is botulinum toxin, the bacteria that causes botulism. Toxicants are man-made toxic chemicals such as pesticides. The phrase "environmental toxins" typically encompasses both toxins and toxicants and will be used throughout this chapter.

Exposure to environmental toxins is a nursing and public health challenge that contributes to adverse health outcomes. While environmental hazards are discussed individually in this chapter, it is important to note that these environmental toxins may have an additive or synergistic role in their effects on human health. For instance, air pollutants such as particulate matter and ozone typically occur as a mixture of pollutants rather than as single air pollutants that affect human health.

Some populations, such as children and pregnant women, are more vulnerable than others to the effects of environmental toxins. Infants and small children may be more susceptible because their bodies and brains are still developing. Unfortunately, the effects of exposure early in childhood may not be realized until later in life as many children do not often experience immediate symptoms when exposed to environmental toxins. An additional factor that places children at risk for exposure to environmental toxins is that they tend to have more hand to mouth behavior, which makes them more likely to be exposed to ingestible toxins (such as lead dust) than older children or adults. (CDC, 2021).

8.2 ENVIRONMENTAL TOXINS IN THE AIR

Air pollution exposure is widespread, and air pollutants may be encountered in both the indoor and outdoor environments. Common air pollutants to which humans are exposed include environmental tobacco smoke, ground level ozone, and particulate matter. The health effects of exposure to environmental tobacco smoke are covered in Chapter 23 of this volume.

8.2.1 OZONE

Ozone (O3) is a highly reactive gas composed of three oxygen atoms. Ozone occurs naturally in the environment but can also be a man-made product that has adverse effects on human health. Stratospheric ozone occurs naturally and reduces the amount of harmful ultraviolet radiation that reaches the Earth's surface. Ground level ozone is formed from man-made processes and is able to be inhaled by humans. Ground level ozone is mainly formed from photochemical reactions between two major classes of air pollutants, volatile organic compounds (VOC) and nitrogen oxides. Significant sources of VOC in the environment are chemical plants, gasoline pumps, and autobody shops. Nitrogen oxides result primarily from high temperature combustion from sources such as power plants, industrial furnaces and boilers, and motor vehicles (EPA, 2021a).

Ground level ozone may affect human health in several ways. It is an irritant that causes damage to the mucous membrane of the respiratory tract. Long-term exposure to ozone has been associated with airway inflammation, compromised lung function, and increased mortality related to diseases of the respiratory system (Breitner et al., 2021; Karakatsani et al., 2017). Those with airway inflammation and compromised lung function may be less likely to participate in exercise and physical activities. Physical activity is important to overall health, and consistent physical activity helps to improve psychological well-being and quality of life (Hale et al., 2021).

Parks are outdoor spaces where people may engage in recreational physical activity, and access to parks and urban green spaces may provide a place to help people counteract a trend toward more sedentary lifestyles. While parks may contribute to health and well-being through decreased psycho-social stress, increased social ties, and increased physical activity, they are also places where people may encounter air pollution. Air pollution in parks is partly dependent on the park's geographical location. Disparities in air pollutants in parks have been found in more disadvantaged communities compared to parks in more affluent neighborhoods. Exposure to ground level ozone was significantly higher in the disadvantaged community parks (Winter et al., 2019). This disparity in exposure to air pollutants may adversely impact the ability of people in disadvantaged neighborhoods to fully participate in physical activities that may improve health and decrease risks for preventable chronic illnesses such as hypertension and obesity.

8.2.2 Particulate Matter

Particulate matter (PM) is a phrase that describes a mixture of solid particles and liquid droplets found in the air. Particles may be visible to the naked eye, such as dust or smoke, or may be so small that they are visible only when using an electron microscope. Information about particulate matter is reported according to the size of the particle being studied, either PM_{10} or $PM_{2.5}$. PM_{10} are inhalable particles, with diameters that are generally 10 micrometers and smaller, whereas $PM_{2.5}$ are considered to be fine inhalable particles, with diameters of 2.5 micrometers and smaller. To provide a scale, a single human hair is typically 50–70 micrometers (EPA, 2021b).

Exposure to particulate matter has been shown to increase the risk for cardiovascular and respiratory diseases (Elliot et al., 2020). As with ground level ozone, air pollution associated with PM may interfere with a person's ability to participate in regular physical activities. Physical activity is a strong modifiable factor associated with cardiovascular disease risk. During outdoor physical activities, increased respiration may increase air pollution dose, potentially attenuating the benefits of physical activity on cardiovascular disease (Elliot et al., 2020).

PM air pollution exposure was associated with increased prevalence of hypertension (Li et al. 2020), a higher risk of weight gain in children and adolescents (de Bont et al. 2019), and an increased risk of obesity and weight gain in a large, predominantly male cohort of U.S. veterans (Bowe et al., 2021). $PM_{2.5}$ has also been found to be a metabolic risk associated with the development of diabetes mellitus (Bowe et al. 2018).

8.3 ENVIRONMENTAL TOXINS IN THE BUILT ENVIRONMENT

Common environmental toxins found in the built environment include bisphenol A (BPA), phthalates, lead, and radon.

8.3.1 Bisphenol A and Phthalates

Bisphenol A (BPA) is an industrial chemical used to make certain plastics. BPA is used in a variety of products in the home, including food/beverage storage containers, toys, and food can linings. Phthalates are chemicals used to make plastics more durable. They may also be used to help other products dissolve (such as hair sprays—allowing them to form a flexible film on hair).

Both BPA and phthalates have been shown to have adverse effects on human health. BPAs and phthalates are known endocrine disruptors—chemicals that interfere with the action of the body's natural hormones. Exposure to BPAs have adverse effects on hormones such as estrogen and thyroid hormone (Vom Saal & Vandenberg, 2020). BPAs have been reported to disrupt appetite regulation and lipid metabolism and are associated with obesity, which places individuals at high risk for chronic disorders such as type 2 diabetes and cardiovascular disease (Amin et al., 2019; Zarean et al., 2018). Phthalates have been associated with being overweight, higher systolic blood pressure, and increased triglyceride level—all of which are associated with an adverse cardiac profile (Silva et al., 2021).

8.3.2 LEAD

Lead is a naturally occurring element found throughout the environment. In the home, it may be found in paint, leaded crystal glasses, ceramics, and plumbing materials. Lead may also be found in soil from past emissions related to the use of leaded gasoline (Markowitz, 2019) and from contaminated sites such as former lead smelters (EPA, 2021c).

In children, the main source of lead poisoning is from ingestion of lead-based paint chips or dust particles from lead-based paint. Children can also come into contact with lead from foreign spices and traditional medicines that have been contaminated with lead (Markowitz, 2019). Drinking water can also be a source of exposure to lead, as seen in the Flint, Michigan, water crisis, where lead from aging pipes leached in the city's water supply, exposing nearly 100,000 people to elevated levels of lead in their residential drinking water (Sadler, LaChance, & Hanna-Attisha, 2017).

Occupational exposures are the main source of lead exposures for adults. Adults who perform renovation or repair work that disturbs painted surfaces in older homes and buildings are at risk for lead exposure. Individuals who participate in hobbies where lead is used, such as stained glass making, are also at risk for increased lead exposure (EPA, 2021c).

When ingested or inhaled, lead can have adverse effects on the human body. Lead is a known neurotoxin, and its neurotoxicological effects are irreversible. In children, exposure to elevated levels of lead may result in learning and behavior problems as well as problems hearing. In adults, exposure to elevated levels of lead may result in decreased kidney function and increased blood pressure (EPA, 2021c).

8.3.3 RADON

Radon is a naturally occurring radioactive gas produced by the breakdown of uranium in rock, soil, and water. Radon gas is invisible, tasteless, and odorless. It is a known carcinogen. After smoking, radon is the second-leading cause of lung cancer (Vienneau et al., 2017). Radon is potentially one of the worst environmental hazards in the home environment. Humans are exposed to radon when the radon gas passes through cracks and openings in walls and foundations and into spaces such as basements and lower levels of homes, where individuals inhale radon. Inhaled radon deposits in an individual's respiratory tract, where they decay and irradiate lung tissues (Vienneau et al., 2017).

In addition to the underlying geology of the environment, there are several factors that determine whether someone is at risk for developing lung cancer from radon exposure: the dose (measure of radon in the home), host factors (smoking status), and the duration of exposure (time spent in the house) (Nwako & Cahill, 2020). Radon exposure has also been associated with the development of cancers besides lung cancer. Researchers noted a statistically significant increased risk of death from malignant melanoma and skin cancer in adults associated with exposure to radon (Vienneau et al., 2017).

8.4   ENVIRONMENTAL TOXINS IN FOOD AND DRINK

Environmental toxins found in food and drink include arsenic, lead, mercury, and pesticides.

8.4.1 ARSENIC

Arsenic is a naturally occurring element present in the Earth's crust. It is found in organic and inorganic forms. The inorganic forms are toxic to humans. Arsenic has been discovered in ground water and in the food supply—mainly in rice and poultry. Much of the contamination in groundwater is a result of the use of arsenic-based pesticides and wood preservatives. Although inorganic arsenic-based pesticides have not been used in the United States for decades, the residues still exist in soil today. Pesticides and fertilizers with organic forms of arsenic are still used in farming (Streit, 2021).

Due to groundwater contamination and the continued use of organic arsenic-based pesticides, many plant foods grown in soil will contain some arsenic. Contaminated water used for crop irrigation may be an additional contributor to arsenic in foods. Thus, contamination in both soil and water is responsible for arsenic in foods (Nachman, et al., 2019).

Rice is often grown in areas with soil previously treated with large amounts of inorganic arsenic-based pesticides, potentially causing rice to contain high amounts of inorganic arsenic. Additionally, products derived from rice, such as rice milk, rice bran, brown rice syrup, and rice cereal for babies are also sources of inorganic arsenic in the food supply (Streit, 2021). People with celiac disease may have increased dietary arsenic exposure due to a rice-based, gluten-free diet (Nachman, et al., 2019).

Arsenic exposure has several established adverse health effects. It is an endocrine disruptor that affects glucose homeostasis and has been associated with type 2 diabetes (Konkel, 2020). Inorganic arsenic has been associated with increased blood pressure and has been identified as a known human carcinogen. Arsenic may be associated with atherosclerosis and may impede the function of high-density lipoproteins (Streit, 2021). Elevated levels of arsenic exposure in ground water have been shown to significantly increase the risk of developing peripheral neuropathy (Pizzorno & Crinnion, 2017).

8.4.2 Lead

Although lead was mentioned in the previous section on the built environment, it deserves mention as an environmental toxin that is potentially present in drinking water and some food products. Lead in contaminated soil may eventually move from the soil into groundwater—posing a potential concern for families with well water. Older private wells (more than 25 years old) may contain leaded-brass components that may cause lead to seep into the drinking water (CDC, 2015). Lead may also enter drinking water through corrosion of pipes and other plumbing materials that bring water to the home. Homes built before 1986 are more likely to have lead pipes, fixtures, and solder (EPA, 2021c).

Lead may enter the food supply if lead in contaminated soil is absorbed by plants grown for fruits and vegetables. Additionally, lead can leach into food from being stored in food containers contaminated with lead (United States Food and Drug Administration, 2020). Lead has also been found in spices such as turmeric that have been imported to the United States (Kappel et al., 2021).

8.4.3 Mercury

Mercury is a naturally occurring element found in the Earth's crust. It exists in three forms: elemental mercury, inorganic mercury compounds, and organic compounds such as methylmercury. Humans are exposed to mercury in several ways: through their occupations (e.g. dentistry); contact with products that contain mercury (e.g. dental amalgams); or from environmental contamination (EPA, 2021d).

Dietary consumption of contaminated shellfish and fish is a significant source of mercury exposure. Shellfish and large, predatory species of fish (e.g. tuna, swordfish, grouper, mackerel) have been found to be the most highly contaminated seafoods. Fish-consumption advisories have been issued for pregnant women and women of childbearing age to avoid mercury neurotoxic effects on the fetus (Hu, Singh, & Chan, 2018). Rice, mentioned previously as a source of arsenic exposure, may also be grown in sites heavily contaminated with mercury, representing an additional source of mercury exposure for some communities (Basu et al., 2018).

Like other naturally occurring environmental toxins discussed in this chapter, exposure to mercury has adverse effects on human health. Similar to lead, mercury is a neurotoxin. It affects the nervous system causing such symptoms as tremors, weakness, and mental disturbances (Bagheri Hosseinabadi et al., 2020). In addition to its toxic effects on the neurological system, exposure to mercury has also been associated with hypertension (Hu, Singh, & Chan, 2018) and an elevated risk of developing colorectal cancer (Kim, et al., 2020).

8.4.4 PESTICIDES

A pesticide is a broad term used to describe a substance used to destroy insects or other organisms deemed harmful to cultivated plants. Pesticides can include herbicides, which help destroy weeds; insecticides, for controlling the insect population; and fungicides, which prevent the growth of molds and mildew. Because pesticides are often used in agriculture, humans are exposed to chemicals from pesticides in the food supply (National Institute of Environmental Health Sciences, 2021). Some individuals, such as those who work on farms, are exposed to pesticides during the course of their daily work—through skin and mucous membrane exposure. Organic farming systems allow use of some biologically based pesticides that have not been shown to have the same problematic health effects as chemical-based pesticides (Benbrook & Davis, 2020).

While pesticides can be helpful in protecting crops in the farming industry, they can be harmful to the human body. Pesticides are often fat-soluble and can accumulate in the human body, resulting in adverse health effects. Pesticides can act as endocrine disruptors and have also been associated with the development of autoimmune disorders and some cancers such as Hodgkin's lymphoma (Latifovic et al., 2020), renal cell carcinoma (Andreotti, et al., 2020), and liver cancer in those that apply pesticides to crops (National Institutes of Health, 2021). Parkinson's disease is a known consequence of organochlorine pesticide exposures (Kessman & Rais, 2020).

8.5 ENVIRONMENTAL HEALTH DISPARITIES

In the United States, low-income individuals and communities of color often face disproportionate burdens of exposure to environmental toxins. Compared to those in more affluent areas, individuals in low-income communities often live in neighborhoods with poorer air quality, more environmental hazards, and fewer health-promoting environmental amenities, such as parks (Winter et al., 2019).

People in low-income areas disproportionately face deteriorating housing conditions and corroded plumbing, which puts them at risk of lead poisoning—as such homes are more likely to have lead in paint and plumbing (Sadler et al., 2017). These same individuals are likely to be from communities and households that are facing complex challenges of inadequate housing, unemployment, lack of access to quality health care, improper nutrition, and other issues that pose risk factors for exposure to environmental toxins (Whitehead & Buchanan, 2019). Individuals in more affluent areas may be better equipped to shield against exposure to environmental hazards through improved nutrition, home improvements of lead in paint and the elimination of radon, decreased exposure to environmental toxins in air and soil, or the ability to afford water alternatives to avoid drinking contaminated water (Sadler, et al., 2017).

Differences in exposures to environmental toxins may contribute to health disparities in environmentally sensitive health conditions such as hypertension, cancer, and asthma (Schaider, et al., 2019). While treatment of health issues that accompany increased exposures to environmental toxins is of great significance, addressing the underlying causes that may contribute to exposure disparities and produce environmental inequities is important as well (Whitehead & Buchanan, 2019).

8.6 CONCLUSION

Environmental toxins are ubiquitous and cannot be totally avoided. Individuals may be exposed to environmental toxins both inside their homes (lead and radon) and outside of their homes (ground level ozone and particulate matter). Exposures to environmental toxins may be minimized if people are educated on how toxins affect human health and ways to limit contact with environmental hazards. Nurses can apply their knowledge to communicate the risks of exposure to environmental toxins and engage with communities to improve and protect health.

Hypertension, obesity, and type 2 diabetes have long been recognized in a category of potentially preventable chronic issues. As more research is being conducted, it is becoming clearer that in addition to individual lifestyle factors, these conditions may be affected by exposures to endocrine disrupting chemicals and disparities in exposures to environmental toxins. While nutrition and physical activity are encouraged to decrease the incidence and progression of certain chronic illnesses, it is important to take into account environmental toxins that may be present in an individual's food or water sources and air pollution that may be present in their recreational spaces. Bowe et al. (2021) remind health practitioners that discussions about the epidemiology of obesity should consider its association with $PM_{2.5}$.

Many studies mentioned in this chapter researched environmental toxins individually. However, it is important to note that exposures to environmental toxins do not occur in isolation; people will likely be exposed to more than one hazard at the same time. The synergistic effect of these environmental exposures might, in conjunction, exert a larger effect than either environmental toxin would alone.

While empowering individuals with knowledge about environmental toxins is the first step, regulatory advances are essential for effective, measurable interventions to lower exposures to environmental toxins. Nurses can advocate for policies that create standards and enforceable regulations for exposures to environmental toxins. Additionally, nurses can assist policymakers and decision makers prioritize activities to benefit communities disproportionately burdened by contact with multiple environmental health hazards. As exposure to environmental toxins is not a problem limited to the United States, global commitment by governments worldwide is needed to reduce the use of environmental toxins in order to protect human health and the environment.

REFERENCES

Amina, M., Ebrahima, K., Hashemi, M., Shoshtari-Yeganeha, B., Rafieia, N., Mansouriane, M., & Kelishadi, R. (2019). Association of exposure to Bisphenol A with obesity and cardiometabolic risk factors in children and adolescents. *International Journal of Environmental Health Research*, 29, 94–106.

Andreotti, G., Beane-Freeman, L., Shearer, J., Lerro, C., Koutros, S., & Parks, C., ... Hofmann, J. (2020). Occupational pesticide use and risk of renal cell carcinoma in the Agricultural Health Study. *Environmental Health Perspectives*, 128, 067011.

Basu, N., Horvat, M., Evers, D., Zastenskaya, I., Weihe, P., & Tempowski, J. (2018). A state-of-the-science review of mercury biomarkers in human populations worldwide between 2000 and 2018. *Environmental Health Perspectives*, 126, 106001.

Benbrook, C., & Davis, D. (2020). The dietary risk index system: A tool to track pesticide dietary risks. *Environmental Health*, 19, 103.

Bowe, B., Xie, Y., Li, T., Yan, Y., Xian, H., & Al-Aly, Z. (2018). The 2016 global and national burden of diabetes mellitus attributable to $PM_{2.5}$ air pollution. *Lancet Planet Health*, 2, e301–e312.

Bowe, B., Gibson, A., Xie, Y., Yan Y., van Donkelaar, A., Martin, R., & Al-Aly, Z. (2021). Ambient fine particulate matter air pollution and risk of weight gain and obesity in United States veterans: An observational cohort study. *Environmental Health Perspectives*, 129, 047003.

Breitner, S., Steckling-Muschack, N., Markevych, I., Zhao, T., Mertes, H., Nowak, D., & Heinrich, J. (2021). The burden of COPD due to ozone exposure in Germany. *Deutsches Ärzteblatt International*, 118, 491–496.

Centers for Disease Control and Prevention (2015). Lead and drinking water from private wells. www.cdc.gov/healthywater/drinking/private/wells/disease/lead.html

Centers for Disease Control and Prevention. (2021). Childhood lead poisoning prevention: Populations at higher risk. Retrieved from: www.cdc.gov/nceh/lead/prevention/populations.htm

de Bont, J., Casas, M., Barrera-Gómez, J., Cirach, M., Rivas, I., &, Valvi, D. (2019). Ambient air pollution and overweight and obesity in school-aged children in Barcelona, Spain. *Environment International*, 125, 58–64.

Elliott, E., Laden, F., James, P., Rimm, E., Rexrode, K., & Hart, J. (2020). Interaction between long-term exposure to fine particulate matter and physical activity, and risk of cardiovascular disease and overall mortality in U.S. women. *Environmental Health Perspectives*, 128, Article 127012.

Environmental Protection Agency. (2020). Basic information about the built environment. Retrieved from: www.epa.gov/smm/basic-information-about-built-environment

Environmental Protection Agency. (2021a). What is ozone? Retrieved from: www.epa.gov/ozone-pollution-and-your-patients-health/what-ozone

Environmental Protection Agency. (2021b). Particulate matter (PM) basics. Retrieved from: www.epa.gov/pm-pollution/particulate-matter-pm-basics

Environmental Protection Agency. (2021c). Learn about lead. Retrieved from: www.epa.gov/lead/learn-about-lead

Environmental Protection Agency. (2021d). Basic information about mercury. Retrieved from: www.epa.gov/mercury/basic-information-about-mercury

Hale, G., Colquhoun, L., Lancastle, D., Lewis, N., & Tyson, P. (2021). Review: Physical activity interventions for the mental health and well-being of adolescents—a systematic review. *Child & Adolescent Mental Health*, 26, 357–368.

Bagheri Hosseinabadi, M., Khanjani, N., Mobarake, M., & Shirkhanloo, H. (2020). Neuropsychosocial effects of long-term occupational exposure to mercury among chloralkali workers. *Work*, 66(3), 491–498.

Hu, X., Singh, K., & Chan, H. (2018). Mercury exposure, blood pressure, and hypertension: A systematic review and dose–response meta-analysis. *Environmental Health Perspectives*, 126, 076002.

Kappel, M., Kraushaar, V., Mehretu, A., Slater, W., & Marquez, E. (2021). Childhood lead poisoning associated with turmeric spices—Las Vegas, 2019. *Morbidity and Mortality Weekly Report (MMWR)*, 70, 1584–1585.

Karakatsani, A., Samoli, E., Rodopoulou, S., Dimakopoulou, K., Papakosta, D., Spyratos, D., Grivas, G., Tasi, S., Angelis, N., Thirios, A., Tsiotsios, A., & Katsouyanni, K. (2017). Weekly personal ozone exposure and respiratory health in a panel of Greek schoolchildren. *Environmental Health Perspectives*, 125, 077016.

Kessman, J., & Rais, A. (2020). Climate change, pesticides, and health consequences. *Family Doctor*, 8, 36–39.

Kim, H., Lee, J., Woo, H., Kim, D., Oh, J., Chang, H., Sohn, D., Shin, A., & Kim, J. (2020). Dietary mercury intake and colorectal cancer risk: A case-control study. *Clinical Nutrition*, 39, 2106–2113.

Konkel, L. (2020). Arsenic exposure and glucose metabolism: Experimental studies suggest implications for type 2 diabetes. *Environmental Health Perspectives*, 128, 094003.

Latifovic, L., Beane-Freeman, L., Spinelli, J., Pahwal, M., Kachuri1, L., Blair, A., … Harris, S. (2020). Pesticide use and risk of Hodgkin lymphoma: Results from the North American Pooled Project (NAPP). *Cancer Causes & Control*, 31, 583–599.

Li, N., Chen, G., Liu, F., Mao, S., Liu, Y., & Liu S. (2020). Associations between long-term exposure to air pollution and blood pressure and effect modifications by behavioral factors. *Environmental Research*, 182, 109109.

Markowitz, M. (2021). Lead poisoning: An update. *Pediatrics in Review*, 42, 302–315.

Nachman, K., Punshon, T., Rardin, L., Signes-Pastor, A., Murray, C., Jackson, B., … Karagas, M. (2018). Opportunities and challenges for dietary arsenic intervention. *Environmental Health Perspectives*, 126, 084503.

National Institute of Environmental Health Sciences. (2021). Pesticides. Retrieved from: www.niehs.nih.gov/health/topics/agents/pesticides/index.cfm

National Institutes of Health. (2021) Agricultural Health Study: 2021 study update. Retrieved from: https://aghealth.nih.gov/news/2021.html

Nwako, P. & Cahill, T. (2020). Radon gas exposure knowledge among public health educators, health officers, nurses, and registered environmental health specialists: A cross-sectional study. *Journal of Environmental Health*, 82, 22–28.

Pizzorno, J., & Crinnion, W. (2017). Arsenic: The underrecognized common disease-inducing toxin. *Integrative Medicine*, 16, 8–13.

Sadler, R., LaChance, J., & Hanna-Attisha, M. (2017). Social and built environmental correlates of predicted blood lead levels in the Flint water crisis. *American Journal of Public Health*, 107, 763–769.

Schaider, L., Swetschinski, L., Campbell, C., & Rudel, R. (2019). Environmental justice and drinking water quality: Are there socioeconomic disparities in nitrate levels in U.S. drinking water? *Environmental Health*, 18, 3.

Silva, C., Jaddoe, V., Sol, C., El Marroun, H., Martinez-Moral, M., Kannan, K., Trasande, L., & Santos, S. (2021). Phthalate and bisphenol urinary concentrations, body fat measures and cardiovascular risk factors in Dutch school-age children. *Obesity*, 29, 409–417.

Streit, E. (2021). Arsenic in food. *Today's Dietitian*, August/September, 48–52.

United States Food and Drug Administration. (2020). Lead in food, foodwares, and dietary supplements. Retrieved from: www.fda.gov/food/metals-and-your-food/lead-food-foodwares-and-dietary-supplements

Vienneau, D., de Hoogh, K., Hauri, D., Vicedo-Cabrera, A., Schindler, C., Huss, A., & Röösli, M. (2017). Effects of radon and UV exposure on skin cancer mortality in Switzerland. *Environmental Health Perspectives*, 125, 067009.

Vom Saal, F., & Vandenberg, L. (2020). Updates on the health effects of bisphenol A: Evidence of overwhelming harm. *Endocrinology*, 162, 1–25.

Whitehead, L., & Buchanan, S. (2019). Childhood lead poisoning: A perpetual environmental justice issue? *Journal of Public Health Management and Practice*, 25, S115–S120.

Winter, P., Padgett, P., Milburn, L., & Li, W. (2019). Neighborhood parks and recreationists' exposure to ozone: A comparison of disadvantaged and affluent communities in Los Angeles, California. *Environmental Management*, 63, 379–395.

Zarean, M., Poursafa, P. Amin, M., & Kelishadi, R. (2018). Association of endocrine disrupting chemicals, bisphenol a and phthalates, with childhood obesity: A systematic review. *Journal of Pediatrics Review*, 6, e11894.

Part II

The Nurses' Code of Ethics

9 Self-Care, Including the History of the Nurses' Code

Elizabeth Simkus[1], Deborah Chielli[2], and Gia Merlo[3]
[1]Rush University College of Nursing
Chicago, Illinois, USA
[2]Wilkes University, Wilkes-Barre, PA, USA
[3]NYU Meyers College of Nursing
New York, New York, USA
NYU Grossman School of Medicine
New York, New York, USA

CONTENTS

KEY POINTS

- Nurses are faced with a variety of stressors during their careers. Self-care is a way to build resiliency and prevent burnout.
- The Nursing Code of Ethics has been developed as an expression of nursing values, virtues, and responsibilities that guide modern nursing practice. Provision 5 addresses self-care.
- The onus of self-care is not placed solely on the nurse. Nurse leaders, educational institutions, employers, policymakers, and nursing associations/organizations have a vested interest in the health of nurses.

9.1   INTRODUCTION

Nurses are challenged physically, mentally, emotionally, and ethically during their careers. Support for nurses' well-being ought to span from nursing school to retirement (NASEM, 2021). Nurses are not as healthy as the average American as more are overweight, under greater levels of stress, and get fewer hours of sleep (ANA Enterprise, 2021). Nurses provide optimal care when they are healthy themselves (ANA, 2017). Consideration must be taken for their physical health, occupational safety and health, mental and behavioral health, moral well-being, social health and well-being, and the impact of racism and discrimination (NASEM, 2021).

9.2   CURRENT STATE OF NURSES' HEALTH

There are nearly 4 million nurses in the United States, making nursing the largest healthcare profession in the nation (AACN, 2021). Nurses need to practice self-care and be aware of their own well-being if they expect to have the capacity to provide optimal care throughout their careers. However, according to the American Nurses Association's (2017) Health Risk Appraisal, almost 70% of nurses report putting their patients' safety and health before their own. In addition, stress was the number one health and safety risk in the nursing work environment as evidenced by 82% of respondents indicating significant levels of stress at work. This is concerning since stress can lead to reduced capacity for physical, mental, and compassion efforts, which translates to burnout (NurseJournal, 2021). Beyond stress, around half of the respondents reported musculoskeletal pain related to work, not having 100% compliance with using lift or transfer equipment, coming in early, staying late, and/or foregoing a break to complete their work, working 10 or more hours per shift, and experiencing bullying at work. Finally, about one-third of respondents often found their workload to be uncomfortable. With these work conditions, it is not surprising that nurses have a significantly higher rate of missed work due to occupational-related injury or illness compared with other occupations (US Bureau of Labor Statistics, 2018). These statistics are concerning for further increasing the current nursing shortage. When surveyed in March 2021, the percentage of nurses who were either planning on or undecided if they would leave their current position or the profession within the next six months was 40% and 15%, respectively (ANA Enterprise, 2021).

In addition to the work environment impacting nurses' health, individual modifiable risk factors also play a role. Chronic disease is the number one cause of death and disability in the United States (CDC, 2021), and 80% of heart disease, stroke, and type 2 diabetes, while 40% of cancers could be prevented if modifiable risk factors were removed (WHO, n.d.). Nurses themselves engage in some of these modifiable risk factors. According to the aforementioned ANA (2017) survey, only half of the respondents engaged in strength training at least two days per week. Dietary choices fared far worse, with only 35% reporting consuming three daily servings of whole grains and 16% intaking the minimum recommended five servings of fruits and vegetables. Per week, 15% of respondents consume more than 35 ounces of sugar-sweetened beverages. Smoking cigarettes was less of a concern, as 94% reported not smoking and over half of those who did smoke were trying to quit. A lifestyle modification approach by nurses has the power to delay or avoid the onset of chronic disease. Li et al. (2020) published a prospective study with data from the Nurses Health Study and the Health Professionals Follow-Up Study that found that low-risk health behaviors included in many of the pillars of lifestyle medicine have the potential to delay or avoid onset of chronic disease.

9.3   THE CODE AND SELF-CARE: AN ETHICAL OBLIGATION

Each medical profession has an ethical standard by which its members are guided. For nurses, that standard is the Code of Ethics for Nurses with Interpretive Statements, henceforth The Code (ANA, 2015). The Code "establishes the ethical standard for the profession and provides a guide for nurses to use in ethical analysis and decision-making" (ANA, 2015, p. 9). Ethical problems can arise at the societal, political, organizational, or individual/population level (Epstein & Turner, 2015). The Code provides guidance applicable to any nursing practice. It is an expression of nursing values, virtues, and responsibilities that guide modern nursing practice. Overall, the concepts in the nine provisions of the Code include how nurses are required to conduct themselves with patients, other nurses, themselves, the profession, and society. Prior to the American Nurses Association (ANA) Code of Ethics with Interpretive Statements (the Code), nurses used Gretter's Nightingale Pledge, which was comparable to the Hippocratic Oath in medicine (Epstein & Turner, 2015). The history of The Code dates to the late 1800s when the ANA was established, early nursing ethics literature, and the first Nursing Code of Ethics from 1950 (ANA, 2015).

Provision 5 of the Code discusses self-care. Nurses are held to the same responsibilities to themselves as to others, including health promotion, safety, character and integrity, competency, and growth, both personally and professionally. The Code Provision 5 states that "the nurse owes the same duties to self as to others, including the responsibility to promote health and safety" (p. 19).

Linton and Koonmen (2020) note that one factor leading nurses to neglect self-care is the mistaken idea that this is self-indulgent. The authors note that although a number of nursing codes from around the world speak to the duty of caring for self, it is often within the context of supplying safe patient care. In the current ANA Code (2015), according to the authors, self-care is a duty separate from and in addition to duty to care for others. The inclusion of self-care in The Code underscores its importance to nurses and as an ethical duty that, per the authors, is one of the ANA's goals.

Historically, from the early days of modern nursing, nursing's system of ethics was virtue-based with an emphasis on duty to self, according to Fowler (2018). The author cites texts from this time period that speak to the importance of the development and nurturance of a nurse's mental, spiritual, social, and physical well-being. In fact, Fowler (2018), a historian of The Code, states that for "the first 100 years of modern nursing (1860–1965), approximately 100 nursing ethics textbooks (and editions) were published … all addressed a collective duty of 'duties to self' " (p. 153). Then, around 1965, as nursing education moved into colleges and universities, nursing ethics became increasingly duty-based, and the prominence of duty to self was weakened. Duty to self was again prominent in the 2001 revision, then weaker in subsequent revisions until the current 2015 revision of The Code, in which the author "reclaims the full expression of duties to self" from the first 100 years of nursing ethics (Fowler, 2018).

The Code Provision 2 asserts "the nurse's primary commitment is to the patient," whereas Provision 5 affirms "the nurse owes same duties to self as to others, including responsibility to promote health and safety" (ANA, 2015, p. 7). According to Schroeter (2008), the tension between these ethical obligations is intensified, particularly during times of disasters or pandemics, when nurses and others in healthcare must reckon with their capacity to provide quality care, while at the same time maintaining attention to their own self-care. This became increasingly evident during the COVID-19 pandemic when nurses were on the frontlines. The impact of COVID-19 on the Nursing and Midwifery workforce (ICON) study began in 2020. Nurses reported in the survey high rates of burnout, post-traumatic stress disorder, and depression. Burnout is not a new concept. It dates back in the literature to the 1970s and consists of a variety of symptoms, including being emotionally drained, disconnected, and unaccomplished at work (NASEM, 2019). It is imperative for nurses to be aware of their physical, mental, occupational, moral, and spiritual health and to adjust as necessary.

9.4 SELF-CARE AND THE NURSE

According to the World Health Organization (WHO), self-care for an individual includes the ability "to promote health, prevent disease, maintain health, and to cope with illness and disability" (WHO, 2022, p. 1).

At the individual level, components to well-being incorporate personality, resilience, and social support (NASEM, 2021). Current nursing practice needs to recognize the importance of self-care for the stainability of our nursing workforce. Components of self-care include awareness, expression, and preparation (Mills et al., 2017). Awareness of one's physical, mental, and emotional well-being is key to being able to adjust accordingly. The component of expression within self-care can be accomplished via journaling, debriefing, poetry, or mindfulness meditation. Finally, prioritization for self-care is compared to creating a care plan for a patient. The nurse should put in equal effort to create a self-care plan (Mills et al., 2017). Self-care begins before one becomes a nurse. Healthcare students' participation in self-care seemed to reduce their perceived stress and its impact on reported quality of life (Ayala et al., 2018).

Yet, there is little if any attention given in nursing education to instructing students in the how and why of caring for self and in its place in the nursing code (Green, 2020; ANA, 2015).

Based on The Code Provision 5, Green (2020) ran a pilot project in which a nurse educator engaged BSN students with holistic education and activities and then evaluated for self-reported stress reduction by the students. The BSN accelerated program was chosen specifically because of its intensive timeline for adult students, who often also have competing responsibilities and financial stressors.

A study by Nevins and Sherman (2015) with students in a traditional baccalaureate program found that students were very interested in improving their "well-being in the areas of diet, exercise, sleep and hydration" (p. 191) and also in learning more about complementary and alternative modalities. The authors note that nursing students must learn not only about health but also how to apply this in their own lives. The role of faculty, according to the authors, is to both identify impediments to student self-care and incorporate practices that encourage self-care, such as reminding them to hydrate or discussing how to integrate physical activity into each day. The value of students developing self-care practices lies not only in health and performance but also, down the road, in RNs who will then serve as role models and teachers for patients and the public (Nevins & Sherman, 2015).

What works for one nurse for self-care practices may not work for others. It is not a one-size-fits-all approach, and nurses should try various self-care practices to determine what works best for them. Activities may include mindfulness, gratitude, yoga, journaling, listening to music, reading positive affirmations, limiting news or social media, hydration, prioritizing sleep, going outdoors, physical activity, volunteering, being with others, letting go of perfectionism, hobbies, professionally appropriate humor at work, or practice in setting boundaries (Mills et al., 2018 and Steinheiser, 2021). The American Nurses Association Enterprise has created the Healthy Nurse Healthy Nation (HNHN) challenge. The concept of the challenge is to engage nurses, employers, and organizations to improve the health of nurses. Healthy nurses could then be role models for their family, friends, and co-workers. HNHN (2021) focuses on physical activity, nutrition, rest, quality of life, and safety. It has tips for individual self-care, for example, using the 20 seconds during hand washing to say a meditation or affirmation, or to pray or sing a song.

9.5   SYSTEM SUPPORT FOR NURSES' SELF-CARE

Responsibility for well-being and self-care is not placed solely on the nurse. Nurse leaders, educational institutions, employers, policymakers, and nursing associations/organizations have a vested interest in assisting nurses in maintaining their health (NASEM, 2021). In the American Association of Colleges of Nursing (2021) Core Competencies, Domain 10 addresses the need for a nursing curriculum to include content on nurses' self-care and resiliency. At entry-level nursing education, topics of self-care and work-life balance are to be incorporated. At advanced-level nursing education, it needs to be taught that the advanced practice nurse should assess and contribute to a work environment that supports self-care and health. An example of such self-care content at an educational institution is at the University of Minnesota's (2021) Earl E. Bakken Center for Spirituality and Healing. Here they offer graduate programs, for-credit courses, mindfulness programs, online learning, and well-being lecture series.

The American Nurses Association (ANA) Enterprise (n.d.) has a Well-Being Initiative. This initiative offers free online tools and apps to help nurses practice gratitude, expressive writing, a 24/7 confidential line, podcast, app to track healthy habits, and more. Mayo Clinic published "Healing the Professional Culture of Medicine" as a response to the gap in self-care education for clinicians (Shanafelt et al., 2019). It reports the need to have a cultural shift to prevent burnout. Shifts related to self-care include making self-care a necessity, creating support groups, achieving adequate sleep and self-calibration, as well as breaking down mental health stigma. One organization that is attempting to help with this shift is the American College of Lifestyle Medicine. They have created a course on clinician well-being that covers individual physical and mental health as well as strategies to improve the workplace and team culture (ACLM, 2021).

Employers need to create a culture that promotes inclusivity and support for the health and well-being of their staff. It is important for staff experiences to be heard and adjustments made accordingly. An example of this type of systems-level approach is the Center for Clinical Wellness at Rush University Medical Center (RUMC) in Chicago. The center strives to foster a culture of wellness through programming related to burnout, resilience, work satisfaction, and mental health support (Rush, 2021). During the pandemic, RUMC also implemented wellness rounds in the hospital, consisting of system leaders, chaplains, and other specialists.

There are multiple external influencers within the work environment that impact the well-being of nurses, including organizational structure, policies, and work conditions (NASEM, 2021).

Shah et al. (2020) found that more than 60% of nurses who left or were considering leaving their position due to burnout reported being in a stressful work environment and inadequate staffing. Staffing ratios, education on professional boundary setting, consistency in breaks, management team intervention for challenging patients, debriefing after stressful events, and self-care opportunities such as a meditation or relaxation room are examples of external influencers that can fight against burnout (Steinheiser, 2021). The National Student Nurses' 2018 Association created a resolution supporting the implementation of Code Lavender, which is a team-based approach to supporting clinician well-being after stressful events (NSNA, 2018).

Another resource for clinicians and institutions is the National Academy of Medicine (NAM). The NAM has created an action collaborative to provide resources for leadership and staff on clinician well-being and resilience (NAM, 2022). Resources have been divided into six essential elements: Advanced organizational commitment, strengthening leadership behaviors, conducting workplace assessment, examining policies and practices, enhanced workplace efficiency, and cultivating a culture of connection and support. Resources within the elements include toolkits, case examples, courses for continuing education, help with institution proposals, videos, journals, assessment instruments, podcasts, online communities, and COVID-related resources.

Institutions could utilize survey tools to help identify potential burnout. One such tool is the Professional Quality of Life (ProQOL). This is a tool that measures both compassion satisfaction stemming from the positive feelings associated with providing care and compassion fatigue (CF) stemming from the negative feelings. CF results from burnout and secondary traumatic stress (Steinheiser, 2021). Tools such as this would allow institutions to monitor the level of CF and put in place interventions to help counteract it and thus hopefully retain their nursing staff. HNHN (2020) recommends supervisors and employers offer mental health screening, evidence-based programs for prevention and alleviation of anxiety and depression, mental health and resilience interventions, and caregiver response teams with emotional first-aid providers. They should also celebrate victories and appreciate nurses. Policies and procedures are needed to reduce the risk for occupational health hazards, workplace violence, bullying, and incivility. Nurses' health and well-being make an impact on the quality, cost, and safety of the care provided (NASEM, 2021). System-level supports were created out of the identified need to address clinician well-being and prevent burnout. Self-care and system-level programs can assist in building resilience, processing grief, managing stress, and retaining the nursing workforce.

9.6 CONCLUSION

Individuals entering nursing are accepting a challenging and rewarding career. It is the role of the nurse, educational institutions, leaders, employers, policymakers, and professional organizations to promote self-care and well-being of nurses. Nurses have a significant role in the health of the nation since they are the largest and most trusted healthcare profession. Nurses that are healthy and practice self-care can serve as wonderful role models for communities (ANA, 2021) and nursing colleagues.

REFERENCES

American Association of Colleges of Nursing. (2021). *The essentials: Core competencies for professional nursing education.* Retrieved December 18, 2021, from www.aacnnursing.org/AACN-Essentials

American College of Lifestyle Medicine. (2021). *Physician and health professional well-being course.* Retrieved December 26, 2021, from www.lifestylemedicine.org/ACLM/Education/Continuing_Educat ion/Well-Being_Course/ACLM/Education/Physician%20Well-Being/PHPWB.aspx?hkey=d0248dcf-fb55-48a4-a590-baaf0d849129

American Nurses Association (ANA). (2017). *Executive summary American Nurse Association health risk appraisal.* Retrieved December 15, 2021, from www.nursingworld.org/~4aeeeb/globalassets/practicean dpolicy/work-environment/health--safety/ana-healthriskappraisalsummary_2013-2016.pdf

American Nurses Association (ANA). (2015). *The Code of Ethics for nurses with interpretive statements.* Retrieved December 18, 2021, from www.nursingworld.org/coe-view-only

American Nurses Association (ANA) Enterprise. (2021). *Healthy nurse, healthy nation.* Retrieved December 12, 2021, from www.healthynursehealthynation.org/

American Nurses Association (ANA) Enterprise. (2021). *COVID-19 impact assessment survey—the first year.* Retrieved January 5, 2022, from nursingworld.org

American Nurses Association (ANA) Enterprise. (n.d.). *Well-being initiative.* Retrieved December 15, 2021, from www.nursingworld.org/practice-policy/work-environment/health-safety/disaster-preparedness/ coronavirus/what-you-need-to-know/the-well-being-initiative/

Ayala, E. E., Winseman, J. S., Johnesen, R. D., & Mason, H. R. (2018). U.S. medical students who engage in self-care report less stress and higher quality of life. *BMC Medical Education, 18.* https://doi.org/ 10.1186/s12909-018-1296-x

Centers for Disease Control and Prevention (CDC). (2021). *Chronic diseases in America.* Retrieved December 26, 2021, from www.cdc.gov/chronicdisease/resources/infographic/chronic-diseases.htm

Epstein, B. & Turner, M. (2015). The Nursing Code of Ethics: Its value, its history. *Online Journal of Issues in Nursing, 20*(2), 33–41. http://dx.doi.org.wilkes.idm.oclc.org/10.3912/OJIN.Vol20No02Man04.

Fowler, M. (2018). Duties to self: The nurse as a person of dignity and worth. *Creative Nursing, 24*(3). https:// doi.org/10.1891/1946-6560.24.3.152

Green, C. (2020). Teaching accelerated nursing students' self-care: A pilot project. Wiley Nursing Open. https://doi.org/10.1002/nop2.384

Islami, F., Goding Sauer, A., Miller, K. D., Siegel, R. L., Fedewa, S. A., Jacobs, E. J., McCullough, M. L., Patel, A. V., Ma, J., Soerjomataram, I., Flanders, D., Brawley, O. W., Gapstur, S. M., & Jemal, A. (2018). Proportion and number of cancer cases and deaths attributable to potentially modifiable risk factors in the United States. *CA: A Cancer Journal for Clinicians, 68*(1), 31–54. https://doi.org/10.3322/caac.21440

Li, Y. , Schoufour, J., Wang, D. D., Dhana, K., Pan, A., Liu, X., Song, M., Liu, G., Shin, H. J., Sun, Q., Al-Shaar, L., Wang, M., Rimm, E. B., Hertzmark, E., Stampfer, M. J., Willett, W. C., Franco, O. H., & Hu, F. B. (2020). Healthy lifestyle and life expectancy free of cancer, cardiovascular disease, and type 2 diabetes: Prospective cohort study. *BMJ, 368.* https://doi.org/10.1136/bmj.l6669

Linton, M., & Koonmen, J. (2020). Self-care as an ethical obligation for nurses. *Nursing Ethics, 27*(8), 1694–1702. https://doi.org/10.1177/0969733020940371

Mills, J., Wand, T., & Fraser, J. (2017). Palliative care professionals' care and compassion for self and others: A narrative review. *International Journal of Palliative Nursing, 23*(5), 219–229.

Mills, J., Wand, T., & Fraser, J. (2018). Examining self-care, self-compassion and compassion for others: A cross sectional survey of palliative care nurses and doctors. *International Journal of Palliative Nursing, 24*(1), 4–11. https://doi.org/10.12968/ijpn.2018.24.1.4

National Academies of Sciences, Engineering & Medicine. (2019). *Taking action against clinician burnout: A systems approach to professional well-being (2019).* Washington, DC: The National Academies Press. https://doi.org/10.17226/25521

National Academy of Medicine (NAM). (2022). Action Collaborative on Clinician Well-Being and Resilience. https://nam.edu/initiatives/clinician-resilience-and-well-being/

National Student Nurses' Association (NSNA). (2018). *Resolutions 2018.* Retrieved December 25, 2021, from www.nsna.org/resolutions-by-year.html

Nevins, C. M., & Sherman, J. (2016). Self-care practices of baccalaureate nursing students. *Journal of Holistic Nursing, 34*(2), 185–192. https://doi-org.wilkes.idm.oclc.org/10.1177%2F0898010115596432

NurseJournal Staff. (2021). *Nurse burnout*. Retrieved January 5, 2022, from nursejournal.org

Rush University Medical Center (RUMC) (2021). Rush Wellness. Retrieved from www.rush.edu/health-care-professionals/rush-wellness

Schroeter, K. (2008). Duty to care versus duty to self. *Journal of Trauma Nursing: The Official Journal of the Society of Trauma Nurses*, *15*(1), 3–4. http://doi.org/10.1097/01.JTN.0000315779.97341.d3

Shanafelt, T.D, Schein, E., Minor, L.B., Trockel, M., Schein, P., & Kirch, D. (2019). *Healing the professional culture of medicine*. Retrieved December 26, 2021, from www.mayoclinicproceedings.org/action/show Pdf?pii=S0025-6196%2819%2930345-3

Shah, M.K., Gandrakota, N., Cimiotti, J.P., Ghose, N., Moore, M., & Ali, M.K. (2021). Prevalence of and factors associated with nurse burnout in the US. *JAMA Network Open*, *4*(2). http://doi.org/10.1001/jamanetworkopen.2020.36469

Steinheiser, M. (2021). *Compassion fatigue risk among skilled nursing facility nurses*. Retrieved December 15, 2021, from www.myamericannurse.com/compassion-fatigue-risk-among-skilled-nursing-facility-nurses/

University of Minnesota Center for Spirituality & Healing. (2021). *Earl E. Bakken Center for Spirituality & Healing*. Retrieved December 15, 2021, from www.csh.umn.edu/

US Bureau of Labor Statistics. (2018). *Occupational injuries and illnesses among registered nurses*. Retrieved January 10, 2022, from www.bls.gov/opub/mlr/2018/article/pdf/occupational-injuries-and-illnesses-among-registered-nurses.pdf

World Health Organization (WHO). (2022). *What do we mean by self-care?* Retrieved January 10, 2022, from www.who.int/publications/i/item/9789240030909

10 Theories Around Self-Promotion and Self-Management

Maria Grandinetti[1] and Sarah E. Abalos[2]
[1]Wilkes University
Wilkes-Barre, PA, USA
[2]Thiel College
Greenville, PA, USA

CONTENTS

KEY POINTS

- Key concepts in the nursing metaparadigm and grand, middle-range, and practice theories serve as a framework for knowledge of human self-promotion and self-management.
- Nursing theories have the purposes of describing, explaining, and predicting care outcomes based on relationships among their concepts of nursing phenomena.
- Nursing theories continue to have scientific value, as they guide research, education, and professional nursing practice, foster innovation, and reduce health disparities.

DOI: 10.1201/9781003178330-12

10.1 INTRODUCTION

Nursing theory is an integral component of behavioral change, innovation, and cultural competence in nursing. It is fundamentally based on gained knowledge. Knowledge development in nursing was first introduced by Florence Nightingale in the nineteenth century. Nightingale recognized that the cleanliness of an environment for healing leads to the recovery of patients' physical and mental well-being. With this knowledge, her Environmental Theory developed and resulted in healthcare reforms that continue to this day. Nursing theory guides nurses to understand their role and purpose in the healthcare setting. It leads nurses to know the practices of nursing care. The theory also serves to elucidate what is known and helps to determine areas that need further explanation. Nursing theory is continuously evolving because nursing science is constantly developing new evidence and knowledge. The application of theory in practice can result in acquired behavior that can increase the possibility of positive self-care outcomes.

10.1.1 INNOVATION

Applying theory in nursing practice also drives innovation within the discipline. Innovation in nursing is defined as the intersection of critical thinking, data collection, and clinical expertise that leads to the creation of strategies that improve patient care and, ultimately, the overall health and well-being of the population nurses care for (Johnson & Johnson, 2021). Roger's (2003) Diffusion of Innovation Theory and Steps (Table 10.1) is rooted in communication but can be applied to nursing to explain how an innovative idea can be developed into a new model of nursing care.

The discipline of nursing has been shaped and impacted by innovative nurses since its beginnings. Table 10.2 provides some examples of innovation in nursing from the inception of modern nursing through the current Covid-19 pandemic (Johnson & Johnson, 2021).

10.1.2 CULTURAL COMPETENCE

Understanding how culture impacts health and health perception is critical to the provision of patient-centered care and another important function of nursing theory. Cultural competence is the process of learning about the values, beliefs, and traditions of a group and then directly applying that knowledge to improve the delivery of nursing care (Williams & Harrison, 2010). Madeleine Leininger's Theory of Transcultural Nursing can be used to provide patient care that incorporates cultural considerations (Leininger & McFarland, 2002). The theory explains the role of culture in health, establishes how patients respond to illness, suffering, and death, promotes respect of diversity, and improves nurse–patient relationships. Nurses should use culturological assessments

TABLE 10.1
The five steps of Roger's Diffusion of Innovation Theory

Step	Purpose
Relative advantage	Used to determine if the newly developed model of care is superior to current models of care.
Combability	Is the new model of care aligned with the values and needs of the nurses and the patients who will be impacted by the new model of care?
Complexity	Describes the ease and feasibility of implementation of the new model of care.
Triability	Focuses on if and how easily the model of care can be tested before full implementation.
Observability	Describes the new model of care's ability to produce meaningful and tangible results.

Source: Data from Rogers, E. M. (2003). *Diffusion of innovations* (5th ed.). Free Press.

TABLE 10.2
Contributions of nurse innovators: Nightingale to present

Nurse	Time Period	Innovative Contribution to Nursing
Florence Nightingale	1854	Developed hygiene practice still used today.
Elizabeth Kenny	1939	Determined heat and gentle movement were effective in returning limb function to polio patients.
Adda May Allen	1940s	Created a plastic liner for baby bottles to making infant feeding easier.
Sister Jean Ward	1950s	Discovered that exposure to sunlight decrease jaundice in newborns, leading to the development of neonatal phototherapy.
Elise Sorensen	1954	Invented disposable ostomy bags.
Anita Dorr	1968	Invented the crash cart.
Donna Wong Connie Baker	1980s	Developed the Baker-Wong pediatric pain scale.
Teri Barton-Salinas Gail Barton-Hay	2003	Designed color-coded IV lines to ease medication administration and increase patient safety.
Rebecca Koszalinski	2016	Developed the Speak for Myself app, which allows patients who cannot effectively verbalize their needs to communicate with caregivers.
Ellen Smithline	2020	Created a flexible shield for eye protection to be worn over N-95 respirators during the Covid-19 pandemic.

Source: Data from Johnson & Johnson. (2021). *Innovation 101*. https://nursing.jnj.com/innovation-101

to develop plans of care that more fully address patient needs that result from cultural factors. Using the Theory of Transcultural Nursing, an individual's culture can be preserved or maintained, accommodated or negotiated, and repatterned or restructured to assist the individual in achieving the highest levels of health (Leininger & McFarland, 2002). Nurses who understand the impact of culture on health can design strategies to improve health that may be more appealing and sustainable to the individual. Theories in nursing continue to be relevant in contemporary practice as they provide nurses with the wisdom to solve encountered problems.

10.1.3 LEVELS OF NURSING THEORY

There are four levels of nursing theory. They include the nursing metaparadigm, grand theory, middle-range theory, and practice-level theory. The broadest and most abstract level is that of the nursing metaparadigm. Grand theory and middle-range theory follow. The most specific level is that of practice-level theory. A relationship exists between theory development and the foundations for clinical decision-making and critical thinking in nursing practice. All theories are comprised of well-defined key concepts, and relational and non-relational propositions are also included. These propositions vary in how specific and concrete they are.

10.2 THE NURSING METAPARADIGM

A metaparadigm is a set of concepts that can be used to define the phenomenon of a discipline and describes the relationships between those phenomena (Kuhn, 1977). Nursing theory can also be viewed from a broad perspective, taking into consideration domain concepts of interest to the discipline of nursing that make up the nursing metaparadigm. The nursing metaparadigm consists of four domain concepts: person, environment, health, and nursing (Fawcett, 1978). The nursing metaparadigm is the most abstract element of nursing knowledge and the foundation of all nursing theories. Using the metaparadigm to guide knowledge generation provides a systematic approach to the process (Hardy, 1978).

10.2.1 DOMAINS OF THE NURSING METAPARADIGM

In nursing, the concept of person is defined as the individual receiving nursing care (Fawcett, 1993). The concept of person may also include the client's family members, friends, and community. The concept of environment refers to the individuals the client interacts with, the setting in which the client is located, and the nursing care that is being provided. The concept of health is described as the client's level of self-care, self-promotion, self-management, and overall well-being. This concept occurs on a continuum that ranges from sickness to wellness. The concept of nursing encompasses the five phases of the nursing process: assessment, diagnosis, planning, implementation, and evaluation. The definition of the concept of nursing includes all other interactions between a nurse and the client (Fawcett, 1993).

Although the concepts within the nursing metaparadigm are generally addressed in grand nursing theories, different nursing theorists have unique interpretations for the concepts, and a theorist may place more importance on a specific concept of the nursing metaparadigm. Table 10.3 illustrates these differences among Gene Watson's Theory of Human Caring, Dorothea Orem's Theory of Self-Care, and Florence Nightingale's Environmental Theory (Branch et al., 2016).

10.2.2 INTERACTIONS OF THE CONCEPTS IN THE NURSING METAPARADIGM

Donaldson and Crowley (1978) have identified four interactions among the concepts of the nursing metaparadigm. The discipline of nursing is concerned with (1) the principles and laws that govern the life-process, well-being, and optimal functioning of human beings, sick or well, (2) the patterning of human behavior in interaction with the environment in normal life events and critical life situations, (3) the nursing actions or process by which positive changes in health status are affected, and (4) the wholeness or health of human beings, recognizing that they are in continuous interaction with their environments.

10.2.3 LEVELS OF NURSING KNOWLEDGE

All nursing knowledge is the result of the concepts in the metaparadigm and the interaction among those concepts. Nursing philosophy, conceptual models, theories, and empirical indicators are the different nursing knowledge levels derived from the metaparadigm. The levels of nursing knowledge range from the abstract, as with philosophy, to concrete measurements or procedures of empirical indicators.

Nursing theory is the fourth level of nursing knowledge and can be considered less abstract than conceptual models but more abstract than empirical indicators. Theories are comprised of two kinds of propositions. Non-relational propositions are used to define or describe the concepts of a theory. Some concepts that have been used in nursing theory are empowerment, mobility, pain, and caring. Relational propositions are used to link and explain interactions among concepts. Relational propositions often describe how the concepts are connected or the type of relationship through quantifying language such as positive/negative, small/moderate/large, asymmetrical/symmetrical, or concurrent/sequential (Fawcett & Downs, 1992). An example of a relational proposition is high levels of trait anger are related to high blood pressure in overweight children (Nichols et al., 2011). Propositions have been empirically tested and create a rich body of knowledge that describes how nursing practice influences patient health, and how patient's social and physical environments influence their experiences of health (Bender & Feldman, 2015).

TABLE 10.3
Focus and definition of metaparadigm concepts for Watson, Orem, and Nightingale

Theorist	Focus of Theory	Definition of Person	Definition of Health	Definition of Environment	Definition of Nursing
Watson	Nursing	All patients have unique needs, and their wishes, customs, and beliefs must be respected for healing to occur.	Health is a state of balance in a patient's physical, cognitive, and spirituality. Illness prevention is an integral component of health.	Nurses should strive to create an environment that is home-like and comfortable to increase health. Including nature as part of the environment can further increase health.	Caring is essential to nursing. Developing meaningful relationships with patients allows nurses to promote healing.
Orem	Person	Nurses should provide patients with the knowledge and skill to manage their own health.	The development of self-care strategies is essential to improving health.	The environment includes family and friends who provide support to the patient.	Nurses are responsible for teaching patients self-care strategies to aid the healing process.
Nightingale	Environment	Nurses provide patient-centered care that includes attention to a patient's mind, body, and spirit.	Health can be improved through meeting basic medical needs, caring, and cleanliness.	The management of noise, lighting, ventilation, and smells can have a significant impact on a patient's health.	Nursing is responsible for promoting the overall health of the patients, not merely implementing physician's orders.

Source: Data from Branch, C., Deak, H., Hiner, C., & Holzwart, T. (2016). Four nursing metaparadigms. *IU South Bend Undergraduate Research Journal, 16*, 123–132.

10.2.4 LEVELS OF NURSING THEORY

In practice, nurses should know theories ranging from grand theory to practice-level theory. This knowledge will allow the nurse to combine practice knowledge with disciplinary knowledge, thereby providing holistic, client-centered care. The provision of holistic client-centered care, guided by theory, is the fullest expression of nursing.

10.3 GRAND NURSING THEORIES FOR SELF-PROMOTION AND SELF-MANAGEMENT

Grand nursing theories are considered complex, broad, and abstract in scope, making them difficult to test. Grand nursing theory can often be applied to a range of topics and situations. An example of this is Florence Nightingale's Environmental Theory. Nightingale's theory can be used in various settings and across patient populations.

10.3.1 OREM'S THEORY OF SELF-CARE

Dorothea Orem began developing the Theory of Self-Care in the 1950s as a result of her work focused on the education of licensed practical (vocational) nurses. The Theory of Self-Care consists of the concepts of self-care, self-care agency, basic conditioning factors, therapeutic self-care demand, and self-care requisites. Five key concepts comprise Orem's (2001) Theory of Self-Care (Table 10.4).

Orem's Theory of Self-Care (2001) focuses on the performance or practice of activities that individuals accomplish on their behalf to maintain one's life and life functioning, to develop oneself, or to correct a health deviation or condition. Although this theory was initially developed to assist nurses with caring for clients, the theory is a practical approach for clients to achieve and maintain optimal self-health and wellness.

10.3.2 ROGER'S THEORY OF THE SCIENCE OF UNITARY HUMAN BEINGS

Martha Rogers believed that the essence of nursing is service to humanity and that it is "a humanistic science dedicated to compassionate concern for maintaining and promoting health, preventing illness, and caring for and rehabilitating the sick and disabled" (Rogers, 1970, p. vii, ix). Roger's Theory of the Science of Unitary Human Beings (1970) is built on five basic assumptions. The first is that the human being is a unified whole, possessing individual integrity and manifesting characteristics that are more than and different from the sum of the parts. The second is that the individual and the environment are continuously exchanging matter and energy with each other. The third is that the life processes of human beings evolve irreversibly and unidirectionally along with the space-time continuum. The fourth is that patterns identify human beings and reflect their innovative wholeness. And the fifth is that individuals are characterized by the capacity for abstraction and imagery, language, thought sensation, and emotion. Using these five assumptions, Rogers (1970) developed four building blocks of the theory. These include energy fields, which are "the fundamental units of the living and the non-living" (p. 7). Openness is the interaction between human and environmental energy and occurs because both are open systems and allow energy to be continually exchanged. Pan-dimensionality is energy fields that cannot be divided or reduced and have infinite dimensions. And there is a pattern, meaning that energy fields have a pattern represented by a single wave that changes as required by different situations.

Rogers (1970) used these five basic assumptions and these four buildings blocks of the theory to develop three principles. Integrality is defined by Rogers as the inseparability of human beings and their environments within the pan-dimensional universe. This principle can be used to explain

TABLE 10.4
Definitions of the concepts that comprise Orem's Theory of Self-Care

Concept	Definition
1. Self-Care	• The performance of practice of activities that an individual initiates and performs of their own accord to maintain life, health, and well-being. When these activities are executed adequately, an individual can maintain structural integrity, human functioning and proper development.
2. Self-Care agency	• An individual's ability to engage in self-care activities. Primary conditioning factors influence the ability to engage in self-care activities.
3. Basic conditioning factors	• Factors include age, gender, developmental state, sociocultural orientation, healthcare system factors, family system factors, living patterns, environmental factors, and resource adequacy and availability.
4. Therapeuticself-caredemand	• "Self-care actions to be performed for some duration to meet known self-care requisites by using valid methods and related sets of operations and actions" (p. 123).
5. Self-carerequisites	A. General self-care requisites: • The maintenance of sufficient intake of air. • The maintenance of sufficient intake of water. • The maintenance of sufficient intake of food. • The provision of care associated with elimination processes and excrements. • The maintenance of a balance between activity and rest. • The maintenance of a balance between solitude and social interaction. • The prevention of hazards to human life, human functioning, and human well-being. • The promotion of human functioning and development within social groups in accord with human potential, known human limitations, and the human desire to be normal (p. 126). B. Developmental self-care requisites: "Either specialized expressions of universal self-care requisites that have been particularized for developmental processes or they are new self-care requisites derived from a condition … or associated event" (p. 130). Examples of this include adjusting to a major life event or the changes that result from the aging process. C. Health deviation self-care requisites: • Seeking and securing appropriate medical assistance. • Being aware of and attending to the effects and results of pathological conditions. Effectively carrying out medically prescribed diagnostic, therapeutic, and rehabilitative measures. • Being aware of and attending to or regulating the discomforting or deleterious effects of prescribed medical measures. • Modifying the self-concept (and self-image) in accepting oneself as being in a particular state of health and need of specific forms of healthcare. • Learning to live with the effects of pathologic conditions and states and the effects of medical diagnostic and treatment measures in a lifestyle that promotes continued personal development (p. 134).

Source: Data from Orem, D. E. (2001). *Nursing: Concepts in practice* (6th Ed.). Mosby.

déjà vu and clairvoyance. Resonance is explained as human and environmental energy fields that are constantly changing from lower frequency, longer waves to higher frequency, shorter waves. All aspects of humanity and the environment are in constant motion. And helicy, as the "continuous innovative, unpredictable, increasing diversity of the human and environmental field pattern" (Rogers, 1970, p. 8). Using Rogers' theory allows nurses to identify patterns resulting from a client's interaction with the environment. The nurse uses the identified patterns and incorporates their energy fields to develop an individualized plan of care to return the client to optimal levels of health.

10.4 MIDDLE RANGE NURSING THEORIES FOR SELF-PROMOTION AND SELF-MANAGEMENT

Middle-range nursing theories are more concrete than grand nursing theories and often link grand nursing theory to nursing practice. Middle-range theories can describe, explain, or predict the phenomena experienced by nurses in clinical practice. An example of a middle-range theory derived from a grand theory is Jean Watson's Theory of Human Care, which serves as a lead to Katharine Kolcaba's Theory of Comfort. Kolcaba's (2001) theory has "universality" and provides specific guidance to nurses to contribute to the relief or ease a patient requires to transcend and rise above the challenges they are facing.

10.4.1 SWANSON'S THEORY OF CARING AND HEALING

Kristen Swanson's Theory of Caring and Healing (1993) is a middle-range theory and is based on the belief that nurses who demonstrate that they care about a client's well-being are equally essential as the nursing activities that they complete. Swanson's (1993) theory consists of six concepts that are used to improve the well-being of the client (Table 10.5).

TABLE 10.5
Concepts and definitions of Swanson's Theory of Caring and Healing

Concept	Definition
1. Caring	A nurturing way of relating to a valued other to whom one feels a personal sense of commitment and responsibility. Caring is growth and health producing, occurs in relationships to the one cared-for, individualized and intimate, with a sense of commitment, accountability, and duty.
2. Maintaining and belief	Conviction is the basis of all nursing care and requires a fundamental belief in persons and their ability to navigate events and transitions and face the future with meaning.
3. Knowing	Occurs when one perceives events according to the meaning they have in the life of the other.
4. Being-with	Occurs when the nurse is emotionally present with the client and results in the nurse demonstrating that the client's experiences are essential to the nurse.
5. Doing-for	The foundation of nursing practice includes all of the activities carried out by the nurse to assist and improve the client's well-being.
6. Enabling	Facilitating the other's passage through life transitions and unfamiliar events.

Source: Data from Swanson, K. M. (1993). Nursing as informed caring for the well-being of others. *Journal of Nursing Scholarship*, 25(4), 352–357.

10.4.2 Pender's Health Promotion Model

Nola Pender's Health Promotion Model (1982) was derived from social cognitive theory and includes three groups of factors that influence health behavior: individual characteristics, behavior-specific cognitions and affect, and immediate behavioral contingencies. Pender's theory was written to develop and incorporate the promotion of behaviors to improve health and well-being. This theory applies across the life span. Its purpose is to help nurses understand the major determinants of health behaviors as a foundation for behavioral counseling, and the importance of promoting well-being and healthy lifestyles for themselves and for the clients they care for. The model is concerned with individual characteristics and experiences, behavior-specific cognitions and affect, and behavioral outcomes. Pender's (1982) Health Promotion Model is based on five concepts (Table 10.6).

Pender's (1982) Health Promotion Model consists of seven assumptions (Table 10.7).

Nola Pender's Health Promotion Model (1982) is comprised of 14 theoretical propositions to guide nurses to improving health behaviors (Table 10.8).

TABLE 10.6
Concepts of Pender's Health Promotions Model

Concept	Definition
Person	A biophysical organism shaped by the environment that also seeks to create an environment in which human potential can be fully experienced.
Environment	Includes the social, cultural, and physical context in which a person lives.
Nursing	A collaborative effort including patients, families, and communities to facilitate health-enhancing behaviors.
Health	The actualization of human potential through goal-directed behavior, self-care, and relationships with others involve making adjustments that are necessary to optimize the environment.
Illness	Discrete life events that hinder or facilitate health.

Source: Data from Pender, N., J. (1982). *Health promotion in nursing practice*. Appleton-Century-Crofts.

TABLE 10.7
Assumptions of Pender's Health Promotion Model

Assumptions

1. People try to create conditions of living through which they can express their unique human potential.
2. People have the capacity for reflective self-awareness, including assessment of their own competencies.
3. People value positive growth and strive to find a balance between stability and change.
4. People seek to actively regulate their behavior.
5. People interact with their environment, transforming it and themselves over time.
6. Nurses and other health professionals make up a part of the interpersonal environment, which exerts influence on people throughout their lifespan.
7. Self-initiated reconfiguration of the interactive patterns between people and their environments is necessary for a behavior change.

Source: Data from Pender, N., J. (1982). *Health promotion in nursing practice*. Appleton-Century-Crofts.

TABLE 10.8
Theoretical propositions of Pender's Health Promotion Model

Propositions

1. Behavior and characteristics influence beliefs, affect, and enactment of health-promoting behavior.
2. People commit to engaging in behaviors from which they anticipate deriving personally valued benefits.
3. Barriers can constrain commitment to action.
4. Competence to execute a given behavior increases the likelihood of commitment to action and actual performance of the behavior.
5. Greater perceived self-efficacy results in fewer barriers to specific health behavior.
6. Positive effect toward a behavior results in greater perceived self-efficacy.
7. When positive emotions are associated with a behavior, the probability of commitment and action is increased.
8. People are more likely to commit to health-promoting behaviors when others model the behavior, expect it to occur, and provide support to enable it.
9. Families, peers, and healthcare providers are important sources of interpersonal influence that can increase or decrease commitment to health-promoting behavior.
10. Situational influences in the external environment can increase or decrease commitment to or participation in health-promoting behavior.
11. The greater the commitment to a specific plan of action, the more likely health-promoting behaviors are to be maintained over time.
12. Commitment to a plan of action is less likely to result in the desired behavior when competing demands over which persons have little control require immediate attention.
13. Commitment to a plan of action is less likely to result in the desired behavior when other actions are more attractive and thus preferred over the target behavior.
14. People can modify cognitions, affect, interpersonal influences, and situational influences to create incentives for health-promoting behavior.

Source: Data from Pender, N., J. (1982). *Health promotion in nursing practice*. Appleton-Century-Crofts.

Pender's Health Promotion Theory (1982) captures the position nurses hold, to recognize their responsibility to practice themselves and support the teaching of self-promotion and self-management of health and wellness.

10.5 PRACTICE-LEVEL NURSING THEORIES FOR SELF-PROMOTION AND SELF-MANAGEMENT

Practice-level nursing theories have the narrowest scope of all nursing theories and focus on a specific patient population experiencing a particular phenomenon. Although practice-level theories are rooted in grand and middle-range theory, they are detailed enough to serve as the framework for nursing interventions and may predict the outcomes of the interventions.

10.5.1 BANDURA'S SELF-EFFICACY THEORY

Albert Bandura's (1977) Self-Efficacy Theory has been used extensively in positive psychology to promote healthy behaviors such as exercise, a healthy diet, and smoking cessation. The theory is based on the central concept of self-efficacy, which is defined as an individual's optimistic belief in their innate ability, competence, or chance of completing a task and producing a favorable outcome (Bandura, 1977). Five concepts are central to the development of self-efficacy (Table 10.9).

TABLE 10.9
Central concepts for Bandura's Development of Self-Efficacy

Concept	Definition
1. Performance experience	The most important concept in the theory and results from the use of perseverance and resilience to overcome challenges.
2. Vicarious experience	Results when an individual observes a role model and realizes that success is possible.
3. Social persuasion	Occurs when mentors and role models provide the support that increases an individual's belief that they can succeed.
4. Imaginal experience	When an individual envisions achieving success in a specific situation.
5. Physical and emotional states	Impacts how an individual judges their level of self-efficacy and is impacted by factors such as depression, stress, and tension.

Source: Data from Bandura, A. (1977). Self-efficacy: Toward a unifying theory of behavioral change. *Psychological Review*, *84*(2), 191–215. https://psycnet.apa.org/doi/10.1037/0033-295X.84.2.191

10.5.2 BARKER'S TIDAL MODEL THEORY

Phil Barker's Tidal Model Theory (2001) "assumes that nurses need to get close to the people in their care so that they might explore (together) the experience of health and illness" (p. 237). Buchanan-Barker and Barker (2015) have discovered many experiences are universal and provide the language for individuals to describe their experiences using similes and metaphors. The Tidal Model is founded on the metaphor:

> Life is a journey undertaken on an ocean of experience. All human development, including the experience of illness and health, involves discoveries made on a journey across that ocean of experience. At critical points in the life journey, the person may experience storms or even piracy (crisis). At other times the ship may begin to take in water and the person may face the prospect of drowning or shipwreck (breakdown). The person may need to be guided to a haven to undertake repairs or to recover from the trauma (rehabilitation). Only once the ship is made intact, or the person has regained the necessary sea-legs, can the ship set sail again, aiming to put the person back on the life course (recovery).

> *Barker, 2002, p. 45*

The purpose of the Tidal Model is to allow the nurse to care with and not care for the patient (Barker, 2003). There are three central concepts of the Tidal Model (Table 10.10).

10.6 CONCLUSION

Nursing theory serves as a fundamental foundation for nursing practice and allows nurses to generate new knowledge and interventions that can inform and guide practice. The key concepts of person, environment, health, and nursing make up the nursing metaparadigm that serves as a footing of nursing practice and all levels of theory development. Grand theories are the most abstract, while middle-range and practice-level theories are more focused on situations and patient-specific populations. Theories surrounding self-promotion and self-management can serve to encourage positive and self-promoting behavior modifications to assist individuals in making the necessary change to increase their levels of health and well-being.

TABLE 10.10
The central concepts of Barker's Tidal Model

Concept	Definition
1. The process of change	There is no single path to recovery. Instead, individuals should receive support focused on what they need at the moment that will allow the next step in the recovery process to occur.
2. The power of narrative	Life is viewed as a narrative that cannot be separated from an individual's experience. Nurses should develop collaborative relationships with patients that allow patients an opportunity to express what they need to heal and not merely describe the cause of their issues. The power of narrative provides meaning that fosters growth and change.
3. Empowerment	Nurses should empower patients by ensuring emotional and physical safety, assisting the patient in identifying areas needing change, facilitating recovery, and identifying how the available support system can aid in the recovery process.

Source: Data from Barker, P. (2003). The tidal model: Psychiatric colonization, recovery, and the paradigm shift in mental health care. *International Journal of Mental Health Nursing, 12*, 96–102.

REFERENCES

Bandura, A. (1977). Self-efficacy: Toward a unifying theory of behavioral change. *Psychological Review, 84*(2), 191–215. https://psycnet.apa.org/doi/10.1037/0033-295X.84.2.191

Barker, P. (2001). The tidal model: Developing an empowering, person-centered approach to recovery within psychiatric and mental health nursing. *Journal of Psychiatric and Mental Health Nursing, 8*(3), 233–234. https://doi.org/10.1046/j.1365-2850.2001.00391.x

Barker, P. (2002). The tidal model. *Journal of Psychosocial Nursing & Mental Health Services, 40*(7), 42–50.

Barker, P. (2003). The tidal model: Psychiatric colonization, recovery, and the paradigm shift in mental health care. *International Journal of Mental Health Nursing, 12*, 96–102.

Bender, M., & Feldman, M. S. (2015). A practice theory approach to understanding the interdependency of nursing practice and the environment. *Advances in Nursing Science, 38*(2), 96–109. https://doi.org/10.1097/ANS.0000000000000068

Branch, C., Deak, H., Hiner, C., & Holzwart, T. (2016). Four nursing metaparadigms. *IU South Bend Undergraduate Research Journal, 16*, 123–132.

Buchanan-Barker, P., & Barker, P. (2015). Welcome to the tidal model. Retrieved from http://tidal-model.com/

Donaldson, S. K., & Crowley, D. M. (1978). The discipline of nursing. *Nursing Outlook, 26*(2), 113–120.

Hardy, M. E. (1978). Perspectives on nursing theory. *Advances in Nursing Science, 1*(1), 37–48. https://doi.org/10.1097/00012272-197810000-00006

Fawcett, J. (1993). *Analysis and evaluation of nursing theories.* F. A. Davis Company.

Fawcett, J. (1978). The "what" of theory development. *NLN Publications, 15*(1708), 17–33.

Fawcett, J., & Downs, F. S. (1992). *The relationship of theory and research* (2nd ed.). F. A. Davis Company.

Johnson & Johnson. (2021). *Innovation 101.* https://nursing.jnj.com/innovation-101

Leininger, M., & McFarland, M. R. (2002). *Transcultural nursing: Concepts, theories, research, and practice* (3rd ed.). McGraw Hill.

Kolcaba, K. (2001). Evolution of the mid-range theory of comfort for outcomes research. *Nursing Outlook, 49*(2), 86–92. http://doi.org/10.1067/mno.2001.110268

Kuhn, T. S. (1977). The historical structure of scientific discovery. In *The essential tension: Selected studies in scientific tradition and change* (pp. 165–177). University of Chicago Press.

Nichols, K. H., Rice, M., & Howell, C. (2011). Anger, stress, and blood pressure in overweight children. *Journal of Pediatric Nursing, 26*(5), 446–455. https://doi.org/10.1016/j.jpedn.2010.05.002

Orem, D. E. (2001). *Nursing: Concepts in practice* (6th ed.). Mosby.

Pender, N., J. (1982). *Health promotion in nursing practice*. Appleton-Century-Crofts.

Rogers, E. M. (2003). *Diffusion of innovations* (5th ed.). Free Press.

Rogers, M. E. (1970). *An introduction to the theoretical basis of nursing*. F. A. Davis Company.

Swanson, K. M. (1993). Nursing as informed caring for the well-being of others. *Journal of Nursing Scholarship*, *25*(4), 352–357.

Williamson, M., & Harrison, L. (2010). Providing culturally appropriate care: A literature review. *International Journal of Nursing Studies*, *47*, 761–769. http://doi.org/10.1016/j.ijnurstu.2009.12.012

11 Nurse as Patient

Elizabeth Ann Robinson

Santa Barbara Cottage Hospital
Santa Barbara, California, USA

CONTENTS

KEY POINTS

- What is tempered by personal suffering often translates as empathy, trust, and understanding.
- Mourning allows a slowing down to listen and work with the illness, not against it.
- The role of the patient is not passive.

11.1 INTRODUCTION

American cultural anthropologist Susan Sontag famously wrote, "everyone who is born holds dual citizenship in the kingdom of the well and in the kingdom of the sick." Sontag acknowledged and explored both realms. She died of myelodysplastic syndrome, a precursor to rapidly progressive leukemia, when she was 71. Through my own experience, I learned that being a patient is lonely and deeply private and that suffering exacerbated by fear and loss of control leads to withdrawal. The patient faces a dull silence. Chaos, anguish, and uncertainty threaten one's identity and integrity. And at the same time, suffering slows everything down, opens the floodgates to understanding, and deepens the soul, a distinctive process different from intellectual learning. A life-threatening illness is something one never forgets, and it leaves a lasting scar. Carl Jung described the practitioner who had suffered such a plight as the wounded healer. For me, the presence of concerned others who did not deny its existence aided my recovery. As a nurse, as a patient, I discovered that I entered a new domain. I had much to teach and more to learn. Subsumed into darkness, I followed my intuition and the guidance of others. I had a foot in each kingdom, and it affirmed that healing goes both ways.

11.2 EVERY CARDIAC NURSE'S NIGHTMARE: CARDIAC TAMPONADE

While working on the final draft of my book, *The Soul of the Nurse*, giving lectures to doctoral students, and preparing to speak at a memorial for James Hillman, an influential archetypal psychologist, I was not feeling well. Hillman had influenced my research and worldview, so this was an honor for me. I made it through the tribute, and in retrospect, listening to the audio still posted now, there's a gasping sound to my voice. After an evaluation at the emergency department and urgent care twice, I attempted to go on with my life. The physicians said I "looked good." Unusually short of breath, I returned to the ED a few days later on my hands and knees to alleviate inspiratory

DOI: 10.1201/9781003178330-13

chest pain. This time in atrial fibrillation/flutter and full of fluid, as seen on the portable ultrasound machine. After X-ray, echocardiogram, and another spiral CT, I was diagnosed with pericarditis and admitted to the ICU for a harrowing 14 nights. What ensued included seven consultations with specialists, four thoracenteses, and placement and removal of an inferior vena cava filter. As every cardiac nurse knows in this situation, the biggest worry is cardiac tamponade. And this time, I was assessing myself as the patient.

My first encounter with a life-threatening illness came as a healthy 16-year-old when I was diagnosed with nodular sclerosing Hodgkin lymphoma. The hematologist was blunt, even dark in his prognosis, revealing the treatment and sequelae of health issues I would encounter for the rest of my life. He told me the truth, and that's what I wanted. I knew, by his honesty and integrity, he would not abandon me but would travel with me. After a splenectomy and two 5-week courses of radiation treatment, I gradually returned to high school, springboard diving, musical theater, and an active social life.

Eight years later, I took my first job as a Registered Nurse on the oncology unit, the same ward where I recovered from a staging laparotomy for Hodgkin's. I learned essential skills such as inserting nasogastric tubes, foleys, intravenous lines, and chemotherapy administration. I loved the relationships and bonded with my patients and their loved ones. Within nine months, four patients died from Hodgkin lymphoma, and I could no longer separate myself from the patients under my care. Reminded of my mortality day in and day out, I was not living my life fully. So, I transferred to cardiology, where I've stayed in some facet my entire career.

The sequela of medical issues related to radiation treatment my oncologist predicted followed. It was no surprise when I was diagnosed with basal cell carcinoma, thyroid carcinoma, and mitral valve prolapse. And now, here I was, 33 years later, and one week into my ICU stay for pericarditis, when I began to decompensate. I experienced a frightening night of apnea, with oxygen saturation at 70%. In the next room, a stab victim consumed all the nursing staff and physicians' time and energy. I knew I was in trouble and forced myself to stay awake and breathe to maintain my O2 saturation. I understood all too well the enormity of my life-threatening crisis.

I watched monitors, vital signs, and incoming labs. As shards of daylight illuminated my room the next morning, my blood pressure dropped, and my pulse pressure narrowed to 80/60. I summoned my nurse to get another echocardiogram and call in an intensivist to do a physical exam. He confirmed I was in trouble. The on-call cardiologist, whom I had never met, came to talk to me about my options. He admitted to being very tired, having been up all night with the stab victim. We laughed at the absurdity of the procedure; a blind stick aimed toward the left shoulder to drain the fluid that crowded my heart. I appreciated his frankness and even his hesitancy. I told him he was likely not going to get any sleep between now and the middle of the next night, so we ought to go to the Cath Lab now to relieve cardiac tamponade. My argument was that it would be safer in the Cath Lab, a controlled environment with the benefit of fluoroscopy, than when I crashed in the ICU later that night. Also, my favorite echocardiogram technician would assist him. He agreed. As I hugged my husband and walked to the gurney, I caught a glimpse of my nurse with tears in her eyes. She was right there with me.

As they wheeled me through corridors, I asked the Cath Lab staff if the cardiologist had good hands, knowing how important that is, interventional cardiology being my specialty. Unbeknownst to me, the cardiologist was following behind and overheard my question and blurted, "Yes, I have great hands!" It turns out he did. He inserted the long needle under my sternum into my pericardium and drained the fluid, squeezing my heart.

After the procedure, each ICU nurse sat on the edge of my bed and shared their own stories. One veteran nurse told me about her experience with pericarditis and reassured me. Each nurse listened to me and left the monitors facing me to watch my hemodynamics. None of the nurses did a power-play to keep me from being a nurse, and my expertise didn't intimidate any of the nurses, even the new graduates.

The transfer out of the ICU to a monitored hospital room was sublime. A small, elderly porter serenaded me in Spanish as he pushed my wheelchair down to the first floor by the lush gardens and sculptures and through hallways lined with artwork by local artists. His tenderness brought tears to my eyes as he lifted my legs from the wheelchair and gently placed me in my new bed.

The next day I was home, taking my first full shower in over two weeks. Restorative yoga, gentle strength training, massage, walks on the beach, and day trips to art museums were all part of my recovery. When people saw me after the ordeal, they'd ask if I was back to normal. I would pause and think before answering. With acquaintances, it felt like they just wanted me to say, "oh yes," so they could move on. Knowing that my ordeal is a reminder, or trigger, of their own mortality, I would say, "well, it's slow, but I'm getting better." With those who really wanted to know, I'd say, "no, I'll never be the same, and I wouldn't want to be. Even if I regain my vitality, I am changed forever." Something shifts on a deep level when an illness of this magnitude visits.

The worst part of being a patient is the diagnostic tests—the anxiety before the test and the worry awaiting the results. I'm convinced a patient can deal with just about anything once they know the truth. I've had too many biopsies, mammograms, labs, looking for something, often with untimely follow-up. Even during my 2-week ICU stay, the specialists looked for something exotic rather than treating my symptoms. In the end, the diagnosis was idiopathic pericarditis, possibly linked to radiation treatment decades prior or inflammation secondary to viral pneumonia several months before. It progressed because it went untreated. In a retrospective review, the ECG from the first emergency room visit did show subtle changes (slight PR depression and slight ST elevation). The first spiral CT scan showed a small pericardial effusion.

Both of my parents died six years before my ICU stay. Recently, I had an email exchange with one of their close friends. He remembered what it was like for them when I had Hodgkin lymphoma at 16 years old. He said,

> Your illness terrified, devastated, and changed your parents. I can only imagine what it would be to have my child facing a critical illness, battling through the debilitating treatments, and trying to be strong for them while cowering in terror and uncertainty inside myself. Your resilience inspired them. They had profound gratitude that you were alive and that you were so resilient and seemingly so well-adjusted, despite your burdens, trials that no one should face at that age.

I told him that I've always been grateful that my parents allowed my high school experience to be about socializing and sports, and for that, I have great memories. He responded, "I think that was what they wanted you to have, given the mountains you had to climb. Wasn't it a gift that this is your memory of those times?" What a beautiful thing to learn at this stage of life. He let me in on what it was like for my parents.

11.3 IT IS NOT A BATTLE

Nurses tend to be perfectionists and task-oriented, which is quite useful to the role. They become uncomfortable when things slow down. Productivity and efficiency are essential. I want to make a case for slowing down. Like wintertime, there are times to pull in, leave the extroverted world, and go inward.

I've learned that the body is resilient and rebounds from illness, and there are opportunities to learn and adapt with each experience. Accepting personal limitations and help from others, when needed, develops character. Yet, how do we listen and work with the body to create an environment conducive to our particular way of healing? I've learned to stop and listen and never make it a battle. Starting a war against an illness means fighting against one's own body. It can't be a conflict. Otherwise, the body is ravaged by civil war. I cringe each time I read an obituary about someone who "lost their battle" with cancer. Serious illness calls for creativity and kindness. Witnessing, being present, and encouragement are helpful tools. Illness is a time to slow down and listen. This gives one access to unknown inner strength. Many connect to a higher power or something larger that enhances life's meaning.

And, here's my case for "the blues." When melancholy shows up, I embrace it. Deep sadness and grief are afflictions of the soul, symptoms that need attention. Melancholia has taught me to slow down and feel life in its fullness, which includes the joys and sorrows. The word *treatment* has etymological roots in "to haul" or "to drag." The soul does not want to be hauled or dragged through life. Rather than advance, deep sorrow insists on retreat. One is forced downwards toward the instinctual self. The soul wants time to backtrack, linger, and ponder. Mourning goes hand in hand with illness and proclaims the necessity for change. Symptoms are persistent. They sound an alarm and require interaction. I sit quietly and ask, "what do you need? What do you want?" There is always an answer. Healing doesn't mean cure, but rather transition, acceptance, and growth. It is not putting on a cheerful face but allows sadness, pensiveness, and heaviness of heart to prevail. Without mourning, there is no enrichment, no refinement of the soul.

As a nurse, supporting the patient by staying in reality without pretending everything will be all right acknowledges the truth and keeps the patient grounded. At the core, this helps them not give up. We all face the same terror—death. In mythology, we learn that gods and goddesses are jealous of humans because we are mortal and know we have limited time. Sigmund Freud suggested that this human limitation raises the value of enjoyment. Staring into the face of death makes life more precious.

Some nurses are most comfortable when staying busy. Even when the occasion arises to slow down, a new task distracts them. As nurses, we are always on alert for a crisis. There is a particular way each nurse practices, and exactness and compulsiveness are typical safety features. It also brings comfort in the form of control. I notice this when working with nurses and when I'm a patient receiving their care. Occasionally, a nurse is present and slow, willing to discuss the big picture. The exchange is allowed to go both ways. It's powerful and something I wish I could teach nurses; how to slow down when there is an opportunity and look at the exquisite bond available to them.

My academic training has taught me how to make meaning out of suffering through myths and archetypal figures. Collective stories can open the complexities of our shared humanity. For instance, I associate my experience with Hodgkin lymphoma with Persephone, the young maiden abruptly kidnaped by Hades and taken into the underworld. Her time of childhood innocence and girlhood sharply ended. My hematologist at Stanford, like Hades, became my guide. What followed was staging, surgery, radiation treatment, and recovery—a heroine's journey. An initiation that developed into a 40-year friendship until he died. We each said, "I love you," on his deathbed.

Grief work and mourning are different than depression. We must allow time to honor our sorrows. Rather than battle or blame, this tragic sensibility gives freedom for movement in and out of health and illness, joy and vulnerability. Without trying to fix things right away, sadness and the blues connect to humility, and we can stay grounded while the mystery of our life unfolds.

11.4   THE ROLE OF PATIENT

I "lost it" a few times during my ICU stay. I was getting worse, and each consultant focused on causality, not my symptoms. Only when I voiced my frustration, the tide shifted. They heard me. My nursing background saved me. They took measures to treat my symptoms even though the diagnosis was still unclear.

In 1628, William Harvey published *De Motu Cordis*, a book that identified the heart as a mechanical pump. It shifted the paradigm. The heart is no longer the center of our being—our feeling—but a mechanism. How readily we compartmentalize and numb out to avoid feeling. Facing our broken hearts with courage can help clarify individual and collective values. The necessity of grief work is to acknowledge life's complexity. Without a tragic sensibility, we remain isolated and forget what makes us feel deeply, connect to others, and experience the exquisite joy of being alive.

During my ICU stay, I was new to the community. My trusted medical and nursing colleagues were elsewhere and only available by telephone. I had to rely on my gut and trust practitioners I did not know. From the very start, I knew I needed to focus on being a patient. First, I made it clear I did not want any visitors. My job was to focus on my illness. Since I knew my friends would worry, my husband and I composed daily email updates like this one:

Day 3

Elizabeth had a right thoracentesis (lung tap) yesterday, and we are anxiously awaiting the pathology report, which will take a few days. It is likely something to do with one of three scenarios: infection, autoimmune, or malignancy. So, we are in that place of not knowing, which is always the most intense and exhausting. We so appreciate all the calls, emails, and offers to help. We are taking good care of one another and even finding some laughter through it all. The nursing staff is excellent. Elizabeth is more comfortable today and is off oxygen. She is loved by many and bolstered by all the thoughts, prayers, love, and well wishes. We will check emails and voicemails when we can and will keep you posted as we know more.

It made absolutely no sense to me to have social visits. My role, as an ICU patient, was to listen to my body, remain alert, and communicate with nurses, physicians, and others caring for me, available to each consultant 24 hours a day, focused on every piece of information to make the right decisions. I pulled in. I was in trouble and needed all of my faculties and energy. As a patient, my respect for each nurse, physician, aide, technician, housekeeper allows them to be clear-minded and do their best work. I reap the benefits of each person's training, calling, and compassion. I must see them for them to see me.

Nurses commented on the ambiance of my ICU room. I played my favorite music and meditations, focusing on body scans and the chakra system. Essential oils, lotions, and potions were around. Being a good eater, I decided to try everything on the room service menu throughout my stay. Each morning I'd walk to the whiteboard and write my goals for the day, and then my husband gave me a foot and sponge bath. On occasion, the nurse rolled my bed under a window where the sun could shine on me. Florence Nightingale was an advocate of fresh air, clean sheets, quiet, nutrition, pet visitation, and putting the patient in the best condition for nature to heal the body, which also means to soothe and heal the mind and spirit.

There I was, frightened, fully exposed, with specialists looking for either a simple answer or some exotic disease. On a mythical level, I was a sacrificial victim associated with growth, renewal, and water. My body was full of water on admission. It was everywhere. In alchemy, there is a period of flooding after the darkness. I had completed the agonizing push to finish my dissertation the year before. Right after my oral defense, I developed pneumonia and never felt quite right all year, and then the pericarditis developed. In retrospect, it feels this physical manifestation was part of my metamorphosis from a young adult into maturity.

My closest friendships have developed during difficult and transformative times. Showing vulnerability opens new doors. We need souls to witness our suffering. The idea that we can control our lives and live in total health denies the randomness of illness and suffering. The best clinicians ask what the patient feels is going on, listens, takes it into account, and never patronizes.

Schopenhauer's idea, as described by mythologist Joseph Campbell, observes that

once you have reached an advanced age … as you look back over your life, it can seem to have had a plot, as though composed by a novelist. Events that seemed entirely accidental or incidental turn out to have been central in the composition.

112

I find this to be true throughout life's hardships. Things almost always make sense in retrospect. Knowing this helps me when I face what at the time seems insurmountable.

Day 8

Elizabeth was sitting up in a chair this morning when I arrived, and the nurse had washed her hair. She was smiling. She said while brushing her teeth, "Today feels so much different than yesterday." Yesterday she was recovering from an emergency procedure for cardiac tamponade (400 cc/13.5 oz, fluid removed) and placement of an IVC filter. Then she had a run in with a cardiac surgeon who wanted to do a non-emergent-pericardial-window—right now—with no explanation. When she said she wanted to wait and discuss the surgery with her physician team, he stormed off, threw his cell phone, and yelled at the nurses. Elizabeth queried, "Could you imagine me letting that mean man touch my heart?" … Because of a low census, Elizabeth moved to a different ICU room. She walked rather than being transported. Because it's an end room, it has a recessed rectangular window through which she watched a crescent moon at 5 a.m. She asked to have her bed positioned against a window to feel the sunlight and see a bit of nature. Watching Elizabeth interact with the nurses is a treat.

When I got home, I set up all my favorite pillows and blankets with all the windows open in my bedroom, allowing natural light to stream in. My husband shopped at the farmer's market and created beautiful plates of whole fresh food. As I felt better, I read poetry, and we made trips to art museums because art and poetry connect me to my inner life—massage, theater, film, women-friends, and working on things bigger than myself brought meaning. Finding joy and cultivating love helped me the most.

My illnesses have awakened me. The body is profound and the conduit to the soul. I strive for complexity, not perfection. We are each given a particular life, with specific lessons, challenges, and growth and renewal opportunities. Through curiosity, experience, academics, relationships, health, and illnesses, we become more fully who we are.

During the pandemic, I've been working remotely, resisting exposure to the coronavirus. Being high-risk, I was eager to receive the vaccine. As soon as I did, I started the training to work at the vaccination clinic, even though it had been three decades since I'd given an IM injection. My first exposure to anyone outside my household was at the drive-through station, leaning into cars, giving shots. Each patient was so grateful. The intensity, stimulation, and anxiety from every carload penetrated my psyche. I could feel it in my body throughout the day. I felt shaky. After my shift, I walked to my car and sat for a while before heading home. Tears came to my eyes as I began to let in the enormity. Overwhelmed with the collective grief I felt from the day, I welcomed a flow of cleansing tears. What an honor to be a nurse, to be of use in a practical way. Sometimes, I'm a patient. Sometimes, I'm a nurse. I am always both. My role at the clinic is nurse, and what I carry in each encounter is the clarity I acquired as a patient.

11.5   SUGGESTED READING

Becker, E. (2020). *The denial of death*. Souvenir Press.

Bond, D. S. (2001). *Living myth: Personal meaning as a way of life*. Shambhala.

Campbell, J., & Kudler, D. (2018). *Pathways to bliss: Mythology and personal transformation*. Yogi Impressions.

Cowan, L. (2004). *Portrait of the blue lady: The character of melancholy*. Spring Journal Books.

Guggenbuhl-Craig, A. (2009). *Power in the helping professions*. Spring Publications.

Heilbrun, C. (1988). *Writing a woman's life*. Ballantine.

Hillman, J. (2019). *Healing fiction*. Spring Publications.

Jung, C.G. (1969–1989). *The collected works of C. G. Jung* (R. F. Hull, Trans.). Bollingen Series 20. Princeton University Press.

Mitford, J. (1963). *The American way of death*. Simon and Schuster.

Mogenson, G. (2005). *Greeting the angels: An imaginal view of the mourning process*. Baywood.

Nightingale, F. (2001–2012). *The collected works of Florence Nightingale* (1820–1910). 16 vols. (Lynn McDonald, Ed.). Wilfrid Laurier University Press.

Robinson, E.A. (2013). *The soul of the nurse*. SpannRobinson.

Sontag, S. (1988). *Illness as metaphor*. Farrer, Straus, & Giroux.

Woodman, M. (1982). *Addiction to perfection: The still unravished bride*. Inner City Books.

Woodman, M. (2001). *Bone: Dying into life*. Penguin Compass.

12 Effects of Disease on Families and Support Systems

Janine Santora
Capital Health Institute for Neurosciences
Pennington, NJ, USA

CONTENTS

KEY POINTS

- Chronic disease is the leading cause of disability and death in the US, with approximately 70% of all deaths in the US caused by chronic disease.
- Informal caregivers play a fundamental role in homecare. Caregiving occurs across all family types, generations, racial/ethnic groups, gender identities, sexual orientations, education levels, and income levels.
- Disease affects not only the individual with the diagnosis but also those who care for and support the individual. A negative impact on a spouse/significant other or family member's daily activities can occur due to the time dedicated to care for their loved one diagnosed with the disease.

12.1 INTRODUCTION

The effect of disease can reduce quality of life for the individual living with the diagnosis along with the people in their support system (Golics et al., 2013). Health-related quality of life (HRQOL) focuses on how a person's health status impacts their physical, social, and emotional functioning (Healthy people, 2020). According to Golics et al. (2013), previous research has shown that the negative impact of illness regarding emotional functioning can be more significant on family members when compared to patients themselves. The effects of disease can negatively affect families and support systems, impacting their ability to care for a loved one diagnosed with disease (Litterini & Wilson, 2021). Worrying about the future of their loved one can cause emotional distress along with feelings of helplessness and stress. Daily activities of family members and other support can be negatively impacted due to the time dedicated to caring for their loved one who has been diagnosed with disease. Instead of spending time on their own hobbies, interests, and self-care, they dedicate their time to their loved one's health, which may include eating, hygiene, safety, medication management, mobility, medical management, dressing, and managing a household. Family relationships like marriage may become strained due to increased tension and stress of disease. Less time may

DOI: 10.1201/9781003178330-14

be spent with other family members, including other children, spouses, mothers, and fathers. Sleep can also be negatively impacted. Waking up to check on loved ones, losing sleep due to worry, and waking up to assist the loved one living with disease can lead to sleep loss. Taking vacations can be negatively impacted due to doctor's appointments, impact of the illness, or worrying about meeting the medical needs of their loved one while on vacation. There may be a significant financial impact of disease on caregivers due to the loss of income if the caregiver is unable to work due to the commitments of caring for their loved one living with disease. Partners and family members report a negative impact on their social life due to lack of funds, worrying about others' perception of their loved one's illness, and leaving social events early. The impact of disease can be profound and affect all within reach.

12.2　CHRONIC DISEASE

Chronic diseases are conditions that persist for a year or more (University of Michigan, 2021). Chronic disease may limit activities of daily living and require continuing medical care. Heart disease, cancer, stroke, Alzheimer's, diabetes, and chronic lung disease are major chronic diseases. In the United States (US), 6 in 10 adults live with one chronic disease, and 4 in 10 adults live with two or more chronic diseases.

12.2.1　MORTALITY OF CHRONIC DISEASE

Chronic disease is the leading cause of disability and death in the US. Seventy percent of all deaths in the US are caused by chronic disease (CDC, 2021).

Chronic diseases are responsible collectively for 71% of all deaths worldwide (WHO, 2021). Chronic diseases are noncommunicable diseases (NCDs). Worldwide, 41 million individuals die each year from noncommunicable diseases. Worldwide, 15 million individuals between the ages of 30 and 69 years of age die prematurely from noncommunicable diseases, including cardiovascular disease (17.9 million deaths annually), cancers (9.3 million deaths annually), respiratory diseases (4.1 million deaths annually), and diabetes (1.5 million deaths annually), which account for 80% of all premature deaths from noncommunicable diseases. Chronic disease can negatively impact quality of life, shorten life expectancy, increase healthcare costs, and lead to decreased productivity, depression, acute health issues, and symptoms that may require daily management. Chronic diseases pose deleterious health consequences for the individual living with chronic disease along with consequences for the loved ones caring for them, the communities they live in, and the overwhelming impact on healthcare systems.

12.3　INFORMAL CAREGIVERS

Informal caregivers are family members or friends (Prevo et al., 2018). The care of individuals living with chronic disease is a priority in most countries around the world (Szlenk-Czyczerska et al., 2020). The individual's home is the preferred location for treatment and care. Informal caregivers are often unpaid and play a fundamental role in homecare. There is a knowledge deficit related to the support of caregivers despite their growing numbers. Caregiving can be rewarding, but it can also put caregivers at increased risk for negative health consequences. One in five Americans are caregivers, totaling an estimated 53 million adult caregivers in the United States (AARP, 2020). Caregiving occurs across all family types, generations, racial/ethnic groups, gender identities, sexual orientations, education levels, and income levels. Women comprised 61% of caregivers compared to 39% of men. Many caregivers are caring for one person, but up to 24% of caregivers reported caring for two or more ill adults. Caring for the chronically ill can lead to caregiver burden, causing long-term stress due to physical, emotional, social, and economic costs.

12.3.1   Negative Impact of Caregiving

Caregivers often develop disease themselves as a result of exposure to chronic stress (Szlenk-Czyczerska et al., 2020). An important aspect of caregiving is the choice of taking on the caregiver role (AARP, 2020). More than half of caregivers felt they did not have a choice when taking on the responsibility of caregiving (53%), compared to 46% who felt they did have a choice. Among caregivers, 40% lived in the same household as the care recipient, 36% lived within 20 minutes, and 11% lived 1–2 hours away from the care recipient. Caregivers provide care an average of 23.7 hours a week, with 21% of caregivers working a full-time job of 40 hours or more. Caregivers assist with a wide range of activities of daily living (ADLs), including getting in and out of beds and chairs (41%), getting dressed (31%), getting to and from the toilet (27%), bathing and showering (27%), feeding (26%), and dealing with incontinence (18%). One in five caregivers reports difficulty in assisting care recipients with ADLs. Instrumental activities of daily living (IADLs) include transportation, grocery or other shopping, housework, preparing meals, managing finances, giving medications, and arranging outside services. Among caregivers, 99% assist care recipients with IADLs, and 93% assist with two or more IADLs. Caregivers also monitor the severity of the care recipient's condition (71%), communicate with healthcare professionals (65%), and advocate with providers, services, and agencies (56%). The decline of caregiver self-rated health over the past five years may be exacerbated by the stress associated with caregiving (AARP, 2020). Caregivers often reported it was challenging to care for their own health (23%) with 17% of caregivers reported that their caregiver duties caused high physical strain. The emotional and burden was significant with 36% of caregivers reported caregiving to be highly stressful and 21% of caregivers reported feeling alone. Interestingly even with the added stress, 51% of caregivers reported that their caregiving role gave them a sense of purpose or meaning in life.

Financial stress was reported in 18% of the caregivers. The top financial impacts on caregivers included stopped saving (28%), took on more debt (23%), used up personal short-term savings (22%), left bills unpaid/paid them late (19%), and borrowed money from family or friends (15%). Caregiving can negatively impact caregivers that work. The work impacts of caregiving include going in late, leaving early, taking time off (53%), going from working full time to part-time or reduced hours (15%), leave of absence (14%), receiving warnings about performance/attendance (8%), turned down a promotion (7%), gave up work entirely (6%), retired early (5%), or lost job benefits (4%). Among caregivers, 27% reported it was difficult to get affordable services in the community, including in-home health services, transportation, or delivered meals to assist with care. Support for caregivers is critical to prevent the decline of self-reported caregiver health. Caregivers need to attend to their own health, so they can in turn care for others.

12.4   THE FAR REACH OF DISEASE

Diseases have a far-reaching effect on all those that come to know the devastation of illness. When a loved one is diagnosed with disease, those who care about them often experience emotional distress.

Disease can destroy future dreams and change lives. The diagnosis of disease causes a cascade of events from understanding the diagnosis to end-of-life planning. There are barriers preventing the full understanding of a diagnosis, such as language barriers and lack of access to informative resources. Obtaining medicines, medical equipment, and therapy services can negatively impact a family if economic resources are limited or insurance does not cover the needed medical necessities. Disease can cause disabilities that require caregiving, which is often done by an informal caretaker. Having an informal caregiver can alter the relationship between the individual diagnosed and those who care about them. Daughters may bathe, dress, and feed mothers that no longer recognize them. Wives may give up careers to care for their husbands in wheelchairs. Husbands may watch diabetes rob their wives of their eyesight, kidney function, limbs, or ability to walk. Homes may need to be altered and equipped with handicap ramps, safety bars, and equipment in the bathroom, hospital beds, and oxygen tanks, depending on the individual's needs. Bank accounts may be drained to pay for medical care, equipment, therapy, medicines, and copays. Informal caregiving can become an overwhelming full-time job.

12.5   CONCLUSION

The emotional toll of disease on family members and support systems can be overwhelming. Hopes and dreams for the future change due to this unwanted, uninvited new family member, disease. The self-care techniques described throughout this book are applicable to not only the patient and the nurse but also families and support systems. Specifically, the mindfulness skills suggested in Chapter 31 can help loved ones navigate the stress associated with disease.

REFERENCES

American Association of Retired Persons. (2020, May 1). *Caregiving in the U.S. 2020*. AARP. Retrieved May 16, 2021, from www.aarp.org

Centers for Disease Control and Prevention. (2021, April 28). *About chronic diseases*. National Center for Chronic Disease Prevention and Health Promotion (NCCDPHP). Retrieved May 16, 2022, from www.cdc.gov

Golics, C., Basra, M., Salek, & Finlay, A. Y. (2013). The impact of patients' chronic disease on family quality of life: An experience from 26 specialties. *International Journal of General Medicine*, 6, 787–798. https://doi.org/10.2147/ijgm.s45156

Healthy People. (2020, October 8). *Health-related quality of life & well-being*. Retrieved May 9, 2021, from www.healthypeople.gov

Litterini, A. J., & Wilson, C. M. (2021). *Physical activity and rehabilitation in life-threatening illness* (1st ed.). Taylor & Francis.

Prevo, L., Hajema, K., Linssen, E., Kremers, S., Crutzen, R., & Schneider, F. (2018). Population characteristics and needs of informal caregivers associated with the risk of perceiving a high burden: A cross-sectional study. *Inquiry*, 55. http://doi.org/10.1177/0046958018775570

Szlenk-Czyczerska, E., Guzek, M., Bielska, D., Ławnik, A., Polański, P., & Kurpas, D. (2020). Needs, aggravation, and degree of burnout in informal caregivers of patients with chronic cardiovascular disease. *International Journal of Environmental Research and Public Health*, 17(17), 6427. https://doi.org/10.3390/ijerph17176427

University of Michigan. (2021, January 1). *About chronic disease*. Center for Managing Chronic Disease University of Michigan. Retrieved May 16, 2021, from https://cmcd.sph.umich.edu

World Health Organization. (2021, January 1). *Noncommunicable diseases*. World Health Organization. Retrieved May 16, 2021, from www.who.int

13 Health Disparities

*Yvonne Commodore-Mensah[1], Ruth-Alma Turkson-Ocran[2],
Oluwabunmi Ogungbe[1], Samuel Byiringiro[1], and
Diana-Lyn Baptiste[1]*

[1]Johns Hopkins School of Nursing
Baltimore, Maryland, USA
[2]Johns Hopkins School of Medicine
Baltimore, Maryland, USA

CONTENTS

KEY POINTS

- Health disparities are often described in the context of racial and ethnic disparities, although many dimensions of health disparities exist in the United States and globally.
- Social and environmental factors such as socioeconomic status, education, employment, discrimination, and healthcare access contribute to health disparities.
- Nurses are uniquely positioned to address national and global health disparities and influence change through humanitarian interventions, health policy, and research.

13.1 DEFINITION OF HEALTH DISPARITIES

Health disparities are defined as differences in health outcomes that are closely linked with social, economic, and environmental disadvantage—driven by the social conditions in which individuals

DOI: 10.1201/9781003178330-15

live, learn, work, and play (Marmot & Allen, 2014). These conditions are often referred to as social determinants of health (SDoH). The World Health Organization (WHO) defines SDoH as conditions in which people are born, grow, work, live, and age and the wider set of forces and systems shaping the conditions of daily life (World Health Organization, 2011). These forces and systems include economic policies and systems, development agendas, social norms, social policies, and political systems (World Health Organization, 2011). Health equity, however, is achieved "when every person has the opportunity to attain his or her full health potential, and no one is disadvantaged from achieving this potential because of social position or other socially determined circumstances" (Whitehead et al., 2006).

13.2 TYPES OF HEALTH DISPARITIES

Although health disparities are commonly viewed through a race/ethnicity lens, disparities can occur across various dimensions, including age, gender, socioeconomic status, language, geography, physical disability, nativity status (US-born versus foreign-born), sexual orientation, and identity, among others. Notably, these groups are not mutually exclusive—they often intersect. Intersectionality is a term that has been used to describe how multiple dimensions of social inequality, including race, gender, income, and neighborhood, interact (Bauer, 2014; Crenshaw, 1989; Veenstra, 2013) to influence health outcomes.

13.2.1 RACE AND ETHNICITY

There is no biological basis for racial and ethnic groupings that are commonly defined in the literature. Indeed, race and ethnicity are social constructs used to describe populations and influence how they are perceived by others and themselves (Du Bois, 2017). Historical policies and practices, migration patterns, and social perceptions are factors that have shaped the social construction of race and ethnicity (Du Bois, 2017).

In the US, health disparities were documented in a seminal Institute of Medicine report (Institute of Medicine Committee on Understanding and Eliminating Racial and Ethnic Disparities in Health Care, 2003). Almost two decades later, the recommendations presented by the committee have not translated into a narrowing of health disparities. For instance, the Black–White disparity in life expectancy is approximately 3.6 years (Arias et al., 2019). Although this represents a 50% reduction in the gap from the 1980s (Centers for Disease Control and Prevention, 2017), there are persistent disparities in life expectancy across different US states. For example, in the District of Columbia and states such as New Hampshire, Wisconsin, and Maine, the Black–White life expectancy increased between 1990 and 2009 (Harper et al., 2014). Although age-adjusted mortality rates from cardiovascular disease (CVD) have declined from 1999 to 2017, the mortality rate for Black people is more than twice that of Asian or Pacific Islander persons and higher than White persons (Centers for Disease Control Prevention, 2019). Moreover, the prevalence of CVD risk factors such as hypertension, obesity, and diabetes are higher among racial and ethnic minorities, particularly non-Hispanic Black and Hispanic adults (Virani et al., 2020).

Another striking instance of racial and ethnic differences is in maternal health outcomes in developed countries. In the US, mortality rates from pregnancy-related causes are two to three times higher among Black, American Indian, and Alaska Native (AI/AN) women than White women (Petersen et al., 2019). In the United Kingdom, Black women are four times more likely to die during pregnancy and childbirth than White women (Knight et al., 2017). These disparities are preventable and have persisted over time, despite advances in maternal health.

Among men, the mortality rate from prostate cancer is 2.5 times higher in Black men than White men (Dess et al., 2019). During the COVID-19 pandemic, racial and ethnic disparities in cases, hospitalization, and mortality have also been documented. Black persons, Hispanic persons, American

Indian, or Alaskan Native persons are more likely to be hospitalized and die from COVID-19 than Whites in the US (Centers for Disease Control Prevention, 2021).

13.2.2 SEX DIFFERENCES

Sex differences are differences in health status and outcomes based on biological sex, which is usually defined by chromosomal composition and/or hormonal influences rather than environmental (e.g., social and cultural) and psychological (e.g., developmental) factors (Glezerman, 2016). It is important to note that historically, studies examining sex differences have not investigated or reported the gap between sex assigned at birth and gender expression. For these reasons, we focus our discussion on sex differences in health outcomes.

Differences in the health of males and females have been well documented. Sex differences are observed in the pathophysiology, risk, prevalence, manifestation, progression, treatment, response, and mortality for several disease conditions (Mauvais-Jarvis et al., 2020). Due to safety considerations surrounding childbearing, women (particularly of childbearing age) were historically excluded from clinical trials (Clayton, 2016). However, this practice changed in 1993, when the National Institutes of Health (NIH) Revitalization Act of 1993 mandated that women be included in clinical trials. Hypertension and dyslipidemia, for example, are lower in men and premenopausal women (Group et al., 2016). Women have a higher prevalence of diabetes, depression, and anxiety and suffer worse outcomes after myocardial infarction than men (Asleh et al., 2021).

13.2.3 ABILITY STATUS

People with disabilities are an understudied population with respect to health disparities. Globally, more than 1 billion people, or about 15%, live with a disability (World Health Organization, 2020). In the US, one in four noninstitutionalized people has a disability (Okoro et al., 2018). Disability status also intersects with race and ethnicity, gender, and socioeconomic status. People who are disabled (40.3%) are more likely to rate their health as poor than those who are not disabled (9.9%) (Altman & Bernstein, 2008). Persons with disabilities have a higher prevalence of death from cardiovascular disease and lower respiratory diseases (Forman-Hoffman et al., 2015).

13.2.4 GEOGRAPHIC LOCATION

Where a person lives is a good indicator of their health, quality of life, and life span. Additionally, features of the area in which a person lives affect health and quality of life (Institute of Medicine, 2008). Studies have highlighted differences in life expectancy by virtue of differences in zip code that are not explained by biological or genetic differences and that one's zip code matters more than their genetic code (Graham, 2016). Observed geographical health disparities have been attributed to differences in healthcare access, lifestyle, and cultural practices, and regional policies (National Academies of Sciences et al., 2017).

Health disparities have been observed by geographical location (region, state, urban, rural) and zip code (Institute of Medicine, 2002). For example, regardless of race/ethnicity, persons in the Southeastern US have a higher prevalence of stroke and death from hypertension than other US regions (Howard et al., 2007). This area is known as the Stroke Belt. Within this area lies the Stroke Buckle, a region along the coastal "low country" plains of the Carolinas and Georgia, which has even higher stroke rates (Howard & Howard, 2020).

Differences in infant mortality rates, life expectancy, chronic diseases, risk factors for preventable diseases such as smoking, and social determinants of health such as access to healthcare, healthy food, and physical activity are observed by geographical areas. Persons living in geographically remote areas or rural areas experience higher morbidity and mortality rates than persons living in urban areas with higher health ratings (Institute of Medicine, 2002). Living in rural areas has been associated with higher death rates for children and young adults (Institute of Medicine, 2002) and higher death rates from suicide, unintentional motor vehicle-traffic incidents, and ischemic heart disease among men (Institute of Medicine, 2002).

Racial/ethnic minorities also have lower rates of cancer screening and management and higher rates of cardiovascular disease and chronic disease risk factors such as diabetes compared to White persons by geographical region (Institute of Medicine, 2002) and higher mortality rates due to lower survival rates for serious health conditions (e.g., myocardial infarction, stroke) (Institute of Medicine, 2002).

13.3   THE ROOT CAUSES OF HEALTH DISPARITIES

When health disparities are described in the literature, there is often a tendency to summarize findings without discussing the root causes of health disparities. It is now widely accepted that racism, discrimination, and different forms of biases are fundamental drivers of disparities in health outcomes (Boyd et al., 2020; National Academies of Sciences, 2017).

13.3.1   RACISM

Racism of all forms, including interpersonal and structural racism, may be one of the causes of health disparities. At the interpersonal level, persons who report experiences of racism have poorer health outcomes than those who do not report it (Brondolo et al., 2011). For instance, in a multi-ethnic study of atherosclerosis, adults who reported experiencing lifetime discrimination have a higher risk of incident hypertension (Hazard Ratio: 1.35, 95% CI: 1.07, 1.69) than those who reported lower levels of lifetime discrimination (Forde Allana et al., 2021).

Structural racism is defined as the "normalization and legitimization of an array of dynamics—historical, cultural, institutional and interpersonal—that routinely advantage White people while producing cumulative and chronic adverse outcomes for people of color" (Lawrence & Keleher, 2004). Structural racism has recently been acknowledged as the fundamental cause and driver of health disparities in the US (Churchwell et al., 2020). Structural racism, which limits the lives of racially and ethnically diverse populations, operates at the most influential level—the socio-ecological level. This means that the structural mechanisms that generate and reinforce inequities do not require the actions of individual people (Gee & Ford, 2011).

13.3.2   HEALTHCARE ACCESS

The lack of equitable access to healthcare has been a long-standing problem in the US, underscoring the need for healthcare providers to pay close attention to those who have limited access (Arnett et al., 2019). Research shows that limited or no access to health services is associated with poorer health outcomes (Derose et al., 2011). Access to healthcare is highly dependent on social, environmental, and structural factors. Social determinants of health such as race/ethnicity, gender, socioeconomic status (SES), occupation, immigrant status, and rural or urban residence play a significant role in healthcare access and use of quality health services (Singh et al., 2017). There are marked disparities in the access, utilization, and affordability of healthcare. For example, those without health insurance may use the emergency department of hospitals to manage acute and chronic health problems, lacking the continuity of care and preventive health education needed to effectively manage these conditions. Additionally, access to healthcare does not necessarily equate with quality health services.

13.3.3 Racial Residential Segregation

Racial residential segregation, characterized by the physical separation of racial groups by enforced residence in specific neighborhoods, is recognized as a form of institutionalized racism and the root cause of health disparities (Williams & Collins, 2001). Residential separation is a phenomenon that reflects not personal choice but rather a result of public policies that were designed to subjugate racial and ethnic minorities to certain living conditions. In the US, a person's zip code is a more powerful determinant of health than their genetic code (Graham, 2016). Where people live affects their housing conditions, access to transportation, education, healthcare, and employment, among others. Although the discriminatory policies (e.g., mortgage redlining) and practices (blockbusting, steering, etc.) that promoted racial residential segregation have been outlawed for decades in the US, their impact can still be felt today (Collin et al., 2021; Lynch et al., 2021). According to the 2016 US County Health Rankings, Black–White residential segregation is highest in the Northeast and Great Lakes and lowest in the Southeast (University of Wisconsin Population Health Institute, 2015).

Differences in quality of life and life expectancy have been observed between persons who live within a few miles of each other, within the same geographical area. For instance, in Illinois, persons who live in downtown Chicago, an urban area characterized by business and high-rise buildings, have a life expectancy of 83 years (median income of $103,336), while residents who live three train stops away in the Washington Park area have a life expectancy of only 69 years (median household income of $25,385) (Healthbox, 2019). Across major cities such as Baltimore, Cleveland, Washington, DC, and New York, similar disparities in life expectancy have been documented among residents who live a few miles apart (Boing et al., 2020; Hunt et al., 2015).

13.3.4 Lifestyle Behaviors

Engaging in healthy lifestyle behaviors improves health and longevity. Conversely, unhealthy lifestyle behaviors, such as poor diet, physical inactivity, smoking, poor sleep, and alcohol intake, contribute to poor health, increased morbidity, and mortality. Disparities in health-promoting behaviors exist by age, sex, race/ethnicity, and region (Saint Onge & Krueger, 2017). Based on national US data, persons who are Black and Hispanic are less likely to engage in health-promoting behaviors (high levels of physical activity, healthy diet, adequate sleep, low levels of heavy drinking, and smoking) compared to persons who are White (Saint Onge & Krueger, 2017; Morris et al., 2018). Similarly, persons who live in the Western part of the US are more likely to engage in health-promoting behaviors than persons in the South, and persons who are in midlife are more likely to engage in healthier behaviors than persons who are younger or older (Saint Onge & Krueger, 2017). Men are also less likely to engage in health-promoting behaviors compared to women (Morris et al., 2018; Saint Onge & Krueger, 2017).

Disparities in the engagement in health-promoting behaviors are often driven by structural factors. The access to and availability of healthy foods is influenced by inequitable access in the environment, often under the influence of sociopolitical factors, with neighborhoods with low-income persons, minoritized populations, or persons living in rural areas having less healthy food access or living in healthy food deserts (Larson et al., 2009). Persons with access to more nutritious food sources have healthier diets and better health profiles (Larson et al., 2009). Similarly, persons who live in safe neighborhoods with infrastructure that makes it easy to engage in physical activity (e.g., are well lit, have parks, adequate sidewalks, and adequate recreational exercise facilities) are healthier than those who do not (Ammerman et al., 2006; Kohl et al., 2012).

13.4 GLOBAL HEALTH DISPARITIES

Nurses must also advocate for health and wellness for everyone around the globe. Global health disparities are well documented. The majority of African countries have high infant mortality rates, while those in Europe and North America have lower rates (World Health Organization, 2011). The life expectancy of a Malawian child is only 47 years, while that of a Japanese child is 83 years (World Health Organization, 2011). Health disparities exist within and across borders globally. Health conditions eradicated in many wealthy countries continue to claim millions of lives in resource-constrained nations. Factors including political, environmental, and socioeconomic motives fuel these disparities, yet socially and economically disadvantaged people are disproportionately affected. The epidemiological transition may account for global health disparities. The epidemiologic transition refers to the shift of the pattern of mortality and the cause of death from communicable diseases to noncommunicable diseases (NCDs) such as CVD, degenerative diseases, cancers, and mental health ailments (McCracken & Phillips, 2017; Mendoza & Miranda, 2017; Mercer, 2018). The epidemiologic transition is the result of globalization, access to better healthcare, and changes in the standards of living. For instance, the rising rates of CVD in low- and middle-income countries (LMICs) are attributed to change in lifestyle behaviors (Burroughs Pena & Bloomfield, 2015).

Despite the changing patterns of fertility, diseases, and mortality in LMICs experiencing the epidemiologic transition, infectious diseases such as HIV, tuberculosis, and upper respiratory infections have not been eradicated (Santosa & Byass, 2016). Health systems in LMICs are challenged with managing the double burden of both communicable and NCDs. The 10 leading causes of death in LMICs include NCDs such as stroke, ischemic heart diseases, road injuries, and infectious diseases such as lower respiratory infections, diarrheal diseases, HIV/AIDS, and tuberculosis (Mathers et al., 2017). For example, rheumatic heart disease (RHD), a chronic condition resulting from recurrent untreated Group A Streptococcus throat infections and causing rheumatic fever and heart, blood vessel, and joint damage, is more prevalent in LMICs but nearly eradicated in high-income countries despite the effectiveness of penicillin in treating this condition (Byiringiro et al., 2020; Lyons & Stewart, 2011; Watkins et al., 2017).

13.4.1 Solutions to Address Health Disparities

The complexity of health disparities warrants a comprehensive, multi-pronged problem-solving approach. Factors contributing to health go beyond the individual domain and include local, state, regional, national, and global level policies (National Academies of Sciences Engineering and Medicine, 2017b). In the US, health disparities are recognized and addressed by government agencies such as the Centers for Disease Control (CDC) and the US Department of Health and Human Services (USDHHS) through the Health People campaigns.

Every decade, the Healthy People initiative develops a new set of science-based, 10-year national objectives to improve the health of all Americans (US Department of Health and Human Services, Office of Disease Prevention and Health Promotion, 2020). The development of Healthy People 2030 (HP2030) includes establishing a framework for the initiative—the vision, mission, foundational principles, plan of action, and overarching goals of improving general health status, health-related quality of life, SDoH, and health disparities.

Additionally, the CDC and USDHHS propose initiatives to inform and influence health policies that further fill gaps in healthcare and health disparities. More recently, with the emergence of the COVID-19 pandemic, it is suggested that HP2030 shift objectives to prioritizing access to digital health and improving health literacy to reduce health disparities.

Globally, the WHO continues to lead efforts to eliminate global health disparities. The WHO addresses health inequalities across LMICs, focused on eliminating the 17 Sustainable Development Goals, which include common SDoH such as poverty, access to healthcare, education, affordable clean energy, and sustainable cities and communities.

13.4.2 Community-Based Interventions

If communities shape the development and transmission of diseases, those same communities are ideal avenues to promote health and well-being. Community-based interventions are actions, policy programs that are driven by members of a community and have the potential to address health inequities (National Academies of Sciences Engineering and Medicine, 2017b). Communities are the bedrock of health, and different communities experience health disparities differently. However, there are challenges that may be unique to underserved and marginalized populations (National Academies of Sciences Engineering and Medicine, 2017b).

Three major elements of successful community interventions include multi-sector collaboration, health equity as a shared vision and value, and community capacity to shape outcomes (National Academies of Sciences Engineering and Medicine, 2017a). Multi-sector partnerships among various actors, including community members and groups, private sector, non-profit, researchers, public health, government, etc., are essential to achieving health equity(Mattessich & Rausch, 2014; National Academies of Sciences Engineering and Medicine, 2017a). The solutions to health disparities are more likely to have a systemic impact when they are community-driven and involve resources and insights from various perspectives. Community-driven solutions fundamentally rely on a shared goal and vision by members of the community. Achieving health equity needs to be a shared vision to set critical community-based partnerships in motion. Community capacity is the capability of communities to identify common needs and to draw on resources and community actors to build social and political capital to address these needs. The capacity of communities to recognize the issues of health inequities and organize to address these issues fosters authentic community-led action.

13.4.3 Training of Healthcare Personnel

The complexity of health disparities highlights the need for training and retraining of healthcare personnel. It is crucial to adopt a transdisciplinary lens to such training. There is growing acknowledgment of and appreciation for the need to develop a culturally competent healthcare workforce (McGregor et al., 2019). Thus, the integration of cultural competence of curricula devoid of stereotypes into nursing and healthcare curricula is an essential strategy to reducing health inequities (McGregor et al., 2019).

Most cultural competency training has focused on knowledge and skills for responding to sociocultural issues during clinical encounters. Such approaches have been criticized as stereotypical and inaccurate representations of entire populations. As such, cultural competence training should focus on understanding how culture shapes people's lives and lifestyle behaviors, effective integration of cultural competence into healthcare practices, continuous value clarification, and awareness of personal biases and prejudices (Hark & DeLisser, 2011; Purnell, 2012).

13.4.4 Diversifying the Healthcare Workforce

Diversifying the healthcare workforce is a crucial strategy to reducing health disparities. However, significant gaps exist in the successful diversification of the healthcare workforce. Diversifying the healthcare workforce facilitates adequate representation; cultural understanding; and linguistic competency of healthcare providers, professionals, and students for assurance of appropriate, effective, adequate, responsive, and acceptable care (Office of Minority Health, 2011). Furthermore, this approach reduces linguistic and cultural barriers and improves the quality of care.

The Advisory Committee on Minority Health (ACMH) has recommended the development of a healthcare workforce representative and reflective of the communities being served to improve the health of historically underserved communities and ameliorate health disparities (Office of Minority Health, 2011).

13.4.5 ADDRESSING SOCIAL DETERMINANTS OF HEALTH

The conditions in which people live, work, play, and congregate can impact their health and well-being and contribute to health disparities. Poverty, inadequate access to quality education, housing, employment sanitation, potable water, quality, and healthy foods; exposure to neighborhood violence; poor working conditions; and clustering of disadvantage in a particular group of people are examples of SDoH that negatively impact health (Braveman et al., 2011; Thornton et al., 2016). Thus, solutions to health inequities should include interventions that tackle social determinants. These include increasing access to high-quality education, including structured early childhood education and parental support programs (Cohen & Syme, 2013; Karoly et al., 2005); urban planning and community development to drive changes in nutrition; physical activity and safety within communities (Fenton, 2012) high-quality housing to increase low-income families' access to economic opportunities and safer neighborhoods (Cohen & Syme, 2013); and employment interventions to improve quality of life, finances, and social support (Luciano et al., 2014).

REFERENCES

Altman, B. M., & Bernstein, A. (2008). Disability and health in the United States, 2001–2005. https://stacks.cdc.gov/view/cdc/6983

Ammerman, A., Leung, M. M., & Cavallo, D. (2006). Addressing disparities in the obesity epidemic. *North Carolina Medical Journal*, *67*(4), 301–304.

Arias, E., Xu, J., & Kochanek, K. D. (2019). United States Life Tables, 2016. *National Vital Statistics Report*, *68*(4), 1–66.

Arnett, D., Blumenthal, R. S., Albert, M. A., Buroker, A., Goldberger, Z., Hahn, E., Dennison-Himmelfarb, C., Khera, A., Lloyd-Jones, D., McEvoy, J., Michos, E., Miedema, M., Munoz, D., Smith, S., Virani, S., Williams, K., Yeboah, J., & Ziaeian, B. (2019). 2019 ACC/AHA guideline on the primary prevention of cardiovascular disease: A report of the American College of Cardiology/American Heart Association Task Force on clinical practice guidelines. *Circulation*, *140*(11), e596–e646. https://doi.org/10.1161/cir.0000000000000678

Asleh, R., Manemann, S. M., Weston, S. A., Bielinski, S. J., Chamberlain, A. M., Jiang, R., Gerber, Y., & Roger, V. L. (2021). Sex differences in outcomes after myocardial infarction in the community. *The American Journal of Medicine*, *134*(1), 114–121. https://doi.org/10.1016/j.amjmed.2020.05.040

Bauer, G. R. (2014). Incorporating intersectionality theory into population health research methodology: Challenges and the potential to advance health equity. *Social Science & Medicine*, *110*, 10–17.

Boing, A. F., Boing, A. C., Cordes, J., Kim, R., & Subramanian, S. V. (2020). Quantifying and explaining variation in life expectancy at census tract, county, and state levels in the United States. *Proceedings of the National Academy of Sciences of the United States of America*, *117*(30), 17688–17694. https://doi.org/10.1073/pnas.2003719117

Boyd, R. W., Lindo, E. G., Weeks, L. D., & McLemore, M. R. (2020). On racism: A new standard for publishing on racial health inequities. *Health Affairs Blog*, *10*. www.healthaffairs.org/do/10.1377/forefront.20200630.939347/

Braveman, P., Egerter, S., & Williams, D. R. (2011). The social determinants of health: Coming of age. *Annual Review of Public Health*, *32*, 381–398. https://doi.org/10.1146/annurev-publhealth-031210-101218

Brondolo, E., Hausmann, L. R., Jhalani, J., Pencille, M., Atencio-Bacayon, J., Kumar, A., Kwok, J., Ullah, J., Roth, A., Chen, D., Crupi, R., & Schwartz, J. (2011). Dimensions of perceived racism and self-reported health: Examination of racial/ethnic differences and potential mediators. *Annals of Behavioral Medicine*, *42*(1), 14–28. https://doi.org/10.1007/s12160-011-9265-1

Burroughs Pena, M. S., & Bloomfield, G. S. (2015). Cardiovascular disease research and the development agenda in low- and middle-income countries. *Global Heart*, *10*(1), 71–73. https://doi.org/10.1016/j.gheart.2014.12.006

Byiringiro, S., Nyirimanzi, N., Mucumbitsi, J., Kamanzi, E. R., & Swain, J. (2020). Cardiac surgery: Increasing access in low- and middle-income countries. *Current Cardiology Reports*, *22*(7), 37. https://doi.org/10.1007/s11886-020-01290-5

Centers for Disease Control and Prevention. (2017). *Life expectancy at birth and at age 65, by sex: Organisation for Economic Co-operation and Development (OECD) countries, selected years 1980–2015*. www.cdc.gov/nchs/data/hus/2017/014.pdf

Centers for Disease Control Prevention. (2019). *Health, United States spotlight: Racial and ethnic disparities in heart disease*. Retrieved from www.cdc.gov/nchs/hus/spotlight/HeartDiseaseSpotlight_2019_0404.pdf

Centers for Disease Control Prevention. (2021). *Risk for COVID-19 infection, hospitalizations and death by race/ethnicity*. Retrieved on March 16, 2021, from www.cdc.gov/coronavirus/2019-ncov/covid-data/investigations-discovery/hospitalization-death-by-race-ethnicity.html

Churchwell, K., Elkind Mitchell, S. V., Benjamin Regina, M., Carson April, P., Chang Edward, K., Lawrence, W., Mills, A., Odom, T. M., Rodriguez, C. J., Rodriguez, R., Sanchez, E., Sharrief, A. Z., Sims, M., & Williams, O. (2020). Call to action: Structural racism as a fundamental driver of health disparities: A presidential advisory from the American Heart Association. *Circulation, 142*(24), e454–e468. https://doi.org/10.1161/CIR.0000000000000936

Clayton, J. A. (2016). Studying both sexes: A guiding principle for biomedicine. *FASEB J, 30*(2), 519–524. https://doi.org/10.1096/fj.15-279554

Cohen, A. K., & Syme, S. L. (2013). Education: A missed opportunity for public health intervention. *American Journal of Public Health, 103*(6), 997–1001. https://doi.org/10.2105/AJPH.2012.300993

Collin, L. J., Gaglioti, A. H., Beyer, K. M., Zhou, Y., Moore, M. A., Nash, R., Switchenko, J. M., Miller-Kleinhenz, J. M., Ward, K. C., & McCullough, L. E. (2021). Neighborhood-level redlining and lending bias are associated with breast cancer mortality in a large and diverse metropolitan area. *Cancer Epidemiology Biomarkers & Prevention, 30*(1), 53–60. https://doi.org/10.1158/1055-9965.Epi-20-1038

Crenshaw, K. (1989). Demarginalizing the intersection of race and sex: A black feminist critique of antidiscrimination doctrine, feminist theory and antiracist politics. *University of Chicago Legal Forum*, 139. https://philpapers.org/rec/CREDTI

Derose, K. P., Gresenz, C. R., & Ringel, J. S. (2011). Understanding disparities in health care access—and reducing them—through a focus on public health. *Health Affairs (Millwood), 30*(10), 1844–1851. https://doi.org/10.1377/hlthaff.2011.0644

Dess, R. T., Hartman, H. E., Mahal, B. A., Soni, P. D., Jackson, W. C., Cooperberg, M. R., Amling, C. L., Aronson, W. J., Kane, C. J., Terris, M. K., Zumsteg, Z. S., Butler, S., Osborne, J. R., Morgan, T. M., Mehra, R., Salami, S. S., Kishan, A. U., Wang, C., Schaeffer, E. M., … Spratt, D. E. (2019). Association of Black race with prostate cancer—specific and other-cause mortality. *JAMA Oncology, 5*(7), 975–983. https://doi.org/10.1001/jamaoncol.2019.0826

Du Bois, W. E. B. (2017). *Black reconstruction in America: Toward a history of the part which Black folk played in the attempt to reconstruct democracy in America, 1860–1880*. Routledge.

Fenton, M. (2012). Community design and policies for free-range children: Creating environments that support routine physical activity. *Child Obesity, 8*(1), 44–51. https://doi.org/10.1089/chi.2011.0122

Forde Allana, T., Lewis Tené, T., Kershaw Kiarri, N., Bellamy Scarlett, L., & Diez Roux Ana, V. (2021). Perceived discrimination and hypertension risk among participants in the multi-ethnic study of atherosclerosis. *Journal of the American Heart Association, 10*(5), e019541. https://doi.org/10.1161/JAHA.120.019541

Forman-Hoffman, V. L., Ault, K. L., Anderson, W. L., Weiner, J. M., Stevens, A., Campbell, V. A., & Armour, B. S. (2015). Disability status, mortality, and leading causes of death in the United States community population. *Medical Care, 53*(4), 346–354. https://doi.org/10.1097/MLR.0000000000000321

Gee, G. C., & Ford, C. L. (2011). Structural racism and health inequities: Old issues, new directions. *Du Bois Review, 8*(1), 115–132. https://doi.org/10.1017/S1742058X11000130

Glezerman, M. (2016). *Gender medicine: The groundbreaking new science of gender- and sex-related diagnosis and treatment*. Abrams.

Graham, G. N. (2016). Why your ZIP code matters more than your genetic code: Promoting healthy outcomes from mother to child. *Breastfeeding Medicine, 11*, 396–397. https://doi.org/10.1089/bfm.2016.0113

Group, E. U. C. C. S., Regitz-Zagrosek, V., Oertelt-Prigione, S., Prescott, E., Franconi, F., Gerdts, E., Foryst-Ludwig, A., Maas, A. H. E. M., Kautzky-Willer, A., Knappe-Wegner, D., Kintscher, U., Ladwig, K. H., Schenck-Gustafsson, K., & Stangl, V. (2016). Gender in cardiovascular diseases: Impact on clinical manifestations, management, and outcomes. *European Heart Journal, 37*(1), 24–34. https://doi.org/10.1093/eurheartj/ehv598

Hark, L., & DeLisser, H. (2011). *Achieving cultural competency: A case-based approach to training health professionals.* John Wiley & Sons.

Harper, S., MacLehose, R. F., & Kaufman, J. S. (2014). Trends in the black–white life expectancy gap among US states, 1990–2009. *Health Affairs (Millwood), 33*(8), 1375–1382. https://doi.org/10.1377/hlth aff.2013.1273

Healthbox. (2019). *Root causes of health.* Retrieved April 14, 2021, from www.healthbox.com/wp-content/uploads/2019/01/Healthbox-Root-Causes-of-Health-Report.pdf

Howard, G., & Howard, V. J. (2020). Twenty years of progress toward understanding the Stroke Belt. *Stroke, 51*(3), 742–750. https://doi.org/10.1161/strokeaha.119.024155

Howard, G., Labarthe, D. R., Hu, J., Yoon, S., & Howard, V. J. (2007). Regional differences in African Americans' high risk for stroke: The remarkable burden of stroke for Southern African Americans. *Annals of Epidemiology, 17*(9), 689–696. https://doi.org/10.1016/j.annepidem.2007.03.019

Hunt, B. R., Tran, G., & Whitman, S. (2015). Life expectancy varies in local communities in Chicago: Racial and spatial disparities and correlates. *Journal of Racial and Ethnic Health Disparities, 2*(4), 425–433. https://doi.org/10.1007/s40615-015-0089-8

Institute of Medicine. (2002). *Guidance for the National Healthcare Disparities Report.* The National Academies Press. https://doi.org/10.17226/10512

Institute of Medicine. (2008). *Challenges and successes in reducing health disparities: Workshop summary.* The National Academies Press. https://doi.org/10.17226/12154

Institute of Medicine Committee on Understanding and Eliminating Racial and Ethnic Disparities in Health Care. (2003). Unequal treatment: Confronting racial and ethnic disparities in health care. In B. D. Smedley, A. Y. Stith, & A. R. Nelson (Eds.), *Unequal treatment: Confronting racial and ethnic disparities in health care.* Institute of Medicine. https://doi.org/10.17226/12875

Jones, G. C., & Sinclair, L. B. (2008). Multiple health disparities among minority adults with mobility limitations: An application of the ICF framework and codes. *Disability and Rehabilitation, 30*(12–13), 901–915. https://doi.org/10.1080/09638280701800392

Karoly, L. A., Kilburn, M. R., & Cannon, J. S. (2005). *Early childhood interventions: Proven results, future promise.* RAND Corporation. https://doi.org/10.7249/MG341

Knight, M., Kenyon, S., Brocklehurst, P., Neilson, J., Shakespeare, J., & Kurinczuk, J. J. (2017). *Saving lives, improving mothers' care: Lessons learned to inform future maternity care from the UK and Ireland confidential enquiries into maternal deaths and morbidity 2009–2012.* National Perinatal Epidemiology Unit, University of Oxford.

Kohl, H. W., Craig, C. L., Lambert, E. V., Inoue, S., Alkandari, J. R., Leetongin, G., & Kahlmeier, S. (2012). The pandemic of physical inactivity: Global action for public health. *The Lancet, 380*(9838), 294–305. https://doi.org/10.1016/S0140-6736(12)60898-8

Larson, N. I., Story, M. T., & Nelson, M. C. (2009). Neighborhood environments: Disparities in access to healthy foods in the U.S. *American Journal of Preventative Medicine, 36*(1), 74–81. https://doi.org/10.1016/j.amepre.2008.09.025

Lawrence, K., & Keleher, T. (2004). Chronic disparity: Strong and pervasive evidence of racial inequalities: Poverty outcomes: Structural racism. National Conference on Race and Public Policy, Berkeley, CA.

Luciano, A., Bond, G. R., & Drake, R. E. (2014). Does employment alter the course and outcome of schizophrenia and other severe mental illnesses? A systematic review of longitudinal research. *Schizophrenia Research, 159*(2–3), 312–321. https://doi.org/10.1016/j.schres.2014.09.010

Lynch, E. E., Malcoe, L. H., Laurent, S. E., Richardson, J., Mitchell, B. C., & Meier, H. C. S. (2021). The legacy of structural racism: Associations between historic redlining, current mortgage lending, and health. *SSM Population Health, 14*, 100793. https://doi.org/10.1016/j.ssmph.2021.100793

Lyons, J. G., & Stewart, S. (2011). Prevention: Convergent communicable and noncommunicable heart disease. *Nature Reviews Cardiology, 9*(1), 12–14. https://doi.org/10.1038/nrcardio.2011.180

Marmot, M., & Allen, J. J. (2014). Social determinants of health equity. *American Journal of Public Health, 104*(Suppl 4), S517–519. https://doi.org/10.2105/AJPH.2014.302200

Mathers, C., Stevens, G., Hogan, D., Mahanani, W. R., & Ho, J. (2017). Global and regional causes of death: Patterns and trends, 2000–15. In D. T. Jamison, H. Gelband, S. Horton, P. Jha, R. Laxminarayan, C. N. Mock, & R. Nugent (Eds.), *Disease control priorities: Improving health and reducing poverty.*

The International Bank for Reconstruction and Development / The World Bank. https://doi.org/10.1596/978-1-4648-0527-1_ch4

Mattessich, P. W., & Rausch, E. J. (2014). Cross-sector collaboration to improve community health: A view of the current landscape. *Health Affairs (Millwood)*, *33*(11), 1968–1974. https://doi.org/10.1377/hlthaff.2014.0645

Mauvais-Jarvis, F., Bairey Merz, N., Barnes, P. J., Brinton, R. D., Carrero, J.-J., DeMeo, D. L., De Vries, G. J., Epperson, C. N., Govindan, R., Klein, S. L., Lonardo, A., Maki, P. M., McCullough, L. D., Regitz-Zagrosek, V., Regensteiner, J. G., Rubin, J. B., Sandberg, K., & Suzuki, A. (2020). Sex and gender: Modifiers of health, disease, and medicine. *The Lancet*, *396*(10250), 565–582. https://doi.org/10.1016/S0140-6736(20)31561-0

McCracken, K., & Phillips, D. R. Demographic and epidemiological transition. In *International Encyclopedia of Geography* (pp. 1–8). https://doi.org/10.1002/9781118786352.wbieg0063

McGregor, B., Belton, A., Henry, T. L., Wrenn, G., & Holden, K. B. (2019). Improving behavioral health equity through cultural competence training of health care providers. *Ethnicity & Disease*, *29*(Suppl 2), 359–364. https://doi.org/10.18865/ed.29.S2.359

Mendoza, W., & Miranda, J. J. (2017). Global shifts in cardiovascular disease, the epidemiologic transition, and other contributing factors: Toward a new practice of global health cardiology. *Cardiology Clinics*, *35*(1), 1–12. https://doi.org/10.1016/j.ccl.2016.08.004

Mercer, A. J. (2018). Updating the epidemiological transition model. *Epidemiology & Infection*, *146*(6), 680–687. https://doi.org/10.1017/S0950268818000572

Morris, A. A., Ko, Y. A., Hutcheson, S. H., & Quyyumi, A. (2018). Race/Ethnic and sex differences in the association of atherosclerotic cardiovascular disease risk and healthy lifestyle behaviors. *Journal of the American Heart Association*, *7*(10), e008250. https://doi.org/10.1161/JAHA.117.008250

National Academies of Sciences, Engineering, and Medicine. (2017a). The role of communities in promoting health equity. In A. Baciu, Y. Negussie, A. Geller, & J. N. Weinstein (Eds.), *Communities in Action: Pathways to Health Equity*. National Academies Press. www.ncbi.nlm.nih.gov/books/NBK425849

National Academies of Sciences, Engineering, and Medicine. (2017b). The root causes of health inequity. In A. Baciu, Y. Negussie, A. Geller, & J. N. Weinstein (Eds.), *Communities in Action: Pathways to Health Equity*. National Academies Press (US). www.ncbi.nlm.nih.gov/books/NBK425845/

Office of Minority Health. (2011). *Reflecting America's population diversifying a competent health care workforce for the 21st century: A statement of principles and recommendations*. https://minorityhealth.hhs.gov/Assets/pdf/Checked/1/FinalACMHWorkforceReport.pdf

Okoro, C. A., Hollis, N. D., Cyrus, A. C., & Griffin-Blake, S. (2018). Prevalence of disabilities and health care access by disability status and type among adults—United States, 2016. *MMWR Morbidity and Mortality Weekly Rep*, *67*(32), 882–887. https://doi.org/10.15585/mmwr.mm6732a3

Petersen, E. E., Davis, N. L., Goodman, D., Cox, S., Syverson, C., Seed, K., Shapiro-Mendoza, C., Callaghan, W. M., & Barfield, W. (2019). Racial/Ethnic disparities in pregnancy-related deaths—United States, 2007–2016. *MMWR Morbidity and Mortality Weekly Report*, *68*(35), 762–765. https://doi.org/10.15585/mmwr.mm6835a3

Purnell, L. D. (2012). *Transcultural health care: A culturally competent approach* (4th ed.). F.A. Davis.

Saint Onge, J. M., & Krueger, P. M. (2017). Health lifestyle behaviors among U.S. adults. *SSM—Population Health*, *3*, 89–98. https://doi.org/10.1016/j.ssmph.2016.12.009

Santosa, A., & Byass, P. (2016). Diverse empirical evidence on epidemiological transition in low- and middle-income countries: Population-based findings from INDEPTH network data. *PLoS One*, *11*(5), e0155753. https://doi.org/10.1371/journal.pone.0155753

Singh, G. K., Daus, G. P., Allender, M., Ramey, C. T., Martin, E. K., Perry, C., De Los Reyes, A., & Vedamuthu, I. P. (2017). Social determinants of health in the United States: Addressing major health inequality trends for the nation, 1935–2016. *International Journal of Maternal and Child Health and AIDS*, *6*(2), 139–164. https://doi.org/10.21106/ijma.236

Solar, O., & Irwin, A. (2010). A conceptual framework for action on the social determinants of health. Social Determinants of Health Discussion Paper 2 (Policy and Practice). www.who.int/publications/i/item/9789241500852

Thornton, R. L., Glover, C. M., Cene, C. W., Glik, D. C., Henderson, J. A., & Williams, D. R. (2016). Evaluating strategies for reducing health disparities by addressing the social determinants of health. *Health Affairs (Millwood)*, *35*(8), 1416–1423. https://doi.org/10.1377/hlthaff.2015.1357

University of Wisconsin Population Health Institute. (2015). *2016 county health rankings key findings report*. www.countyhealthrankings.org/resources/2016-county-health-rankings-key-findings-report

US Department of Health and Human Services, Office of Disease Prevention and Health Promotion. (2020). *History & development of healthy people*. US Department of Health and Human Services, Office of Disease Prevention and Health Promotion. Retrieved April 14 from www.healthypeople.gov/2020/About-Healthy-People/History-Development-Healthy-People-2020

Veenstra, G. (2013). Race, gender, class, sexuality (RGCS) and hypertension. *Social Science and Medicine*, *89*, 16–24. https://doi.org/10.1016/j.socscimed.2013.04.014

Virani, S. S., Alonso, A., Benjamin, E. J., Bittencourt, M. S., Callaway, C. W., Carson, A. P., Chamberlain, A. M., Chang, A. R., Cheng, S., Delling, F. N., Djousse, L., Elkind, M. S. V., Ferguson, J. F., Fornage, M., Khan, S. S., Kissela, B. M., Knutson, K. L., Kwan, T. W., Lackland, D. T., ... Tsao, C. W. (2020). Heart disease and stroke statistics—2020 update: A report from the American Heart Association. *Circulation*, *141*(9), e139–e596. https://doi.org/10.1161/CIR.0000000000000757

Watkins, D. A., Johnson, C. O., Colquhoun, S. M., Karthikeyan, G., Beaton, A., Bukhman, G., Forouzanfar, M. H., Longenecker, C. T., Mayosi, B. M., Mensah, G. A., Nascimento, B. R., Ribeiro, A. L. P., Sable, C. A., Steer, A. C. Naghavi, M., Mokdad, A. H., Murray, C. J. L., Vos, T., Carapetis, J. R., & Roth, G. A. (2017). Global, regional, and national burden of rheumatic heart disease, 1990–2015. *New England Journal of Medicine*, *377*(8), 713–722. https://doi.org/10.1056/NEJMoa1603693

Whitehead, M., Dahlgren, G. R., & Organization, W. H. (2006). *Levelling up (part 1): A discussion paper on concepts and principles for tackling social inequities in health*. https://apps.who.int/iris/handle/10665/107790

Williams, D. R., & Collins, C. (2001). Racial residential segregation: A fundamental cause of racial disparities in health. *Public Health Reports*, *116*(5), 404–416. https://doi.org/10.1093/phr/116.5.404

World Health Organization. (2020). *Disability and health*. Retrieved April 7, 2021, from www.who.int/news-room/fact-sheets/detail/disability-and-health

Part III

Lifestyle Medicine for Chronic Conditions

14 Preventing, Treating, and Reversing Chronic Disease With Nutritional Interventions

Alexandra Lessem[1] and Caroline Trapp[2]

[1]North Colorado Family Medicine

Greeley, Colorado, USA

[2]University of Michigan School of Nursing

Ann Arbor, MI, USA

Physicians Committee for Responsible Medicine Scientific Advisory Board

CONTENTS

DOI: 10.1201/9781003178330-17

KEY POINTS

- The leading causes of morbidity and mortality in the United States (cardiovascular disease, obesity, diabetes, and cancer) are all exacerbated by a diet high in fat, processed foods, sugar, and animal products and low in fiber, vitamins, and antioxidants.
- The risk of developing these conditions can be reduced by following a healthful, nutrient dense diet with high intake of fruits, vegetables, whole grains, and legumes.
- Treatment, and often reversal, of these diseases can be achieved through dietary changes and adherence to a predominantly plant-based diet.
- Following a healthful diet can have a positive impact on cognition, autoimmune diseases, pain, mood, and many other conditions as well.
- Nurses at all levels of education and across practice settings should utilize their patient education and counseling skills to assist patients to initiate and sustain a dietary pattern that addresses the underlying cause of common chronic diseases.

14.1   INTRODUCTION

There has long been knowledge of the importance of nutrition in health. As early as the 1700s, many practitioners advocated for a predominantly vegetarian diet and recognized the importance of fruits and vegetables for health (Stuart, 2007). Florence Nightingale wrote *Directions for Cooking by Troops in Camp and Hospital* in 1861 to address the nutrition needs of soldiers during the Civil War (Hertzler, 2004). While many of her recommendations are outdated, she advocated for proper nutrition and her influence may have helped reduce malnutrition and food-borne disease among the troops (Hertzler, 2004). As knowledge of nutrition has accumulated, there is a growing understanding of the importance of a healthful diet in preventing and treating the world's most prevalent chronic diseases. As nurses, we have a responsibility to bring this life-saving information to our patient encounters.

Most Americans fall far short of basic nutrition recommendations. Refined flours, fats, and oils comprise 46.6% of total daily calories while fruit and vegetable intake accounts for 7.9%, down from 9.23% in 1970 (DeSilver, 2016). Between 2007 and 2010, 76% of American adults did not meet fruit intake recommendations, and 87% did not meet vegetable intake recommendations (Moore & Thompson, 2015). This has led to a largely preventable explosion of obesity, diabetes, cardiovascular disease, and many other chronic health problems. Nurses have a key role in helping to reverse these trends through advocating for a healthful diet for their patients and themselves.

14.2   CARDIOVASCULAR DISEASE

Cardiovascular disease (CVD) is the leading cause of death for men and women in the United States, accounting for 859,125 deaths in 2017—440,460 among men and 418,665 women (Virani et al., 2020). The prevalence of all types of cardiovascular disease is 48%, including coronary heart disease (CHD), stroke, hypertension (HTN), and heart failure (HF), with HTN being the most prevalent. The costs of CVD are high. In 2014–2015, direct and indirect costs totaled $351.3 billion (Virani et al., 2020).

14.2.1   Nutrition and Cardiovascular Disease Risk

According to a systematic review of the Global Burden of Disease Study, dietary risks were associated with 22.4% of all deaths and 49.2% of CVD deaths in 2016 in the World Health Organization (WHO) European region (Meier et al., 2018). In the United States (US), the top risk factor for CVD is a suboptimal diet, followed by smoking, high body mass index (BMI), elevated blood pressure, elevated fasting blood sugar, and physical inactivity (Murray et al., 2013). Following at least six of the American Heart Association's (AHA's) Life's Simple Seven health metrics, which address these risk factors, is associated with a 76% reduced risk of CVD mortality and 51% reduced risk of all-cause mortality (Yang et al., 2012). However, less than 1% of people meet all seven metrics and only 0.7% to 11.0% meet at least six. Only 0.3% of adults and 0% of children age 12 to 19 meet four out of five dietary recommendations; at least 4.5 cups of fruits and vegetables daily, at least two servings of fish per week, less than 1500 mg of sodium per day, less than 36 oz of sugar sweetened beverages per week, and at least three servings of whole grains per day (Virani et al., 2020).

There is tremendous opportunity to positively impact CVD morbidity and mortality through dietary interventions. Epidemiological studies show a dramatically reduced risk of coronary heart disease (CHD) among those following a predominantly plant-based diet. According to the land-mark Cornell-Oxford China Study, between 1973 and 1975 the US had a CHD mortality rate of 66.8 per 100,000 for men and 18.9 per 100,000 for women as compared to 4.0 per 100,000 for men and 3.4 per 100,000 for women aged 0–64 in China (Campbell et al., 1998). Coronary artery disease mortality was inversely associated with green vegetable and monounsaturated fatty acid intake and positively associated with salt, animal protein intake, and frequency of meat intake (Campbell et al., 1998).

In a recent study utilizing data from the Nurses Health Studies I and II and the Health Professionals' Follow-Up Study, greater adherence to any of four healthful dietary patterns was associated with a 14% to 21% reduced risk of CVD over 5,257,190 person years of follow-up (Shan et al., 2020). Each of the four dietary patterns (Healthy Eating Index–2015 [HEI-2015], Alternate Mediterranean Diet Score [AMED], Healthful Plant-Based Diet Index [HPDI], and Alternate Healthy Eating Index [AHEI]) emphasize greater intake of fruits, vegetables, whole grains, legumes, and omega fatty acids, and reduced intake of processed foods, sugar-sweetened beverages, red meat, and saturated fat. The AMED and HEI-2015 give higher scores to increased seafood intake and all scales generally discourage alcohol, though the AMED allows for moderate wine consumption (Shan et al., 2020).

A similar study followed middle-aged adults from 1987 to 2017 and assessed their dietary quality using a general plant-based dietary index (PDI), HPDI, unhealthy plant-based diet index (UPDI), and pro-vegetarian diet index (Kim et al., 2019). Reduced CVD incidence, CVD mortality, and all-cause mortality were associated with greater adherence to plant-based dietary patterns (Kim et al., 2019). Wang et al. (2020) found greater adherence to a PDI to be associated with lower rates of mortality, myocardial infarction (MI), and acute ischemic stroke among a group of 181,351 veterans over 717,857 person years of follow-up.

14.2.2   Mediterranean Diet and Cardiovascular Disease Risk

The Prevencion con Dieta Mediterranea (PREDIMED) study was a randomized primary prevention trial to investigate the impact of a Mediterranean diet (MeDiet) with supplemental olive oil or nuts on cardiovascular risk among high-risk individuals (Ros et al., 2014). The MeDiet encourages high consumption of plant foods and olive oil, moderate intake of wine, seafood, fermented dairy products, poultry, and eggs, and low consumption of red meat, processed meat, and sweets. Over 4.8 years of follow-up, those randomized to the MeDiet plus nuts or olive oil had a 30% reduced risk of CVD events as compared to the control group advised to follow a low-fat diet (Ros et al., 2014). Intervention participants also had reduced risk of diabetes and metabolic syndrome and positive changes in blood lipids and other markers. A study comparing a green Mediterranean diet with supplemental green tea and a daily *Wolffia globosa* protein shake in place of animal protein at dinner with a traditional Mediterranean diet showed a greater improvement in LDL cholesterol, diastolic blood pressure, insulin resistance, and 10-year Framingham risk score among those following the green Mediterranean diet (Tsaban et al., 2020). Similarly, a 36-week randomized crossover trial comparing a Mediterranean diet with a low-fat vegan diet found the vegan diet performed better for weight loss, LDL cholesterol, and insulin resistance, while the Mediterranean diet outperformed the vegan diet for blood pressure reduction (Barnard et al., 2022).

14.2.3 The Portfolio Diet for Cholesterol Management

In a separate study, a portfolio diet with high intake of specific foods thought to be effective for lowering cholesterol was shown to be comparable to statin medication and superior to a low-fat diet. Cholesterol levels were compared after following a diet high in the portfolio foods (plant sterols, soy protein, almonds, and soluble fiber) or a very low-fat diet either with or without lovastatin 20 mg daily for four weeks each (Jenkins et al., 2005). At the end of the study period, LDL reductions were $-8.5 \pm 1.9\%$, $-33.3 \pm 1.9\%$, and $-29.6 \pm 1.3\%$ for low-fat diet alone, low-fat diet plus lovastatin, and portfolio diet respectively (Jenkins et al., 2005). A systematic review and meta-analysis of studies combining the Portfolio Diet and the National Cholesterol Education Program (NCEP) Step II diet found the addition of the portfolio diet reduced LDL by an additional 17% as compared to the Step II diet alone (Chiavaroli et al., 2018).

14.2.4 Nutrition and Cardiovascular Disease Treatment

In addition to reducing the risk of CVD, nutrition can be used to improve outcomes among those with established CVD. In the Lifestyle Heart Trial, participants with known CAD who followed a low-fat vegetarian diet, participated in stress-reduction classes, stopped smoking, and engaged in moderate physical activity had regression in coronary artery stenosis at one and five years, while those in the control group had progression of their disease (Ornish et al., 1990; Ornish et al., 1998). Esselstyn (2014) saw similar results in a series of studies in which participants with documented severe CAD were followed for up to 10 years. Those who followed a low-fat vegetarian diet had CAD stenosis regression and a substantially reduced risk of cardiovascular event recurrence: 0.6% as compared to 62% (Esselstyn et al., 1995; Esselstyn et al., 2014). Participants reported subjective improvement in angina symptoms and activity tolerance. The Lyon Diet Heart Study investigated the impact of a Mediterranean diet on recurrence rates of CVD events among 424 patients who had recently survived an MI. After a mean of 46 months of follow-up, all-cause and cardiovascular mortality, recurrent MI, and other cardiac events or symptoms were significantly reduced among those following the Mediterranean diet as compared to those following a control diet, with risk ratios ranging from 0.23 (95% CI 0.11–0.48) to 0.51 (95% CI 0.35–0.73). Higher total cholesterol and blood pressure increased recurrence risk (Lorgeril et al., 1999).

14.2.5 Nutrition and Hypertension

The impact of diet on HTN is well established with evidence supporting the Dietary Approaches to Stop Hypertension (DASH) diet. This dietary pattern promotes greater intake of fruits, vegetables, and whole grains and reduced intake of sweets, sugar-sweetened beverages, sodium, and foods high in saturated fat such as fatty meats, full-fat dairy products, and tropical oils (NHLBI, n.d.). A systematic review and meta-analysis of 20 studies investigating the impact of the DASH diet on blood pressure (BP) found a 5.2 mmHg decrease in systolic BP and 2.6 mmHg decrease in diastolic BP among those following the diet. The changes were of greater magnitude among those with higher baseline BP or BMI (Siervo et al., 2015). The DASH diet also reduced total and low-density lipoprotein (LDL) cholesterol and resulted in a 13% reduced 10-year Framingham CVD risk score (Siervo et al., 2015).

Another systematic review and meta-analysis looking at seven clinical trials and 32 observation studies investigating vegetarian diets and BP found consumption of a vegetarian diet was associated with a 4.8 to 6.9 mmHg lower systolic BP and 2.2 to 4.7 mmHg lower diastolic BP as compared to an omnivorous diet (Yokoyama et al. 2014). This is in line with another systematic review and meta-analysis looking at 41 clinical trials of plant-predominant dietary patterns and blood pressure. This review found many plant-predominant diets (DASH, Mediterranean, lacto-ovo vegetarian, and Nordic) were associated with decreased blood pressure as compared to control diets. The greatest decrease was for the DASH diet with a mean SBD decrease of −5.53 mmHg (95% CI −7.95, −3.12; Gibbs et al., 2020). Decreasing or controlling blood pressure is important because the risk of having a cardiovascular event increases as blood pressure goes up. For every increase of 20 mmHg systolic or 10 mmHg diastolic pressure, the risk of death from CVD doubles (Basile & Bloch, 2021) and lower blood pressures result in reduced risk.

14.3 OBESITY

Obesity is another significant health problem in the United States, and increasingly around the world. According to the National Health and Nutrition Examination Study (NHANES), the obesity rate for 2017–2018 was 42.4%, an increase of 26% since 2008 (Warren et al., 2020). Only Colorado and Washington, DC, have obesity rates of less than 25%, both at 23.8%, in comparison to 2000 when no state was above 25% (Warren et al., 2020). Colorado was the last state to surpass 20% in 2011 (Virani et al., 2020). The childhood obesity rate is rising rapidly. From 1976–1980 to 2017–2018, the obesity rate for children ages 2–19 rose from 5.5% to 19.3%, a more than three-fold increase (Warren et al., 2020). As with adults, obesity rates are higher among Black and Latinx children as well as those with lower socioeconomic status (Warren et al., 2020). Most children with obesity will become adults with obesity, so prevention is key to reduce the risk of obesity-related health problems such as CVD, HTN, type 2 diabetes mellitus (DM), obstructive sleep apnea (OSA), venous thromboembolism (VTE), atrial fibrillation, dementia, and increased mortality (Virani et al., 2020). Approximately $1429 more is spent on annual medical costs for those with obesity as compared to those without (Virani et al., 2020).

14.3.1 NUTRITION AND OBESITY RISK

As with CVD, the prevalence of obesity can be reduced through greater adherence to a healthful, predominantly plant-based diet. An analysis of 55,459 women in the Swedish Mammography Cohort found a 48% to 65% lower prevalence of overweight or obesity among semi-vegetarians, lactovegetarians, and vegans as compared to omnivorous women (Newby et al., 2005). The Adventist Health Study 2, which collected data from 22,434 male and 38,469 women Seventh-Day Adventist members, found vegans to have the lowest mean BMI (23.6 kg/m^2) and nonvegetarians the highest (28.8 kg/m^2). Diabetes prevalence among vegans was also substantially less than among nonvegetarians (2.9% versus 7.6%; Tonstad et al., 2009).

14.3.2 NUTRITION AND WEIGHT GAIN WITH AGE

Weight gain over time appears to be less in people adherent to a more plant-based diet. In a group of 21,966 men and women followed for five years, weight gain was less among vegans (284 g in men and 303 g in women) than meat-eaters (406 g in men and 423 g in women; $P<0.05$ for both sexes). Participants who gained the least weight were those who changed their diet to a more plant-predominant one, while those who changed to a more meat-predominant dietary pattern gained the most (Rosell et al., 2006). In a review of three prospective cohort studies (Nurses Health Study 1 and 2, and Health Professionals Follow-Up Study), weight gain was less among those scoring higher on a general plant-based dietary index and healthful plant-based index, while an unhealthful plant-based index was associated with greater weight gain over four years (Satija et al., 2019). Plant predominant dietary patterns may be protective against obesity in children as well, though evidence is lacking or inconsistent and more research is needed (Newby, 2009).

14.3.3 Nutrition and Weight Loss

Intervention studies have generally found that the type of diet is not as important as adherence in promoting weight loss (Gibson & Sainsbury, 2017), although there may be benefit to plant-predominant diets. A systematic review and meta-analysis of 12 clinical trials comparing vegetarian and vegan diets with omnivorous diets for weight loss found the greatest weight loss over an average of 18 weeks was among those following a vegan diet with a greater loss of 2.52 kg (Huang et al., 2016). In a 22-week intervention study in which participants were randomized to a low-fat vegan group or control group, the intervention group participants lost an average of 5.1 kg while those in the control group gained 0.1 kg ($p < 0.0001$), and those in the intervention group also had reduced waist circumference, waist to hip ratio, and were more likely to lose at least 5% of total body weight (Ferdowsian et al., 2010). In a similar 18-week study, intervention participants lost an average of 4.3 kg while control group participants gained 0.08 kg ($p < 0.001$; Mishra et al., 2013), and in a 16-week trial comparing a low-fat vegan diet to a control group, the vegan group lost weight, fat mass, and visceral fat volume while the control group did not (Kahleova et al., 2018). A trial comparing five different weight loss dietary interventions (vegan, vegetarian, pesco-vegetarian, semi-vegetarian, and omnivorous) found the greatest weight loss among vegan participants with an average loss of 7.5% of starting body weight as compared to 3.1 to 3.2% among the other groups (Turner-McGrievy et al., 2015). Plant-based diets can also reduce obesity-associated inflammatory markers, helping to reduce the risks associated with obesity such as CVD (Bolori et al., 2019; Fernandez, 2019). Weight loss maintenance was found to be greater among those more adherent to a Mediterranean diet as compared to less adherent participants (Poulimeneas et al., 2020).

Other reviews, however, have found that weight loss is similar among different diets, whether based on nutrient manipulation (high-fat, low-fat, low-carbohydrate, etc.), specific food restriction (vegan, Paleo, ketogenic, etc.), or timing of eating (i.e., timed or intermittent fasting; Freire, 2020), and a weight loss plan should be based on patient-specific, cultural, and societal factors with consideration of adequate nutrient intake (Koliaki et al., 2018). Any dietary pattern for weight loss must create a caloric deficit, but there is a lot of flexibility in how to achieve this. While ketogenic or other highly restrictive or very low-calorie diets can be beneficial for short-term weight loss, and useful as a jump-start to increase motivation, there are concerns about potential adverse cardiovascular effects and nutritional deficiencies due to high reliance on fatty, animal-derived foods, avoidance of whole grains and legumes, which provide fiber and other nutrients, or long-term caloric deprivation (Freire, 2020; Koliaki et al., 2018). Healthful, nutrient-dense dietary patterns such as plant-based or Mediterranean are good choices for long-term weight loss and maintenance, and "the optimal diet to treat obesity should be safe, efficacious, healthy and nutritionally adequate, culturally acceptable and economically affordable, and should ensure long-term compliance and maintenance of weight loss" (Koliaki et al., 2018, p. 1). Adherence can be improved through strategies to control an increased drive to eat, tailoring diets to each person, and promoting self-monitoring of intake (Gibson & Sainsbury, 2017).

14.4 DIABETES

Diabetes mellitus (DM) is becoming an ever-greater risk to millions of Americans. From 2013 to 2016, there were 1.26 million adults 20 years of age and older diagnosed with DM, or 9.8% of the total US population (Virani et al., 2020). An additional 9.4 million people are believed to be living with undiagnosed DM and 91.8 million have prediabetes (37.6% of the US population). Long thought to be an adult disease, children are now being diagnosed with type 2 DM with some regularity. Between 2001 and 2009, the prevalence among children increased 30.7% along with the increase in childhood obesity rates (Virani et al., 2020). Diabetes treatment cost $327 billion in 2017, 25% of all healthcare spending. Personal medical costs are 2.3 times higher among those diagnosed with DM than for those without DM, an average of $16,752 per year (Virani et al., 2020).

14.4.1 Diabetes Pathophysiology

Type 2 DM is directly impacted by weight and nutrition status. Traditionally, diabetes was thought to develop from excess sugar and carbohydrate intake. Evidence now shows that in most cases sustained over-consumption of calories and subsequent growth in adipose tissue leads to type 2 DM. Insulin resistance in muscle tissue occurs long before diagnosed diabetes and has been shown to be due to dysfunctional glucose transporter protein type 4 (GLUT-4) function from excess adipose tissue and associated oxidative stress (Boden et al., 2015) as well as increased intramyocellular lipid droplets in the skeletal muscle cells (Meex et al., 2019). GLUT-4 is the primary membrane transport protein to allow glucose into muscle and adipose cells and is essential for glucose homeostasis (Vargas et al., 2021). When the peripheral cells begin to show insulin resistance, the body responds by increasing insulin production, which leads to increased fat in the liver and pancreas, eventually leading to beta cell destruction and need for exogenous insulin (Taylor et al., 2019). Through reversing this trend, largely through very calorie deficient diets, the cycle can be interrupted, and diabetes reversed (Taylor, 2008; Taylor et al., 2019).

14.4.2 Nutrition and Diabetes Risk

There is a substantially reduced risk of developing diabetes for those following a healthful diet without excessive caloric intake. Satija et al. (2016) found that healthful plant-based diets were associated with an approximately 50% reduced risk of diabetes, while unhealthful plant-based diets (high in processed foods and sweets) were associated with a 16% increased risk as compared to a standard diet. The PREDIMED trial found that participants in the MedDiet groups had a 52% reduced risk of developing diabetes over four years as compared to the control group (Salas-Salvado et al., 2011). A systematic review and meta-analysis of nine studies including 307,099 participants found greater adherence to a plant-based diet to be associated with a 23% reduced risk of type 2 DM incidence (Qian et al., 2019), and Chiu et al. (2018) found following a vegetarian diet to be associated with a 35% lower risk of developing diabetes over five years. Changing from an omnivorous diet to a vegetarian one during the study period resulted in a 53% reduced risk among Taiwanese adults (Chiu et al., 2018). Vegan participants in the Adventist Health Study 2 had a two-year diabetes incidence rate of 0.54% as compared to 2.12% among nonvegetarians. Diabetes risk was also reduced among lacto-ovo and semi-vegetarian participants (Tonstad et al., 2013).

Lifestyle and dietary changes can be superior to medication in the prevention of diabetes. The Diabetes Prevention Program (DPP) trial was conducted between 1996 and 1999 with 3,234 study participants at high risk of developing diabetes due to elevated BMI and/or elevated glucose (prediabetes). In the DPP, participants were randomized to one of three groups: Control, metformin, or lifestyle. After an average follow-up of 2.8 years, participants in the intensive lifestyle group who followed a low-fat, low-calorie diet and engaged in physical activity with goal weight loss of at least 7% of baseline weight had a 58% lower incidence of diabetes as compared to the control group, while the metformin group had a 31% lower incidence (Diabetes Prevention Program Research Group, 2002).

14.4.3 Nutrition and Diabetes Treatment

Nutrition can be helpful in treating established diabetes as well. A systematic review looking at 11 studies completed between 1999 and 2017, including a total of 433 participants with mean duration of 23.2 weeks, showed that plant-based diets were associated with improvements in HbA1C levels as well as many quality-of-life measures, cholesterol levels, and general health as compared to various comparison diets (Toumpanakis et al., 2018). Overall, HbA1C levels declined by 0.55% in intervention group participants and 0.19% in control group participants. More participants in the intervention groups were able to reduce or discontinue diabetes medication and lost more weight than those in the control groups (Toumpanakis et al., 2018). Dietary adherence was generally greater among intervention group participants.

14.4.4 PROFESSIONAL SOCIETY GUIDELINES AND RECOMMENDATIONS

The American Association of Clinical Endocrinologists and American College of Endocrinology confirm this evidence in their consensus statement on type 2 diabetes management. This statement stresses the importance of lifestyle optimization for all patients and states "all patients should strive to attain and maintain an optimal weight through a primarily plant-based meal plan high in polyunsaturated and monounsaturated fatty acids, with limited intake of saturated fatty acids and avoidance of trans fats" (Garber et al., 2020, p. 109). It is the position of the American College of Lifestyle Medicine that sufficiently intensive lifestyle interventions are capable of producing significant clinical improvements, including remission of type 2 diabetes. They recommend moderate exercise coupled with a whole food, plant-based dietary pattern that emphasizes fruits and vegetables, legumes, and whole grains and includes nuts and seeds while eliminating or minimizing animal foods such as red meat, poultry, fish, eggs, and dairy, as well as refined foods that included added sugars and oils (Kelly et al., 2020).

14.4.5 PATIENT VIGNETTE

Mr. G. was diagnosed at age 40 with T2DM and high blood pressure. His father had died of complications of T2DM after three years of renal dialysis. Despite Mr. G's efforts, his disease progressed to the point where he required insulin injections. As a busy high school teacher, he feared having to organize his life around blood sugar testing and insulin administration. As an alternative, he agreed to the suggestion of his nurse practitioner to attend group classes offered through his primary care practice to learn how to prepare nutrient-dense, plant-based meals. He and his wife attended, and though she did not change her diet, she supported his efforts and he succeeded in losing 60 pounds and avoided the need for insulin injections. Eight years later, he remains completely free of diabetes and hypertension, off all medications, and credits his nurse practitioner for helping him to avoid his father's fate.

14.5 CANCER

Cancer is the second leading cause of death in the US behind cardiovascular disease, accounting for approximately 606,880 deaths in 2019. The most common cancers are breast, prostate, lung and bronchus, and colorectal (Siegel et al., 2019). Annual individual medical costs for cancer treatment range from $41,800 to $239,400 depending on the stage and type of cancer, leading to national costs of $160 billion for direct care and $18 billion for oral prescription drugs in 2015. Costs are projected to increase 34% by 2030 to $221 billion and $25 billion (Mariotto et al., 2020).

14.5.1 NUTRITION AND CANCER RISK

Many cancers are impacted by nutrition. The Adventist Health Study 2 (Tantamango-Bartley et al., 2013; Tantamango-Bartley et al., 2016) showed a reduced risk of overall cancer, female, gastrointestinal, and prostate cancers among those following a vegan diet as compared to those following an omnivorous diet. European studies have shown a reduced risk of stomach cancer, lymphatic and blood cancers, multiple myeloma, and overall cancer in those following a vegan diet (Key et al., 2014).

14.5.2   Nutrition and Cancer Outcomes

Researchers have shown improved outcomes among those diagnosed with cancer who follow a healthful diet. Men with biopsy confirmed prostate cancer choosing active surveillance had a relative increase in telomere length after five years of an intensive lifestyle intervention including a low-fat, plant-based diet as compared to a control group (Ornish et al., 2013). Another small group of men with recurrent prostate cancer had improved prostate specific antigen (PSA) levels after six months of following a plant-based diet with median doubling time increasing from 11.9 to 112.3 months (Saxe et al., 2006). A review of these and other studies concluded "with no adverse effects noted and no contraindications, dietary intervention [with a plant-based diet] would offer a cost-effective way to reduce the risk of prostate cancer, and to treat those cases where watchful waiting is prescribed" (Rose & Strombom, 2018, p. 5).

A systematic review and meta-analysis of 117 studies including 209,597 cancer survivors showed that higher intake of vegetables and fish were inversely associated with mortality while higher intake of alcohol was positively associated with mortality (Schwedhelm et al., 2016). Greater adherence to a healthful diet emphasizing a high intake of fruit, vegetables, whole grains, poultry, and low-fat dairy was associated with a 32% reduced mortality risk. Following a Western diet with high intake of red and processed meat, refined grains, sweets, and high-fat dairy products was associated with a 46% increased mortality risk (Schwedhelm et al., 2016). A review of several studies found predominantly plant-based diets to improve survival and treatment outcomes among those with breast, prostate, or colorectal cancer (Madigan & Karhu, 2018). A review of nutrition guidelines for breast cancer patients found cruciferous vegetables and garlic to be particularly beneficial for reducing breast cancer growth and that avoidance of proinflammatory foods such as refined carbohydrates and saturated fat is important to maximize treatment response (Limon-Miron et al., 2017). Proceedings from the 2017 American College of Nutrition Annual Meeting conclude "nutrient dense dietary patterns characterized by higher intakes of plant foods with lower intakes of added sugars, refined grains and starch, as well as saturated and trans fats are likely to contribute to cancer prevention" (Wallace et al., 2019). The American Institute for Cancer Research (AICR) recommends the New American Plate in which 2/3 of the plate is filled with plant-based foods and the other 1/3 of the plate may be filled with animal-based foods such as seafood, poultry, and dairy foods with occasional lean red meat (AICR, 2021).

14.6   OTHER CONDITIONS

Healthful dietary patterns are useful for many other conditions in addition to the major chronic diseases discussed above.

14.6.1   Nutrition and Autoimmune, Inflammatory, and Painful Conditions

Many autoimmune disorders appear to be positively impacted by a more healthful diet. Patients with multiple sclerosis have reported lower levels of disability, pain, severe fatigue, cognitive impairment, and depression when consuming greater amounts of plant-based foods and lesser amounts of meat and sugar (Fitzgerald et al., 2018), and a diet high in meat, processed foods, sugar, and fat is associated with higher rates of multiple sclerosis, inflammatory bowel disease, inflammatory arthritis, and systemic lupus erythematosus (Stancic, 2017). Increased fiber intake can reduce the risk of osteoarthritis and decrease knee pain in those with established arthritis (Dai et al., 2017). Plant-based diets can decrease migraine headache pain (Bunner et al., 2014), dysmenorrhea (Barnard et al., 2000), and delay the onset of menopause, reducing breast cancer risk (Boutot et al. 2017).

14.6.2   Impact of Nutrition on Cognitive and Mental Health

There is substantial evidence showing the positive effects of predominantly plant-based diets on mental and cognitive health. Women in the highest quintile of cruciferous and green leafy vegetable intake had slower cognitive decline over two years as compared with those in the lowest quintile (Kang et al., 2005). Both genders of adults aged 58–99 years of age had slower cognitive decline with greater green leafy vegetable intake over an average of 4.7 years (Morris et al., 2018). A systematic review found a diet high in fruit, vegetables, fish, and whole grains to be associated with a reduced risk of depression (Lai et al., 2014), and individual studies have shown plant-based diets to be associated with reduced stress (Beezhold & Johnston, 2012) and anxiety (Beezhold et al. 2015) and overall improved emotional well-being (Agarwal et al., 2015; Lessem et al., 2018).

14.7   ONGOING RESEARCH

Many studies are ongoing, which will hopefully shed more light on the role of nutrition in chronic disease management, and are described next.

14.7.1   Personalized Medicine

Personalized medicine is becoming increasingly important as understanding of genetics, epigenetics, and the microbiome becomes greater (Wallace et al., 2019). Participants in the 2019 Lifestyle Medicine Research Summit confirmed the health benefits of a predominantly plant-based diet for chronic disease and emphasized the need for additional studies to "advance the understanding of plant-predominant eating on the prevention and treatment of a wide array of diseases" (Vodovotz et al., 2020, p. 7), focusing particularly on disadvantaged and underserved populations.

14.7.2   Project Baseline and the Women's Health Initiative

Several large-scale research studies are underway to better understand many aspects of health and disease. Project Baseline is cosponsored by the Stanford School of Medicine, Duke School of Medicine, the American Heart Association, and Google to gather clinical and lifestyle data from diverse participants and study their impact on cardiovascular disease, diabetes, mood, and overall health (www.projectbaseline.com/). The aim of the project is to develop "new tools and capabilities for learning about health and preventing, treating, and reducing disease" (www.projectbaseline.com/). The Women's Health Initiative (WHI) is a large-scale ongoing study of over 161,000 participants aimed at better understanding how to prevent heart disease, breast and colorectal cancer, and osteoporosis in postmenopausal women (www.whi.org). Recent WHI studies have found an increased risk of CVD and all-cause mortality among postmenopausal women with higher cholesterol and egg intake (Chen et al., 2020) and the presence of three or four nutrition-related cardiometabolic risk factors (waist circumference, hypertension, high cholesterol, and type 2 diabetes) to be associated with increased all-cause, CVD, and cancer-specific mortality among postmenopausal women diagnosed with cancer over 10 years of follow-up (Simon et al., 2021). As these and other large studies continue to collect data, the evidence supporting a healthful diet for disease prevention and treatment will surely continue to accumulate.

14.8   CONCLUSION

There is ample evidence showing the importance of a healthful diet for chronic disease prevention and treatment. While there is some variety in specific dietary patterns recommended, all beneficial patterns are based on greater intake of fruits, vegetables, whole grains, and legumes and lesser intake of animal products, added fat, and added sugar. If even a small proportion of American citizens were to change to a plant-predominant dietary pattern, the impact on chronic disease rates would be significant. Improved diet quality is associated with a reduced risk of all-cause mortality (Sotos-Prieto et al., 2017; Kim et al., 2018), as is higher intake of fruits and vegetables (Wang et al., 2014). Nurses should encourage all patients to increase their intake of plant-based foods and decrease their intake of animal products and highly processed foods and counsel on the reasons for doing so. Additional support can be provided by connecting patients to community and online resources to support therapeutic dietary change for chronic disease prevention and treatment.

REFERENCES

Agarwal, U., Mishra, S., Xu, J., Levin, S., Gonzales, J., & Barnard, N. D. (2015). A multicenter randomized controlled trial of a nutrition intervention program in a multiethnic adult population in the corporate setting reduces depression and anxiety and improves quality of life: The GEICO study. *American Journal of Health Promotion, 29*(4), 245–254. https://doi.org/10.4278/ajhp.130218-QUAN-72

American Institute of Cancer Research (2021). Cancer prevention recommendation. Retrieved from www.aicr.org

Barnard, N. D., Alwarith, J., Rembert, E., Brandon, L., Nguyen, M., Goergen, A., Horne, T., do Nascimento, G. F., Lakkadia, K., Tura, A., Holubkov, R, & Kahleova, H. (2022). A Mediterranean diet and low-fat vegan diet to improve body weight and cardiometabolic risk factors: A randomized, cross-over trial. *Journal of the American College of Nutrition, 41*(2), 127–130. https://doi.org/10.1080/07315724.2020.1869625

Barnard, N. D., Scialli, A. R., Hurlock, D., & Bertron, P. (2000). Diet and sex-hormone binding globulin, dysmenorrhea, and premenstrual symptoms. *Obstetrics and Gynecology, 95*(2), 245–250.

Basile, J. & Bloch, M. J. (2021). Overview of hypertension in adults. In G. L. Bakris & W. B. White (Eds.), *UpToDate*. Retrieved from www.uptodate.com

Beezhold, B. L., & Johnston, C. S. (2012). Restriction of meat, fish, and poultry in omnivores improves mood: A pilot randomized controlled trial. *Nutrition Journal, 11*(1), 9. https://doi.org/10.1186/1475-2891-11-9

Beezhold, B., Radnitz, C., Rinne, A., & DiMatteo, J. (2015). Vegans report less stress and anxiety than omnivores. *Nutritional Neuroscience, 18*(7), 289–296. http://doi.org/10.1179/1476830514Y.0000000164

Boden, G., Homko, C., Barrero, C. A., Stein, T. P., Chen, X., Cheung, P., Fecchio, C., Koller, S., & Merali, S. (2015). Excessive caloric intake acutely causes oxidative stress, GLUT4 carbonylation, and insulin resistance in healthy men. *Science translational medicine, 7*(304), 304re7–304re7. https://doi.org/10.1126/scitranslmed.aac4765

Bolori, P., Setaysh, L., Rasaei, N., Jarrahi, F., Yekaninejad, M., & Mirzaei, k. (2019). Adherence to a healthy plant diet may reduce inflammatory factors in obese and overweight women—a cross-sectional study. *Diabetes & Metabolic Syndrome: Clinical Research & Reviews, 13*(4), 2795–2802. https://doi.org/10.1016/j.dsx.2019.07.019

Boutot, M. E., Purdue-Smithe, A., Whitcomb, B. W., Szegda, K. L., Manson, J. E., Hankinson, S. E., Rosner, B. A., & Bertone-Johnson, E. R. (2017). Dietary protein intake and early menopause in the nurses' health study II. *American Journal of Epidemiology, 187*(2), 1–22. https://doi.org/10.1093/aje/kwx256

Bunner, A. E., Agarwal, U., Gonzales, J. F., Valente, F., & Barnard, N. D. (2014). Nutrition intervention for migraine: A randomized crossover trial. *The Journal of Headache and Pain, 15*, 69. https://doi.org/10.1186/1129-2377-15-69

Campbell, T. C., Parpia, B., & Chen, J. (1998). Diet, lifestyle, and the etiology of coronary artery disease: The Cornell China study. *The American Journal of Cardiology, 82*(10), 18–21. https://doi.org/10.1016/S0002-9149(98)00718-8

Chen, G. C., Chen, L. H., Mossavar-Rahmani, Y., Kamensky, V., Shadyab, A. H., Haring, B., Wild, R. A., Silver, B., Kuller, L. H., Sun, Y., Saquib, N., Howard, B., Snetselaar, L. G., Neuhouser, M. L., Allison, M. A., Van Horn, L., Manson, J. E., Wassertheil-Smoller, S., & Qi, Q. (2020). Dietary cholesterol and egg intake in relation to incident cardiovascular disease and all-cause and cause-specific mortality in postmenopausal women. *The American Journal of Clinical Nutrition, 113*(4), 948–959.

Chiavaroli, L., Nishi, S. K., Khan, T. A., Braunstein, C. R., Glenn, A. J., Mejia, S. B., Rahelić, D., Kahleová, H., Salas-Salvadó, J., Jenkins, D. J. A., Kendall, C. W. C. & Sievenpiper, J. L. (2018). Portfolio dietary pattern and cardiovascular disease: A systematic review and meta-analysis of controlled trials. *Progress in Cardiovascular Diseases*, *61*(1), 43–53. https://doi.org/10.1016/j.pcad.2018.05.004

Chiu, T. H., Pan, W. H., Lin, M. N., & Lin, C. L. (2018). Vegetarian diet, change in dietary patterns, and diabetes risk: A prospective study. *Nutrition & Diabetes*, *8*(1), 1–9. https://doi.org/10.1038/s41387-018-0022-4

Dai, Z., Niu, J., Zhang, Y., Jacques, P., & Felson, D. T. (2017). Dietary intake of fibre and risk of knee osteo-arthritis in two US prospective cohorts. *Annals of the Rheumatic Diseases*, *76*(8), 1411–1419. https://doi.org/10.1136/annrheumdis-2016-210810

DeSilver, D. (2016). What's on your table? How America's diet has changed over the decades. Retrieved from www.pewresearch.org/fact-tank/2016/12/13/whats-on-your-table-how-americas-diet-has-changed-over-the-decades/

Diabetes Prevention Program Research Group. (2002). Reduction in the incidence of type 2 diabetes with life-style intervention or metformin. *New England Journal of Medicine*, *346*(6), 393–403. https://doi.org/10.1056/NEJMoa012512

Esselstyn, C. B., Ellis, S. G., Medendorp, S. V., & Crowe, T. D. (1995). A strategy to arrest and reverse coronary artery disease: A 5-year longitudinal study of a single physician's practice. *Journal of Family Practice*, *41*(6), 560–569. Retrieved from www.mdedge.com/jfponline

Esselstyn, C. B., Gendy, G., Doyle, J., Golubic, M., & Roizen, M. F. (2014). A way to reverse CAD? *Journal of Family Practice*, *63*(7), 356–364. Retrieved from www.mdedge.com/jfponline

Ferdowsian, H. R., Barnard, N. D., Hoover, V. J., Katcher, H. I., Levin, S. M., Green, A. A., & Cohen, J. L. (2010). A multicomponent intervention reduces body weight and cardiovascular risk at a GEICO corporate site. *American Journal of Health Promotion*, *24*(6), 384–387. https://pubmed.ncbi.nlm.nih.gov/20594095/

Fernandez, M. L. (2019). Plant-based diet quality is associated with changes in plasma adiposity biomarker concentrations in women. *The Journal of Nutrition*, *149*(4), 551–552. https://doi.org/10.1093/jn/nxy317

Fitzgerald, K., Tyry, T., Salter, A., Cofield, S., Cutter, G., Fox, R., & Marrie, R. (2018). Diet quality is associated with disability and symptom severity in multiple sclerosis. *Neurology*, *90*(1), e11. https://doi.org/10.1212/WNL.0000000000004768

Freire, R. (2020). Scientific evidence of diets for weight loss: Different macronutrient composition, intermittent fasting, and popular diets. *Nutrition*, *69*, 110549, 1–11. https://doi.org/10.1016/j.nut.2019.07.001

Garber, A. J., Handelsman, Y., Grunberger, G., Einhorn, D., Abrahamson, M. J., Barzilay, J. I., Blonde, L., Bush, M. A., DeFronzo, R. A., Garber, J. R., Garvey, W. T., Hirsch, I. B., Jellinger, P. S., McGill, J. B., Mechanick, J. I., Perreault, L., Rosenblit, P. D., Samson, S., & Umpierrez, G. E. (2020). Consensus statement by the American Association of Clinical Endocrinologists and American College of Endocrinology on the comprehensive type 2 diabetes management algorithm–2020 executive summary. *Endocrine Practice*, *26*(1), 107–139. https://doi.org/10.4158/CS-2019-0472

Gibbs, J., Gaskin, E., Ji, C., Miller, M. A., & Cappuccio, F. P. (2021). The effect of plant-based dietary patterns on blood pressure: A systematic review and meta-analysis of controlled intervention trials. *Journal of Hypertension*, *39*(1), 23–37. https://doi.org/10.1097/HJH.0000000000002604

Gibson, A. A., & Sainsbury, A. (2017). Strategies to improve adherence to dietary weight loss interventions in research and real-world settings. *Behavioral Sciences*, *7*(3), 44. https://doi.org/10.3390/bs7030044

Hertzler, A. (2004). Florence Nightingale's influence on civil war nutrition. *Nutrition Today*, *39*(4), 157–160.

Huang, R. Y., Huang, C. C., Hu, F., & Chavarro, J. (2016). Vegetarian diets and weight reduction: A meta-analysis of randomized controlled trials. *Journal of General Internal Medicine*, *31*(1), 109–116. https://doi.org/10.1007/s11606-015-3390-7

Jenkins, D. J., Kendall, C. W., Marchie, A., Faulkner, D. A., Wong, J. M., de Souza, R., Emam, A., Parker, T. L., Vidgen, E., Trautwein, E. A., Lapsley, K. G., Josse, R. G., Leiter, L. A., Singer, W., & Connelly, P. W. (2005). Direct comparison of a dietary portfolio of cholesterol-lowering foods with a statin in hypercholesterolemic participants. *The American Journal of Clinical Nutrition*, *81*(2), 380–387. https://doi.org/10.1093/ajcn.81.2.380

Kahleova, H., Fleeman, R., Hlozkova, A., Holubkov, R., & Barnard, N. D. (2018). A plant-based diet in overweight individuals in a 16-week randomized clinical trial: metabolic benefits of plant protein. *Nutrition & Diabetes*, *8*(1), 1–10. https://doi.org/10.1038/s41387-018-0067-4

Kang, J. H., Ascherio, A., & Grodstein, F. (2005). Fruit and vegetable consumption and cognitive decline in aging women. *Annals of Neurology*, *57*(5), 713–720. https://doi.org/10.1002/ana.20476

Kelly, J., Karlsen, M., & Steinke, G. (2020). Type 2 diabetes remission and lifestyle medicine: A position statement from the American College of Lifestyle Medicine. *American Journal of Lifestyle Medicine*, *14*(4), 406–419. https://doi.org/10.1177/1559827620930962

Key, T. J., Appleby, P. N., Crowe, F. L., Bradbury, K. E., Schmidt, J. A., & Travis, R. C. (2014). Cancer in British vegetarians: Updated analyses of 4998 incident cancers in a cohort of 32,491 meat eaters, 8612 fish eaters, 18,298 vegetarians, and 2246 vegans. *The American Journal of Clinical Nutrition, 100 Suppl*, *1*(1), 385S. https://doi.org/10.3945/ajcn.113.071266

Kim, H., Caulfield, L. E., & Rebholz, C. M. (2018). Healthy plant-based diets are associated with lower risk of all-cause mortality in US adults. *The Journal of Nutrition*, *148*(4), 624–631. https://doi.org/10.1093/jn/nxy019

Kim, H., Caulfield, L. E., Garcia-Larsen, V., Steffen, L. M., Coresh, J., & Rebholz, C. M. (2019). Plant-based diets are associated with a lower risk of incident cardiovascular disease, cardiovascular disease mortality, and all-cause mortality in a general population of middle-aged adults. *Journal of the American Heart Association*, *8*(16), e012865. https://doi.org/10.1161/JAHA.119.012865

Koliaki, C., Spinos, T., Spinou, M., Brinia, M. E., Mitsopoulou, D., & Katsilambros, N. (2018, September). Defining the optimal dietary approach for safe, effective and sustainable weight loss in overweight and obese adults. *Healthcare*, *6*(3), 73. Multidisciplinary Digital Publishing Institute. https://doi.org/10.3945/ajcn.113.069880

Lai, J. S., Hiles, S., Bisquera, A., Hure, A. J., McEvoy, M., & Attia, J. (2014). A systematic review and meta-analysis of dietary patterns and depression in community-dwelling adults. *The American Journal of Clinical Nutrition*, *99*(1), 181–197. https://doi.org/10.3945/ajcn.113.069880

Lessem, A., Gould, S. M., Evans, J., & Dunemn, K. (2020). A whole-food plant-based experiential education program for health care providers results in personal and professional changes. *Journal of the American Association of Nurse Practitioners*, *32*(12), 788–794. https://doi.org/10.1097/JXX.0000000000000305

Limon-Miron, A., Lopez-Teros, V., & Astiazaran-Garcia, H. (2017). Dietary guidelines for breast cancer patients: A critical review. *Advances in Nutrition*, *8*(4), 613–623. https://doi.org/10.3945/an.116.014423

De Lorgeril, M., Salen, P., Martin, J. L., Monjaud, I., Delaye, J., & Mamelle, N. (1999). Mediterranean diet, traditional risk factors, and the rate of cardiovascular complications after myocardial infarction: Final report of the Lyon Diet Heart Study. *Circulation*, *99*(6), 779–785.

Madigan, M., & Karhu, E. (2018). The role of plant-based nutrition in cancer prevention. *Journal of Unexplored Medical Data*, *3*(9). http://dx.doi.org/10.20517/2572-8180.2018.05

Mariotto, A. B., Enewold, L., Zhao, J., Zeruto, C. A., & Yabroff, K. R. (2020). Medical care costs associated with cancer survivorship in the United States. *Cancer Epidemiology and Prevention Biomarkers*, *29*(7), 1304–1312. https://doi.org/10.1158/1055-9965.EPI-19-1534

Meex, R. C., Blaak, E. E., & van Loon, L. J. (2019). Lipotoxicity plays a key role in the development of both insulin resistance and muscle atrophy in patients with type 2 diabetes. *Obesity Reviews*, *20*(9), 1205–1217. https://doi.org/10.1111/obr.12862

Meier, T., Gräfe, K., Senn, F., Sur, P., Stangl, G. I., Dawczynski, C., März, W., Kleber, M. E., & Lorkowski, S. (2019). Cardiovascular mortality attributable to dietary risk factors in 51 countries in the WHO European Region from 1990 to 2016: a systematic analysis of the Global Burden of Disease Study. *European Journal of Epidemiology*, *34*, 37–55. https://doi.org/10.1007/s10654-018-0473-x

Mishra, S., Xu, J., Agarwal, U., Gonzales, J., Levin, S., & Barnard, N. D. (2013). A multicenter randomized controlled trial of a plant-based nutrition program to reduce body weight and cardiovascular risk in the corporate setting: The GEICO study. *European Journal of Clinical Nutrition*, *67*(7), 718. https://doi.org/10.1038/ejcn.2013.92

Moore, L. V., & Thompson, F. E. (2015). Adults meeting fruit and vegetable intake recommendations—United States, 2013. *MMWR. Morbidity and Mortality Weekly Report*, *64*(26), 709–713. Retrieved from www.ncbi.nlm.nih.gov/pubmed/26158351

Morris, M. C., Wang, Y., Barnes, L. L., Bennett, D. A., Dawson-Hughes, B., & Booth, S. L. (2018). Nutrients and bioactives in green leafy vegetables and cognitive decline. *Neurology*, *90*, 1. https://doi.org/10.1212/WNL.0000000000004815

Murray, C. J., Abraham, J., Ali, M. K., Alvarado, M., Atkinson, C., Baddour, L. M., ... & Lopez, A. D. (2013). The state of US health, 1990–2010: Burden of diseases, injuries, and risk factors. *Jama*, *310*(6), 591–606. https://doi.org/10.1001/jama.2013.13805

Newby, P. K. (2009). Plant foods and plant-based diets: protective against childhood obesity? *The American Journal of Clinical Nutrition, 89*(5), 1572S–1587S. https://doi.org/10.3945/ajcn.2009.26736G

Newby, P. K., Tucker, K. L., & Wolk, A. (2005). Risk of overweight and obesity among semivegetarian, lacto-vegetarian, and vegan women. *American Journal of Clinical Nutrition, 81*, 1267–74.

NHLBI (n.d.). DASH Eating Plan. *National Heart Lung and Blood Institute*, U.S. Department of Health and Human Services. Retrieved February 22, 2021, from www.nhlbi.nih.gov/health-topics/dash-eating-plan

Ornish, D., Brown, S. E., Billings, J. H., Scherwitz, L. W., Armstrong, W. T., Ports, T. A., McLanahan, S. M., Kirkeeide, R. L., Gould, K. L., & Brand, R. J. (1990). Can lifestyle changes reverse coronary heart disease?: The lifestyle heart trial. *The Lancet, 336*(8708), 129–133. https://doi.org/10.1016/0140-6736(90)91656-U

Ornish, D., Lin, J., Chan, J. M., Epel, E., Kemp, C., Weidner, G., Marlin, R., Frenda, S. J., Magbanua, M. J. M., Daubenmeir, J., Estay, I., Hills, N. K., Chainani-Wu, N., Carroll, P. R., & Blackburn, E. H. (2013). Effect of comprehensive lifestyle changes on telomerase activity and telomere length in men with biopsy-proven low-risk prostate cancer: 5-year follow-up of a descriptive pilot study. *Lancet Oncology, 14*(11), 1112–1120. https://doi.org/10.1016/S1470-2045(13)70366-8

Ornish, D., Scherwitz, L. W., Billings, J. H., Gould, K. L., Merritt, T. A., Sparler, S., Armstrong, W. T., Ports, T. A., Kirkeeide, R. L., Hogeboom, C., & Brand, R. J. (1998). Intensive lifestyle changes for reversal of coronary heart disease. *Jama, 280*(23), 2001–2007. https://doi.org/10.1001/jama.280.23.2001

Poulimeneas, D., Anastasiou, C. A., Santos, I., Hill, J. O., Panagiotakos, D. B., & Yannakoulia, M. (2020). Exploring the relationship between the Mediterranean diet and weight loss maintenance: The MedWeight study. *British Journal of Nutrition, 124*(8), 874–880. https://doi.org/10.1017/S0007114520001798

Qian, F., Liu, G., Hu, F. B., Bhupathiraju, S. N., & Sun, Q. (2019, July 22). Association between plant-based dietary patterns and risk of type 2 diabetes: A systematic review and meta-analysis. *JAMA Internal Medicine, 179*(10), 1335–1344. https://doi.org/10.1001/jamainternmed.2019.2195

Ros, E., Martínez-González, M. A., Estruch, R., Salas-Salvadó, J., Fitó, M., Martínez, J. A., & Corella, D. (2014). Mediterranean diet and cardiovascular health: Teachings of the PREDIMED study. *Advances in Nutrition, 5*(3), 330S–336S. https://doi.org/10.3945/an.113.005389

Rose, S., & Strombom, A. (2018). A plant-based diet prevents and treats prostate cancer. *Cancer Therapy & Oncology International Journal, 11*(3), 70–76. https://doi.org/10.19080/CTOIJ.2018.11.555813

Rosell, M., Appleby, P., Spencer, E., & Key, T. (2006). Weight gain over 5 years in 21 966 meat-eating, fish-eating, vegetarian, and vegan men and women in EPIC-Oxford. *International Journal of Obesity, 30*(9), 1389–1396. https://doi.org/10.1038/sj.ijo.0803305

Salas-Salvadó, J., Bulló, M., Babio, N., Martínez-González, M. Á., Ibarrola-Jurado, N., Basora, J., Estruch, R., Covas, M. I., Corella, D., Arós, F., Ruiz-Gutiérrez, V., Ros, E., & PREDIMED Study Investigators. (2011). Reduction in the incidence of type 2 diabetes with the Mediterranean diet: Results of the PREDIMED-Reus nutrition intervention randomized trial. *Diabetes Care, 34*(1), 14–19. https://doi.org/10.2337/dc10-1288

Satija, A., Bhupathiraju, S. N., Rimm, E. B., Spiegelman, D., Chiuve, S. E., Borgi, L., Willett, W. C., Manson, J. E., Sun, Q., & Hu, F. B. (2016). Plant-based dietary patterns and incidence of type 2 diabetes in US men and women: Results from three prospective cohort studies. *PLoS Medicine, 13*(6), e1002039. https://doi.org/10.1371/journal.pmed.1002039

Saxe, G. A., Major, J. M., Nguyen, J. Y., Freeman, K. M., Downs, T. M., & Salem, C. E. (2006). Potential attenuation of disease progression in recurrent prostate cancer with plant-based diet and stress reduction. *Integrative Cancer Therapies, 5*(3), 206–213. https://doi.org/10.1177/1534735406292042

Schwedhelm, C., Boeing, H., Hoffmann, G., Aleksandrova, K., & Schwingshackl, L. (2016). Effect of diet on mortality and cancer recurrence among cancer survivors: a systematic review and meta-analysis of cohort studies. *Nutrition Reviews, 74*(12), 737–748.

Shan, Z., Li, Y., Baden, M. Y., Bhupathiraju, S. N., Wang, D. D., Sun, Q., Rexrode, K. M., Rimm, E. B., Qi, L., Willett, W. C., Manson, J. E., Qi, Q., & Hu, F. B. (2020). Association between healthy eating patterns and risk of cardiovascular disease. *JAMA Internal Medicine, 180*(8), 1090–1100. https://doi.org/10.1001/jamainternmed.2020.2176

Siegel, R. L., Miller, K. D., & Jemal, A. (2019). Cancer statistics, 2019. *CA: A Cancer Journal for Clinicians, 69*(1), 7–34. https://doi.org/10.3322/caac.21551

Siervo, M., Lara, J., Chowdhury, S., Ashor, A., Oggioni, C., & Mathers, J. C. (2015). Effects of the Dietary Approach to Stop Hypertension (DASH) diet on cardiovascular risk factors: A systematic review and meta-analysis. *British Journal of Nutrition, 113*(1), 1–15. https://doi.org/10.1017/S0007114514003341

Simon, M. S., Hastert, T. A., Barac, A., Banack, H. R., Caan, B. J., Chlebowski, R. T., Foraker, R., Hovsepyan, G., Liu, S., Luo, J., Manson, J. E., Neuhouser, M. L., Okwuosa, T. M., Pan, K., Qi, L., Ruterbusch, J. J., Shadyab, A. H., Thomson, C. A., Wactawski-Wende, J., ... Beebe-Dimmer, J. L. (2021). Cardiometabolic risk factors and survival after cancer in the Women's Health Initiative. *Cancer, 127*(4), 598–608. https://doi.org/10.1002/cncr.33295

Sotos-Prieto, M., Bhupathiraju, S. N., Mattei, J., Fung, T. T., Li, Y., Pan, A., Willett, W. C., Rimm, E. B., & Hu, F. B. (2017). Association of changes in diet quality with total and cause-specific mortality. *New England Journal of Medicine, 377*(2), 143–153. https://doi.org/10.1056/NEJMoa1613502

Stancic, S. (2017, May). The potential for lifestyle medicine and plant-based nutrition to address autoimmune diseases: Might the key to managing autoimmune disease be found on our dinner plate? Paper presented at the 4th Annual Plant-Based Prevention of Disease Conference, Albuquerque, NM.

Stuart, T. (2007). *The bloodless revolution: A cultural history of vegetarianism from 1600 to modern times.* New York, NY: W. W. Norton and Company.

Tantamango-Bartley, Y., Jaceldo-Siegl, K., Fan, J., & Fraser, G. (2013). Vegetarian diets and the incidence of cancer in a low-risk population. *Cancer Epidemiology, Biomarkers & Prevention, 22*(2), 286–294. https://doi.org/10.1158/1055-9965.EPI-12-1060

Tantamango-Bartley, Y., Knutsen, S. F., Knutsen, R., Jacobsen, B. K., Fan, J., Beeson, W. L., Sabate, J., Hadley, D., Jaceldo-Siegl, K., Penniecook, J., Herring, P., Butler, T., Bennett, H., & Fraser, G. (2016). Are strict vegetarians protected against prostate cancer? *The American Journal of Clinical Nutrition, 103*(1), 153–160. https://doi.org/10.3945/ajcn.114.106450

Taylor, R. (2008). Pathogenesis of type 2 diabetes: tracing the reverse route from cure to cause. *Diabetologia, 51*(10), 1781–1789. https://doi.org/10.1007/s00125-008-1116-7

Taylor, R., Al-Mrabeh, A., & Sattar, N. (2019). Understanding the mechanisms of reversal of type 2 diabetes. *The Lancet Diabetes & Endocrinology, 7*(9), 726–736. https://doi.org/10.1016/S2213-8587(19)30076-2

Toumpanakis, A., Turnbull, T., & Alba-Barba, I. (2018). Effectiveness of plant-based diets in promoting well-being in the management of type 2 diabetes: A systematic review. *BMJ Open Diabetes Research and Care, 6*(e000534). https://doi.org/10.1136/bmjdrc-2018-000534

Tsaban, G., Meir, A. Y., Rinott, E., Zelicha, H., Kaplan, A., Shalev, A., Katz, A., Rudich, A., Tirosh, A., Shelef, I., Youngster, I., Lebovitz, S., Israeli, N., Shabat, M., Brikner, D., Pupkin, E., Stumvoll, M., Thiery, J., Ceglarek, U., ... Shai, I. (2020). The effect of green Mediterranean diet on cardiometabolic risk: A randomised controlled trial. *Heart, 107*(13), 1–8. https://doi.org/10.1136/heartjnl-2020-317802

Turner-McGrievy, G. M., Davidson, C. R., Wingard, E. E., Wilcox, S., & Frongillo, E. A. (2015). Comparative effectiveness of plant-based diets for weight loss: A randomized controlled trial of five different diets. *Nutrition, 31*(2), 350–358. https://doi.org/10.1016/j.nut.2014.09.002

Vargas, E., Podder, V., Carrillo, S. M. A. (2021). *Physiology, glucose transporter type 4.* StatPearls . StatPearls Publishing. Retrieved from www.ncbi.nlm.nih.gov/books/NBK537322/

Virani, S. S., Alanso, A., Benjamin, E. J., Bittencourt, M. S., Callaway, C. W., Carson, A. P., Chamberlain, A. M., Chang, A. R., Cheng, S., Delling, F. N., Djousse, L., Elkind, M. S. V., Ferguson, J. F., Fornage, M., Khan, S. S., Kissela, B. M., Knutson, K. L., Kwan, T. W., Lackland, D. T., ... Tsao, C.W. (2020). Heart disease and stroke statistics—2020 update: A report from the American Heart Association. *Circulation, 141*, e1–e148. https://doi.org/10.1161/CIR.0000000000000757

Vodovotz, Y., Barnard, N., Hu, F. B., Jakicic, J., Lianov, L., Loveland, D., Buysse, D., Szigethy, E., Finkel, T., Sowa, G., Verschure, P., Williams, K., Sanchez, E., Dysinger, W., Maizes, V., Junker, C., Phillips, E., Katz, D., Drant, S. ... Parkinson, M. D. (2020). Prioritized research for the prevention, treatment, and reversal of chronic disease: Recommendations from the lifestyle medicine research Summit. *Frontiers in Medicine, 7*(585744), 1–20. https://doi.org/10.3389/fmed.2020.585744

Wallace, T. C., Bultman, S., D'Adamo, C., Daniel, C. R., Debelius, J., Ho, E., Eliassen, H., Lemanne, D., Mukherjee, P., Seyfried, T. N., Tian, Q., & Vahdat, L. T. (2019). Personalized nutrition in disrupting cancer—Proceedings from the 2017 American College of Nutrition Annual Meeting. *Journal of the American College of Nutrition, 38*(1), 1–14. https://doi.org/10.1080/07315724.2018.1500499

Wang, X., Ouyang, Y., Liu, J., Zhu, M., Zhao, G., Bao, W., & Hu, F. B. (2014). Fruit and vegetable consumption and mortality from all causes, cardiovascular disease, and cancer: Systematic review and dose-response meta-analysis of prospective cohort studies. *BMJ*, *349*, 1–14. https://doi.org/10.1136/bmj.g4490

Warren, M., Beck, S., & Delgado, D. (2020). The state of obesity: Better policies for a healthier America. Trust for America's Health. Retrieved from www.tfah.org

Yang, Q., Cogswell, M. E., Flanders, W. D., Hong, Y., Zhang, Z., Loustalot, F., Gillespie, C., Merritt, R., & Hu, F. B. (2012). Trends in cardiovascular health metrics and associations with all-cause and CVD mortality among US adults. *Jama*, *307*(12), 1273–1283. https://doi.org/10.1001/jama.2012.339

Yokoyama, Y., Nishimura, K., Barnard, N. D., Takegami, M., Watanabe, M., Sekikawa, A., Okamura, T., & Miyamoto, Y. (2014). Vegetarian diets and blood pressure: A meta-analysis. *JAMA Internal Medicine*, *174*(4), 577–587. https://doi.org/10.1001/jamainternmed.2013.14547

Wang, D., Li, Y., Ho, Y., Nguyen, X., Song, R., Hu, F. B., Willett, W., Wilson, P. W. F., Cho, K., Gaziano, J. M., & Djousse, L. (2020). Plant-based diet and the risk of cardiovascular disease and mortality: The Million Veteran program. *Current Developments in Nutrition*, *4*(Suppl 2). https://doi.org/10.1093/cdn/nzaa061_130

15 Hypertension

Matthew Petersen[1], Steven Brady[1], Eileen M. Handberg[2,3], and Monica Aggarwal[2]

[1]Department of Medicine, University of Florida
Gainesville, Florida, USA

[2]Division of Cardiology, University of Florida
Gainesville, Florida, USA

[3]One Florida PCOR.net Clinical Data Research Network

CONTENTS

KEY POINTS

- Many factors contribute to hypertension, including weight, physical activity, state of mind, inflammatory state within the body, and diet.
- Hypertension is one of the most prevalent and significant cardiovascular risk factors in the United States.
- Aerobic exercise and mindfulness exercises have been shown to reduce blood pressure.

DOI: 10.1201/9781003178330-18

- Diets that are rich in fruits and vegetables and low in salt, processed foods, and red meats lower cardiovascular risk and blood pressure.
- Many nutrients and supplements can help play a role in blood pressure control.

15.1   INTRODUCTION

The prevalence of cardiovascular disease (CVD) remains high globally due to an increase in cardiovascular risk factors such as hypertension and obesity (WHO, 2020). With the 2017 hypertension guidelines, almost 50% of the United States (US) population is now considered hypertensive and nearly 70% of the population is overweight or obese (CDC, 2021, Muntner et al., 2018). Less than half of those with hypertension are aware of their condition, and many others are inadequately treated. Untreated hypertension not only leads to significant individual health consequences, including CVD, stroke, and renal failure, but also puts a significant financial burden on the health system as a whole (Kirkland et al., 2018). Though broad-based pharmaceuticals have significantly reduced the mortality rate of CVD in the US, the prevalence of risk factors and economic burden of CVD remain exceedingly high.

Data from the Medical Expenditure Panel Survey (MEPS) suggest that hypertension is the single-most costly contributor to CVD, with an estimated direct cost of $69.9 billion in 2010 (Heidenreich et al., 2011). On an individual level, patients with hypertension are estimated to spend approximately $2000 more in healthcare expenses annually compared with patients without hypertension. Furthermore, patients with hypertension were found to spend roughly two and a half times more on inpatient care, two times more on outpatient care, and three times more on prescription medications compared with their normotensive peers (Heidenreich et al., 2011). While the physical and financial burden of hypertension is alarming, the good news is that hypertension is a very treatable and, even more importantly, a preventable condition.

15.1.1   Etiologies of Hypertension

The etiology of hypertension is multifactorial in nature, with both modifiable and non-modifiable risk factors that contribute to its development. For the purposes of this chapter, hypertension will refer to primary essential hypertension and will not address the nuances of secondary causes of high blood pressure (BP) such as primary aldosteronism, sleep apnea, pheochromocytoma, Cushing's disease, vasculopathies/aortopathies, or thyroid disorders.

Genetic predisposition explains a significant, however relatively small, effect on hypertension. Multiple genes have been discovered that influence BP; however, it is estimated that these genetic variations only account for about 3.5% of BP variability in the population (Whelton et al., 2018). Although hypertension has a familial component, obesity, sedentary lifestyle, alcohol intake, and poor dietary habits are well-recognized modifiable risk factors.

Increased alcohol intake has been shown to have a direct relationship with increased BP (Pareek & Olsen 2017). Although there are some conflicting data on whether a low amount of alcohol consumption is protective, studies agree that a large amount of alcohol consumption, defined as >2 drinks per day, has a negative impact on BP. Animal models have explored the etiology of alcohol-related hypertension, and current research suggests that effects of alcohol on BP are multifactorial (Puddey et al., 2019). Proposed mechanisms include dysregulation of the autonomic nervous system and the renin-angiotensin-aldosterone-system (RAAS), inappropriate sensing in the body's baroreceptors, and inappropriate smooth muscle activity (Puddey et al., 2019). Alcohol intake also increases caloric intake, more likely predisposing development of obesity and metabolic syndromes.

Excessive calorie intake and obesity are major factors contributing to hypertension (Savica et al., 2010). This increase in obesity and its related comorbidities is driven in part by poor dietary habits. The common diet, the standard American diet (SAD), includes an increased consumption of fried foods, fatty meats, dairy products, salts, refined processed grains, and added sugars (Grotto & Zied, 2010). In addition to increasingly unhealthy foods, Americans have been consuming only fractions of the recommended fruits, vegetables, and whole grains (Grotto & Zied, 2010). Study of the SAD reveals increased caloric consumption over the last 50 years, as well as increased consumption of fast food and nutrient-poor food, with an overall reduction of nutrient-dense foods. A direct relationship between weight, body mass index (BMI), central fat distribution, and an individual's BP has been observed, with increase in BMI yielding an almost linear increase in BP on a population scale (Dawber et al., 1951; Savica et al., 2010). Increased adipose (fat cells) can lead to increased BP through multiple factors, including activating the RAAS, increasing inflammation, and disrupting vasoregulation and endothelial function (Brandes, 2014; Furukawa et al., 2004; Hall et al., 2015; Savica et al., 2010). The RAAS is a neurohormonal regulation system whereby pressure sensors and chemoreceptors in the kidneys and blood vessels sense changes in serum sodium levels and BP and adjust BP to maintain pressure homeostasis. Dysregulation of this control system can lead to inappropriate retention of sodium and fluid, elevating BPs. Fortunately, weight loss can reverse this dysregulation (Dornfeld et al., 1987). The obese patient is also more likely to have increased inflammatory cytokines, oxidative damage, and increased sympathetic drive (Furukawa et al., 2004; Hall et al., 2015; Savica et al., 2010), all of which are associated with increased BP. These elevated inflammatory signals and the body's increased sympathetic drive (fight response) can inhibit the blood vessels' ability to regulate their own BP by causing endothelial dysfunction (Brandes, 2014). Each blood vessel is lined with endothelium, a thin layer of cells that has the ability to locally influence pressure changes in the vessels by producing a compound called nitric oxide (NO). Obesity and chronic inflammation can inhibit the endothelial lining's ability to produce NO and impair the endothelium's ability to regulate BP (Brandes, 2014). Reducing excess calories and weight loss can be valuable tools in combating hypertension. The American College of Cardiology (ACC)/ American Heart Association (AHA) Guideline recommends weight loss as a BP control strategy for all patients with obesity and hypertension (class 1A recommendation) (Whelton et al., 2018).

15.1.2 CLASSIFICATION

The ACC/AHA updated the hypertension guidelines in 2017 to reflect a notable increased morbidity at lower than previously thought BPs (Table 15.1). Each higher level is associated with an increased risk of developing CVD (Whelton et al., 2018).

The definition of these classifications of BP was justified by the increasing risk of CVD among adults in each category. Those with stage 1 hypertension have been shown through observational data and randomized control trials (RCTs) to have a higher risk of developing CVD (Guo et al., 2013;

TABLE 15.1
Blood pressure categories*

Category	Systolic Blood Pressure (mmHg)		Diastolic Blood Pressure (mmHg)
Normal blood pressure	< 120	and	< 80
Elevated blood pressure	120–129	and	< 80
Stage 1 hypertension	130–139	or	80–89
Stage 2 hypertension	≥ 140	or	≥ 90

*Stages of normal blood pressure, elevated blood pressure, stage 1 hypertension, and stage 2 hypertension. All readings should be obtained by blood pressure cuff readings on three separate occasions separated by at least 5 minutes (Whelton et al., 2018).

Sundstrom et al., 2015). Patients with stage 2 hypertension, in particular, have a well-established increased risk of developing CVD, including major cardiac events, stroke, renal disease, and other vascular disease (Guo et al., 2013; Huang et al., 2014). Furthermore, control of BP with a goal of <120/80 mmHg has been shown to reduce the incidence of heart attack, stroke, heart failure, and death due to cardiovascular causes (Wright et al., 2015). It is thus beneficial to have patients' BP well controlled with the goal of reducing the risk of complications, particularly CVD, stroke, and renal disease. With a high percentage of Americans having elevated BP and hypertension, there is significant room for improvement in the treatment and prevention of this disease.

15.2 LIFESTYLE-BASED THERAPIES TO TREAT HYPERTENSION

In addition to medical therapies to treat BP, it is important to consider lifestyle-based interventions that have been shown to result in significant reductions in BP. These lifestyle-based interventions include increasing the amount and type of physical activity, stress reduction, and many dietary interventions that provide opportunities for hypertensive patients to adopt changes that match their lifestyle, culture, and palate. In addition, there is a lot of confusion around nutritional and vitamin supplement use, and these will be reviewed here.

15.3 EXERCISE

Routine physical activity is one of the most important modifiable risk factors for preventing the development of hypertension. Though the mechanisms by which exercise lowers BP are not quite clear, there is a direct correlation between exercise and BP reduction. A single exercise session (i.e., cycling for 30 minutes), for example, can reduce both systolic (SBP) and diastolic BP (DBP) by 5–8 mmHg for 11–12 hours and 6–8 mmHg for 6–8 hours, respectively (Wallace, 2003). Proposed mechanisms by which exercise reduces BP include increased production of local vasodilatory molecules, such as nitric oxide, during exercise, leading to post-exercise hypotension (Halliwill, 2001; Laughlin et al., 2001; MacDonald, 2002). Post-exercise hypotension is a phenomenon of decreased resting BP immediately following an exercise session, likely due to increased NO production and decreased total peripheral resistance after exercise. Since BP, or mean arterial pressure, is equivalent to the product of cardiac output and total peripheral resistance, in theory one of these factors must decrease to cause an overall reduction in BP. As cardiac output does not decrease with exercise, decreased total peripheral resistance, therefore, is thought to be the primary driver behind BP reduction with exercise (MacDonald, 2002). NO is produced by NO synthase, an enzyme found in the endothelial cells lining the body's vasculature. During exercise, NO is released from the vascular endothelium, leading to local vasodilation, and studies have even suggested that chronic exercise can induce upregulation of NO synthase and therefore an increase in the total amount of circulating NO (Laughlin et al., 2001).

While some individuals may benefit from a strategically built exercise regimen, simply walking daily has been shown to reduce BP (Iwane et al., 2000; Mandini et al., 2018). One study analyzed the effects of walking 10,000 or more steps per day over the course of 12 weeks in both hypertensive and non-hypertensive individuals, and concluded that those who walked over 10,000 steps daily were found to have a statistically significant reduction in blood pressure (from 149.3±2.7 / 98.5±1.4 mmHg to 139.1±2.9 / 90±1.9 mmHg) compared with those who did not (Iwane et al., 2000). Another study analyzed the effect of a supervised walking program at least five days weekly for six months and its effect on blood pressure. Participants started with 15 to 30 minutes of daily walking and gradually increased both walking speed and duration to a uniform duration of 300 walking minutes weekly by the second month of the study. The results demonstrated a statistically significant net reduction in both SBP and DBP with a more drastic reduction seen in individuals with a higher baseline BP. For example, those with a resting SBP >160 mmHg at the start of the study were found to have an average reduction in SBP and DBP of −21.3±9.4 mmHg and −7.3±8.3 mmHg, respectively, while those with a baseline SBP between 130 and 139 mmHg were found to have an average reduction in SBP and DBP of −5.3±5.4 mmHg and −2.2±8.7 mmHg, respectively (Mandini et al., 2018). These studies demonstrate that routine walking can safely and effectively lower BP in individuals with hypertension.

In addition to routine aerobic exercise, the AHA also recommends moderate- to high-intensity muscle-strengthening activity, such as resistance training or weight training, at least two days per week (AHA, 2018). Resistance training is activity in which muscles contract against an opposing resistant force with the goal of increasing muscular strength, power, and/or endurance (Cornelissen & Smart, 2013). While the degree of BP reduction with cardiopulmonary exercise is greater when compared with that of resistance training alone in hypertensive individuals, there remains a role for resistance training in both treatment and prevention of hypertension (Kelley & Kelley, 2000; Wallace, 2003; Whelton et al., 2002). A meta-analysis of RCTs reviewing the effect of resistance exercise on BP in both hypertensive and non-hypertensive participants demonstrated a mean decrease in both SBP and DBP of −3±3 mmHg and −3±2 mmHg, respectively (Kelley & Kelley, 2000).

The amount of exercise an individual should perform on a daily or weekly basis is widely debated with varied recommendations from major professional organizations. The AHA recommendation is that adults should perform at least 150 minutes of moderate-intensity aerobic exercise or 75 minutes of vigorous aerobic activity per week, preferably spread throughout the week. Examples of moderate- and high-intensity aerobic activities are listed in Table 15.2 (AHA, 2018).

15.4 MINDFULNESS

Stress is detrimental to overall physical health and is becoming an increasingly identified contributor to the development of hypertension. Stress stimulates the sympathetic nervous system to secrete large amounts of catecholamines, such as epinephrine, which cause systemic vasoconstriction and subsequently elevated BP (Kulkarni et al., 1998). We typically think of the sympathetic nervous system as the primary driver of the "fight or flight" response. Alternatively, the parasympathetic nervous system, primarily responsible for the body's "rest and digest" functions, offsets the sympathetic nervous system by reducing levels of circulating catecholamines. With chronic stress, the human body is heavily shifted toward a sympathetic-predominant state, and over time this leads to chronically elevated levels of catecholamines and subsequently elevated BP (Aggarwal et al., 2017). Several techniques can reduce stress and allow the body to shift its autonomic balance in favor of the "rest and digest" phase.

Mindfulness is defined by the Oxford Learner's Dictionaries as "a mental state achieved by concentrating on the present moment, while calmly accepting the feelings and thoughts that come to

TABLE 15.2
Moderate- and high-intensity aerobic exercises

Moderate-Intensity Exercises	High-Intensity Exercises
Brisk walking (≥ 2.5 miles per hour)	Hiking uphill or with a heavy backpack
Water aerobics	Running
Dancing	Swimming laps
Gardening	Aerobic dancing
Doubles tennis	Heavy yard work
Biking < 10 miles per hour	Singles tennis
	Cycling ≥ 10 miles per hour
	Jumping rope

you, used as a technique to help you relax" or, simply put, "paying attention on purpose" (Kabat-Zinn, 2005). Meditation, specifically Transcendental Meditation (TM), is a key component of mindfulness. TM is a meditative technique in which individuals perform a silent mantra while sitting with closed eyes for approximately 20 minutes twice daily. TM is recommended by the AHA as a nondietary, nonpharmaceutical method for lowering BP (*Class IIb, Level of Evidence B*) (Brook et al., 2013). The first RCT studying the effects of TM on BP, psychological distress, and coping in college students was published in 2009. Participants performed TM for 20 minutes twice daily while sitting comfortably with closed eyes. The study showed a reduction in both systolic (−2.0 mmHg) and diastolic (−1.2 mmHg) BP in the TM group compared with a slight increase in SBP (+0.4 mmHg) and DBP (+0.5 mmHg) in the control group. Though the reduction in BP was not statistically significant, there were significant improvements in total psychological distress, anxiety, depression, anger/hostility, and coping (Nidich et al., 2009). A 2008 meta-analysis found that TM was associated with a significant reduction in SBP and DBP of approximately −4.7 and −3.2 mmHg, respectively (Anderson et al., 2008). Furthermore, a subgroup analysis of the studies that included hypertensive adults was completed and demonstrated similar results. This BP reduction technique comes at no cost, has no pharmacologic side effects, and ideally should be widely implemented in the treatment and prevention of hypertension.

15.5 DIET

Several dietary patterns have been shown to be beneficial in reducing BP (Horvath et al., 2008).

15.5.1 Dietary Approaches to Stop Hypertension (DASH) Diet

One of the first landmark diet studies examining blood pressure and cardiovascular health was the Dietary Approaches to Stop Hypertension (DASH) diet study in 1997, a large prospective study of 459 adults who had moderately elevated BPs and were monitored while eating an intervention diet versus control diet. The intervention diet was primarily composed of fruits, vegetables, low-fat dairy, and moderate amounts of fish, poultry, and whole grains. The control group consumed a regulated diet that was typical to that of many Americans, matched for macronutrient and mineral consumption averages of Americans at that time. This study found that the group consuming the DASH diet for three weeks was found to have lower BPs with an average of 11 and 3 mmHg reduction in SBP and DBP, respectively, in those with previous hypertension (Appel et al., 1997). The 2017 ACC/AHA hypertension guidelines give a class 1A recommendation for a heart-healthy diet such as the DASH to all patients with elevated BP or hypertension (Whelton et al., 2018). *Patients with high BP should utilize a DASH diet to help lower BP.*

15.5.2 The Mediterranean Diet (MedDiet)

The MedDiet is a diet that consists mostly of fruits, vegetables, primarily fish sources of protein, whole grains, and olive oil as its primary source of fat. It has been studied for its effects on CVD and risk factors for development of CVD. Although limited RCTs have directly examined the effects of the MedDiet on BP, one Australian RCT of 137 patients who were randomized to a usual diet vs a MedDiet with plant-based foods, abundant olive oil, and minimal red meat and processed foods for six months showed a small but significant 1.1 mmHg mean BP reduction in the MedDiet group (Davis et al., 2017). Another European-based multicenter RCT of over 1200 patients randomized individuals into groups with tailored standardized dietary advice with a goal to increase adherence to a MedDiet vs control who continued with their habitual diet. This study found a 5.5 mmHg reduction in SBP, with a greater effect seen in males (Jennings et al., 2019). Olive oil, a common component of the MedDiet and other "heart healthy" diets, is thought to lower blood pressure due to its high content of oleic acid and polyphenol antioxidants (Massaro et al., 2020). *The MedDiet is beneficial for BP and overall outcomes, driven primarily by reduction in strokes.*

15.5.3 WHOLE-FOOD PLANT-BASED (WFPB)

The WFPB diet consists of fruits, vegetables, whole grains, nuts, and legumes, with no animal products or refined grains. This diet has also been shown to have beneficial BP effects (Campbell et al., 2019). An RCT of 690 subjects randomized to increased fruit and vegetable intake of at least five servings a day versus a regular control diet for six months found that the increased fruit and vegetable intake resulted in lower SBP and DBP of 4 and 1.5 mmHg, respectively, with a correlated rise in plasma antioxidant levels in the blood, suggesting a possible mechanism of BP lowering with a diet rich in fruits and vegetables (John et al., 2002). In a cohort study of 78 participants who completed an eight-week dietary intervention of a WFPB diet, patients were able to lower BMI by an average of 12 lbs. and reduce SBP by 7 mmHg and DBP by 7 mmHg (Campbell et al., 2019). Another cohort study of 151 adults that consumed a WFPB showed SBP means of 113 mmHg in women and 120 mmHg in long-term outcomes (2–10 years), with 95% of participants achieving goal blood pressure targets (Jakse et al., 2019). One particularly large cohort study of over 73,000 participants followed for a mean of almost six years found a reduced all-cause mortality in those who were vegetarian (HR 0.88. 95% CI, 0.8–0.97) (Orlich et al., 2013). Further analysis of this cohort displayed a lower BP in the vegan-vegetarians in the cohort, with a mean SBP and DBP that was 6.8 mmHg and 6.9 mmHg, respectively, lower than that of the nonvegetarians (Pettersen et al., 2012). The prevalence of hypertension in the vegan-vegetarian subgroup was only about one-third of that of the nonvegetarian diet group (odds ratio of having hypertension of 0.37 compared with the nonvegetarian) (Orlich & Fraser, 2014). These cohort studies show the short- and long-term benefits of a WFPB diet on BP as well as mortality and longevity. *The WFPB diet focuses on fruits and vegetables, high fiber, and unprocessed foods. This dietary pattern is beneficial in BP and overall cardiovascular health and is recommended as a dietary modification for those with hypertension and/or cardiovascular disease.*

15.5.4 SODIUM REDUCTION

The standard American dietary pattern (SAD) is typically very high in sodium content, and most Americans eating this dietary pattern consume over 3 grams of sodium daily (Grotto & Zied, 2010). By changing a patient's diet to one based on the MedDiet, WFPB, or DASH dietary patterns discussed above, sodium consumption is significantly reduced by removing processed food and adding back fruits, vegetables, whole grains, and legumes (Grotto & Zied, 2010). Salt restriction is part of the American Heart Association (AHA) guidelines. However, the appropriate level of sodium intake in the diet has been controversial. In review of dietary studies like the DASH study, excess salt intake as part of the SAD has been linked to elevated BP (Sacks et al., 2001). The DASH follow-up study further evaluated the specific effects of sodium along with dietary change on BP. The study examined 412 participants randomized to either a SAD or the DASH diet, and within each diet group, subjects were instructed to consume 30 days each of high (150 mmol/day), intermediate (100 mmol/day), and low (50 mmol/day) levels of sodium. The results showed a decrease in SBP by around 2 mmHg in the control group and 1.3 mmHg in the DASH group when reducing sodium intake from the high to intermediate level. When reducing sodium from the intermediate to low level, there was an even further decrease in SBP of 4.6 mmHg and 1.7 mmHg in the control group and DASH group, respectively, suggesting that daily sodium reduction had benefits beyond dietary changes (Sacks et al., 2001). While studies show that there is a problem with too much sodium in the diet, too little sodium also appears to be an issue. More recent reviews and meta-analyses of cohort studies in healthy non-hypertensive patients have shown a U-shaped relationship between sodium intake and all-cause mortality, suggesting that too little sodium and too much sodium can be detrimental in healthy individuals (Graudal et al., 2014). The ACC/AHA guidelines call for limited salt intake in all patients with hypertension (class 1A recommendation) up to 1.5 grams daily (Whelton et al., 2018). *All patients with hypertension should aim for reduced dietary sodium intake with a goal of <1.5 grams of sodium daily.*

15.5.5 ALCOHOL REDUCTION

A recent meta-analysis and systematic review examined the effects of heavier alcohol consumption on BP. After reviewing 36 trials with 2865 participants (86% of them men), the authors concluded that in those who drank >2 alcoholic beverages a day, a reduction in alcohol consumption was associated with a 5 and 4 mmHg reduction in SBP and DBP respectively on average (Roerecke et al., 2017). The BP lowering effect of reducing alcohol intake was even more robust in participants who drank >6 alcoholic drinks a day (Roerecke et al., 2017). The ACC/AHA currently recommends that those with hypertension should consume no more than two standard alcoholic drinks a day for men, and no more than one standard alcoholic drink a day for women (Whelton et al., 2018). *For those with high BP, it is recommended to reduce alcohol consumption to under two drinks per day in men and under one drink per day in women for better BP control.*

15.6 NUTRIENTS AND SUPPLEMENTS AND HYPERTENSION

15.6.1 NITRATES

Nitrates are compounds that can be found in many dietary food sources. Dietary nitrates found in salt-preserved meats have been linked to increased incidence of gastric cancers; however, nitrate-containing vegetables have been linked to reduced gastric cancer risk (Terry et al., 2001). Nitrates from vegetable sources appear to have the ability to increase the amount of NO produced within the body, which increases the efficiency of vasoregulation and vasodilation. This increased ability to vasodilate via the NO mechanism, when augmented by dietary nitrates, is thought to lower BP (d'El-Rei et al., 2016, Kapil et al., 2015). One RCT of 68 hypertensive patients who received 250 ml of dietary nitrates in the form of beetroot juice vs a placebo demonstrated a mean reduction in BP of 7.7 mmHg SBP and 2.4 mmHg DBP, with good tolerance among the participants (Kapil et al., 2015). This improved BP regulation with dietary nitrates has been shown to have beneficial cardiovascular effects as well (d'El-Rei et al., 2016). Foods with high natural nitrate content include root vegetables and leafy greens, such as celery, chard, beetroot, spinach, and arugula (d'El-Rei et al., 2016, Hord et al., 2009). Doses used in trials range from 155 to 1484 mg/day of dietary nitrates, with varying degrees of BP benefit. One review acknowledged the benefits but, due to the mixed size, doses, and populations of current RCTs, called for larger RCTs to investigate the matter further (d'El-Rei et al., 2016). *Dietary nitrates can show benefit in lowering BP in hypertensive patients; however, optimal level of consumption is unknown and more research needs to be done. Focus on plant-based sources of nitrates is optimal.*

15.6.2 VITAMIN D

Vitamin D is a steroid prohormone that is produced by keratinocytes within the epidermis when exposed to ultraviolet radiation. Vitamin D can also be obtained through food products such as fish, mushrooms, and fortified milks. Deficiency in vitamin D has been linked to hypertension and CVD (Anderson et al., 2010, Judd & Tangpricha, 2009). Using vitamin D supplementation to treat hypertension, however, has not shown to be definitively beneficial. In several recent meta-analyses of 12 RCTs that included almost 2500 subjects, supplementation of vitamin D in those with hypertension did not show any significant change in blood pressure (Farapti et al., 2020). *Vitamin D supplementation is currently recommended for vitamin D deficiency and bone health; however, there is not enough data to support vitamin D supplementation for BP control.*

15.6.3 FLAVONOIDS

Flavonoids are a group of antioxidants found in various fruits, vegetables, wine, and teas. The antioxidant effects of this group of molecules have been associated with anti-inflammation and improved endothelial function. In rat studies, supplemental epicatechin, a type of flavonoid, was shown to reduce BP by NO-induced vasodilation (Galleano et al., 2013). There is limited human data, however. These molecules can be found in an abundance of healthy dietary sources, and it is recommended to obtain these potentially beneficial molecules through a well-rounded diet rich in fruits and vegetables. *Increased consumption of healthy dietary sources of flavonoids can be beneficial for endothelial function.*

15.6.4 MAGNESIUM

Magnesium is an elemental electrolyte that is utilized in a variety of cellular functions and is considered an essential nutrient. Magnesium can lower BP by blocking natural calcium channels in the cells of vascular smooth muscle, which inhibits constriction of these muscles. Magnesium can be found in food sources such as dark green leafy vegetables and whole grains or can be ingested as a supplement. Supplementation of magnesium has been shown in several meta-analyses of RCTs, one examining 20 RCTs with over 1000 subjects and another 34 RCTs with over 2000 subjects, to modestly lower SBP and DBP by approximately 2–4 mmHg (Jee et al., 2002, Zhang et al., 2016). *Magnesium supplementation has been shown to have a statistically significant but weak effect of lowering BP. Sources of magnesium in the diet are cashews, almonds, bananas, avocado, pumpkin seeds, spinach, and whole wheat.*

15.6.5 POTASSIUM

Potassium is an essential element and electrolyte in the body and is responsible for controlling many cellular functions from neuronal activity to BP regulation. Lower consumption of dietary potassium is associated with increased BP, stroke, and CVD (D'Elia et al., 2011; Dyer, et al., 1994). Oral potassium supplementation has been shown in multiple meta-analyses of RCTs to have beneficial effects on BP, lowering SBP and DBP by 3–6 mmHg and 2–3 mmHg, respectively (Cappuccio & MacGregor, 1991; Aburto et al., 2013). The largest benefits were seen in individuals with hypertension, with less benefit seen in those with normal BP. No adverse effects were noted with regard to renal function, lipid levels, or catecholamine concentrations with supplementation of up to 120 mmol per day (Aburto et al., 2013). Based on the current SAD, the average American consumes only about half the recommended amount of potassium (Grotto & Zied, 2010). Many foods are rich in potassium and can be an ample source of dietary potassium, including potatoes, carrots, tomatoes, beans, and salmon (USDHHS, 2015). The ACC/AHA guidelines currently recommend (class 1A recommendation) potassium supplementation, preferably through dietary sources, for adults with elevated BP and hypertension unless contraindicated by the presence of kidney disease or concomitant use of medications that can increase potassium (Whelton et al., 2018). The ACC/AHA outlines a goal of 3500–5000 mg per day of potassium consumption with an approximate impact of around 4–5 mmHg improvement in blood pressure in hypertensive patients (Whelton et al., 2018). *Patients with hypertension should increase potassium intake to a goal of 3500–5000 mg daily, ideally through dietary sources, to improve BP control. Due to narrow homeostatic range of potassium and potentially dangerous adverse effects of increased potassium, we recommend laboratory monitoring of levels, review of current medication, and discussion with a healthcare provider prior to supplementation.*

15.6.6 CALCIUM

The current research pertaining to calcium and BP is mixed, and supplemental use of calcium for BP benefit is controversial. Dietary calcium has been associated with BP reduction in short- but not long-term longitudinal observational studies (Witteman et al., 1989). Meta-analyses of calcium supplementation showed a small effect on BP, lowering SBP by 1.2–1.4 mmHg with no effect on DBP (Bucher et al., 1996; Griffith et al., 1999). A recent review, however, highlighted that observational studies and RCTs have suggested that vitamin D and calcium supplementation have the potential for adverse outcomes and cardiovascular harm as well as an increased risk of myocardial infarction and stroke (Michos et al., 2021). The authors call for cautious use of calcium supplementation and suggest that optimal calcium intake should be from dietary sources. At this time, these small effects of dietary supplemental calcium on BP do not support its regular use as a primary BP-lowering strategy and could increase the risk of harmful cardiovascular outcomes. *Currently there is no strong evidence supporting the use of calcium supplementation as a primary strategy for BP control. There is some evidence suggesting that calcium supplementation could increase the risk of adverse cardiovascular outcomes.*

15.6.7 OMEGA 3 FATTY ACIDS

Omega 3 fatty acids are a group of polyunsaturated fatty acids found mostly in marine food sources. Thorough literary research has been devoted to the relationship between supplemental omega 3 fatty acids, such as eicosapentaenoic acid (EPA) and docosahexaenoic acid (DHA), and BP. A recent large meta-analysis of RCTs showed that compared with placebo, supplementation of EPA and DHA provided a modest BP benefit, lowering SBP and DBP by an average of 1.5 mmHg and 1 mmHg, respectively. Stronger effects were seen in a subgroup analysis of untreated hypertensive patients with an average reduction in SBP of 4.5 mmHg and DBP of 3 mmHg (Miller et al., 2014). Omega 3 fatty acids have a significant role in cardiovascular disease. Recent data from the REDUCE-IT trial showed that supplementation with highly purified EPC (Icosapentyl Ethyl) was associated with a significant reduction in a combined cardiovascular endpoint in patients with CVD or with diabetes and additional cardiovascular risk factors. A notable effect was seen in patients with high and normal triglycerides (Bhatt et al., 2019). Omega 3 fatty acids can be obtained from fatty fish such as salmon or anchovies, as well as plant sources such as algal oil, walnuts, and flax seed. Plant-based sources include chia seeds, flax seeds, walnuts, and soybeans. Omega 3 fatty acids can also be supplemented in pill form, but non-prescription formulas have significant variety in the EPA and DHA concentrations and, therefore, care should be used in finding the best supplement. *Omega 3 fatty acid supplementation can lower BP and provide other significant cardiovascular benefits.*

15.6.8 ARGININE

Arginine is an amino acid that has been of interest because of its ability to use enzymes called NO synthases to increase the availability of NO, thereby potentially contributing to the beneficial vasodilatory effects of NO. There have been some mixed results in the research in this area, however. One meta-analysis of 11 RCTs showed that supplementation with arginine did lower SBP and DBP by a mean 5.39 mmHg and 2.66 mmHg, respectively (Dong et al., 2011). However, another study looked at arginine supplementation in 153 patients following an acute ST-segment elevation myocardial infarction (STEMI). Participants were randomized post-STEMI to receive L-arginine 3 g three times daily vs placebo. Six patients (8.6%) in the experimental group died during the six-month follow-up compared with no deaths observed in the placebo group (Schulman et al., 2006). This study was discontinued due to lack of benefit and increased mortality in patients who recently suffered a myocardial infarction, and as a result, L-arginine supplementation is not recommended in those patients (Schulman et al., 2006). *Although some data show a modest reduction in BP with arginine supplementation, large studies and analyses are necessary in order to recommend arginine supplementation as a first-line therapy for BP control. Of note, there is potential harm with arginine when given to patients that recently suffered an acute STEMI and therefore it should be avoided in this cohort.*

15.6.9 TAURINE

Taurine is an amino acid that has been studied for BP control, and there is some evidence that showed a benefit of taurine supplementation regarding BP control. One RCT of 178 patients with hypertension were administered taurine supplementation vs placebo for 12 weeks. Patients in the experimental group were observed to have a decrease in BP with a reduction of 7.2 mmHg for SBP and 4.7 mmHg for DBP (Sun et al., 2016). *Despite this promising trial, more studies are needed prior to recommending taurine for BP control.*

15.6.10 COENZYME Q10

Coenzyme Q10 (CoQ10) is an antioxidant and electron transporter found in every tissue in the human body. It is vital to mitochondria and energy production in the cell and is found in highest concentrations in cardiac tissue. Supplementation with CoQ10 for the benefit of BP control has mixed results. One meta-analysis examined 12 clinical trials (three of which were RCTs) and showed an average decrease in SBP of 16 mmHg and DBP of 8 mmHg in the treatment group with no significant change in the placebo group (Rosenfeldt et al., 2007). A Cochrane review in 2016, however, recommended against the use of CoQ10 supplementation for the management of hypertension due to the small number of RCTs reviewed in their study, questionable reliability of the data, and a small pooled benefit (Ho et al., 2016). *Despite some promising preliminary data, there are not enough data and RCTs currently to recommend Coenzyme Q10 for BP management.*

15.6.11 TEA

Because of the popularity of tea consumption around the world, its effects on BP are potentially widespread. The effect of tea on BP is hypothesized to be due to the endothelial effects of the flavonoids that are found in many teas. Large meta-analyses of RTCs, one with 25 studies including 1476 subjects and another with 24 RCTs including 1697 subjects, have shown a significant but small improvement in SBP and DBP of approximately 1–2 mmHg with chronic tea consumption, independent of caffeine dose (Liu et al., 2014; Xu et al., 2020). Most of the studies support green tea as having a larger benefit over black tea on BP-lowering effects, also with long-term tea drinking required (usually over 12 weeks) before an effect can be seen (Liu et al., 2014; Xu et al., 2020). *Tea consumption appears to have a significant, yet very modest benefit in reducing BP, and a large quantity of tea consumed over a long period of time is required to show benefit.*

15.6.12 POMEGRANATE JUICE

The potential BP benefit of pomegranate juice is thought to be due to high concentrations of tannins, which are antioxidants found within the fruit juice. In one small cohort study of patients with hypertension, consuming 50 mL of pomegranate juice daily for two weeks showed reduction in angiotensin-converting enzyme (ACE) activity by 36% (Aviram & Dornfeld, 2001). ACE is a key target in many of the most effective antihypertensive medications. The inhibition of ACE by pomegranate juice led to a 5% reduction in BP in this study (Aviram & Dornfeld, 2001). *The dose frequency of pomegranate juice consumption for optimal BP management is still unknown, and more research needs to be done in this area, with a particular need for RCTs. Consuming pomegranates is reasonable as part of a plant-based diet.*

15.6.13 Cocoa

Cocoa is a main ingredient of chocolate. Darker chocolates have higher concentrations of cocoa and flavanols. One study of 20 patients with hypertension not on medical therapy randomized subjects to dark vs white chocolate. This study found that ingesting dark chocolate daily for two weeks showed significant reduction of SBP by 12 mmHg and DBP by 8 mmHg (Grassi et al., 2005). Other studies, such as a slightly larger RCT of 44 patients with untreated hypertension who received 18 weeks of dark vs white chocolate, also show BP improvements with dark chocolate consumption, but the BP reduction was more modest at 3 mmHg and 1.9 mmHg for SBP and DBP, respectively (Taubert et al., 2007). In addition to the beneficial effects on BP, consumption of cocoa products and chocolate has been shown to reduce cardiovascular risk markers and risk of developing CVD. In two meta-analyses, one of 42 short-term RCTs and another of 19 RCTs, chocolate consumption was found to improve insulin resistance, BP, and LDL and HDL cholesterol levels (Hooper et al., 2012; Lin et al., 2016). Another meta-analysis including over 400,000 subjects found a reduction in relative risk of CVD, stroke, and myocardial infarction with consumption of 20 g/week of chocolate (Ren et al., 2019). It is important to note that most studies showing the benefits of cocoa/chocolate utilized chocolate with high cocoa percentages and lower milk and sugar content (i.e., dark chocolate), and that many of these benefits were lessened with milk chocolate (Corti et al., 2009). *Dark chocolate appears to have a significant, yet modest benefit in lowering BP in patients with hypertension. Regular consumption of cocoa under 100 g/week does appear to have a benefit in reduction of CVD and stroke. Caution is needed to minimize excess sugar and milk in the chocolate.*

15.7 CONCLUSION

High BP is a key modifiable risk factor for heart disease, stroke, and kidney disease and is the cause of a high burden of disease. BP can be lowered through a variety of different lifestyle and dietary modifications, including exercise, mindfulness practices, diets with reduced fat, salt, and processed food consumption; and a variety of nutrients that together can improve the body's ability to naturally regulate its BP.

Table 15.3 summarizes the data supporting non-pharmacological interventions of blood pressure.

TABLE 15.3
Summary of data supporting non-pharmacological interventions of blood pressure

Strong Data Supporting Benefit (Effect)	Weak Data Supporting Benefit (Effect)	Data Showing No Benefit
DASH diet (strong)	Nitrate supplementation (moderate)	Vitamin D supplementation
Whole food plant-based diet (moderate)	Flavonoid supplementation (modest)	Calcium supplementation
Mediterranean Diet (modest)	Arginine supplementation (moderate)* potentially harm in STEMI	
Sodium reduction below 1.5 g/day (moderate)	Taurine supplementation (moderate)	
Potassium intake 3.5–5 g/day (modest)	Pomegranate juice (moderate)	
Tea consumption (modest)	Cocoa consumption (modest–moderate)	
Magnesium supplementation (modest)		
Omega 3 fatty acid supplementation (modest)		

REFERENCES

Aburto, N. J., Hanson, S., Gutierrez, H., Hooper, L., Elliott, P., & Cappuccio, F. P. (2013). Effect of increased potassium intake on cardiovascular risk factors and disease: Systematic review and meta-analyses. *BMJ, 346*, f1378.

Aggarwal, M., Aggarwal, B., & Rao, J. (2017). Integrative medicine for cardiovascular disease and prevention. *Medical Clinics of North America, 101*, 895–923.

AHA. (2018). Recommendations for physical activity in adults and kids. www.heart.org/en/healthy-living/fitness/fitness-basics/aha-recs-for-physical-activity-in-adults

Anderson, J. L., May, H. T., Horne, B. D., Blair, T. L., Hall, N. L., Carlquist, J. F., Lappé, D. L., Muhlestein, J. B., & Intermountain Heart Collaborative Study Group. (2010). Relation of vitamin D deficiency to cardiovascular risk factors, disease status, and incident events in a general healthcare population. *American Journal of Cardiology, 106*, 963–968.

Anderson, J. W., Liu, C., & Kryscio, R. J. (2008). Blood pressure response to transcendental meditation: A meta-analysis. *American Journal of Hypertension, 21*, 310–316.

Appel, L. J., Moore, T. J., Obarzanek, E., Vollmer, W. M., Svetkey, L. P., Sacks, F. M., Bray, G. A., Vogt, T. M., Cutler, J. A., Windhauser, M. M., Lin, P. H., & Kranja, N. (1997). A clinical trial of the effects of dietary patterns on blood pressure. DASH Collaborative Research Group. *New England Journal of Medicine, 336*, 1117–1124.

Aviram, M., & Dornfeld, L. (2001). Pomegranate juice consumption inhibits serum angiotensin converting enzyme activity and reduces systolic blood pressure. *Atherosclerosis, 158*, 195–198.

Bhatt, D. L., Steg, P. G., Miller, M., Brinton, E. A., Jacobson, T. A., Ketchum, S. B., Doyle, R. T., Juliano, R. A., Jiao, L., Granowitz, C., Tardif, J-C., & Ballantyne, C. M. (2019). Cardiovascular risk reduction with icosapent ethyl for hypertriglyceridemia. *New England Journal of Medicine, 380*, 11–22.

Brandes, R. P. (2014). Endothelial dysfunction and hypertension. *Hypertension, 64*, 924–928.

Brook, R. D., Appel, L. J., Rubenfire, M., Ogedegbe, G., Bisognano, J. D., Elliot, W. J., Fuchs, F. D., Hughes, J. W., Lackland, D. T., Staffileno, B. A., Townsend, R. R., & Rajagopalan, S. (2013). Beyond medications and diet: Alternative approaches to lowering blood pressure: a scientific statement from the American Heart Association. *Hypertension, 61*, 1360–1383.

Bucher, H. C., Cook, R. J., Guyatt, G. H., Cook, D. J., Hatala, R., & Hunt, D. L. (1996). Effects of dietary calcium supplementation on blood pressure: A meta-analysis of randomized controlled trials. *JAMA, 275*, 1016–1022.

Campbell, E. K., Fidahusain, M., & Campbell Ii, T. M. (2019). Evaluation of an eight-week whole-food plant-based lifestyle modification program. *Nutrients, 11*, 1–12.

Cappuccio, F. P., & MacGregor, G. A. (1991). Does potassium supplementation lower blood pressure? A meta-analysis of published trials. *Journal of Hypertension, 9*, 465–473.

CDC. (2021). Underlying cause of death 1999–2019. CDC WONDER database. https://wonder.cdc.gov/wonder/help/ucd.html

Cornelissen, V. A., & Smart, N. A. (2013). Exercise training for blood pressure: A systematic review and meta-analysis. *Journal of the American Heart Association, 2*, e004473.

Corti, R., Flammer, A. J., Hollenberg, N. K., & Luscher, T. F. (2009). Cocoa and cardiovascular health. *Circulation, 119*, 1433–1441.

d'El-Rei, J., Cunha, A. R., Trindade, M., & Neves, M. F. (2016). Beneficial effects of dietary nitrate on endothelial function and blood pressure levels. *International Journal of Hypertension*, 6791519.

D'Elia, L., Barba, G., Cappuccio, F. P., & Strazzullo, P. (2011). Potassium intake, stroke, and cardiovascular disease a meta-analysis of prospective studies. *Journal of the American College of Cardiology, 57*, 1210–1219.

Davis, C. R., Hodgson, J. M., Woodman, R., Bryan, J., Wilson, C., & Murphy, K. J. (2017). A Mediterranean diet lowers blood pressure and improves endothelial function: Results from the MedLey randomized intervention trial. American *Journal of Clinical Nutrition, 105*, 1305–13.

Dawber, T. R., Meadors, G. F., & Moore, Jr., F. E. (1951). Epidemiological approaches to heart disease: The Framingham Study. *American Journal of Public Health and the Nation's Health, 41*, 279–281.

Dong, J. Y., Qin, L. Q., Zhang, Z., Zhao, Y., Wang, J., Arigoni, F., & Zhang, W. (2011). Effect of oral L-arginine supplementation on blood pressure: A meta-analysis of randomized, double-blind, placebo-controlled trials. *American Heart Journal, 162*, 959–965.

Dornfeld, L. P., Maxwell, M. H., Waks, A., & Tuck, M. (1987). Mechanisms of hypertension in obesity. *Kidney International Supplements*, *22*, S254–258.

Dyer, A. R., Elliott, P., & Shipley, M. (1994). Urinary electrolyte excretion in 24 hours and blood pressure in the INTERSALT Study. II. Estimates of electrolyte-blood pressure associations corrected for regression dilution bias. The INTERSALT Cooperative Research Group. *American Journal of Epidemiology*, *139*, 940–951.

Farapti, F., Fadilla, C., Yogiswara, N., & Adriani, M. (2020). Effects of vitamin D supplementation on 25(OH) D concentrations and blood pressure in the elderly: a systematic review and meta-analysis. *F1000Res 9*, 633.

Furukawa, S., Fujita, T., Shimabukuro, M., Iwaki, M., Yamada, Y., Nakajima, Y., Nakayama, O., Makishima, M., Matsuda, M., & Shimomura, I. (2004). Increased oxidative stress in obesity and its impact on metabolic syndrome. *Journal of Clinical Investigation*, *114*, 1752–1761.

Galleano, M., Bernatova, I., Puzserova, A., Balis, P., Sestakova, N., Pechanova, O., & Fraga, C. G. (2013). (-)-Epicatechin reduces blood pressure and improves vasorelaxation in spontaneously hypertensive rats by NO-mediated mechanism. *IUBMB Life*, *65*, 710–715.

Grassi, D., Necozione, S., Lippi, C., Croce, G., Valeri, L., Pasqualetti, P., Desideri, G., Blumberg, J. B., & Ferri, C. (2005). Cocoa reduces blood pressure and insulin resistance and improves endothelium-dependent vasodilation in hypertensives. *Hypertension*, *46*, 398–405.

Graudal, N., Jurgens, G., Baslund, B., & Alderman, M. H. (2014). Compared with usual sodium intake, low- and excessive-sodium diets are associated with increased mortality: A meta-analysis. *American Journal of Hypertension*, *27*, 1129–1137.

Griffith, L. E., Guyatt, G. H., Cook, R. J., Bucher, H. C., & Cook, D. J. (1999). The influence of dietary and nondietary calcium supplementation on blood pressure: An updated metaanalysis of randomized controlled trials. *American Journal of Hypertension*, *12*, 84–92.

Grotto, D., & Zied, E. (2010). The Standard American Diet and its relationship to the health status of Americans. *Nutrition in Clinical Practice*, *25*, 603–612.

Guo, X., Zhang, X., Guo, L., Li, Zhao, Zheng, L. Yu, S., Yang, H., Zhou, X., Zhang, X., Sun, Z., Li, J., & Sun, Y. (2013). Association between pre-hypertension and cardiovascular outcomes: A systematic review and meta-analysis of prospective studies. *Current Hypertension Reports*, *15*, 703–716.

Hall, J. E., do Carmo, J. M., da Silva, A. A., Wang, Z., & Hall, M. E. (2015). Obesity-induced hypertension: Interaction of neurohumoral and renal mechanisms. *Circulation Research*, *116*, 991–1006.

Halliwill, J. R. (2001). Mechanisms and clinical implications of post-exercise hypotension in humans. *Exercise and Sport Sciences Review*, *29*, 65–70.

Heidenreich, P. A., Trogdon, J. G., Khavjou, O. A., Buter, J., Dracup, K., Ezekowitz, M. D., Finkelstein, E. A., Hong, Y., Johnston, S. C., Khera, A. Lloyd-Jones, D. M., Nelson, S. A., Nichol, G., Orenstein, D., Wilson, P. W. F., Woo, Y. J., American Heart Association Advocacy Coordinating Committee, Stroke Council, Council on Cardiovascular Radiology and Intervention, … Interdisciplinary Council on Quality of Care and Outcomes Research. (2011). Forecasting the future of cardiovascular disease in the United States: A policy statement from the American Heart Association. *Circulation*, *123*, 933–944.

Ho, M. J., Li, E. C., & Wright, J. M. (2016). Blood pressure lowering efficacy of coenzyme Q10 for primary hypertension. *Cochrane Database of Systematic Reviews*, *3*, CD007435.

Hooper, L., Kay, C., Abdelhamid, A., Kroon, P. A., Cohn, J. S., Rimm, E. B., & Cassidy, A. (2012). Effects of chocolate, cocoa, and flavan-3-ols on cardiovascular health: A systematic review and meta-analysis of randomized trials. *American Journal of Clinical Nutrition*, *95*, 740–751.

Hord, N. G., Tang, Y., & Bryan, N. S. (2009). Food sources of nitrates and nitrites: The physiologic context for potential health benefits. *American Journal of Clinical Nutrition*, *90*, 1–10.

Horvath, K., Jeitler, K., Siering, U., Stich, A. K., Skipka, G., Gratzer, T. W., & Siebenhofer, A. (2008). Long-term effects of weight-reducing interventions in hypertensive patients: Systematic review and meta-analysis. *Archives for Internal Medicine*, *168*, 571–580.

Huang, Y., Cai, X., Li, Y., Su, L., Mai, W., Wang, S., Hu, Y., Wu, Y., & Xu, D. (2014). Prehypertension and the risk of stroke: A meta-analysis. *Neurology*, *82*, 1153–1161.

Iwane, M., Arita, M., Tomimoto, S., Satani, O., Matsumoto, M., Miyashita, K., & Nishio, I. (2000). Walking 10,000 steps/day or more reduces blood pressure and sympathetic nerve activity in mild essential hypertension. *Hypertension Research*, *23*, 573–580.

Jakse, B., Jakse, B., Pinter, S., Jug, B., Godnov, U., Pajek, J., & Mis, N. F. (2019). Dietary intakes and cardiovascular health of healthy adults in short-, medium-, and long-term whole-food plant-based lifestyle program. *Nutrients, 12*(1), 55.

Jee, S. H., Miller, E. R., Guallar, E., Singh, V. K., Appel, L. J., & Klag, M. J. (2002). The effect of magnesium supplementation on blood pressure: A meta-analysis of randomized clinical trials. *American Journal of Hypertension, 15*, 691–696.

Jennings, A., Berendsen, A. M., de Groot, L. C. P. G. M., Feskens, E. J. M., Brzozowska, A., Sicinska, E., Pietruszka, B., Meunier, N., Caumon, E., Malpuech-Brugère, C., Santoro, A., Ostan, R., Franceschi, C., Gillings, R., O'Neill, C. M., Fairweather-Tait, S. J., Minihane, A-M., & Cassidy, A. (2019). Mediterranean-style diet improves systolic blood pressure and arterial stiffness in older adults. *Hypertension, 73*, 578–586.

John, J. H., Ziebland, S., Yudkin, P., Roe, L. S., Neil, H. A. W., & Oxford Fruit and Vegetable Study Group. (2002). Effects of fruit and vegetable consumption on plasma antioxidant concentrations and blood pressure: A randomised controlled trial. *Lancet, 359*, 1969–1974.

Judd, S. E., & Tangpricha, V. (2009). Vitamin D deficiency and risk for cardiovascular disease. *American Journal of the Medical Sciences, 338*, 40–44.

Kabat-Zinn, J. (2005). *Full catastrophe living: Using the wisdom of your body and mind to face stress, pain, and illness* (15th anniversary ed.). Piatkus Books.

Kapil, V., Khambata, R. S., Robertson, A., Caulfield, M. J., & Ahluwalia, A. (2015). Dietary nitrate provides sustained blood pressure lowering in hypertensive patients: A randomized, phase 2, double-blind, placebo-controlled study. *Hypertension, 65*, 320–327.

Kelley, G. A., & Kelley, K. S. (2000). Progressive resistance exercise and resting blood pressure: A meta-analysis of randomized controlled trials. *Hypertension, 35*, 838–843.

Kirkland, E. B., Heincelman, M., Bishu, K. G., Schumann, S. O., Schreiner, A., Axon, R. N., Mauldin, P. D., & Moran, W. P. (2018). Trends in healthcare expenditures among US adults with hypertension: National estimates, 2003–2014. *Journal of the American Heart Association, 7*(11), 1–9.

Kulkarni, S., O'Farrell, I., Erasi, M., & Kochar, M. S. (1998). Stress and hypertension. *WMJ, 97*, 34–38.

Laughlin, M. H., Pollock, J. S., Amann, J. F., Hollis, M. L., Woodman, C. R., & Price, E. M. (2001). Training induces nonuniform increases in eNOS content along the coronary arterial tree. *Journal of Applied Physiology (1985), 90*, 501–510.

Lin, X., Zhang, I., Li, A., Manson, J. E., Sesso, H. D., Wang, L., & Liu, S. (2016). Cocoa flavanol intake and biomarkers for cardiometabolic health: A systematic review and meta-analysis of randomized controlled trials. *Journal of Nutrition, 146*, 2325–2333.

Liu, G., Mi, X. N., Zheng, X. X., Xu, Y. L., Lu, J., & Huang, X. H. (2014.) Effects of tea intake on blood pressure: A meta-analysis of randomised controlled trials. *British Journal Nutrition, 112*, 1043–1054.

MacDonald, J. R. (2002). Potential causes, mechanisms, and implications of post exercise hypotension. *Journal of Human Hypertension, 16*, 225–236.

Mandini, S., Conconi, F., Mori, E., Myers, J., Grazzi, G., & Mazzoni, G. (2018). Walking and hypertension: Greater reductions in subjects with higher baseline systolic blood pressure following six months of guided walking. *PeerJ, 6*, e5471.

Massaro, M., Scoditti, E., Carluccio, M. A., Calabriso, N., Santarpino, G., Verri, T., & De Caterina, R. (2020). Effects of olive oil on blood pressure: Epidemiological, clinical, and mechanistic evidence. *Nutrients, 12*(6), 1548. https://doi.org/10.3390/nu12061548

Michos, E. D., Cainzos-Achirica, M., Heravi, A. S., & Appel, L. J. (2021). Vitamin D, calcium supplements, and implications for cardiovascular health: JACC focus seminar. *Journal of the American College of Cardiology, 77*, 437–449.

Miller, P. E., Van Elswyk, M., & Alexander, D. D. (2014). Long-chain omega-3 fatty acids eicosapentaenoic acid and docosahexaenoic acid and blood pressure: A meta-analysis of randomized controlled trials. *American Journal of Hypertension, 27*, 885–896.

Muntner, P., Carey, R. M., Gidding, S., Jones, D. W., Taler, S. J., Wright, J. T. Jr., & Whelton, P. K. (2018). Potential US population impact of the 2017 ACC/AHA high blood pressure guideline. *Circulation, 137*, 109–118.

Nidich, S. I., Fields, J. Z., Rainforth, M. V., Pomerantz, R., Cella, D., Kristeller, J., Salerno, J. W., & Schneider, R. H. (2009). A randomized controlled trial of the effects of transcendental meditation on quality of life in older breast cancer patients. *Integrative Cancer Therapies, 8*, 228–234.

Orlich, M. J., & Fraser, G. E. (2014). Vegetarian diets in the Adventist Health Study 2: A review of initial published findings. *American Journal of Clinical Nutrition, 100 Suppl, 1*, 353S–258S.

Orlich, M. J., Singh, P. N., Sabaté, J., Jaceldo-Seigl, K., Fan, J., Knutsen, S., Beeson, W. L., & Fraser, G. E. (2013). Vegetarian dietary patterns and mortality in Adventist Health Study 2. *JAMA Internal Medicine, 173*, 1230–1238.

Pareek, M., & Olsen, M. H. (2017). Alcohol and blood pressure. *Lancet Public Health, 2*, e63–e4.

Pettersen, B. J., Anousheh, R., Fan, J., Jaceldo-Seigl, K., & Fraser, G. E. (2012). Vegetarian diets and blood pressure among white subjects: Results from the Adventist Health Study-2 (AHS-2). *Public Health Nutrition, 15*, 1909–1916.

Puddey, I. B., Mori, T. A., Barden, A. E., & Beilin, L. J. (2019). Alcohol and hypertension—new insights and lingering controversies. *Current Hypertension Reports, 21*, 79.

Ren, Y., Liu, Y., Sun, X. Z., Wang, B-Y., Zhao, Y., Liu, D-C., Zhang, D-D., Liu, X-J., Zhang, R-Y., Sun, H-H., Liu, F-Y., Chen, X., Cheng, C., Liu, L-L., Zhou, Q-G., Zhang, M., & Hu, D-S. (2019). Chocolate consumption and risk of cardiovascular diseases: A meta-analysis of prospective studies. *Heart, 105*, 49–55.

Roerecke, M., Kaczorowski, J., Tobe, S. W., Gmel, G., Hasan, O. S. M., & Rehm, J. (2017). The effect of a reduction in alcohol consumption on blood pressure: A systematic review and meta-analysis. *Lancet Public Health, 2*, e108–e120.

Rosenfeldt, F. L., Haas, S. J., Krum, H., Hadj, A., Ng, K., Leong, J-Y., & Watts, G. F. (2007). Coenzyme Q10 in the treatment of hypertension: A meta-analysis of the clinical trials. *Journal of Human Hypertension, 21*, 297–306.

Sacks, F. M., Svetkey, L. P., Vollmer, W. M., Appel, L. J., Bray, G. A., Harsha, D., Obarzanek, E., Conlin, P. R., Miller, E. R., Simons-Morton, D. G., Karanja, N., & Lin, P. H. (2001). Effects on blood pressure of reduced dietary sodium and the Dietary Approaches to Stop Hypertension (DASH) diet. DASH-Sodium Collaborative Research Group. *New England Journal of Medicine, 344*, 3–10.

Savica, V., Bellinghieri, G., & Kopple, J. D. 2010. The effect of nutrition on blood pressure. *Annual Review of Nutrition, 30*, 365–401.

Schulman, S. P., Becker, L. C., Kass, D. A., Champion, H. C., Terrin, M. L., Forman, S., Ernst, K. V., Kelemen, M. D., Townsend, S. N., Capriotti, A., Hare, J. M., Gerstenbilth, G. (2006). L-arginine therapy in acute myocardial infarction: the Vascular Interaction With Age in Myocardial Infarction (VINTAGE MI) randomized clinical trial. *JAMA, 295*, 58–64.

Sun, Q., Wang, B., Li, Y., Sun, F., Li, P., Xia, W., Zhou, X., Li, Q., Wang, X., Chen, J., Zeng, X., Zhao, Z., He, H., Liu, D., & Zhu, Z. (2016). Taurine supplementation lowers blood pressure and improves vascular function in prehypertension: Randomized, double-blind, placebo-controlled study. *Hypertension, 67*, 541–549.

Sundstrom, J., Arima, H., Jackson, R., Turnbull, F., Rahimi, K., Chalmers, J., Woodward, M., Neal, B., & Blood Pressure Lowering Treatment Trialists' Collaboration. (2015). Effects of blood pressure reduction in mild hypertension: A systematic review and meta-analysis. *Annals of Internal Medicine, 162*, 184–191.

Taubert, D., Roesen, R., Lehmann, C., Jung, N., & Schomig, E. (2007). Effects of low habitual cocoa intake on blood pressure and bioactive nitric oxide: a randomized controlled trial. *JAMA, 298*, 49–60.

Terry, P., Terry, J. B., & Wolk, A. (2001). Fruit and vegetable consumption in the prevention of cancer: An update. *Journal of Internal Medicine, 250*, 280–290.

USDHHS. (2015). U.S. Department of Health and Human Services and U.S. Department of Agriculture. December 2015. 2015—2020 Dietary Guidelines for Americans (8th ed.). https://health.gov/our-work/food-nutrition/previous-dietary-guidelines/2015

Wallace, J. P. (2003). Exercise in hypertension. A clinical review. *Sports Medicine, 33*, 585–598.

Whelton, P. K., Carey, R. M., Aronow, W. S., Casey, D. E. Jr., Collins, K. J., Himmelfarb, C. D., DePalma, S. M., Gidding, S., Jamerson, K. A., Jones, D. W., MacLaughlin, E. J., Muntner, P., Ovbigele, B., Smith, S. C. Jr., Spencer, C. C., Stafford, R. S., Taler, S. J., Thomas, R. J., Williams, K. A. Sr., … Wright, J. T. Jr. (2018). 2017 ACC / AHA / AAPA / ABC / ACPM / AGS / APhA / ASH / ASPC / NMA / PCNA guideline for the prevention, detection, evaluation, and management of high blood pressure in adults: A report of the American College of Cardiology/American Heart Association Task Force on clinical practice guidelines. *Journal of the American College of Cardiology, 71*, e127–e248.

Whelton, S. P., Chin, A., Xin, X., & He, J. (2002). Effect of aerobic exercise on blood pressure: A meta-analysis of randomized, controlled trials. *Annals of Internal Medicine, 136*, 493–503.

WHO. 2020. The top 10 causes of death. World Health Organization Fact Sheet. www.who.int/news-room/
fact-sheets/detail/the-top-10-causes-of-death.

Witteman, J. C., Willett, W. C., Stampfer, M. J., Colditz, G. A., Sacks, F. M., Speizer, F. E., Rosner, B., &
Hennekens, C. H. (1989). A prospective study of nutritional factors and hypertension among US women.
Circulation, *80*, 1320–1327.

Wright, J. T., Jr., Williamson, J. D., Whelton, P. K., Snyder, J. K., Sink, K. M., Rocco, M. V., Reboussin, D. M.,
Rahman, M., Oparil, S., Lewis, C. E., Kimmel, P. L., Johnson, K. C., Goff, D. C., Jr., Fine, L. J., Cutler,
J. A., Cushman, W. C., Cheung, A. K., & Ambrosius, W. T. (2015). A randomized trial of intensive versus
standard blood-pressure control. *New England Journal of Medicine*, *373*, 2103–2116.

Xu, R., Yang, K., Ding, J., & Chen, G. (2020). Effect of green tea supplementation on blood pressure: A systematic review and meta-analysis of randomized controlled trials. *Medicine (Baltimore)*, *99*, e19047.

Zhang, X., Li, Y., Del Gobbo, L. C., (2016). Effects of magnesium supplementation on blood pressure: A meta-
analysis of randomized double-blind placebo-controlled trials. *Hypertension*, *68*, 324–333.

16 Impact of Lifestyle on Cardiometabolic Syndrome and Type 2 Diabetes

Cindy Lamendola[1] and Jane Nelson Worel[2]
[1]Stanford University
Stanford, California, USA
[2]Preventive Cardiovascular Nurses Association
Madison, Wisconsin, USA

CONTENTS

KEY POINTS

- It is important to understand the different definitions, consequences, and the prevalence of cardiometabolic syndrome.
- It is important to be able to identify the related cardiometabolic diseases and understand some of the known pathophysiology.
- Understanding the impact of lifestyle management on cardiometabolic risk factors to help reduce metabolic risk and disease is significant.

16.1 INTRODUCTION

Cardiometabolic syndrome (CMS) is a clustering of cardiovascular (CV) risk factors initially described by Gerald Reaven, MD in 1988 in his Banting lecture (Reaven, 1988). Reaven identified the clustering

DOI: 10.1201/9781003178330-19

of risk factors, associated with resistance to insulin-mediated glucose uptake (insulin resistance), as Syndrome X, which later was known as the insulin resistance syndrome. Insulin resistance syndrome identified a group of individuals with an increased risk for developing cardiovascular disease (CVD) and/or type 2 diabetes (T2D). An abundance of research in this area followed, over a period from 1990 to 2005 there have been several definitions and names to identify this syndrome (Grundy, 2002).

Reaven's research on the pathophysiology of insulin resistance discusses the variability of insulin resistance within a population of people without T2D as 50% due to influences in genetics and 50% due to influences in lifestyle, specifically physical inactivity, and obesity (Reaven, 1988; Reaven, 2000). Others have suggested a different pathophysiology with obesity as the modulator of insulin resistance and the clustering of CV risk factors (Alberti et al., 2009). Understanding the significance of this syndrome to identifying individuals who will be at increased risk for CVD and T2D has been an integral part of the National Heart, Lung, and Blood Institute (NHLBI) and the American Heart Association (AHA) cholesterol-lowering guidelines identified as the metabolic syndrome (Grundy et al. 2002; Grundy et al., 2005).

16.1.1 DIFFERENT DEFINITIONS OF INSULIN RESISTANCE, METABOLIC SYNDROME (ALBERTI ET AL., 2009)

There are multiple definitions of insulin resistance and metabolic syndrome (MS), including the World Health Organization (WHO) definition (see Box 16.1), the National Cholesterol Education Guidelines (see Box 16.2), and the International Diabetes Federation (IDF) (see Box 16.3).

BOX 16.1   WHO (WORLD HEALTH ORGANIZATION) 1999

Presence of insulin resistance or glucose ≥ 110 mg/dL (6.1 mmol/L), 2 h glucose 140 mg/L (7.8 mmol) required along with any two or more of the following:

1. **HDL cholesterol:** Men < 35 mg/dL (0.90 mmol/L), women: < 39 mg/dL in women (1.0 mmol/L).
2. **Triglycerides:** ≥ 150 mg/dL (1.7 mmol/L).
3. **Waist/hip ratio:** Men > 0.9, women: > 0.85; or BMI > 30 kg/m².
4. **Blood pressure:** ≥ 140/90 mmHg.

BOX 16.2   NATIONAL CHOLESTEROL EDUCATION GUIDELINES III DEFINITION OF METABOLIC SYNDROME 2005

These criteria defined metabolic syndrome as present when 3 of these 5 components are present:

1. **Elevated waist circumference:** Men ≥102 cm (≥ 40 inches), women ≥ 88 cm (≥ 35 inches).
2. **Elevated triglycerides:** ≥ 150 mg/dL (1.7 mmol/L) or drug treatment.
3. **Low HDL-C (High Density Lipoprotein-cholesterol):** Men < 40 mg/dL (1.03 mmol/L), women < 50 mg/dL (1.3 mmol/L) or on drug treatment.
4. **Elevated blood pressure systolic:** ≥ 130 mm Hg, or diastolic ≥ 85 mm Hg, or both or drug treatment.
5. **Elevated fasting glucose:** ≥ 100 mg/dL or drug treatment.

BOX 16.3 INTERNATIONAL DIABETES FEDERATION (IDF) 2005

European: Men waist ≥ 94 cm or women ≥ 80 cm; Asians: Men ≥ 90 cm, women ≥ 180 cm; Japanese: Men ≥ 85 cm, women 9 ≥ 90 cm along with the presence of two or more of the following:

1. **Blood glucose:** > greater than 100 mg/dL (5.6 mmol/L) or diagnosed diabetes.
2. **HDL cholesterol:** Men < 40 mg/dL (1.03 0 mmol/L), women < 50 mg/dL (1.3 mmol/L or drug treatment for low HDL-C.
3. **Blood triglycerides:** ≥ 150 mg/dl (1.7 mmol/L) or drug treatment.
4. **Blood pressure:** > 130/85 mmHg or drug treatment.

Although there are differences in agreement of pathophysiology and definitions, there is agreement that the resulting consequence of a clustering of risk factors increases the risk for CVD as well as T2D and now affects adults in the US and globally (Saklayen, 2018; Kelli et al. 2015). The focus of identifying people at risk is twofold: First, to offer tools to decrease one's risk of developing the risk factors in the first place and, second, to control risk factors that are already identified (Reaven, 2004; Reaven, 2003; Ginsberg & MacCallum, 2009).

16.2   INCIDENCE AND PREVALENCE OF METABOLIC SYNDROME (MS)

Assessing incidence and prevalence of MS can be difficult depending on the definition used. In 2009, several organizations joined together to discuss the differences of the definitions and if any one risk factor should be required as the main component of the criteria of the syndrome. They agreed upon a definition using a harmonized criteria where three out of five risk factors were used to define MS instead of using one major component, impaired glucose tolerance, or waist measurement, with two other criteria necessary for the definition (Alberti et al., 2009). The waist circumference criteria were left open to be specific to the population and country definitions (see Box 16.4).

BOX 16.4   DEFINITION OF METABOLIC SYNDROME (MS) USING A HARMONIZED CRITERIA

Elevated waist circumference	Population- and country-specific definitions
Elevated triglycerides	≥ 150 mg/dL (1.7 mmol/L) or drug treatment as an alternate indicator
Low HDL-C (high density lipoprotein- cholesterol)	Men < 40 mg/dL (1.03 mmol/L) and women < 50 mg/dL (1.3 mmol/L) or drug treatment as an alternate indicator
Elevated blood pressure	Systolic ≥ 130 and/or diastolic ≥ 85 mm Hg or antihypertensive drug treatment in a patient with a history of hypertension as an alternate indicator
Elevated fasting glucose	≥ 100 mg/dL or drug treatment for elevated glucose as an alternate indicator. Most patients with type 2 diabetes mellitus will have the metabolic syndrome by the proposed criteria

Source: Alberti et al. (2009)

The 2017 National Health and Nutrition Examination Survey (Moore et al., 2017) used the harmonized criteria for metabolic syndrome and the definition of waist circumference from the National Cholesterol Education Guidelines III Definition of Metabolic Syndrome (Grundy et al., 2005). Importantly, individuals with T2D were included in the outcome data. In US adults (those $\geq$ 18 years old), the prevalence of MS increased more than 35% from 1988–1994 to 2007–2012; increasing from 25% to 34% of all adults in the US who met the criteria for metabolic syndrome. In 2007–2012, non-Hispanic black men were less likely to have MA than non-Hispanic white men. It was the opposite in women, with MS more likely in non-Hispanic black women than in non-Hispanic white women. In that same period, low education level and advanced age was independently associated with MS.

The authors concluded the prevalence of MS increased during the span of time from 1988 to 2012 for every sociodemographic group, resulting in more than one-third of US adults, approximately 66 million, who met the criteria for MS. With this increase, they noted the highest burden was among non-Hispanic black people and adults with low socioeconomic status. It is interesting to note the increase in MS in the US was not just related to in an increase in obesity, since the prevalence remained constant even in the non-obese individuals (Moore, 2017).

Regarding advancing age contributing to the incidence of MS, other factors were felt to contribute to this finding. In this population, there may be decreases in physical activity (more sedentary behavior) related to health issues such as osteoarthritis or other chronic conditions that may contribute to functional disability and increased weight (Reaven, 2003; Moore, 2017; Strath et al., 2007; Mankowski et al., 2015; Denys et al., 2009). These are important issues to remember and focus on when we assess our aging population as we continue to promote lifestyle changes.

Lower socioeconomic status (assessed by age, race/ethnicity, education, and poverty to income ratio) was also associated with MS and is another important factor to remember as we assess and care for patients as well as advocate for public health measures to increase safer and healthier environments (Moore, 2017; Havranek et al., 2015). Results were consistent across several studies, despite variance in criteria used to define insulin resistance and metabolic syndrome (Beltrán-Sánchez et al., 2013; Ford, 2005; Ford et al., 2002). More recently, from 2003 to 2012, Aguilar found the overall prevalence of the MS in the US was 33% (Aguilar et al., 2015).

In the 2021 American Heart Association (AHA) heart disease and stroke statistics (Virani et al., 2021a) based on NHANES from 2007 to 2014, the overall prevalence of MS was 34.3% and similar for both males and females (35.3% and 33.3%, respectively). For black people, based on the Jackson Hole study, CMS prevalence was present in 40% of females and 27% of males (Virani et al., 2021a).

16.2.1 Prevalence of Diabetes and Prediabetes

The prevalence of diabetes is as follows:

- **Total:** 34.2 million people have diabetes (10.5% of the US population).
- **Diagnosed:** 26.9 million people, including 26.8 million adults.
- **Undiagnosed:** 7.3 million people (21.4% are undiagnosed).

Overall prevalence is 90–95% for type 2 diabetes and 5–10% for type 1 diabetes.
The prevalence of prediabetes is as follows:

- **Total:** 88 million people aged 18 years or older have prediabetes (34.5% of the adult US population).
- **65 years or older:** 24.2 million people aged 65 years or older have prediabetes.

TABLE 16.1
Diagnosis of prediabetes and diabetes

Criterion	Value for Prediabetes	Value for Diabetes	
Fasting Plasma Glucose	100–125 mg/dL (5.6–6.9 mmol/L)	≥ 126 mg/dL (7.0 mmol/L)	Fasting = no caloric intake for at least 8 h
2-h post glucose during Oral Glucose Tolerance Test	144–199 mg/dL (7.8–11.0 mmol/L)	≥ 200 mg/dL (11.1mmol/L)	Glucose load = equivalent of 75 G anhydrous glucose dissolved in water
Hemoglobin A1c	5.7–6.4% (39–47 mmol/mol)	≥ 6.5% (48 mmol/mol)	Must be performed using NGSP certified standardized to the DCCT assay
Classic symptoms of hyperglycemia or hyperglycemia crisis	Not applicable	Random plasma glucose ≥ 200 mg/dL (11.1 mmol/L)	
		If unequivocal hyperglycemia is not present, the diagnosis of diabetes requires two abnormal test results from the same sample or in two separate test samples.	

Age-adjusted data for 2017–2018 among US adults aged ≥18 indicate that the highest prevalence of diagnosed diabetes was among the following people: American Indians/Alaska Natives (14.7%), people of Hispanic origin (12.5%), and non-Hispanic blacks (11.7%), followed by non-Hispanic Asians (9.2%) and non-Hispanic whites (7.5%) (CDC, 2020).

16.2.2 DIAGNOSIS OF PREDIABETES AND DIABETES (AMERICAN DIABETES ASSOCIATION (ADA PROFESSIONAL PRACTICE COMMITTEE, 2022B)

Note: Hemoglobin (Hgb) A1c and glycemia can be altered in certain conditions such as sickle cell disease, anemia, pregnancy—second or third trimesters and postpartum period—HIV, hemodialysis, and other conditions. Only criteria using plasma blood glucose should be used to diagnose diabetes.

When using the oral glucose tolerance test to screen for diabetes, a carbohydrate intake of at least 150 g/day should be assured for three days prior to testing.

For prediabetes: In all three tests, risk is continuous, extending below the lower limit of the range and becoming disproportionately greater at the higher end of the range (ADA Professional Practice Committee, 2022b). Table 16.1 summarizes the criterion for the diagnosis of prediabetes and diabetes.

How do we decide who is at risk for developing prediabetes or T2D? With the information and data discussed above regarding clustering of risk factors and associated metabolic disorders and diseases seen in patients with CMS as well as populations most at risk, the list for screening asymptomatic adults for prediabetes and diabetes in the ADA guidelines should not be surprising.

The ADA has recommended the following criteria for screening for diabetes or prediabetes in asymptomatic adults (ADA Professional Practice Committee, 2022b): "Testing should be considered in adults with overweight or obesity (BMI ≥ 25 kg/m2 or ≥ 23 kg/m2 in Asian Americans) who have one or more of the following" risk factors noted in Box 16.5.

> **BOX 16.5   ADA SCREENING CRITERIA**
>
> - First-degree relative with diabetes
> - High-risk race/ethnicity (e.g., African American, Latino, Native American, Asian American, Pacific Islander)
> - History of CVD
> - Hypertension (≥ 140/90 mmHg or on therapy for hypertension)
> - HDL cholesterol level <35 mg/dL (0.90 mmol/L) and/or a triglyceride level >250 mg/dL (2.82 mmol/L)
> - Women with polycystic ovarian syndrome
> - Physical inactivity
> - Other clinical conditions associated with insulin resistance (e.g., severe obesity, acanthosis nigricans)

Testing may be more frequent for certain patient populations. Patients with prediabetes, defined as (A1C ≥ 5.7% (39 mmol/mol), impaired glucose tolerance (IGT), or impaired fasting glucose (IFG), should be tested yearly. Women who were diagnosed with gestational diabetes mellitus should have lifelong testing at least every three years. For all other patients, testing should begin at age 35 years. If results are normal, testing should be repeated at a minimum of three-year intervals, with consideration of more frequent testing depending on initial results and risk status. They also recommend testing people with HIV (ADA Professional Practice Committee, 2022b).

16.3   PATHOPHYSIOLOGY

The pathophysiology of insulin resistance, and its related clustering of risk factors including T2D, is complex and not agreed upon by all. In Figure 16.1, insulin resistance is identified as the culprit, impacted by genetic and lifestyle with related clustering of risk factors; others would put obesity in the center and insulin resistance as one of the consequences/risk factors for CMS (Reaven 1988; Reaven 2004; Grundy 2007; Beverly & Budoff, 2020; Reaven 1995).

All would agree on the importance of identifying and treating these risk factors. Lack of treatment can result in stroke and vascular disease, non-alcoholic fatty liver disease (NAFLD), obstructive sleep apnea (OSA), polycystic ovarian syndrome (PCOS), and some cancers (Einhorn et al., 2003). Briefly, as mentioned earlier, Reaven identified the clustering of risk factors, associated with resistance to insulin-mediated glucose uptake (insulin resistance) and resulting in hyperinsulinemia, which interacts on other tissues; these result in abnormal glucose, atherogenic dyslipidemia, elevated triglycerides and low high-density lipoprotein-cholesterol HDL-C, hypertension and risk factors, and linked to insulin resistance syndrome and CMS diseases (Reaven, 1988; Reaven, 1995).

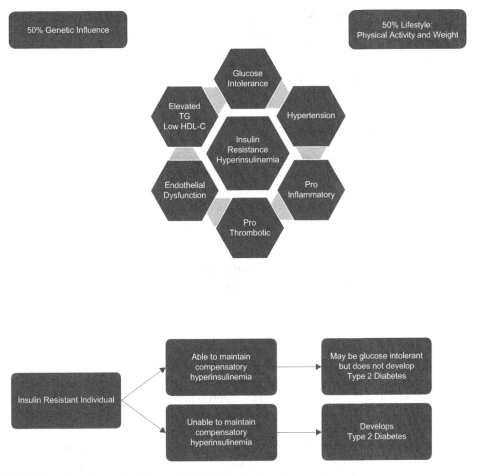

FIGURE 16.1   Clustering of cardiometabolic risk factors based on insulin resistance

(Adapted from Reaven, G. (1995). Pathophysiology of insulin resistance in human disease. *Physiological Reviews*, *75*, 473–486.)

16.4   PATIENT ASSESSMENT

BOX 16.6   ASSESSING THE PATIENT WITH CARDIOMETABOLIC SYNDROME

Past medical/surgical history, pregnancy history, gestational diabetes

Social history includes tobacco, alcohol, nutrition, and physical activity history

Family history includes T2D, CVD, HTN, cancers

Medication: Reconciliation-prescribed and over the counter

Physical assessment: Look for acanthosis nigricans, skin tags (signs of hyperinsulinemia)

Vital signs: Blood pressure, heart rate, height, weight, body mass index (BMI), and waist circumference

Lab tests:
• Lipoprotein panel
• Complex metabolic panel
• Fasting plasma glucose, HgA1c, oral glucose tolerance test if needed
• Thyroid-stimulating hormone (TSH)

Once you have identified your patient with cardiometabolic syndrome, the next step is to provide education and tools to help them engage in a lifestyle to reduce their risk for metabolic disorders and risk for metabolic disease. Research has shown that physical activity and weight loss can improve insulin sensitivity, reduce cardiometabolic risk factors, and, when combined with a heart-healthy diet, improve dyslipidemias (McAuley et al. 2014; McLaughlin et al., 2001; McLaughlin, 2003; Backes et al., 2008; Reaven, 2005).

16.5 LIFESTYLE MANAGEMENT

Lifestyle intervention, for the prevention and management of CMS, includes a heart-healthy diet, exercise and physical activity, management of obesity, and cessation of tobacco use. While each of these interventions stand alone in enhancing cardiometabolic risk reduction, they interrelate with each other, having an additive effect. The National Diabetes Prevention Program (DPP) was developed in 2010 (CDC, 2021) in response to overwhelming evidence from a major multi-center clinical research trial, that lifestyle intervention in those with prediabetes can cut their risk of developing T2D by 58% in the population at large and 71% for those over 60 years old (Diabetes Prevention Program Research Group, 2002). Furthermore, these actions are cost effective and scalable in diverse community settings across the country (CDC, 2021).

16.5.1 HEART-HEALTHY DIET

An individualized eating plan, based on an accepted heart-healthy dietary pattern, will help to improve glycemic control, achieve and maintain a healthy weight, and manage other cardiovascular risk factors such as hypertension and dyslipidemia. Accepted, evidence-based heart-healthy eating plans include the Mediterranean, Dietary Approaches Stop Hypertension (DASH), and low carbohydrate and plant-based vegetarian/vegan diets (American Diabetes Association, 2022; Arnett et al., 2019).

Dietary trial evidence suggests that there is not a "one-size-fits-all" approach to diet in reducing cardiometabolic risk (American Diabetes Association (ADA, 2022). Macronutrient distribution should be based on an individualized assessment of current eating habits, preferences, and metabolic goals as there is no ideal percentage of calories from carbohydrate, protein, and fat to prevent diabetes and reduce cardio metabolic risk. Most important is the overall quality of food consumed, with an emphasis on whole grains, legumes, nuts, fruits, and vegetables with limited refined and processed food (ADA, 2022). It is especially important to select an eating plan that is acceptable to the individual and aligns with their socio-cultural background, personal preferences, and current lifestyle and living situation.

Low and very low carbohydrate diets (<10 % of calories from carbohydrates), along with alcohol and fat restriction, have been shown to reduce triglyceride levels by more than 70% in those with hypertriglyceridemia (Virani et al., 2021b). While counseling patients on carbohydrate restriction, it is also important to recommend a healthy intake of dietary fiber, replacing white bread, rice, and pasta with whole grain counterparts.

A reduction in overall carbohydrate intake has the most impact on hyperglycemia in those with diabetes (Evert et al., 2019). A low or very low carbohydrate diet may be recommended for those not meeting glycemic targets or who wish to reduce their glucose lowering medications. Low carbohydrate diets do provide challenges in terms of sustainability and medical safety and are best done under the supervision of a health care team who can provide close monitoring. The DPP dietary intervention included a reduction in fat and calorie consumption to promote and maintain a weight loss goal of 7% of their body weight (CDC, 2021).

Medical nutrition therapy (MNT) is an important component of diabetes management and a referral to a registered dietitian (RD) who specializes in diabetes specific MNT is recommended

(Evert et al., 2019). Reductions in blood glucose with MNT ranged between 50 and 100 mg/dL (Pastors et al., 2002). The DASH diet is rich in vegetables, fruits, and low-fat dairy, along with a reduction of sodium. It has led to reductions in blood pressure of 7–11 mm Hg and is recommended for the prevention and management of hypertension (Arnett et al., 2019; DASH Sodium Collaborative Research Group, 2001). An RD would also be an important resource for those who have comorbid conditions, such as hypertension or chronic kidney disease, and need specific diets including sodium, protein, or potassium restrictions. Nurses and other health care team members are encouraged to provide education and support to persons with cardio metabolic syndrome and diabetes by emphasizing the consumption of non-starchy vegetables and whole foods while limiting highly processed foods, refined grains, and added sugars.

A reasonable approach to meal planning is the diabetes plate method, which focuses on appropriate portion sizes. Using a 9-inch plate, fill 1/2 the plate with non-starchy vegetables, 1/4 of the plate with lean protein, and 1/4 the plate with grains or starches (ADA, 2021). While carbohydrate counting may be needed for some to achieve glycemic control, the plate method provides a practical approach that is easy to teach and generally well understood. The diabetes plate was developed using an approach first introduced by the US Department of Agriculture. Nurses can freely use the resources available at myplate.gov to guide patients with cardiometabolic risk factors in healthy eating plans and portion control (US Department of Agriculture, 2022).

16.5.2 Physical Activity

The relationship between regular physical activity (PA) and cardiometabolic health has been well established. Regular PA is associated with lower cardiovascular and overall mortality risks in the general population as well as those with diabetes mellitus (DM) (Arnett et al., 2019; PAGC, 2018). Multiple national guidelines point to risk reduction and health promotion benefits of an active lifestyle; however, approximately half of adults in the United States do not meet the minimum physical activity recommendations (Virani et al., 2021b; Arnett et al., 2019). This is similarly true for those with diabetes; however, there is some variability based on race. Hispanic Americans had the highest percentage to meet the recommended minutes of PA per week while just 44.2% of whites and 42.6% of African Americans meet the guidelines (Arnett et al., 2019). Health care professionals are encouraged to routinely assess and prescribe physical activity during clinical encounters with all patients. This is especially true for those with or at risk for CMS and DM and it is important for DM care management teams to identify individual approaches to helping those with DM achieve PA goals.

Aerobic exercise such as brisk walking or bicycling is a cornerstone of ASCVD risk reduction. It has been shown to improve hypertension, blood lipids, and blood glucose control, as well as contribute to weight loss and improved wellbeing (Arnett et al., 2019; ADA, 2021; PAGC, 2018). Strong evidence from meta-analysis has demonstrated significant reduction in systolic BP by 2–5 mm Hg (PAGC, 2018). A meta-analysis of individuals with CMS demonstrated significantly lower fasting glucose levels (3 mg/dL) as well as improved Diastolic BP, waist circumference, and HDL-C (Virani et al., 2021a). Engaging in 150 min/week of moderate-intensity physical activity, as part of the DPP, was found to improve insulin sensitivity, BP, blood lipids, waist circumference, and body mass index (BMI) (ADA, 2022; ADA, 2021). Resistance exercise, including the use of weights, resistance bands, and body weight, also has health benefits, including improved glycemic control in individuals with prediabetes and DM, and possibly BP lowering along with improved physical functioning (ADA, 2022; Arnett et al., 2019; ADA, 2021). Avoiding long periods of sitting is also encouraged and may help lower postprandial glucose levels (ADA, 2022; Arnett et al., 2019; ADA, 2021). Physical activity during pregnancy has been associated with reduced risk of gestational DM (ADA, 2022). While those with type I DM benefit from physical activity, its role in blood glucose management has not been well established nor has its role in preventing microvascular complications related to DM (ADA, 2021).

In general, physical activity and exercise is safe; however, sedentary individuals are advised to start slowly and gradually progress an exercise program. For example, ten-minute walks may be an appropriate starting place, with encouragement to increase duration and walking speed over time, to achieve at least 30 minutes of aerobic PA most days of the week. Daily exercise, or at least not allowing for a two-day or more lapse in exercise, helps to combat insulin resistance in type 1 and 2 DM (ADA, 2021). Screening for coronary artery disease (CAD), prior to starting an exercise program, is not necessary in asymptomatic individuals (Arnett et al., 2019). This includes those with CMS or DM; however, performing a careful history and ASCVD risk assessment is essential, with special attention to atypical CAD symptoms such as excessive fatigue or a decrease in activity tolerance (ADA, 2021). Exercise programs should be tailored to an individual's age, interests, and any comorbid conditions; for example, those with orthopedic problems such as osteoarthritis may prefer non-weight bearing activity such as recumbent cycling or water-based exercise. Individuals with DM-related complications, including peripheral neuropathy or retinopathy, would benefit from careful consideration and referral to physical therapist or exercise professional with expertise in adaptive exercise programs (ADA, 2021).

16.5.3 Weight Management

Weight management plays an important role in diabetes prevention as well as the treatment of T2D. Strong evidence suggests that modest and sustained weight loss helps improve glycemic control with a reduction in fasting glucose of approximately 17 mg/dL or glycated hemoglobin of 1.2% (Rothberg et al., 2017; Case et al., 2002). This may help reduce the need for glucose-lowering medications in individuals with DM and who are overweight or obese. In addition, weight loss improves BP with significant reduction of systolic BP by 6–8 mmHg. (Rothberg et al., 2017). Improved triglycerides and blood lipids are also associated with weight (Virani et al., 2021b; Rothberg et al., 2017; Case et al., 2002). Evidence-based recommendations for obesity management include dietary, behavioral, pharmacologic, and surgical interventions. A nonjudgmental approach and the use of patient-centered communication and motivational interviewing techniques can help to identify personal patient preferences and beliefs, establish realistic goals, and address barriers to weight loss.

Clinically significant benefits of weight loss may be achieved with a ≥ 3–5% reduction in body weight (Arnett et al., 2019; ADA Professional Practice Committee, 2022a). More intensive weight loss goals may be pursued, in motivated patients, and may result in greater health improvements. Successful lifestyle programs for weight management, target a 500–750 kcal/day energy deficit by reducing dietary caloric intake and increasing energy expenditure through physical activity (ADA Professional Practice Committee, 2022a). A typical weight loss program would suggest a daily caloric intake of 1200–1500 kcal for women and 1500–1800 kcal for men, adjusted according to an individual's starting body weight (ADA Professional Practice Committee, 2022a).

Dietary interventions for weight loss may vary based on individual preferences, comorbid conditions, and health status, as long they achieve the necessary calorie deficit to achieve weight loss. Referral to trained dietary and weight loss professionals or organizations, who can provide regular counseling and support through individual and/or group intervention, will likely result in greater weight loss success and ongoing weight maintenance. Under the direction of weight management professionals, intensive weight loss regimens, including very low-calorie diets and meal replacement plans, may be undertaken for short periods of time to achieve a faster pace and larger magnitude weight loss (ADA Professional Practice Committee, 2022a).

In counseling about lifestyle change for cardiometabolic risk reduction, it is important for clinicians to be aware of health disparities in which individuals experience barriers to health based on their race, ethnicity, disability, gender, and so on. Socioeconomic factors may impact a person's access to healthy foods and safe places to engage in physical activity as well as environmental exposures and access to health care.

16.5.4 SMOKING CESSATION

Tobacco use is the leading preventable cause of disease, disability, and death in the US. It is a major risk factor for the development of ASCVD. Smoking and exposure to secondhand smoke are associated with greater risk of death from coronary heart disease (Arnett et al., 2019). Systematic reviews have linked active smoking to insulin resistance and an increased risk of T2D (Bush et al., 2016). Tobacco use, together with insulin resistance, results in elevated triglycerides and other atherogenic lipoproteins (Farin et al., 2007). Smokers have an increased risk of developing T2D by 30–44% when compared to nonsmokers (Bush et al., 2016). Tobacco use in those with diabetes results in higher glucose and Hgb A1C levels, making diabetes more difficult to manage.

All major health promotion and prevention guidelines recommend complete smoking cessation. Documenting smoking status has become a part of our routine vital sign documentation upon intake for all health care visits (Arnett et al., 2019). Guidelines also provide recommendations for behavioral counseling and pharmacologic intervention to assist in smoking cessation. One consequence of tobacco cessation may be weight gain. In most cases, this weight gain is not clinically significant when compared to the benefits of smoking cessation; however, nurses are advised to counsel patients on strategies to avoid weight gain while engaged in tobacco cessation interventions. These include starting or increasing physical activity, low-calorie substitutes to smoking such as sugarless gum, mints, or vegetables, and referrals for medications that may help to delay weight gain as well as recommend tobacco cessation medications that help delay weight gain, such as nicotine replacement therapy. It is also important to reassure smokers that some weight gain after quitting smoking is common but usually self-limiting with appropriate lifestyle changes (Bush et al., 2016).

Tobacco use risk reduction is discussed in more detail in Chapter 23 of this volume.

16.6 CONCLUSION

Cardiometabolic syndrome is a cluster of risk factors that results in cardiometabolic disorders and diseases such as CVD and T2D and affects at least 34% of the adult population in the United States. Table 16.2 summarizes the impact of lifestyle interventions on cardiometabolic risk factors. It is important that we know how to identify our patients both at risk and with this syndrome. We need

TABLE 16.2
Impact of lifestyle interventions on cardiometabolic risk factors

Intervention/ Risk Factors	Heart Healthy Diet	Physical Activity	Weight Loss	Smoking Cessation
	Mediterranean, DASH, low carbohydrate, MNT, and plant-based diets	*≥ 150 min/week moderate intensity or 75 min/week vigorous activity*	*≥ 5% initial weight*	*Complete cessation*
Blood Pressure	Improvement with DASH ↓7–11 mm Hg	↓ systolic BP ~ 2–5 mm Hg	↓ systolic BP ~ 6–11 mm Hg	Improvement
Triglycerides	Improvement with low carb; varies depending on baseline levels and diet ↓ > 70%	Up to 30% ↓ depending on exercise variables	↓~ 10–20% ↓~ 94 mg/d	Improvement
Glucose	With MNT ↓ 50–100 mg/dL or Hgb A1C 0.9–1.9%	Reduction in glucose varies with activity/ intensity and time ~ 3 mg/dL	↓ glucose 17 mg/dL or Hgb A1C ~ 1.7%	Improvement

to understand the impact of lifestyle intervention and provide them with education and tools for effective behavior change to reduce their risk in both primary and secondary prevention of these disorders and cardiometabolic diseases.

REFERENCES

2018 Physical Activity Guidelines Advisory Committee. (2018). *Physical activity guidelines advisory committee scientific report*. Washington, DC: US Dept of Health and Human Services. https://health.gov/our-work/nutrition-physical-activity/physical-activity-guidelines/current-guidelines/scientific-report

Aguilar, M., Bhuket, T., Torres, S., Liu, B., Wong, R. J. (2015). Prevalence of the metabolic syndrome in the United States, 2003–2012. *JAMA, 313*(19), 1973–1974.

Alberti, K. G., Eckel, R. H., Grundy, S. M., Zimmet, P. Z., Cleeman, J. I., Donato, K. A., Fruchart, J. C., James, W. P., Loria, C. M., Smith, S. C., Jr, International Diabetes Federation Task Force on Epidemiology and Prevention, National Heart, Lung, and Blood Institute, American Heart Association, World Heart Federation, International Atherosclerosis Society, & International Association for the Study of Obesity. (2009). Harmonizing the metabolic syndrome: A joint interim statement of the International Diabetes Federation Task Force on Epidemiology and Prevention; National Heart, Lung, and Blood Institute; American Heart Association; World Heart Federation; International Atherosclerosis Society; and International Association for the Study of Obesity. *Circulation, 120*(16), 1640–1645. https://doi.org/10.1161/CIRCULATIONAHA.109.192644

American Diabetes Association Professional Practice Committee. (2022). Obesity and weight management for the prevention and treatment of type 2 diabetes: Standards of medical care in diabetes. *Diabetes Care, 45*(Suppl. 1), S113–124. https://doi.org/10.2337/dc22-s008

American Diabetes Association Professional Practice Committee. (2022). Classification and diagnosis of diabetes: Standards of Medical Care in Diabetes—2022. *Diabetes Care, 45*(Suppl. 1), S17–S38.

American Diabetes Association. (2021). Facilitating behavior change and well-being to improve health outcomes: Standards of medical care in diabetes. *Diabetes Care, 44*(Suppl. 1j), s53–S72. https://doi.org/10.2337/dc21-S005

American Diabetes Association. (2022). Prevention or delay of type 2 diabetes and associated comorbidities: Standards of medical care in diabetes 2022. *Diabetes Care, 45*(Suppl. 1), S39–S45. https://doi.org/10.2337/dc22-S003

Arnett, D., Blumenthal, R. S., Albert, M. A., Buroker, A., Goldberger, Z., Hahn, E., Dennison-Himmelfarb, C., Khera, A., Lloyd-Jones, D., McEvoy, J., Michos, E., Miedema, M., Munoz, D., Smith, S., Virani, S., Williams, K., Yeboah J., & Ziaeian, B. (2019). ACC/AHA Guideline on the primary prevention of cardiovascular disease. *Circulation, 140*, e596–e646. www.ahajournals.org/doi/10.1161/CIR.0000000000000678

Backes, A. C., Abbasi, F., Lamendola, C., McLaughlin, T. L., Reaven, G., & Palaniappan, L. P. (2008). Clinical experience with a relatively low carbohydrate, calorie-restricted diet improves insulin sensitivity and associated metabolic abnormalities in overweight, insulin resistant South Asian Indian women. *Asia Pacific Journal of Clinical Nutrition, 17*(4), 669–671.

Beltrán-Sánchez, H., Harhay, M. O., Harhay, M. M., & McElligott, S. (2013). Prevalence and trends of metabolic syndrome in the adult U.S. population, 1999–2010. *Journal of the American College of Cardiology, 62*(8), 697–703.

Beverly, J. K., & Budoff, M. J. (2020). Atherosclerosis: Pathophysiology of insulin resistance, hyperglycemia, hyperlipidemia, and inflammation. *Journal of Diabetes, 12*, 102–104.

Bush, T., Lovejoy, J., Deprey, M., & Carpenter, K. M. (2016). The effect of tobacco cessation on weight gain, obesity, and diabetes risk. *Obesity, 24*, 1834–1841. https://doi.org/10.1002/oby.21582

Case, C. C., Jones, P. H., Nelson, K., Obrian Smith, E., & Ballantyne, C. M. (2002). Impact of weight loss on the metabolic syndrome. *Diabetes, Obesity, and Metabolism, 6*, 407–414. http://dx.doi.org/10.1046/j.1463-1326.2002.00236.x

Centers for Disease Control and Prevention. (2021). *National diabetes prevention program*. www.CDC.gov/diabetes/prevention

Centers for Disease Control and Prevention. (2020). *National diabetes statistics report, 2020*. Centers for Disease Control and Prevention, US Department of Health and Human Services.

Dash Sodium Collaborative Research Group. (2001). Effects on blood pressure of reduced dietary sodium and the Dietary Approaches to Stop Hypertension (DASH) Diet. *NEJM, 344*, 3–10. www.nejm.org/doi/full/10.1056/nejm200101043440101

Denys, K., Cankurtaran, M., Janssens, W., & Petrovic. M. (2009). Metabolic syndrome in the elderly: An overview of the evidence. *Acta Clinica Belgica, 64*(1), 23–34.

Einhorn, D., Reaven, G. M., Cobin, R. H., Ford, E., Ganda, O. P., Handelsman, Y., Hellman, R., Jellinger, P. S., Kendall, D., Krauss, R. M., Neufeld, N. D., Petak, S. M., Rodbard, H. W., Seibel, J. A., Smith, D. A., & Wilson, P. W. (2003). American College of Endocrinology position statement on the insulin resistance syndrome. *Endocrine Practice: Official Journal of the American College of Endocrinology and the American Association of Clinical Endocrinologists, 9*(3), 237–252.

Evert, A., Dennison, M., Gardner, C., Garvey, T., Lau, K., MacLeod, J., Mitri, J., Pereira, R., Rawlings, K., Robinson, S., Saslow, L., Uelmen, S., Urbanski, P., & Yancy, W. (2019). Nutrition therapy for adults with diabetes or prediabetes: A consensus report. *Diabetes Care, 42*, 731–754. https://doi.org/10.2337%2Fdci19-0014

Farin, H., Abbasi F., Kim S., Lamendola, C., McLaughlin, T., & Reaven, G. (2007). The relationship between insulin resistance and dyslipidaemia in cigarette smokers. *Diabetes, Obesity, and Metabolism, 9*, 65–69 https://doi-org.laneproxy.stanford.edu/10.1111/j.1463-1326.2006.00574.x

Ford, E. S., Giles, W. H., & Dietz, W. H. (2002). Prevalence of the metabolic syndrome among US adults: Findings from the third National Health and Nutrition Examination Survey. *JAMA, 287*(3), 356–359.

Ford, E. S. (2005). Prevalence of the metabolic syndrome defined by the International Diabetes Federation among adults in the U.S. *Diabetes Care, 28*(11), 2745–2749.

Ginsberg, H. N., MacCallum, P. R. (2009). The obesity, metabolic syndrome, and type 2 diabetes mellitus pandemic: Part I. Increased cardiovascular disease risk and the importance of atherogenic dyslipidemia in persons with the metabolic syndrome and type 2 diabetes mellitus. *Journal of the Cardiometabolic Syndrome, 4*(2), 113–119.

Grundy, S. M., Cleeman, J. I., Daniels, S. R., Donato, K. A., Eckel, R. H., Franklin, B. A., Gordon, D. J., Krauss, R. M., Savage, P. J., Smith, S. C., Jr, Spertus, J. A., Costa, F., American Heart Association, & National Heart, Lung, and Blood Institute. (2005). Diagnosis and management of the metabolic syndrome: An American Heart Association/National Heart, Lung, and Blood Institute scientific statement. *Circulation, 112*(17), 2735–2752.

Grundy, S. M. (2007) Metabolic syndrome: A multiplex cardiovascular risk factor. *Journal of Clinical Endocrinology & Metabolism, 92*(2), 399–404.

Grundy, S. M. (2002, October 17). National Cholesterol Education Program (NCEP)—The National Cholesterol Guidelines in 2001, Adult Treatment Panel (ATP) III. Approach to lipoprotein management in 2001 National Cholesterol Guidelines. *American Journal of Cardiology, 90*(8A), 11i–21i.

Havranek, E. P., Mujahid, M. S., Barr, D. A., Blair, I. V., Cohen, M. S., Cruz-Flores, S., Davey-Smith, G., Dennison-Himmelfarb, C. R., Lauer, M. S., Lockwood, D. W., Rosal, M., Yancy, C. W., American Heart Association Council on Quality of Care and Outcomes Research, Council on Epidemiology and Prevention, Council on Cardiovascular and Stroke Nursing, Council on Lifestyle and Cardiometabolic Health, & Stroke Council (2015). Social determinants of risk and outcomes for cardiovascular disease: A scientific statement from the American Heart Association. *Circulation, 132*(9), 873–898. https://doi-org.laneproxy.stanford.edu/10.1161/CIR.0000000000000228

Kelli, H. M., Kassas, I., & Lattouf, O. M. (2015). A global epidemic. *Journal of Diabetes and Metabolism, 6*(3), 513.

Mankowski, R. T., Aubertin-Leheudre, M., Beavers, D. P., Botoseneanu, A., Buford, T. W., Church, T., Glynn, N. W., King, A. C., Liu, C., Manini, T. M., Marsh, A. P., McDermott, M., Nocera, J. R., Pahor, M., Strotmeyer, E. S., Anton, S. D., & LIFE Research Group (2015). Sedentary time is associated with the metabolic syndrome in older adults with mobility limitations—The LIFE Study. *Experimental Gerontology, 70*, 32–36. https://doi-org.laneproxy.stanford.edu/10.1016/j.exger.2015.06.018

McAuley, P. A., Chen, H., Lee, D. C., Artero, E. G., Bluemke, D. A., &Burke, G. L. (2014). Physical activity, measures of obesity, and cardiometabolic risk: The Multi-Ethnic Study of Atherosclerosis (MESA). *Journal of Physical Activity and Health, 4*, 831–837.

McLaughlin, T., Abbasi, F., Kim, H. S., Lamendola, C., Schaaf, P., & Reaven, G. (2001). Relationship between insulin resistance, weight loss, and coronary heart disease risk in healthy, obese women. *Metabolism, 50*(7), 795–800.

McLaughlin, T. L. (2003, September–October). Insulin resistance syndrome and obesity. *Endocrine Practice*, *9*(Suppl. 2), 58–62.

Moore, J. X., Chaudhary, N., & Akinyemiju, T. (2017). Metabolic syndrome prevalence by race/ethnicity and sex in the United States, National Health and Nutrition Examination Survey, 1988–2012. *Preventing Chronic Disease*, *14*, 160287.

Pastors, J., Warshaw, J., Daly, A., Franz, M., & Kulkarni, K. (2002). The evidence for the effectiveness of medical nutrition therapy in diabetes management. *Diabetes Care*, *25*(3), 608–613. https://doi.org/10.2337/diacare.25.3.608

Reaven, G. M. (1988). Banting lecture 1988. Role of insulin resistance in human disease. *Diabetes*, *37*(12), 1595–1607.

Reaven, G. (1995). Pathophysiology of insulin resistance in human disease. *Physiological Reviews*, *75*, 473–486.

Reaven, G. M. (2000). Diet and Syndrome X. *Current Atherosclerosis Reports*, *2*(6), 503–507.

Reaven, G. M. (2003). The insulin resistance syndrome. *Current Atherosclerosis Reports*, *5*(5), 364–371.

Reaven, G. M. (2004). Insulin resistance: Cardiovascular disease, and the metabolic syndrome: How well do the emperor's clothes fit? *Diabetes Care*, *27*(4), 1011–1012.

Reaven, G. M. (2005). The insulin resistance syndrome: definition and dietary approaches to treatment. *Annual Review of Nutrition*, *25*, 391–406.

Rothberg, A., McEwen L., Kraftson A., Ajluni, N., Fowler C., Nay C., Miller N., Burant, C., & Herman, W. (2017). Impact of weight loss on waist circumference and the components of the metabolic syndrome. *BMJ Open Diabetes Research & Care*, *5*(1), e000341. https://drc.bmj.com/content/5/1/e000341

Saklayen, M. G. (2018). The global epidemic of the metabolic syndrome. *Current Hypertension Reports*, *20*(2), 12.

Strath, S., Swartz, A., Parker, S., Miller, N., Cieslik, L. (2007). Walking and metabolic syndrome in older adults. *Journal of Physical Activity and Health*, *4*(4), 397–410.

The Diabetes Prevention Program (DPP) Research Group. (2002). The Diabetes Prevention Program (DPP): Description of lifestyle intervention. *Diabetes Care*, *25*(12), 2165–2171. https://diabetesjournals.org/care/article/25/12/2165/22085/The-Diabetes-Prevention-Program-DPP-Description-of

US Department of Agriculture. (2022). *My Plate*. www.Myplate.gov

Virani S., Alonso A., Aparicio H., Benjamin E., Bittencourt, M., Callaway, C. Carson, A., Chamberlain, A., Cheng, S., Delling F., Elkind M., Evenson, K., Ferguson J., Gupta D., Khan s., Kissela B., Knutson K., Lee C., Lewis T., … Wang, N. (2021a). Heart disease and stroke statistics—2021 update: A report from the American Heart Association. *Circulation*, *143*(8), e254–e743. www.ahajournals.org/doi/10.1161/CIR.0000000000000950

Virani, S., Morris, P., Agarwala, A., Ballantyne, C., Birtcher, K., Kris-Etherton, P., Ladden-Stirling, A., Miller, M., Orringer, C., & Stone, N. (2021b). 2021ACC expert consensus decision pathway on the management of ASCVD risk reduction in patients with persistent hypertriglyceridemia. *JACC*, *78*(9), 960–993. https://doi.org/10.1016/j.jacc.2021.06.011

17 Obesity and Weight Management

Marcia L. Stefanick

Stanford Prevention Research Center

Stanford University School of Medicine

Stanford, California, USA

CONTENTS

KEY POINTS

- Obesity, i.e., excess fat accumulation, is highly prevalent in the United States and globally.
- Visceral obesity leads to obesity-related comorbidities, e.g., coronary heart disease (CHD), type 2 diabetes mellitus, an unfavorable lipid profile, hypertension, stroke, gallbladder disease, sleep apnea, certain cancers, and osteoarthritis.
- Obesity in pregnancy poses serious health risks for both the mother and fetus and excess weight gain during pregnancy should be avoided.
- Screening for obesity is recommended in children aged 6 years and older and in adults with the offer or referral for those who have obesity to comprehensive, intensive behavioral interventions to promote improvements in weight status.
- An initial weight loss goal of 10% of baseline body weight over a six-month period with a combination of caloric restriction, increased physical activity, and behavioral therapy is recommended for adults.

17.1 INTRODUCTION: DEFINITIONS AND PREVALENCE (US) OF OBESITY

In 1998, the National Heart Lung and Blood Institute (NHLBI) published the Obesity Education Initiative (OEI): Clinical Guidelines on the Identification, Evaluation, and Treatment of Overweight and Obesity in Adults, which established clinical body weight (status) definitions for adults based on body mass index (BMI), i.e., weight (in kg) divided by height (in meters) squared (NHLBI, 1998). "Normal weight" was and is now defined as having a BMI of 18.5 to 24.9 kg/m^2; "underweight" as a BMI below 18.5 kg/m^2; "overweight" as a BMI of 25 to 29.9 kg/m^2; and, "obesity" as a BMI

DOI: 10.1201/9781003178330-20

of 30 kg/m^2 or greater, with cut-points for Class 1 obesity (BMI = 30–34.9 kg/m^2), Class 2 obesity (BMI = 35–39.9 kg/m^2) and Class 3 (severe) obesity (BMI ≥ 40 kg/m^2). (Of note, the World Health Organization [WHO] set 22.9 kg/m^2 as the upper cut-point for "normal weight" in Asian populations (WHO, 2000), despite wide variation in body type and composition across the many diverse Asian peoples, as is true of all populations. This cut-point, however, is currently rarely applied to people who identify as Asian American in US reports.)

Prior to the widespread dissemination of the NHLBI OEI guidelines and in the WHO 1995 technical report, obesity was defined as "a condition with excessive fat accumulation in the body to the extent that the health and well-being are adversely affected." (WHO, 1995). Accumulation of body fat, however, was and remains difficult to measure accurately, and there is no easily available method for routine clinical use (Pi-Sunyer, 2000). The facts that BMI, which is based on total body weight, cannot distinguish fat mass from lean mass, ectopic fat (visceral and liver) from subcutaneous fat, or other differences in body composition, including metabolic factors inherent to an individual's natural physique or somatotype (of which three extremes have been defined: Endomorphic, or round, fat type; mesomorphic, or muscular type; ectomorphic, or slim, linear type) or effects of steroid and other hormones, including leptin, that underlie sex differences in regional adiposity, which include "essential fat" stores that are important to premenopausal women's reproductive health (Mauvais-Jarvis, 2017; Mathew, 2018), means that a person who does not have "excess" body fat may be classified as "obese" with a BMI of 30 kg/m^2 or higher.

Based on the BMI cut-point, more than 35% of men and 40% of women were obese in the United States in 2018 (USPSTF, 2017), which was before stay-at-home mandates that have been associated with atypical weight gain, with greater weight gain in individuals with obesity in the US (Lin et al., 2021; Seal et al., 2022). National Health and Nutrition Examination Survey (NHANES), 2017–2018, data suggest that the age-adjusted prevalence of severe obesity in US adults aged 20 and older was 9.2% and was higher in women than men and highest in non-Hispanic Black adults compared with other race and Hispanic-origin groups, while the proportion of overweight and obese was lowest in Asian American men and women (Hales et al., 2020). Furthermore, the prevalence of both obesity and severe obesity had increased substantially among adults from 1999–2000 through 2017–2018 (Hales et al., 2020).

In 2006, the US Preventive Services Task Force (USPSTF) deemed age- and sex-adjusted BMI percentile, plotted on growth charts (such as those developed by the Centers for Disease Control and Prevention, CDC, based on US-specific, population-based norms for children 2 years and older), as an acceptable measure for detecting overweight and obesity in children and adolescents, because of its reliability and feasibility for use in primary care and its association with adult obesity (USPSTF, 2006). Defining "obesity" as the 95th percentile or higher of age- and sex-adjusted BMI and "overweight" as the 85th–94th percentile, for year 2000 CDC growth charts, approximately 17% of children and adolescents aged 2 to 19 years had obesity in 2017, and an additional 15% were "overweight" (USPSTF, 2017).

Of clinical importance, overweight and obesity are associated with a wide range of health issues, referred to as obesity-related comorbidities (discussed below), which are generally more common in people with greater fat storage in visceral versus subcutaneous white adipose tissue regions, commonly referred to as an "android" versus "gynoid" fat pattern, respectively, in recognition of generally greater visceral fat accumulation and larger waist-to-hip girth ratio in men compared to most women at a given BMI. Yet, a substantial proportion of women, particularly those with a specific genetic predisposition, have an "android" obesity pattern, which is associated with a much higher prevalence of obesity-related comorbidities than women with a gynoid fat pattern at a similar BMI (Deepa et al., 2006; Despres, 2006; Yang et al., 2021). Although the 1998 OEI guidelines recommended consideration of waist circumference to assess CV risk, as a surrogate for higher visceral fat stores, in conjunction with BMI, waist girth is rarely measured in clinical settings and its usefulness was challenged early on, when analyses of a large multi-racial/multi-ethnic sample from the Third NHANES determined that over 98% of adults would receive the same treatment recommendations whether waist was included or not (Kiernan et al., 2000).

In addition to a high prevalence of obesity-related comorbidities, people with obesity face a pervasive, resilient form of social stigma that can also cause physical and psychological harm, as well as affect clinical care (Rubino et al., 2020). Recognizing that physiologic systems for regulating food intake are well developed for responding to hunger, but poorly developed for curbing overeating, and evolved when physical activity levels were much higher and sedentary behavior was much lower for routine daily functioning than current activity levels, treatment guidelines should consider an individual's daily living environment, as well as community factors that influence eating and physical activity (Kumanyika, 2017). Yet, obesity is generally approached in a clinical setting as a problem for the individual with obesity, rather than as the serious public health problem it has become over the past half century.

17.2 OBESITY-RELATED COMORBIDITIES AND REGIONAL ADIPOSITY

The 1998 NHLBI OEI guidelines (NHLBI, 1998) and subsequent reports (Powell-Wiley et al., 2021; Lauby-Secretan et al., 2016) have laid out the evidence that obesity, defined as BMI ≥ 30 kg/m^2, is strongly associated with coronary heart disease (CHD) and specific CHD risk factors, e.g., type 2 diabetes mellitus (and insulin resistance and glucose intolerance), an unfavorable lipid profile (specifically low HDL-cholesterol and high triglycerides), and hypertension, as well as stroke, gall bladder disease, sleep apnea and respiratory problems, certain cancers (including endometrial, postmenopausal breast, colorectal, esophageal, renal/kidneys, meningioma, pancreatic, gastric cardia, liver, multiple myeloma, ovarian, gallbladder, and thyroid), and osteoarthritis. Over the past decade, great progress has been made in understanding the complexity of adipose tissue and its important role in healthy metabolism, as well as in metabolic disorders caused by excess fat (Goosens, 2017; Kahn et al., 2019).

The World Obesity Federation has argued that obesity is a chronic relapsing disease process, with food, particularly foods that are high in energy density, such as fat or in sugar-sweetened beverages, as the primary agent affecting the host, and that an abundance of food, low physical activity, and several other environmental factors that interact with the genetic susceptibility of the host, produce a positive energy balance that results in excess fat storage and a variety of metabolic, hormonal, and inflammatory products from enlarged adipocytes and ectopic fat that produce damage in the arteries, heart, liver, muscle, and pancreas (Bray et al., 2017). Figure 17.1 presents a model (reproduced from Bray et al., 2017) of the relations of obesity to the diseases associated with it and the pathophysiological factors that are principally involved with the development of each disease, many of which may interact and become involved in more complex causal pathways.

17.2.1 METABOLICALLY UNHEALTHY OBESITY (MUO) VERSUS METABOLICALLY HEALTHY OBESITY (MHO)

Early research on body fat distribution and regional adiposity provided evidence of a large variation in individual risk to developing obesity-related comorbidities that cannot be explained by total fat stored (Vague, 1956), with "abdominal obesity," due to intra-abdominal adiposity, cited as the most prevalent cause of metabolic syndrome (see below) and related cardiometabolic risk (Despres, 2006). Visceral fat, which is released into the portal circulation, thereby affecting liver processes, is associated with more adverse metabolic risk factors, including high blood pressure, dyslipidemia, and high blood sugar, compared to subcutaneous adipose tissue (including fat depots in the buttocks, hips, thighs, upper arms, and breasts), which releases fat into the systemic circulation. Recognition that multiple cardiovascular risk factors of endogenous origin aggregate in an individual led to the

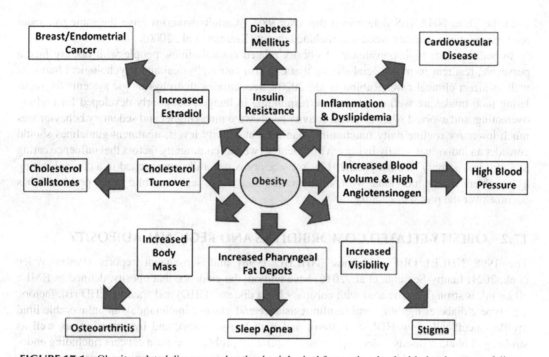

FIGURE 17.1 Obesity-related diseases and pathophysiological factors involved with development of disease

(Reprinted with permission from Bray, G. A., Kim, K. K., Wilding, J. P. H., & World Obesity Federation. (2017). Obesity: A chronic relapsing progressive disease process. A position statement of the World Obesity Federation. *Obesity Reviews*, 18(7), 715–723.)

concept of the metabolic syndrome, which is defined as having at least three of the following: Waist circumference greater than 102 cm in men or 88 cm in women; triglyceride level greater than 150 mg/dL or on drug treatment for elevated triglycerides; high-density lipoprotein cholesterol (HDL-C) less than 40 mg/dL in men or less than 50 mg/dL in women or on drug treatment for low HDL-C; systolic blood pressure at least 130 mmHg or diastolic blood pressure at least 85 mm Hg or taking antihypertensive medications; or fasting plasma glucose level at least 100 mg/dL or taking diabetes medications (Grundy et al., 2005).

Whereas about 80–90% of individuals with obesity have metabolically unhealthy phenotypic traits, including high liver fat content, insulin resistance, higher markers of inflammation, and adipose tissue dysfunction, as well as lower cardiorespiratory fitness, compared to normal weight persons, about 10–20% of individuals with obesity have been regarded as metabolically healthy by virtue of having normal glucose and lipid metabolism parameters and no hypertension, even though these individuals have higher risk than healthy lean individuals (Blüher, 2020). As seen in Figure 17.2, transabdominal Magnetic Resonance Imaging (MRI) scans have provided evidence of about a 2.6-fold higher visceral fat deposition associated with MUO compared to MHO (Blüher, 2020). MHO, however, is likely a transient phenotype as suggested by a median 12.2-year longitudinal analysis among nearly 7000 participants of the Multi-Ethnic Study of Atherosclerosis, in which almost half of MHO participants developed MetS and had a significantly increased Odds Ratio of CVD (OR=1.60, 95% CI 1.27–2.25) compared to MHO persons who did not develop MetS (Mongraw-Chaffine et al., 2019). Weight loss and lifestyle management for CVD risk factors (see Figure 17.2) is therefore recommended for all individuals with obesity, regardless of MUO or MHO status (Blüher, 2020).

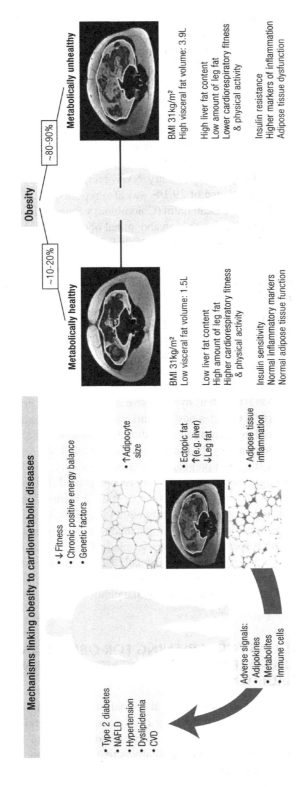

FIGURE 17.2   Mechanisms and phenotypic traits linking obesity to cardiometabolic diseases

(Reprinted with permission from Blüher, M. (2020). Metabolically healthy obesity. *Endocrine Review, 41*(3).)

17.2.2 Normal Weight Obesity (NWO) Syndrome

Another challenge to the simplistic concept that obesity can be diagnosed based on weight and height is Normal Weight Obesity (NWO), which is characterized by excess body fat in individuals with "normal weight" BMI (18.5–24.9 kg/m^2) who have a high degree of metabolic dysregulation, including a higher risk of developing metabolic syndrome, cardiometabolic dysfunction, i.e., increased insulin resistance, hypertension, and/or dyslipidemia, and who also have low-grade proinflammatory status and increased oxidative stress (Oliveros et al., 2014; Franco et al., 2016). The term NWO was initially associated with low lean mass and CVD risk (DeLoreno et al., 2006), but subsequent research has focused on higher visceral fat in persons with NWO, which is estimated to affect about 30 million Americans (Franco et al., 2016). In a Korean study of over 5000 men and nearly 7000 women, using BMI cut-points of 18.5–22.9 kg/m^2 for "normal weight" and percent body fat assessed by dual-energy X-ray absorptiometry, NWO prevalence was 36% in men and 29% in women (Kim et al., 2014). A prevalence of 29.1% was also reported for NWO, using the BMI 18.5–24.9 kg/m^2 cut-points, in 1354 American Latin (Colombian) young adults (61% of whom were women), and the condition was associated with high abdominal obesity and increased CV risk, high blood pressure, low HDL-C, and low muscular strength early in life (Correa-Rodriguez et al., 2020).

17.3 WEIGHT MANAGEMENT OF PREGNANT WOMEN AND WOMEN OF REPRODUCTIVE AGE

Nearly 25% of women in the US who become pregnant have obesity, with the highest prevalence among racial and ethnic minority groups (Ogunwole et al., 2021). As women should attempt to conceive at a normal weight for better obstetric outcomes, young women of reproductive age with obesity are a special group to consider in clinical settings. Mounting evidence of negative health consequences of inadequate or excessive weight gain during pregnancy, for both mother (e.g., adverse pregnancy outcomes (APOs), such as hypertensive disorders during pregnancy, gestational diabetes, and development of type 2 diabetes postpartum) and fetus (e.g., small- or large-for-gestational weight and possible altered gene expression leading to metabolic abnormalities; Ogunwole et al., 2021), led to new 2009 guidelines by the Institute of Medicine and National Research Council for weight gain in women with singleton pregnancies (Rasmussen et al., 2009). Based on WHO/NHLBI BMI cutoff points for pre-pregnancy BMI, it is recommended that weight gain differ by body weight status as follows: Underweight (28–40 lb., i.e., about 1 lb. or 0.5 kg per week); normal weight (25–35 lb., i.e., 1 lb. or 0.4 kg per week); overweight (15–25 lb., i.e., 0.66 lb. or 0.3 kg per week); and obese (11–20 lb., with per week gain not specified (Rasmussen et al., 2009). (Although data were insufficient to construct specific guidelines for class II or class III obesity; weight loss in pregnant women with severe obesity may be reasonable.) In addition, a strong association of gestational weight gain (GWG) and childhood obesity make preconception, gestational, and postpartum weight management of both clinical importance and public health significance (Rogozinska et al., 2019).

17.4 RECOMMENDATIONS FOR SCREENING FOR OBESITY AND BEHAVIORAL (LIFESTYLE-BASED) INTERVENTIONS FOR WEIGHT LOSS AND MANAGEMENT

Population-wide obesity is linked to physiologically abnormal eating and physical activity patterns that have become normative for a large proportion of US individuals who live in obesogenic environments with heavily marketed high-calorie, nutrient-poor foods and beverages and who have daily routines that make it difficult to be physically active and promote sedentary behavior. Furthermore, marked disparities in patterns of obesity by race and ethnicity and others with social disadvantages that lead to even more limited options for healthy eating and physical activity will require comprehensive policy, systems, and environmental changes to shift the range and balance of behavioral options toward an obesity-protective direction (Kumanyika, 2019).

Among recommendations from a 2012 Institute of Medicine expert committee for accelerating progress in obesity prevention is that health care and health service providers, employers, and insurers should increase the support structure for achieving better population health and obesity prevention by providing standardized care and advocating for healthy community environments; ensuring coverage of, access to, and incentives for routine obesity prevention, screening, diagnosis, and treatment; encouraging active living and healthy eating at work; encouraging healthy weight gain during pregnancy and breastfeeding, and promoting breastfeeding-friendly environments (IOM, 2012).

With high levels of obesity in young children, high numbers of children in out-of-home care, and data suggesting a link between early care and education (ECE) participation and overweight/obesity, identifying promising intervention characteristics associated with successful behavioral and anthropometric outcomes is critical. A systematic review of obesity prevention interventions in center-based ECE settings provided evidence that multi-component, multi-level ECE interventions with parental engagement are most likely to be effective (Ward et al., 2017). In 2017, the US Preventive Services Task Force reviewed the evidence on screening for obesity in children and adolescents and concluded, with a B recommendation (meaning there is high certainty that the net benefit is moderate or moderate certainty that the net benefit is moderate to substantial), that clinicians should screen children and adolescents aged 6 years and older (using BMI plotted on growth charts such as those developed by the CDC) and offer or refer those who have obesity to comprehensive, intensive behavioral interventions ($\geq$ 26 contact hours over 2 to 12 months) to promote improvements in weight status (USPSTF, 2017).

Effective interventions had multiple components, including sessions targeting both parent and child; individual sessions for both family and group; offering information about healthy eating, safe exercising, and reading food labels; encouraging stimulus control, e.g., limiting access to tempting foods and screen time, goal setting, self-monitoring, contingent rewards, and problem solving; and supervised physical activity sessions (USPSTF, 2017). While more intensive interventions usually involved referral outside the primary care office, providers included primary care clinicians, exercise physiologists, physical therapists, dietitians, diet assistants, psychologists, and social workers (USPSTF, 2017).

The 2018 update on the 2012 USPSTF recommendation for screening for obesity in adults also focused on behavioral interventions to prevent obesity-related morbidity and mortality in adults (USPSTF, 2017). Due to adequate evidence that such interventions can lead to significant improvements in weight status and reduce the incidence of type 2 diabetes among adults with obesity and elevated plasma glucose levels, the USPSTF recommends, also as a B recommendation, that clinicians offer or refer adults with a BMI of 30 kg/m^2 or greater to intensive, multicomponent behavioral interventions. The interventions deemed to be effective were designed to help participants achieve or maintain a $\geq$ 5% weight loss through a combination of dietary changes and increased physical activity; most lasted for one to two years; the majority had $\geq$ 12 sessions in the first year; most focused on problem solving to identify barriers, self-monitoring of weight, peer support, and relapse prevention; and the interventions also provided tools to support weight loss or weight loss maintenance (e.g.,, pedometers, food scales, or exercise videos).

Prior to releasing these recommendations, the USPSTF convened an expert forum to inform the evaluation of 11 Behavioral Counseling Interventions (BCI), which can be delivered in primary care setting, or patients can be referred to other clinical or community partners, such as to a specialized pediatric obesity clinic or referral to weight loss programs (Krist et al., 2015). Although no single intervention has been found to affect people's lifestyle behaviors successfully and consistently, evidence of synergistic effect of interventions that target multiple levels—e.g., environmental, policy, community, clinical, and individual (Sallis, 2018) and support from clinicians through conversations about lifestyle and referrals to specialists or community programs—increase patients' likelihood to engage in lifestyle change (Jebb et al., 2011; Williams et al., 2021). Potential roles for clinicians included assessing and briefly advising patients; seeking agreement on goals; referring patients for intensive assistance; providing intensive assistance for selected patients; reinforcing community counseling; holding patients accountable to change; personalizing the counseling experience; integrating counseling into health care needs; and longitudinal care after BCI completion (Krist et al., 2015). (Potential roles for counselors and spanning personnel in the clinical-community shared care model were also presented [Krist et al., 2015].)

A healthy diet, physical activity, limiting sedentary behavior, and getting adequate sleep are recommended for all people, regardless of body weight status. Most persons with obesity can lose weight by lifestyle (diet and physical activity); however, successful long-term weight loss is difficult to achieve and most regain their lost weight over time. As addressed in a 2019 National Institute of Diabetes and Digestive and Kidney Diseases workshop titled "The Physiology of the Weight-Reduced State," the neurohormonal, physiological, and behavioral factors that promote weight recidivism are complex (Aronne et al., 2021). Nonetheless, current NHLBI recommendations for a healthy weight (NHLBI, 2022) are consistent with the weight loss recommendations from the 1998 NHLBI OEI guidelines (NHLBI, 1998) and include setting an initial weight loss goal of 10% of baseline body weight over a six-month period and, if successful, attempting further weight loss if warranted. Although the 1998 guidelines recommended caloric restriction of 300–500 kcal/day for persons with a BMI of 27–34.9 kg, for weight loss of 0.5–1 lb./week (0.22–0.45 kg/wk) and caloric restriction of 500–1000 kcal/day for persons with a BMI of ≥ 35 kg, for weight loss of 1–2 lb./week (0.45–0.91 kg/wk), current recommendations promote a caloric deficit of 500–1000 kcal/day for all, with 1–2 lb. loss per week (NHLBI, 2022). The goal of healthy weight loss is the loss of fat mass, particularly visceral fat, and maintenance of lean mass, particularly muscle (which determines basal metabolic rate and thus caloric needs at rest), not total body weight loss. Slow, steady weight loss increases the likelihood of losing mostly fat weight and maintaining lean mass; whereas, rapid weight loss and weight loss by diet alone generally results in loss of substantial lean mass as well, whereas subsequent weight gain is predominantly fat mass gain.

Dietary recommendations for weight loss emphasize low-calorie diets (NHLBI, 2022), i.e., limiting high calorie foods and sweetened beverages, with no specific recommendation for diet composition. At least two large trials have demonstrated clinically meaningful weight change with reduced-calorie diets that met guidelines for cardiovascular health, regardless of which macronutrients they emphasized, with neither finding substantial differences in weight loss between low-fat and low-carbohydrate diets and one comparing diets of average versus high protein (Sachs et al., 2009; Gardner et al., 2018).

The 1998 and current NHLBI guidelines also recommend physical activity as an integral part of a comprehensive weight loss therapy and weight control program because of evidence that physical activity modestly contributes to weight loss in overweight and obese adults, may decrease abdominal fat, increases cardiorespiratory fitness, and may help with maintenance of weight loss (NHLBI, 1998; NHBLI, 2022). Initially, moderate levels of physical activity for 30 to 45 minutes, three to five days a week, should be encouraged, but all adults should set a long-term goal to accumulate at least 30 minutes of moderate-intensity physical activity on most and preferably all days of the week. Minimum guidelines for aerobic physical activity (150 min of moderate or 75 min of vigorous physical activity per week) can improve cardiovascular health; however, these levels are generally inadequate for clinically significant weight loss or weight maintenance without caloric restriction. In fact, patients seeking to lose weight without change in their dietary habits need to be counseled that higher levels of physical activity (225–420 min/week) are necessary to achieve clinically significant weight loss, as well as higher levels (200–300 min/week) for weight maintenance (Swift et al., 2018). Resistance training in combination with other weight loss intervention strategies, including aerobic training, may assist with weight loss or maintenance; however, alone, it is unlikely to produce sufficient negative energy balance to result in clinically significant weight loss compared to aerobic training (Swift et al., 2018).

The 1998 NHLBI guidelines also recommended behavioral therapy, including self-monitoring, stress management, stimulus control, problem solving, contingency management, cognitive restructuring, and social support (NHLBI, 1998), and behavioral therapy continues to be recognized as a useful adjunct for weight loss and maintenance in current recommendations (NHLBI, 2022). A recent scientific statement from the American Heart Association presents evidence of effective behavioral intervention programs for cardiovascular disease (CVD) prevention and risk management, including programs that target diet and nutrient quality, promote physical activity, and present multicomponent interventions targeting both diet and physical activity that are feasible for adoption in primary care settings (Laddu et al., 2021). The statement describes the feasibility for health care professionals to offer or refer patients for effective behavioral counseling and presents an overview of equitable resources available to facilitate the widespread adoption and implementation of programs that facilitate clinic–community partnerships and the practical integration of patient-centered behavioral counseling within diverse care and community settings (Laddu et al., 2021).

17.5 CONCLUSION

Obesity and obesity comorbidities are highly prevalent in the United States and globally. Abdominal (visceral) adiposity, including in persons considered "normal weight" by body mass index cut-points, is particularly problematic and strongly associated with current and future metabolic risk factors linked to cardiovascular disease, cancer, and other chronic diseases. Weight management of women of reproductive age with obesity and pregnant women is a special clinical and public health issue because of health consequences for the fetus as well as the mother. Screening for obesity in clinical settings is highly recommended because of effective, evidence-based behavioral counseling programs that can be provided in primary care and community settings or to which patients should be referred. Indeed, primary health care professionals are viewed as the gatekeepers to delivering intensive behavioral counseling to at-risk patients, and they are encouraged to adopt and implement such programs.

REFERENCES

Aronne, L. J., Hall, K. D., Jakicic, J. M., Leibel, R. L., Lowe, M. R., Rosenbaum, M., & Klein, S. (2021). Describing the weight-reduced state: Physiology, behavior, and interventions. *Obesity (Silver Spring)*, *29*(Suppl. 1), S9–S24.

Blüher, M. (2020). Metabolically healthy obesity. *Endocrine Review*, *41*(3), 1–16.

Bray, G. A., Kim, K. K., Wilding, J. P. H., & World Obesity Federation. (2017). Obesity: A chronic relapsing progressive disease process. A position statement of the World Obesity Federation. *Obesity Reviews*, *18*(7), 715–723.

Correa-Rodríguez, M., González-Ruíz, K., Rincón-Pabón, D., Izquierdo, M., García-Hermoso, A., Agostinis-Sobrinho, C., Sánchez-Capacho, N., Roa-Cubaque, M. A., & Ramírez-Vélez, R. (2020). Normal-weight obesity is associated with increased cardiometabolic risk in young adults. *Nutrients*, *12*(4), 1–13.

De Lorenzo, A., Martinoli, R., Vaia, F., & Di Renzo, L. (2006). Normal weight obese (NWO) women: an evaluation of a candidate new syndrome. *Nutrition, Metabolism, & Cardiovascular Diseases*, *16*(8), 513–523.

Deepa, R., Sandeep, S., & Mohan, V. (2006). Abdominal obesity, visceral fat and type 2 diabetes- Asian Indian phenotype. In V. Mohan & G. H. R. Rao (Eds.), *Type 2 diabetes in South Asians: Epidemiology, risk factors and prevention* (pp. 138–152). Jaypee Brothers Medical Publishers (P) Ltd.

Despres, J-P. (2006). Abdominal obesity: The most prevalent cause of the metabolic syndrome and related cardiometabolic risk. *European Heart Journal Supplements*, *8*(Suppl. B), B4–B12.

Franco, L. P., Morais, C. C., & Cominetti, C. (2016). Normal-weight obesity syndrome: diagnosis, prevalence, and clinical implications. *Nutrition Reviews*, *74*(9), 558–570. https://doi.org/10.1093/nutrit/nuw019

Gardner, C. D., Trepanowski, J. F., Del Gobbo, L. C., Hauser, M. E., Rigdon, J., Ioannidis, J. P. A., Desai, M., & King, A.C. (2018). Effect of low-fat vs low-carbohydrate diet on 12-month weight loss in overweight adults and the association with genotype pattern or insulin secretion: The DIETFITS randomized clinical trial. *JAMA, 319*(7), 667–679.

Goossens, G. H. (2017). The metabolic phenotype in obesity: Fat mass, body fat distribution, and adipose tissue function. *Obesity Facts, 10*(3), 207–215.

Grundy, S. M., Cleeman, J. I., Daniels, S. R., Donato, K. A., Eckel, R. H., Franklin, B. A., Gordon, D. J., Krauss, R. M., Savage, P. J., Smith, S. C., Spertus, J. A., Costa, F., American Heart Association, & National Heart, Lung, and Blood Institute. (2005). *Circulation, 112*(17), 2735–2752.

Hales, C. M., Carroll, M. D., Fryar, C. D., & Ogden, C. L. (2020). Prevalence of obesity and severe obesity among adults: United States, 2017–2018. *NCHS Data Brief, 360*, 1–8.

Institute of Medicine. (2012). *Accelerating progress in obesity prevention: Solving the weight of the nation.* National Academies Press.

Jebb, S. A., Ahern, A. L., Olson, A. D., Aston, L. M., Holzapfel, C., Stoll, J., Amann-Gassner, U., Simpson, A. E., Fuller, N. R., Pearson, S., Lau, N. S., Mander, A. P., Hauner, H., & Caterson, I. D. (2011). Primary care referral to a commercial provider for weight loss treatment versus standard care: a randomised controlled trial. *The Lancet, 378*(9801), 1485–1492. https://doi.org/10.1016/S0140-6736(11)61344-5

Kahn, C. R., Wang, G., & Lee, K. Y. (2019). Altered adipose tissue and adipocyte function in the pathogenesis of metabolic syndrome. *Journal of Clinical Investigation, 129*(10), 3990–4000.

Kiernan, M., & Winkleby, M. A. (2000). Identifying patients for weight-loss treatment: An empirical evaluation of the NHLBI obesity education initiative expert panel treatment recommendations. *Archives of Internal Medicine, 160*(14), 2169–2176. https://doi.org/10.1001/archinte.160.14.2169

Kim, M. K., Han, K., Kwon, H. S., Song, K. H., Yim, H. W., Lee, W. C., & Park, Y. M. (2014). Normal weight obesity in Korean adults. *Clinical Endocrinology, 80*(2), 214–220. https://doi.org.proxy.library.nyu.edu/10.1111/cen.12162

Krist, A. H., Baumann, L. J., Holtrop, J. S., Wasserman, M. R., Stange, K. C., & Woo, M. (2015). Evaluating feasible and referable behavioral counseling interventions. *American Journal of Preventive Medicine, 49*(3), S138–S149. https://doi.org/10.1016/j.amepre.2015.05.009

Kumanyika, S. (2017). Getting to equity in obesity prevention: A new framework. NAM Perspectives. Discussion Paper, National Academy of Medicine, Washington, DC. https://doi.org/10.31478/201701c

Kumanyika, S. K. (2019). A framework for increasing equity impact in obesity prevention. *American Journal of Public Health, 109*(10), 1350–1357. https://doi.org/10.2105/AJPH.2019.305221

Laddu, D., Ma, J., Kaar, J., Ozemek, C., Durant, R. W., Campbell, T., Welsh, J., & Turrise, S. (2021). Health behavior change programs in primary care and community practices for cardiovascular disease prevention and risk factor management among midlife and older adults: A scientific statement from the American Heart Association. *Circulation, 144*(24), e533–e549.

Lauby-Secretan, B., Scoccianti, C., Loomis, D., Grosse, Y., Bianchini, F., & Straif, K. (2016). Body fatness and cancer—viewpoint of the IARC Working Group. *New England Journal of Medicine, 375*, 794–798.

Lin, A. L., Vittinghoff, E., Olgin, J. E., Pletcher, M. J., & Marcus, G. M. (2021). Body weight changes during pandemic-related shelter-in-place in a longitudinal cohort study. *JAMA Network Open, 4*(3), e212536.

Mathew, H., Castracane, V. D., & Mantzoros, C. (2018). Adipose tissue and reproductive health. *Metabolism: Clinical and Experimental, 86*, 18–32.

Mauvais-Jarvis, F. (Ed.). (2017). *Sex and gender factors affecting metabolic homeostasis, diabetes and obesity.* Springer. https://doi.org/10.1007/978-3-319-70178-3

Mongraw-Chaffin, M., Bertoni, A. G., Golden, S. H., Mathioudakis, N., Sears D. D., Szklo, M., Anderson, C. A. M. (2019). Association of low fasting glucose and HbA1c with cardiovascular disease and mortality: The MESA Study. Journal of the Endocrine Society, *3*(5), 892–901. https://doi.org/10.1210/js.2019-00033

NHLBI. (2022). *Aim for a healthy weight.* National Heart, Lung, and Blood Institute. Retrieved January 2, 2022, from www.nhlbi.nih.gov/health/educational/lose_wt/recommen.htm

NHLBI Obesity Education Initiative Expert Panel on the Identification, Evaluation, and Treatment of Obesity in Adults (US). (1998). Clinical guidelines on the identification, evaluation, and treatment of overweight and obesity in adults the evidence report. *Obesity Research, 6*(Suppl. 2), 51S–209S.

Ogunwole, S. M., Zera, C. A., & Stanford, F. C. (2021). Obesity management in women of reproductive age. *JAMA, 325*(5), 433–434.

Oliveros, E., Somers, V. K., Sochor, O., Goel, K., & Lopez-Jimenez, F. (2014). The concept of normal weight obesity. *Progress in Cardiovascular Diseases*, *56*(4), 426–433. https://doi.org/10.1016/j.pcad.2013.10.003

Pi-Sunyer, F. X. (2000). Obesity: Criteria and classification. *Proceedings of the Nutrition Society*, *59*(4), 505–509.

Powell-Wiley, T. M., Poirier, P., Burke, L. E., Després, J. P., Gordon-Larsen, P., Lavie, C. J., Lear, S. A., Ndumele, C. E., Neeland, I. J., Sanders, P., St-Onge, M. P., American Heart Association Council on Lifestyle and Cardiometabolic Health, Council on Cardiovascular and Stroke Nursing, Council on Clinical Cardiology, Council on Epidemiology and Prevention, & Stroke Council. (2021). Obesity and cardiovascular disease: A scientific statement from the American Heart Association. *Circulation*, *143*(21), e984–e1010.

Rasmussen, K. M., Catalano, P. M., & Yaktine, A. L. (2009). New guidelines for weight gain during pregnancy: What obstetrician/gynecologists should know. *Current Opinion in Obstetrics and Gynecology*, *21*(6), 521–526.

Rogozińska, E., Zamora, J., Marlin, N., Betrán, A. P., Astrup, A., Bogaerts, A., Cecatti, J. G., Dodd, J. M., Facchinetti, F., Geiker, N. R. W., Haakstad, L. A. H., Hauner, H., Jensen, D. M., Kinnunen, T. I., Mol, B. W. J., Owens, J., Phelan, S., Renault, K. M., Salvesen, K. Å., ... Thangaratinam, S. (2019). Gestational weight gain outside the Institute of Medicine recommendations and adverse pregnancy outcomes: Analysis using individual participant data from randomised trials. *BMC Pregnancy and Childbirth*, *19*(1), 322.

Rubino, F., Puhl, R. M., Cummings, D. E., Eckel, R. H., Ryan, D. H., Mechanick, J. I., Nadglowski, J., Ramos Salas, X., Schauer, P. R., Twenefour, D., Apovian, C. M., Aronne, L. J., Batterham, R. L., Berthoud, H. R., Boza, C., Busetto, L., Dicker, D., De Groot, M., Eisenberg, D., ... Dixon, J. B. (2020). Joint international consensus statement for ending stigma of obesity. *Nature Medicine*, *26*(4), 485–497.

Sacks, F. M., Bray, G. A., Carey, V. J., Smith, S. R., Ryan, D. H., Anton, S. D., McManus, K., Champagne, C. M., Bishop, L. M., Laranjo, N., Leboff, M. S., Rood, J. C., de Jonge, L., Greenway, F. L., Loria, C. M., Obarzanek, E., & Williamson, D.A. (2009). Comparison of weight-loss diets with different compositions of fat, protein, and carbohydrates. *New England Journal of Medicine*, *360*(9), 859–73.

Sallis, J. F. (2018). Needs and challenges related to multilevel interventions: Physical activity examples. *Health Education and Behavior*, *45*(5), 661–667.

Seal, A., Schaffner, A., Phelan, S., Brunner-Gaydos, H., Tseng, M., Keadle, S., Alber, J., Kiteck, I., & Hagobian, T. (2022). COVID-19 pandemic and stay-at-home mandates promote weight gain in US adults. *Obesity (Silver Spring)* , *30*(1), 240–248.

Swift, D. L., McGee, J. E., Earnest, C. P., Carlisle, E., Nygard, M., & Johannsen, N. M. (2018). The effects of exercise and physical activity on weight loss and maintenance. *Progress in Cardiovascular Disease*, *61*(2), 206–213.

US Preventive Services Task Force. (2006). Screening and interventions for overweight in children and adolescents: Recommendation statement. *American Family Physician*, *73*(1), 115–119.

US Preventive Services Task Force, Grossman DC, Bibbins-Domingo K, Curry SJ, Barry MJ, Davidson KW, Doubeni CA, Epling JW, Kemper AR, Krist AH, Kurth AE, Landefeld CS, Mangione CM, Phipps MG, Silverstein M, Simon MA, Tseng CW. (2017). Screening for Obesity in Children and Adolescents US Preventive Services Task Force Recommendation Statement JAMA. 2017 Jun 20; *317*(23), 2417–2426.

Vague, J. (1956). The degree of masculine differentiation of obesities: A factor determining predisposition to diabetes, atherosclerosis, gout, and uric calculous disease. *American Journal of Clinical Nutrition*, *4*, 20–34.

Ward, D. S., Welker, E., Choate, A., Henderson, K. E., Lott, M., Tovar, A., Wilson, A., & Sallis, J. F. (2017). Strength of obesity prevention interventions in early care and education settings: A systematic review. *Preventative Medicine*, *95*(Suppl.), S37–S52. https://doi.org/10.1016/j.ypmed.2016.09.033

Williams, A. R., Wilson-Genderson, M., & Thomson, M. D. (2021). A cross-sectional analysis of associations between lifestyle advice and behavior changes in patients with hypertension or diabetes: NHANES 2015–2018. *Preventative Medicine*, *145*, 106426.

World Health Organization. (2000). *Obesity: Preventing and managing the global epidemic: Report of a WHO consultation*. WHO technical report series, 894. World Health Organization.

Nutrition and Food Safety. (1995). Overweight adults. In *Physical status: The use and interpretation of anthropometry*, 312–4. WHO technical report series, 854. World Health Organization.

Yang, Y., Xie, M., Yuan, S., Zeng, Y., Dong, Y., Wang, Z., Xiao, Q., Dong, B., Ma, J., & Hu, J. (2021). Sex differences in the associations between adiposity distribution and cardiometabolic risk factors in overweight or obese individuals: A cross-sectional study. *BMC Public Health*, *21*(1), 1232.

18 Dyslipidemia

Susan Halli-Demeter[1] and Lynne T. Braun[2]

[1]Preventive Cardiovascular Nurses Association, Madison, Wisconsin, USA

[2]Rush University, Rush Heart Center for Women

Chicago, Illinois, USA

CONTENTS

KEY POINTS

- Dyslipidemia is a major risk factor for ASCVD, particularly elevated LDL-C and triglycerides.
- Key contributors to dyslipidemia are genetics, unhealthy dietary choices, sedentary lifestyle, tobacco use, and stress.
- Lifestyle intervention is the cornerstone of cardiovascular disease prevention, even for patients with ASCVD who require medications that alter lipids and reduce risk for ASCVD events.

DOI: 10.1201/9781003178330-21

- Dietary interventions, e.g., low saturated fat, Mediterranean, vegetarian, and plant-based, are associated with improved lipid parameters and reduced ASCVD events.
- Soluble fiber and plant stanols/sterols may be adjuncts for additional LDL-C lowering.
- Regular exercise as recommended by the 2018 Physical Activity Guidelines is essential to improve dyslipidemia, plasma glucose, BMI, and waist circumference.
- Tobacco avoidance, limiting alcohol intake, and stress reduction are also important for healthy lifestyle practices.

18.1   INTRODUCTION

18.1.1   DEFINITION OF DYSLIPIDEMIA

Dyslipidemia occurs when genetic and/or environmental conditions alter lipoprotein production, catabolism, or clearance from circulation, resulting in abnormal cholesterol or triglyceride in the blood. Dyslipidemia is characterized by increased low-density lipoprotein cholesterol (LDL-C), low high-density lipoprotein cholesterol (HDL-C) (< 40 mg/dL in a male and < 50 mg/dL in a female), and/or elevated triglycerides. Moderately high LDL-C is defined as an LDL-C ≥ 160 mg/dL and severe hypercholesterolemia is defined as an LDL-C ≥ 190 mg/dL. The presence of triglycerides 175–499 mg/dL is defined as moderate hypertriglyceridemia and triglycerides > 500 mg/dL is classified as severe hypertriglyceridemia (Grundy et al., 2019).

18.1.2   DYSLIPIDEMIA IS A RISK FACTOR FOR CARDIOVASCULAR DISEASE

A wide variety of data have proven that serum cholesterol contributes to atherosclerotic cardio-vascular disease (ASCVD) (Grundy et al., 2019). The term "atherosclerosis" was first defined by pathologist Felix Marchand in 1904, with "athero" meaning gruel or porridge and sclerosis meaning hardening (of the artery) (Gotto, 2005). By 1949, biophysicist John Gofman and colleagues found that the LDL-C was associated with increased risk for ASCVD in patients with familial hypercholesterolemia (FH) (Gotto, 2005). U.S. population studies suggest that optimal total cholesterol levels are around 150 mg/dL (3.8 mmol/L) and LDL-C of about 100 mg/dL (2.6 mmol/L) (Grundy et al., 2019). Low rates of ASCVD are seen in adults with LDL-C levels in this range. Randomized clinical trials with individuals on lipid lowering therapy, particularly statin medications, have concluded that "lower is better" with regard to LDL-C (Grundy et al., 2019). For each 1.8 mg/dL reduction in LDL-C, there is an approximate 1% risk reduction in major cardiovascular events (myocardial infarction, stroke, hospitalization for unstable angina or revascularization (Cannon et al., 2006). Lowering LDL-C through lifestyle and prescription medication lowers the risk for ASCVD, although these interventions may not eradicate it completely. Researchers have also investigated the involvement of low HDL-C and elevated triglycerides. In the Framingham Heart Study, an inverse relationship was observed between low HDL-C and cardiovascular events where a 1 mg/dL increase in HDL lowered heart disease risk by 1% (Gotto, 2005). Approximately 27% of adults have triglyceride levels > 176 mg/dL. In a study comparing individuals with non-fasting triglyceride levels of 580 mg/dL versus 70 mg/dL, there was a 5.1-fold increased risk for myocardial infarction (MI), 3.2-fold increased risk for ischemic heart disease and ischemic stroke, and 2.2-fold for all-cause mortality (Nordestgaard, 2016). Additionally, triglyceride-rich lipoproteins are associated with inflammation and elevated C-reactive protein, which also is found in metabolic syndrome, overweight-obese status, and ultimately ASCVD (Nordestgaard, 2016; Reiner, 2017).

18.1.3   GENETIC VERSUS ENVIRONMENTAL CONTRIBUTIONS TO DYSLIPIDEMIA

Some individuals have a genetic predisposition for familial hypercholesterolemia (FH) (Type IIa hyperlipidemia), familial combined hyperlipidemia (Type IIb hyperlipidemia), familial dysbetalipoproteinemia (Type III hyperlipidemia), and familial hypertriglyceridemia (Type IV hyperlipidemia). Genetic testing can assist in confirming the diagnosis of FH. Other conditions, such as thyroid disease, diabetes, impaired fasting glucose, chronic kidney disease, metabolic syndrome, polycystic ovarian syndrome, obesity, human immunodeficiency virus (HIV), anorexia nervosa, autoimmune disorders (lupus and Cushing's disease), liver disease (cirrhosis and fatty liver disease), pregnancy, and conditions that increase female hormones, can affect the lipid profile, and must be evaluated and treated. Medications can also adversely affect the lipid panel; these include corticosteroids, anabolic steroids, steroid hormones, beta blockers, amiodarone, loop and thiazide diuretics, Sodium-glucose Cotransporter-2 (SGLT2) inhibitors, antiviral therapy, immunosuppressants, antipsychotics, anticonvulsants, retinoids, and growth hormone. Environmental factors that can contribute to dyslipidemia include a high saturated/trans-fat and/or high sugar diet, physical inactivity, physical stress, excessive alcohol, and tobacco use.

18.1.4 OVERALL ROLE OF LIFESTYLE IN THE MANAGEMENT OF DYSLIPIDEMIA

Lifestyle management is especially important in the management of dyslipidemia when evidence of metabolic syndrome is present. Metabolic syndrome increases the risk of cardiovascular disease, diabetes, and all-cause death and is comprised of three of the following risk factors: elevated waist circumference, elevated triglycerides, reduced HDL-C, elevated glucose, and elevated blood pressure (Grundy et al., 2019). Metabolic syndrome is often linked to central weight gain and is reversible with lifestyle modification and weight loss.

18.1.5 WHEN TO ADVISE PHARMACOLOGIC MANAGEMENT

The American College of Cardiology/American Heart Association (ACC/AHA) 2018 Guideline on the Management of Blood Cholesterol (Grundy et al., 2019) provides evidence-based recommendations for cholesterol management in primary and secondary prevention. Pharmacologic management with a high-intensity statin is highly recommended for patients with clinical ASCVD and/or those with a diagnosis of FH or an LDL-C ≥ 190 mg/dL. Additionally, individuals 20–39 years of age with an LDL-C of ≥ 160 mg/dL and family history of premature ASCVD should be considered for statin treatment. The ASCVD pooled risk equation is used to estimate ten-year risk in individuals without known ASCVD or diabetes who are aged 40–75 years. Patients at intermediate risk of 7.5 to < 20%, especially with the presence of risk enhancing factors, should be considered for statin treatment, especially when the clinician–patient risk discussion favors treatment. See Table 18.1. Some individuals carry an intermediate risk and the decision to initiate pharmacologic therapy is uncertain. Further evaluation with a computed tomography (CT) coronary calcium score may help the decision-making process, especially in those with any evidence of coronary calcium and age over 55 years (Grundy et al., 2019). Those with 0 calcium and no significant risk factors can consider moving forward with lifestyle strategies outlined in this chapter. Statins remain the first line treatment for dyslipidemia when pharmacologic management is necessary.

18.2 EVIDENCE FOR SELECTED DIETARY PATTERNS IN THE MANAGEMENT OF DYSLIPIDEMIA

18.2.1 REDUCED SATURATED FAT DIET

The 2018 AHA/ACC Guideline on the Management of Blood Cholesterol continues to support the 2013 guidelines by recommending consumption of a diet rich in vegetables, fruits, whole grains, legumes, healthy protein sources (low-fat dairy and poultry, nuts, and seafood) with limited red meat, non-tropical vegetable oils, and reduced intake of sweets and sweetened beverages (Grundy et al., 2019). Reducing total cholesterol to less than 200 mg/day and saturated fat to less than 7% of

TABLE 18.1
Risk-enhancing factors for clinician–patient risk discussion(Table view)

Risk-Enhancing Factors

Family history of premature ASCVD (males, age < 55 y; females, age < 65 y)

Primary hypercholesterolemia (LDL-C, 160–189 mg/dL [4.1–4.8 mmol/L)] non–HDL-C 190–219 mg/dL [4.9–5.6 mmol/L])*

Metabolic syndrome (increased waist circumference, elevated triglycerides [> 150 mg/dL], elevated blood pressure, elevated glucose, and low HDL-C [< 40 mg/dL in men; < 50 in women mg/dL] are factors; tally of 3 makes the diagnosis)

Chronic kidney disease (eGFR 15–59 mL/min/1.73 m² with or without albuminuria; not treated with dialysis or kidney transplantation)

Chronic inflammatory conditions such as psoriasis, RA, or HIV/AIDS

History of premature menopause (before age 40 y) and history of pregnancy-associated conditions that increase later ASCVD risk such as preeclampsia

High-risk race/ethnicities (e.g., South Asian ancestry)

Lipid/biomarkers: Associated with increased ASCVD risk

Persistently* elevated, primary hypertriglyceridemia (≥ 175 mg/dL);

If measured:

1. Elevated high-sensitivity C-reactive protein (≥ 2.0 mg/L)
2. Elevated Lp(a): A relative indication for its measurement is family history of premature ASCVD. An Lp(a) ≥ 50 mg/dL or ≥ 125 nmol/L constitutes a risk-enhancing factor especially at higher levels of Lp(a).
3. Elevated apoB ≥ 130 mg/dL: A relative indication for its measurement would be triglyceride ≥ 200 mg/dL. A level ≥ 130 mg/dL corresponds to an LDL-C ≥ 160 mg/dL and constitutes a risk-enhancing factor.
4. ABI < 0.9

*Optimally, 3 determinations.

AIDS indicates acquired immunodeficiency syndrome; ABI, ankle-brachial index; apoB, apolipoprotein B; ASCVD, atherosclerotic cardiovascular disease; eGFR, estimated glomerular filtration rate; HDL-C, high-density lipoprotein cholesterol; HIV, human immunodeficiency virus; LDL-C, low-density lipoprotein cholesterol; Lp(a), lipoprotein (a); and RA, rheumatoid arthritis.

Source: Grundy, S. M., Stone, N. J., Bailey, A. L., Beam, C., Birtcher, K. K., Blumenthal, R. S., Braun, L. T., de Ferranti, S., Faiella-Tommasino, J., Forman, D. E., Goldberg, R., Heidenreich, P. A., Hlatky, M. A., Jones, D. W., Lloyd-Jones, D., Lopez-Pajares, N., Ndumele, C. E., Orringer, C. E., Peralta, C. A., … Yeboah, J. (2019). 2018 AHA / ACC / AACVPR / AAPA / A BC / ACPM / ADA / AGS / APhA / ASPC/NLA / PCNA guideline on the management of blood cholesterol: A report of the American College of Cardiology/American Heart Association Task Force on clinical practice guidelines. *Circulation, 139*(25), e1082–e1143. https://doi.org/10.1161/cir.0000000000000625

consumed energy reduced LDL-C by 9–12% compared to baseline diet (Katcher et al., 2009; Van Horn et al., 2008). Avoidance of trans fatty acids (TFA) is advised, as they can raise serum LDL concentrations and have been strongly associated with adverse cardiovascular outcomes (Wojda et al., 2021; Yu et al., 2018). Small intervention studies have found lower total cholesterol, LDL-C, apolipoprotein B, and triglycerides with consumption of tree nuts versus controls (Yu et al., 2018). A meta-analysis by Afshin and colleagues found that approximately 28 g of nuts consumed four times a week had an inverse relationship with fatal and nonfatal ischemic heart disease and diabetes but not stroke (Afshin et al., 2014). They also found that 100 g of legumes four times a week was inversely associated with total ischemic heart disease but not significantly associated with stroke or diabetes (Afshin et al., 2014). An inverse relationship was noted with the intake of apples, pears, citrus fruits, green leafy/cruciferous vegetables, salads, and cardiovascular disease (Aune et al., 2017). Another study by the same author found a 90 g/day increase in whole grain consumption (three servings) was associated with a reduced risk of heart/cardiovascular disease and total cancer, and mortality from all causes, respiratory and infectious diseases, diabetes, and all non-cardiovascular, non-cancer causes. These reductions were observed with up to 210–225 g/day (7 to 7.5 servings per day) of whole grain (Aune et al., 2016). Reductions in cardiovascular disease and all-cause mortality were found with whole grain bread and cereal in addition to bran; however, refined grains, white rice, total rice, and total grains did not show substantial evidence for an association. Galli and colleagues found that 1 g/day of omega 3, or consumption of fatty fish twice a week, had protective effects on the cardiovascular system. Omega 3 has the greatest impact on lowering triglyceride levels, especially with doses of 2 g/day or greater (Galli & Risé, 2009). A meta-analysis found that 1–4 servings of fish per week had a significant effect on the prevention of coronary heart disease (CHD) mortality (Zheng et al., 2012).

18.2.2 MEDITERRANEAN DIET

A Mediterranean diet pattern consists of unprocessed fruits and vegetables, minimal red meat, and use of monounsaturated fatty acids (MUFAs). The PREDIMED Study showed the increased use of MUFAs may lower cardiovascular risk and triglyceride levels, especially when substituting olive oil for other vegetable oils or incorporating a serving of nuts (Sofi et al., 2018; Wojda et al., 2021). When the PREDIMED cohort was reanalyzed post hoc, those in the top two quintiles with the highest vegetarian score had a significant 41% reduction in mortality (Arnett et al., 2019). A study by Gomez Marin et al. (2018) revealed that participants with type 2 diabetes who followed a Mediterranean diet rich in olive oil for three years had a significant triglyceride reduction of 17.3% area under the curve (AUC) (p=0.003) compared to baseline with improvement in postprandial lipemia and remnant cholesterol. Another study also noted a reduction in triglycerides in addition to an increase in HDL-C in patients with type 2 diabetes following the Mediterranean diet and found it to be the most effective in overall reduction of diabetic dyslipidemia (Neuenschwander et al., 2019). Adherence to the Mediterranean diet had an inverse association with cardiometabolic disorders and polypharmacy in over 500 Italian adults aged 50–89 years in one study (Vicinanza et al., 2018). Subjects with low to moderate adherence to a Mediterranean diet had a higher prevalence of arterial hypertension, dyslipidemia, and diabetes compared to those with high adherence (p < 0.001). Conversely, a review of 30 randomized controlled trials (over 12,000 patients) evaluating the benefit of the Mediterranean diet in primary and secondary prevention of cardiovascular disease events and risk factors found some uncertainty regarding its effects (Rees et al., 2019). They found low to moderate quality of evidence supporting the benefits of the Mediterranean diet in cardiovascular risk factors in primary prevention and low quality evidence in reduction of cardiovascular and total mortality (Rees et al., 2019).

18.2.3 CARBOHYDRATE RESTRICTION

Carbohydrate restricted diets can range from mild restriction (45–65% total daily energy) to a very low carbohydrate diet (< 10% total daily energy (Kirkpatrick et al., 2019). Low and very low-carbohydrate diets with high saturated fatty acid content can increase LDL-C; however, genetic factors can play a role in the variability of the LDL-C response (Kirkpatrick et al., 2019). Low and moderate-low carbohydrate diets tend to see more improvements in triglycerides and HDL-C compared to very low-carbohydrate options, though the HDL increase may wane with weight loss or negative energy balance. Very low carbohydrate diets are contraindicated in those with a history of hypertriglyceridemia-associated acute pancreatitis, severe hypertriglyceridemia or inherited severe hypercholesterolemia (Kirkpatrick et al., 2019; Martínez-González et al., 2014). Extreme low and high carbohydrate diets consumed over the long term have been associated with increased all-cause cardiovascular and cancer mortality in the general population (Kirkpatrick et al., 2019).

18.2.4 VEGETARIAN

In 1990, Dean Ornish and colleagues evaluated the progression of atherosclerosis in non-medicated individuals with coronary atherosclerosis who followed a low-fat vegetarian diet, engaged in moderate exercise, managed stress, and quit smoking versus usual care over a period of one year (Ornish et al., 1990). The average diameter of arterial stenosis regressed from 40% to 37.8% in the experimental group and progressed from 42.7% to 46.1% in the control group. Furthermore, in baseline lesions greater than 50%, the average diameter regressed from 61.1% to 55.8% in the experimental group and progressed from 61.7% to 64.4% in the control group (Ornish et al., 1990). The Cardiovascular Prevention with Vegetarian Diet (CARDIVEG) study compared the Mediterranean diet to a vegetarian diet in overweight, low to moderate risk cardiovascular subjects and found better LDL-C reduction with the vegetarian diet by 9.10 mg/dL (p=0.01) in addition to a triglyceride reduction of 12.70 mg/dL (p< 0.01) (Sofi et al., 2018). Both diets had equal effectiveness in reducing body weight, BMI, and fat mass. The PREDIMED study found that high cardiovascular risk omnivorous subjects who followed a food plan emphasizing plant-based foods were at reduced risk for all-cause mortality (Martínez-González et al., 2014).

18.2.5 PLANT-BASED

Studies show that diets high in plant-based foods such as fruits, nuts, and whole grains are associated with a reduced risk of coronary artery disease and stroke due to being rich in mono- and polyunsaturated fatty acids, n-3 fatty acids, antioxidant vitamins, minerals, phytochemicals, fiber, and plant protein (Hu, 2003; Patel et al., 2017). Esselstyn and colleagues found that patients with established cardiovascular disease who followed a plant based diet for 3.7 years had significantly low rates of cardiovascular events compared to those nonadherent to the diet plan (Esselstyn et al., 2014). Data from the Atherosclerosis Risk in Communities (ARIC) study had similar findings with a 19% and 11% lower risk of cardiovascular disease mortality and all-cause mortality in those more adherent to a healthy plant-based diet (H. Kim et al., 2019). Less healthy plant-based foods such as juices, sweetened beverages, refined grains, potatoes/fries, and sweets were associated with higher heart disease risk (Satija et al., 2017). One study compared a low carbohydrate, high vegetable protein diet to a high carbohydrate lacto-ovo vegetarian diet and found similar weight loss with both diets but greater reductions with LDL-C, total cholesterol, HDL-C, and apolipoprotein B-apolipoprotein A1 ratios in the low carbohydrate group (Jenkins et al., 2009).

18.3 DIETARY SUPPLEMENTS

Banach and colleagues (2018) explored the role of nutraceuticals in reducing LDL-C in patients who develop statin-associated muscle symptoms (SAMS). Nutraceuticals can also possibly improve endothelial dysfunction and arterial stiffness in addition to having anti-inflammatory and antioxidative properties. Table 18.2 summarizes the dose, LDL-C lowering, and class/level of evidence for dietary supplements.

18.3.1 RED YEAST RICE (RYR)

Red yeast rice has several bioactive components, with the most abundant being monacolin K, an HMG CoA reductase inhibitor that is structurally identical to lovastatin (Banach et al., 2019). There have been some case reports of rhabdomyolysis, hepatitis, and skin disorders even at low doses; however, in clinical trials the side effects are similar to lovastatin, and average LDL-C lowering in dosages of 1200–4800 mg per day is 36–91 mg/dL (Banach et al., 2019; Banach et al., 2018). The US Food and Drug Administration has prohibited the sale of RYR products containing monacolin K because it is considered an unapproved drug, though there are several RYR products on the market

TABLE 18.2
Dose and effects of nutraceuticals for LDL-C lowering

Product	Class/Level of Recommendation	Dose	LDL Lowering Ranges (Mean mg/dL or %)
Artichoke	IIa/B	1800 mg/day	11–23%
Berberine	I/A	300 mg/day	25 mg/dL, 24%
Bergamot	IIa/B	1300 mg/day	61 mg/dL
Fibers	IIa/A	3–20 g/day	Up to 20%
Garlic	IIa/A	5–6 g/day	9 mg/dL, 20%
Green tea	IIa/A	170–1200 mg/day	7.4 mg/dL
Lupin	IIa/A	25 g/day	4–12%
Plant stanols and sterols	IIa/A	1–3.0 g/day	12 mg/dL, 16%
PUFAs	I/A	1–5 g EPA/DHA/day	Primarily triglycerides
Red yeast rice	I/A	1200–4800 mg/day	36-91 mg/dL
Spirulina	IIa/A	1–10 g/day	41.3 mg/dL
Soy protein	IIa/A	35 mg/day – 25 g/day	< 5 mg/dL

Source: Banach, M., Patti, A. M., Giglio, R. V., Cicero, A. F. G., Atanasov, A. G., Bajraktari, G., Bruckert, E., Descamps, O., Djuric, D. M., Ezhov, M., Fras, Z., Haehling, S., Katsiki, N., Langlois, M., Latkovskis, G., Mancini, J., Mikhailidis, P., Mitchenko, O., & Rizzo, M. (2018). The role of nutraceuticals in statin intolerant patients. *Journal of the American College of Cardiology*, 72(1), 96–118. https://doi.org/10.1016/j.jacc.2018.04.040

and their strength and benefit remain uncertain due to lack of quality control and standardization (Burke, 2015). A study that analyzed 28 brands of RYR found 26 of the brands had 0.09–5.48 mg per 1200 mg of RYR (P. A. Cohen et al., 2017). RYR may be something to consider in patients who will not initiate a statin or have a history of statin-associated side effects, although benefit is uncertain.

18.3.2 PLANT STANOLS/STEROLS

Plant stanols/sterols at 2 g/day can potentially inhibit cholesterol absorption in the intestine and reduce LDL-C by 8–10% (12% at 3 g/day) and triglycerides by 6–9% (Gylling et al., 2014; Trautwein et al., 2018). In a rare genetic disorder called sitosterolemia, plant sterols accumulate in the blood and tissues with decreased biliary excretion. Sitosterolemia has been associated with premature ASCVD in case reports and has led to the hypothesis that plant sterols can increase cardiovascular risk in non-sitosterolemia individuals (Köhler et al., 2017). There are no randomized controlled trials to support the clinical benefit of plant stanols/sterols and consideration should be given when advising these supplements to patients.

18.3.3 FIBER

Soluble fiber such as psyllium, flaxseed, pectin, guar gum, and beta glucans help lower cholesterol by binding with bile acids during the formation of micelles and potentially stimulating bile acid synthesis, reducing hepatic cholesterol content, aiding in upregulating LDL-C receptors, and increasing LDL-C clearance (Santini & Novellino, 2017). The recommended daily allowances for men and women aged 19–50 years old is 38 g/day and 25 g/day. Additionally, several observational studies and a meta-analysis demonstrated the inverse relationship of the intake of dietary fiber and cardiovascular disease (Soliman, 2019).

18.3.4 OMEGA 3 FATTY ACIDS (N-3 FAS)

n-3 FAs are useful in the management of hypertriglyceridemia at a dose of 2–4 g/day. There are dietary supplements and prescription formulations; however, dietary supplements are not reviewed or approved by the FDA for treatment of hypertriglyceridemia (Skulas-Ray et al., 2019). In the GISSI Prevenzione Trial, open-label n-3 PUFAs (eicosapentaenoic acid (EPA) 1.08 g/day) plus vitamin E were given to post MI patients with elevated triglyceride levels. The use of PUFAs reduced triglycerides by 3.4%; however, vitamin E increased the triglycerides by 2.9% (Ng et al., 1999). Prescription omega 3s have not been studied as monotherapy; however, their average triglyceride reduction is approximately 27% (Skulas-Ray et al., 2019). In the Reduction of Cardiovascular Events with Icosapent Ethyl Intervention (REDUCE IT) trial, individuals on a statin with triglycerides 135–499 mg/dL, LDL-C 40–100 mg/dL, and history of ASCVD or diabetes received prescription icosapent ethyl at 4 g/day or placebo. In addition to a reduction in triglycerides, a significant 25% reduction in the primary composite endpoint of cardiovascular death, non-fatal MI, non-fatal stroke, coronary revascularization, or hospitalization for unstable angina ($p = 0.000001$) was observed (Bhatt et al., 2020).

18.3.5 COENZYME Q10 (CoQ10)

Statin-associated muscle symptoms (SAMS) are reported in up to 25% of patients on statin therapy (Parker et al., 2013). There is thought that statins can deplete CoQ10 in the muscle and, by replacing it with supplementation, there may be a reduction in myalgias and improvement in statin tolerance. However, there is conflicting data to support this and studies that have failed to show improvement in muscle symptoms with CoQ10 (Banach et al., 2015; Taylor et al., 2015). As a result of these findings, CoQ10 was not recommended for routine use in patients on statins for treatment of SAMS in the 2018 ACC/AHA Cholesterol Guideline (Grundy et al., 2019).

18.4 EXERCISE AS AN ADJUNCT IN THE MANAGEMENT OF DYSLIPIDEMIA

18.4.1 INTRODUCTION/FITT PRINCIPLE

The 2018 Physical Activity Guidelines recommend at least 150–300 minutes a week of moderate-intensity or 75–150 minutes per week of vigorous-intensity aerobic activity, or an equivalent combination of the two. Muscle strengthening activities should be performed at least twice a week. Sitting less and moving more will likely benefit all individuals and those performing the least will benefit the most with modest increases in moderate or vigorous activity (Piercy et al., 2018). Physical activity can help improve chronic conditions such as dyslipidemia. Consider the FITT principle when recommending an exercise program (frequency, intensity, time, and type of exercise).

18.4.2 AEROBIC EXERCISE

The 2018 AHA/ACC Cholesterol Guideline recommends 30 to 40 minutes of moderate to vigorous intensity exercise, 3–4 sessions per week (Grundy et al., 2019). Many studies show that HDL-C is more sensitive to aerobic exercise than LDL-C and triglyceride levels. A meta-analysis (Kodama et al., 2007) found the minimal amount of exercise to increase HDL-C by a mean 2.53 mg/dL was 120 minutes/week or 900 kcal of energy expenditure per week. Univariate regression analysis suggested that every ten-minute prolongation of exercise per session correlated with an approximate 1.4 mg/dL increase in HDL-C. There was no significant association between exercise frequency or intensity. Exercise appeared to have more of an impact when total cholesterol was greater than

220 or BMI was less than 28 kg/m². Aerobic exercise tends to reduce triglyceride levels; however, elevated baseline triglyceride levels influence the effect of exercise on triglycerides (Wang & Xu, 2017). The effect of aerobic exercise on LDL-C is inconsistent but appears to reduce the concentration of small LDL particles. There appears to be no impact of aerobic activity on lipoprotein(a), and there is varying data on its effect on apolipoprotein B (Wang & Xu, 2017).

18.4.3 RESISTANCE TRAINING

A study by Gordon et al. (2014) summarized the impact of resistance training on lipid markers from various studies and found an approximate 3% reduction in total cholesterol, 6% reduction in triglycerides, 1% increase in HDL-C, 4.5% reduction in LDL-C, and a 6% reduction in non-HDL. Additionally, improvements in two-hour blood glucose levels during a glucose tolerance test, fasting insulin levels, total cholesterol, HDL-C, and LDL-C were seen in chronically disabled, nondiabetic, stroke patients who engaged in lower body resistance training three times a week for eight weeks (Zou et al., 2015).

18.4.4 YOGA

A meta-analysis on the effect of yoga and the parameters of metabolic syndrome only found positive effects on waist circumference and systolic blood pressure and no effect on diastolic blood pressure, fasting glucose, HDL-C, or triglycerides (Cramer et al., 2016). Two studies evaluating the impact of yoga in subjects with diabetes, however, showed reductions in total cholesterol, triglycerides, and LDL-C with improvement of HDL-C (Nagarathna et al., 2019; Shantakumari et al., 2013).

18.5 SUBSTANCE USE AND IMPACT ON DYSLIPIDEMIA AND CV RISK FACTORS

18.5.1 TOBACCO USE

Tobacco use is the leading preventable cause of disability, disease, and death in the United States (Arnett et al., 2019). Forty percent of tobacco related deaths are due to cardiovascular disease (Athyros et al., 2013). Smoking can increase triglycerides, fibrinogen, and C reactive protein and lower HDL-C (Balhara, 2012). It has negative impacts on adipose tissue and accelerates atherosclerosis. Smokers tend to have a higher waist circumference and increased evidence of metabolic syndrome compared to non-smokers, which can persist despite tobacco cessation, although it tends to improve but not to a level as low as non-smokers (Balhara, 2012). The Coronary Diet Intervention with Olive Oil and Cardiovascular Prevention (CORDIOPREV) study found the prevalence of undesirable postprandial hypertriglyceridemia to be 68% in current smokers, 58% in ex-smokers, 49% in long-term ex-smokers, and 48% in never smokers (p < 0.001) (Leon-Acuña et al., 2019). In a case-controlled study, hookah smoking, a non-cigarette tobacco product, was found to be an independent risk factor for first ever ischemic stroke (Tabrizi et al., 2020).

18.5.2 ELECTRONIC CIGARETTES (E-CIGARETTES)

Smokeless tobacco has a varying effect on the lipid panel. E-cigarette use may increase the risk of pulmonary and cardiovascular diseases and release particulates, nicotine, and toxic gases into the air. A study by Kim and colleagues found that e-cigarette use was significantly related to abdominal obesity, metabolic syndrome, and hypertriglyceridemia (T. Kim et al., 2020).

18.5.3 CANNABIS USE

There is sparse and inconsistent high-quality evidence showing an effect of cannabis on lipoproteins. Marginal favorable effects on HDL-C and triglycerides have been observed from smoking cannabis (Lazarte & Hegele, 2019). A review of synthetic cannabinoids found a frequent side effect of tachycardia and less frequent reports of stroke and MI (K. Cohen et al., 2019). One study did identify that among cannabis users, the incidence of MI is 4.8 times higher than baseline one hour following cannabis use and should be avoided in individuals with a history of cardiovascular disease (K. Cohen et al., 2019).

18.5.4 ALCOHOL USE

A study by Du et al. (2017) looked at alcohol consumption in 2200 young adults aged 25–36 years and found moderate alcohol use of 10–20 g/day was at less risk for metabolic syndrome compared to light drinking (0–10 g/day), with better lipid results but not glucose nor blood pressure (Du et al., 2017). The CORDIOPREV study did not find significant differences in alcohol consumption and postprandial hypertriglyceridemia (Leon-Acuña et al., 2019). A J-shaped relationship exists with alcohol consumption and triglyceride levels and this relationship is heightened in obese individuals (Klop et al., 2013). Cross-sectional studies show a positive association between alcohol intake and HDL-C levels. In a Chinese prospective study of 71,379 healthy adults, moderate alcohol consumption (women 0.5–1.0 serving per day; men 1.0–2.0 servings per day) was associated with the slowest decrease in HDL-C over a six-year period (Huang et al., 2017). It's important to recognize that high alcohol intake is also associated with cardiovascular disease (including arrhythmia and cardiomyopathy), hypertension, diabetes, stroke, peripheral arterial disease, fatty liver disease, and pancreatitis (Fernández-Solà, 2015; Klop et al., 2013).

18.6   STRESS AND LIPIDS

Excessive stress may have a detrimental effect on lipids; however, people often cope with stress by engaging in unhealthy behaviors, thus contributing to adverse changes in lipid levels. A recent study (Assadi, 2017) determined the effect of psychological and physical stress on lipid profiles. Results showed that psychological stress was associated with greater triglycerides and LDL-C and with lower HDL-C, although when participants engaged in moderate to heavy physical work, the risk for lipid disorders was reduced. One study investigated people with severe anxiety and depression on tricyclic antidepressants and whether lifestyle factors or biologic stress systems were associated with underlying central obesity or dyslipidemia. The findings suggested that increased obesity and dyslipidemia in those with severe depression and anxiety may be associated with increased C reactive protein and smoking (van Reedt Dortland et al., 2013).

18.7   CONCLUSION

Dyslipidemia is a major risk factor for ASCVD, particularly elevated LDL-C and triglycerides. Additionally, patients with metabolic syndrome, characterized by obesity, elevated fasting glucose, hypertension, low HDL-C, and elevated triglycerides, are at particularly high risk for ASCVD and diabetes. Key contributors to dyslipidemia are genetics, unhealthy dietary choices, sedentary lifestyle, tobacco use, and stress. Lifestyle intervention is the cornerstone of cardiovascular disease prevention, which includes the management of dyslipidemia and metabolic syndrome. For patients with ASCVD who require medications that alter lipids and reduce risk for ASCVD events, lifestyle interventions remain critically important. Dietary interventions discussed in this chapter, e.g., low saturated fat, Mediterranean, vegetarian, and plant-based, are associated with improved lipid parameters and reduced ASCVD events. Soluble fiber and plant stanols/sterols may be adjuncts for additional LDL-C lowering. Regular exercise as recommended by the 2018 Physical Activity Guidelines is essential to improve dyslipidemia, plasma glucose, BMI, and waist circumference.

REFERENCES

Afshin, A., Micha, R., Khatibzadeh, S., & Mozaffarian, D. (2014). Consumption of nuts and legumes and risk of incident ischemic heart disease, stroke, and diabetes: a systematic review and meta-analysis. *American Journal of Clinical Nutrition*, *100*(1), 278–288. https://doi.org/10.3945/ajcn.113.076901

Arnett, D., Blumenthal, R. S., Albert, M. A., Buroker, A., Goldberger, Z., Hahn, E., Dennison-Himmelfarb, C., Khera, A., Lloyd-Jones, D., McEvoy, J., Michos, E., Miedema, M., Munoz, D., Smith, S., Virani, S., Williams, K., Yeboah, J., & Ziaeian, B. (2019). 2019 ACC/AHA guideline on the primary prevention of cardiovascular disease: A report of the American College of Cardiology/American Heart Association Task Force on clinical practice guidelines. *Circulation*, *140*(11), e596–e646. https://doi.org/10.1161/cir.0000000000000678

Assadi, S. N. (2017). What are the effects of psychological stress and physical work on blood lipid profiles? *Medicine (Baltimore)*, *96*(18), e6816. https://doi.org/10.1097/md.0000000000006816

Athyros, V. G., Katsiki, N., Doumas, M., Karagiannis, A., & Mikhailidis, D. P. (2013). Effect of tobacco smoking and smoking cessation on plasma lipoproteins and associated major cardiovascular risk factors: A narrative review. *Current Medical Research and Opinion*, *29*(10), 1263–1274. https://doi.org/10.1185/03007995.2013.827566

Aune, D., Giovannucci, E., Boffetta, P., Fadnes, L. T., Keum, N., Norat, T., Greenwood, D. C., Riboli, E., Vatten, L. J., & Tonstad, S. (2017). Fruit and vegetable intake and the risk of cardiovascular disease, total cancer and all-cause mortality—a systematic review and dose-response meta-analysis of prospective studies. *International Journal of Epidemiology*, *46*(3), 1029–1056. https://doi.org/10.1093/ije/dyw319

Aune, D., Keum, N., Giovannucci, E., Fadnes, L. T., Boffetta, P., Greenwood, D. C., Tonstad, S., Vatten, L. J., Riboli, E., & Norat, T. (2016). Whole grain consumption and risk of cardiovascular disease, cancer, and all cause and cause specific mortality: Systematic review and dose-response meta-analysis of prospective studies. *BMJ*, *353*, i2716. https://doi.org/10.1136/bmj.i2716

Balhara, Y. P. (2012). Tobacco and metabolic syndrome. *Indian Journal of Endocrinology and Metabolism*, *16*(1), 81–87. https://doi.org/10.4103/2230-8210.91197

Banach, M., Bruckert, E., Descamps, O. S., Ellegård, L., Ezhov, M., Föger, B., Fras, Z., Kovanen, P. T., Latkovskis, G., März, W., Panagiotakos, D. B., Paragh, G., Pella, D., Pirillo, A., Poli, A., Reiner, Ž., Silbernagel, G., Viigimaa, M., Vrablík, M., & Catapano, A. L. (2019). The role of red yeast rice (RYR) supplementation in plasma cholesterol control: A review and expert opinion. *Atherosclerosis Supplements*, *39*, e1–e8. https://doi.org/10.1016/j.atherosclerosissup.2019.08.023

Banach, M., Patti, A. M., Giglio, R. V., Cicero, A. F. G., Atanasov, A. G., Bajraktari, G., Bruckert, E., Descamps, O., Djuric, D. M., Ezhov, M., Fras, Z., Haehling, S., Katsiki, N., Langlois, M., Latkovskis, G., Mancini, J., Mikhailidis, P., Mitchenko, O., & Rizzo, M. (2018). The role of nutraceuticals in statin intolerant patients. *Journal of the American College of Cardiology*, *72*(1), 96–118. https://doi.org/10.1016/j.jacc.2018.04.040

Banach, M., Serban, C., Sahebkar, A., Ursoniu, S., Rysz, J., Muntner, P., Toth, P. P., Jones, S. R., Rizzo, M., Glassner, S. P., Lip, G. Y. H., Dragan, S., & Mikhailidis, D. P. (2015). Effects of coenzyme Q10 on statin-induced myopathy: a meta-analysis of randomized controlled trials. *Mayo Clinic Proceedings*, *90*(1), 24–34. https://doi.org/10.1016/j.mayocp.2014.08.021

Bhatt, D. L., Miller, M., Brinton, E. A., Jacobson, T. A., Steg, P. G., Ketchum, S. B., Doyle, R. T., Jr., Juliano, R. A., Jiao, L., Granowitz, C., Tardif, J-C., Olshansky, B., Chung, M. K., Gibson, C. M., Giugliano, R. P., Budoff, M. J., & Ballantyne, C. M. (2020). REDUCE-IT USA: Results From the 3146 patients randomized in the United States. *Circulation*, *141*(5), 367–375. https://doi.org/10.1161/circulationaha.119.044440

Burke, F. M. (2015). Red yeast rice for the treatment of dyslipidemia. *Current Atherosclerosis Reports*, *17*(4), 495. https://doi.org/10.1007/s11883-015-0495-8

Cannon, C. P., Steinberg, B. A., Murphy, S. A., Mega, J. L., & Braunwald, E. (2006). Meta-analysis of cardiovascular outcomes trials comparing intensive versus moderate statin therapy. *Journal of the American College of Cardiology*, *48*(3), 438–445. https://doi.org/10.1016/j.jacc.2006.04.070

Cohen, K., Weizman, A., & Weinstein, A. (2019). Positive and negative effects of cannabis and cannabinoids on health. *Clinical Pharmacology and Therapeutics*, *105*(5), 1139–1147. https://doi.org/10.1002/cpt.1381

Cohen, P. A., Avula, B., & Khan, I. A. (2017). Variability in strength of red yeast rice supplements purchased from mainstream retailers. *European Journal of Preventive Cardiology*, *24*(13), 1431–1434. https://doi.org/10.1177/2047487317715714

Cramer, H., Langhorst, J., Dobos, G., & Lauche, R. (2016). Yoga for metabolic syndrome: A systematic review and meta-analysis. *European Journal of Preventive Cardiology*, *23*(18), 1982–1993. https://doi.org/10.1177/2047487316665729

Du, D., Bruno, R., Dwyer, T., Venn, A., & Gall, S. (2017). Associations between alcohol consumption and cardio-metabolic risk factors in young adults. *European Journal of Preventive Cardiology*, *24*(18), 1967–1978. https://doi.org/10.1177/2047487317724008

Esselstyn, C. B., Jr., Gendy, G., Doyle, J., Golubic, M., & Roizen, M. F. (2014). A way to reverse CAD? *Journal of Family Practice*, *63*(7), 356–364b.

Fernández-Solà, J. (2015). Cardiovascular risks and benefits of moderate and heavy alcohol consumption. *Nature Reviews Cardiology*, *12*(10), 576–587. https://doi.org/10.1038/nrcardio.2015.91

Galli, C., & Risé, P. (2009). Fish consumption, omega 3 fatty acids and cardiovascular disease. The science and the clinical trials. *Nutrition and Health*, *20*(1), 11–20. https://doi.org/10.1177/026010600902000102

Gomez-Marin, B., Gomez-Delgado, F., Lopez-Moreno, J., Alcala-Diaz, J. F., Jimenez-Lucena, R., Torres-Peña, J. D., Garcia-Rios, A., Ortiz-Morales, A. M., Yubero-Serrano, E. M., del Mar Malagon, M., Lai, C. Q., Delgado-Lista, J., Ordovas, J. M., Lopez-Miranda, J., & Perez-Martinez, P. (2018). Long-term consumption of a Mediterranean diet improves postprandial lipemia in patients with type 2 diabetes: The Cordioprev randomized trial. *American Journal of Clinical Nutrition*, *108*(5), 963–970. https://doi.org/10.1093/ajcn/nqy144

Gordon, B., Chen, S., & Durstine, J. L. (2014). The effects of exercise training on the traditional lipid profile and beyond. *Current Sports Medicine Reports*, *13*(4), 253–259. https://doi.org/10.1249/JSR.0000000000000073

Gotto, A. M. (2005). Evolving concepts of dyslipidemia, atherosclerosis, and cardiovascular disease. *Journal of the American College of Cardiology*, *46*(7), 1219–1224. https://doi.org/10.1016/j.jacc.2005.06.059

Grundy, S. M., Stone, N. J., Bailey, A. L., Beam, C., Birtcher, K. K., Blumenthal, R. S., Braun, L. T., de Ferranti, S., Faiella-Tommasino, J., Forman, D. E., Goldberg, R., Heidenreich, P. A., Hlatky, M. A., Jones, D. W., Lloyd-Jones, D., Lopez-Pajares, N., Ndumele, C. E., Orringer, C. E., Peralta, C. A., ... Yeboah, J. (2019). 2018 AHA / ACC / AACVPR / AAPA /A BC / ACPM / ADA / AGS / APhA / ASPC/ NLA / PCNA guideline on the management of blood cholesterol: A report of the American College of Cardiology/American Heart Association Task Force on clinical practice guidelines. *Circulation*, *139*(25), e1082–e1143. https://doi.org/10.1161/cir.0000000000000625

Gylling, H., Plat, J., Turley, S., Ginsberg, H. N., Ellegård, L., Jessup, W., Jones, P. M., Lütjohann, D., Maerz, W., Masana, L., Silbernagel, G., Staels, B., Borén, J., Catapano, A. L., De Backer, G., Deanfield, J., Descamps, O. S., Kovanen, P. T., Riccardi, G., ... Chapman, M. J. (2014). Plant sterols and plant stanols in the management of dyslipidaemia and prevention of cardiovascular disease. *Atherosclerosis*, *232*(2), 346–360. https://doi.org/10.1016/j.atherosclerosis.2013.11.043

Hu, F. B. (2003). Plant-based foods and prevention of cardiovascular disease: an overview. *American Journal of Clinical Nutrition*, *78*(3 Suppl.), 544s–551s. https://doi.org/10.1093/ajcn/78.3.544S

Huang, S., Li, J., Shearer, G. C., Lichtenstein, A. H., Zheng, X., Wu, Y., Jin, C., Wu, S., & Gao, X. (2017). Longitudinal study of alcohol consumption and HDL concentrations: a community-based study. *American Journal of Clinical Nutrition*, *105*(4), 905–912. https://doi.org/10.3945/ajcn.116.144832

Jenkins, D. J., Wong, J. M., Kendall, C. W., Esfahani, A., Ng, V. W., Leong, T. C., Faulkner, D. A., Vidgen, E., Greaves, K. A., Paul, G., & Singer, W. (2009). The effect of a plant-based low-carbohydrate ("Eco-Atkins") diet on body weight and blood lipid concentrations in hyperlipidemic subjects. *Archives of Internal Medicine*, *169*(11), 1046–1054. https://doi.org/10.1001/archinternmed.2009.115

Katcher, H. I., Hill, A. M., Lanford, J. L., Yoo, J. S., & Kris-Etherton, P. M. (2009). Lifestyle approaches and dietary strategies to lower LDL-cholesterol and triglycerides and raise HDL-cholesterol. *Endocrinology & Metabolism Clinics of North America*, *38*(1), 45–78. https://doi.org/10.1016/j.ecl.2008.11.010

Kim, H., Caulfield, L. E., Garcia-Larsen, V., Steffen, L. M., Coresh, J., & Rebholz, C. M. (2019). Plant-based diets are associated with a lower risk of incident cardiovascular disease, cardiovascular disease mortality, and all-cause mortality in a general population of middle-aged adults. *Journal of the American Heart Association, 8*(16), e012865. https://doi.org/10.1161/jaha.119.012865

Kim, T., Choi, H., Kang, J., & Kim, J. (2020). Association between electronic cigarette use and metabolic syndrome in the Korean general population: A nationwide population-based study. *PLoS One, 15*(8), e0237983. https://doi.org/10.1371/journal.pone.0237983

Kirkpatrick, C. F., Bolick, J. P., Kris-Etherton, P. M., Sikand, G., Aspry, K. E., Soffer, D. E., Willard, K-E., & Maki, K. C. (2019). Review of current evidence and clinical recommendations on the effects of low-carbohydrate and very-low-carbohydrate (including ketogenic) diets for the management of body weight and other cardiometabolic risk factors: A scientific statement from the National Lipid Association Nutrition and Lifestyle Task Force. *Journal of Clinical Lipidology, 13*(5), 689–711.e681. https://doi.org/10.1016/j.jacl.2019.08.003

Klop, B., do Rego, A. T., & Cabezas, M. C. (2013). Alcohol and plasma triglycerides. *Current Opinions on Lipidology, 24*(4), 321–326. https://doi.org/10.1097/MOL.0b013e3283606845

Kodama, S., Tanaka, S., Saito, K., Shu, M., Sone, Y., Onitake, F., Shimano, H., Yamamato, S., Kondo, K., Ohashi, Y., Yamada, N., & Sone, H. (2007). Effect of aerobic exercise training on serum levels of high-density lipoprotein cholesterol: a meta-analysis. *Arch Intern Med, 167*(10), 999–1008. https://doi.org/10.1001/archinte.167.10.999

Köhler, J., Teupser, D., Elsässer, A., & Weingärtner, O. (2017). Plant sterol enriched functional food and atherosclerosis. *British Journal of Pharmacology, 174*(11), 1281–1289. https://doi.org/10.1111/bph.13764

Lazarte, J., & Hegele, R. A. (2019). Cannabis effects on lipoproteins. *Current Opinions on Lipidology, 30*(2), 140–146. https://doi.org/10.1097/mol.0000000000000575

Leon-Acuña, A., Torres-Peña, J. D., Alcala-Diaz, J. F., Vals-Delgado, C., Roncero-Ramos, I., Yubero-Serrano, E., Tinahones, F. J., Castro-Clerico, M., Delgado-Lista, J., Ordovas, J., M., Lopez-Miranda, J., & Perez-Martinez, P. (2019). Lifestyle factors modulate postprandial hypertriglyceridemia: From the CORDIOPREV study. *Atherosclerosis, 290*, 118–124. https://doi.org/10.1016/j.atherosclerosis.2019.09.025

Martínez-González, M. A., Sánchez-Tainta, A., Corella, D., Salas-Salvadó, J., Ros, E., Arós, F., Gómez-Gracia, E., Fiol, M., Lamuela-Raventós, R. M., Schröder, H., Lapetra, J., Serra-Majem,, L., Pinto, X., Ruiz-Gutierrez, V., & Estruch, R. (2014). A provegetarian food pattern and reduction in total mortality in the Prevención con Dieta Mediterránea (PREDIMED) study. *American Journal of Clinical Nutrition, 100 Suppl 1*, 320s–328s. https://doi.org/10.3945/ajcn.113.071431

Nagarathna, R., Tyagi, R., Kaur, G., Vendan, V., Acharya, I. N., Anand, A., Singh, A., & Nagendra, H. R. (2019). Efficacy of a validated yoga protocol on dyslipidemia in diabetes patients: NMB-2017 India trial. *Medicines (Basel), 6*(4). https://doi.org/10.3390/medicines6040100

Neuenschwander, M., Hoffmann, G., Schwingshackl, L., & Schlesinger, S. (2019). Impact of different dietary approaches on blood lipid control in patients with type 2 diabetes mellitus: A systematic review and network meta-analysis. *European Journal of Epidemiology, 34*(9), 837–852. https://doi.org/10.1007/s10654-019-00534-1

Ng, W., Tse, H. F., & Lau, C. P. (1999). GISSI-Prevenzione trial. *Lancet, 354*(9189), 1555–1556; author reply 1556–1557. https://doi.org/10.1016/s0140-6736(05)76584-3

Nordestgaard, B. G. (2016). Triglyceride-rich lipoproteins and atherosclerotic cardiovascular disease: New insights from epidemiology, genetics, and biology. *Circulation Research, 118*(4), 547–563. https://doi.org/10.1161/circresaha.115.306249

Ornish, D., Brown, S. E., Scherwitz, L. W., Billings, J. H., Armstrong, W. T., Ports, T. A., McLanahan, S. M., Kirkeeide, R. L., Gould, K. L., & Brand, R. J. (1990). Can lifestyle changes reverse coronary heart disease? The Lifestyle Heart Trial. *Lancet, 336*(8708), 129–133. https://doi.org/10.1016/0140-6736(90)91656-u

Parker, B. A., Capizzi, J. A., Grimaldi, A. S., Clarkson, P. M., Cole, S. M., Keadle, J., Chipkin, S., Pescatello, L. S., Simpson, K., White, C. M., & Thompson, P. D. (2013). Effect of statins on skeletal muscle function. *Circulation, 127*(1), 96–103. https://doi.org/10.1161/circulationaha.112.136101

Patel, H., Chandra, S., Alexander, S., Soble, J., & Williams, K. A., Sr. (2017). Plant-based nutrition: An essential component of cardiovascular disease prevention and management. *Current Cardiology Reports, 19*(10), 104. https://doi.org/10.1007/s11886-017-0909-z

Piercy, K. L., Troiano, R. P., Ballard, R. M., Carlson, S. A., Fulton, J. E., Galuska, D. A., George, S. M., & Olson, R. D. (2018). The physical activity guidelines for Americans. *Jama, 320*(19), 2020–2028. https://doi.org/10.1001/jama.2018.14854

Rees, K., Takeda, A., Martin, N., Ellis, L., Wijesekara, D., Vepa, A., Das, A., Hartley, L., & Stranges, S. (2019). Mediterranean-style diet for the primary and secondary prevention of cardiovascular disease. *Cochrane Database of Systematic Reviews, 3*(3), Cd009825. https://doi.org/10.1002/14651858.CD009825.pub3

Reiner, Ž. (2017). Hypertriglyceridaemia and risk of coronary artery disease. *Nature Revies Cardiology, 14*(7), 401–411. https://doi.org/10.1038/nrcardio.2017.31

Santini, A., & Novellino, E. (2017). Nutraceuticals in hypercholesterolaemia: an overview. *British Journal of Pharmacology, 174*(11), 1450–1463. https://doi.org/10.1111/bph.13636

Satija, A., Bhupathiraju, S. N., Spiegelman, D., Chiuve, S. E., Manson, J. E., Willett, W., Rexrode, K. M., Rimm, E. B., & Hu, F. B. (2017). Healthful and unhealthful plant-based diets and the risk of coronary heart disease in U.S. adults. *Journal of the American College of Cardiology, 70*(4), 411–422. https://doi.org/10.1016/j.jacc.2017.05.047

Shantakumari, N., Sequeira, S., & El deeb, R. (2013). Effects of a yoga intervention on lipid profiles of diabetes patients with dyslipidemia. *Indian Heart Journal, 65*(2), 127–131. https://doi.org/10.1016/j.ihj.2013.02.010

Skulas-Ray, A. C., Wilson, P. W. F., Harris, W. S., Brinton, E. A., Kris-Etherton, P. M., Richter, C. K., Jacobson, T. A., Engler, M. B., Miller, M., Robinson, J. G., Blum, C. B., Rodriguez-Levya, D., de Ferranti, S. D., & Welty, F. K. (2019). Omega-3 fatty acids for the management of hypertriglyceridemia: A science advisory from the American Heart Association. *Circulation, 140*(12), e673–e691. https://doi.org/10.1161/cir.0000000000000709

Sofi, F., Dinu, M., Pagliai, G., Cesari, F., Gori, A. M., Sereni, A., Becatti, M., Fiorillo, C., Marcucci, R., & Casini, A. (2018). Low-calorie vegetarian versus Mediterranean diets for reducing body weight and improving cardiovascular risk profile: CARDIVEG study (cardiovascular prevention with vegetarian diet). *Circulation, 137*(11), 1103–1113. https://doi.org/10.1161/circulationaha.117.030088

Soliman, G. A. (2019). Dietary fiber, atherosclerosis, and cardiovascular disease. *Nutrients, 11*(5). https://doi.org/10.3390/nu11051155

Tabrizi, R., Borhani-Haghighi, A., Lankarani, K. B., Heydari, S. T., Bayat, M., Vakili, S., Maharlouei, N., Hassanzadeh, J., Zafarmand, S. S., Owjfard, M., Avan, A., & Azarpazhooh, M. R. (2020). Hookah smoking: A potentially risk factor for first-ever ischemic stroke. *Journal of Stroke and Cerebrovascular Disease, 29*(10), 105138. https://doi.org/10.1016/j.jstrokecerebrovasdis.2020.105138

Taylor, B. A., Lorson, L., White, C. M., & Thompson, P. D. (2015). A randomized trial of coenzyme Q10 in patients with confirmed statin myopathy. *Atherosclerosis, 238*(2), 329–335. https://doi.org/10.1016/j.atherosclerosis.2014.12.016

Trautwein, E. A., Vermeer, M. A., Hiemstra, H., & Ras, R. T. (2018). LDL-cholesterol lowering of plant sterols and stanols—which factors influence their efficacy? *Nutrients, 10*(9). https://doi.org/10.3390/nu10091262

Van Horn, L., McCoin, M., Kris-Etherton, P. M., Burke, F., Carson, J. A., Champagne, C. M., Karmally, W., & Sikand, G. (2008). The evidence for dietary prevention and treatment of cardiovascular disease. *Journal of American Diet Association, 108*(2), 287–331. https://doi.org/10.1016/j.jada.2007.10.050

van Reedt Dortland, A. K., Vreeburg, S. A., Giltay, E. J., Licht, C. M., Vogelzangs, N., van Veen, T., de Geus, E. J. C., Penninx, B., W. J. H., & Zitman, F. G. (2013). The impact of stress systems and lifestyle on dyslipidemia and obesity in anxiety and depression. *Psychoneuroendocrinology, 38*(2), 209–218. https://doi.org/10.1016/j.psyneuen.2012.05.017

Vicinanza, R., Troisi, G., Cangemi, R., De Martino, M. U., Pastori, D., Bernardini, S., Crisciotti, F., di Violante, F., Frizza, A., Cacciafesta, M., Pignatelli, P., & Marigliano, V. (2018). Aging and adherence to the Mediterranean diet: Relationship with cardiometabolic disorders and polypharmacy. *Journal of Nutrition, Health, & Aging, 22*(1), 73–81. https://doi.org/10.1007/s12603-017-0922-3

Wang, Y., & Xu, D. (2017). Effects of aerobic exercise on lipids and lipoproteins. *Lipids in Health and Disease, 16*(1), 132. https://doi.org/10.1186/s12944-017-0515-5

Wojda, A., Janczy, A., & Małgorzewicz, S. (2021). Mediterranean, vegetarian and vegan diets as practical outtakes of EAS and ACC/AHA recommendations for lowering lipid profile. *Acta Biochimica Polonica, 68*(1). https://doi.org/10.18388/abp.2020_5515

Yu, E., Malik, V. S., & Hu, F. B. (2018). Reprint of: Cardiovascular disease prevention by diet modification: JACC health promotion series. *Journal of the American College of Cardiology, 72*(23 Pt B), 2951–2963. https://doi.org/10.1016/j.jacc.2018.10.019

Zheng, J., Huang, T., Yu, Y., Hu, X., Yang, B., & Li, D. (2012). Fish consumption and CHD mortality: An updated meta-analysis of seventeen cohort studies. *Public Health Nutrition*, *15*(4), 725–737. https://doi.org/10.1017/s1368980011002254

Zou, J., Wang, Z., Qu, Q., & Wang, L. (2015). Resistance training improves hyperglycemia and dyslipidemia, highly prevalent among nonelderly, nondiabetic, chronically disabled stroke patients. *Archives of Physical Medicine and Rehabilitation*, *96*(7), 1291–1296. https://doi.org/10.1016/j.apmr.2015.03.008

19 Autoimmune Disease

Nanette Morales[1], Jessica Landry[2],
Christy McDonald Lenahan[2], and Janine Santora[3]
[1]Ochsner Hospital and Clinic
New Orleans, Louisiana, USA
[2]School of Nursing, University of Louisiana
Lafayette, Louisiana, USA
[3]Capital Health Institute for Neurosciences
Pennington, NJ, USA

CONTENTS

DOI: 10.1201/9781003178330-22

KEY POINTS

- Autoimmune disease (AD) is when the human body turns against itself, causing chronic inflammation that damages body organs and tissues.
- Lifestyle habits associated with increased systemic inflammation are strongly linked to the development of autoimmune disease.
- Genetic susceptibility and environmental triggers can precede the development of AD.
- Although traditionally managed with conventional pharmaceuticals, lifestyle therapies are a remarkable preventative and therapeutic approach to AD treatment.

19.1 INTRODUCTION

Autoimmune diseases (AD) cause the human body to turn against itself, causing chronic inflammation that damages body organs and tissues (National Institute of Environmental Health Sciences [NIEHS], 2021). Chronic inflammation leads to chronic disease, which causes a multitude of symptoms, lowers quality of life, and impacts life expectancy. Chronic diseases are the leading cause of morbidity and mortality (Bodai, 2017). The prevalence of AD in the US is 50 million people (Leech et al., 2020). In comparison, cancer affects 14.5 million people and heart disease affects 22 million people. The direct and indirect cost burden of ADs is estimated to range between $86 and $100 billion annually (AARDA & NCAPG, 2011). Epidemiological data support evidence to show the steady rise in AD in westernized societies over the last 30 years (Lerner et al., 2016). The rise in AD in westernized societies has led researchers to believe environmental factors may have a stronger influence on the development of autoimmune disorders than genetic factors.

19.2 PATHOPHYSIOLOGY

An immune system that functions properly protects humans from invading hosts that cause disease or infection (Lerner et al., 2016). The immune system consists of proteins and cells that recognize invaders and implement an inflammatory response to destroy the invading pathogens. The immune system uses inflammation as a central component to eliminate pathogens and repair tissue (Kopp, 2019). Once activated, the immune system secretes pro-inflammatory cytokines, triggering the production of free radicals until the body is healed. The immune system recognizes pathogens as foreign due to a protein called human leukocyte antigen, which is present on the surface of every cell in the human body. A malfunctioning immune system will attack its own cells, leading to chronic inflammation, which leads to chronic disease.

What happens when our own bodies turn against us and attack healthy cells that are no longer recognized as one's own? If a person's immune system goes into overdrive attacking healthy cells, it can manifest as AD (Kopp, 2019). In AD, the body's immune response breaks down and forms auto-antibodies against normal cells, which causes a cascade of inflammation-causing damage to healthy cells. AD can wreak havoc on the entire human body, including the digestive system, glands, organs, nervous system, skin, joints, and muscles.

19.3 SPECIFIC AUTOIMMUNE DISORDERS

AD can be systemic or target body organs (Leech et al., 2020). Organ-specific ADs produce an immune response to a specific tissue or organ (Ray et al., 2012). Examples of organ-specific ADs include type 1 diabetes (T1D), myasthenia gravis, Addison's disease, and autoimmune hepatitis (Ray et al., 2012). Systemic ADs produce an immune response to multiple organs and result in chronic activation of adaptive immune cells (T and B lymphocytes). Examples of systemic ADs include rheumatoid arthritis (RA), systemic lupus erythematosus (SLE), and multiple sclerosis (MS) (Ray et al., 2012).

There are approximately 100 ADs (Richard-Eaglin & Smallheer, 2018). Women are three times more likely to be affected by AD than men (Houghton, 2021). Evidence suggests that individuals diagnosed with a primary AD are at higher risk for developing multiple ADs. Some of the most prevalent ADs will be described next.

19.3.1 Rheumatoid Arthritis (RA)

RA is a form of autoimmune polyarthritis that attacks the joints (Richard-Eaglin & Smallheer, 2018). RA damages bones and cartilage, lowers the white blood count, causes subcutaneous nodules, and can also affect the eyes. The hallmark of RA is swelling of the joints, most often in the hands and feet (Alwarith et al., 2019). RA can cause debilitating symptoms such as joint stiffness, loss of function, chronic pain, and fatigue, particularly in the morning after long rest periods. If RA is untreated, an individual's mortality risk increases. RA is more prevalent in women and affects approximately 1% of the population.

19.3.2 Systemic Lupus Erythematosus (SLE)

SLE is a systemic AD that can attack various parts of the body, including skin, organs, and joints (Richard-Eaglin & Smallheer, 2018). SLE can cause a multitude of symptoms, including fatigue, joint pain, end-stage renal disease, pericarditis, anemia, psychosis, and malar rash. SLE is classified into three patterns: (1) quiescent, which indicates the disease is present but not active, (2) intermittent, which involves flare-up episodes and remission, and (3) chronically active, which involves organs. SLE can be caused by genetic susceptibility and environmental exposures (Rojas et al., 2018).

19.3.3 Celiac Disease

Celiac disease is an AD that attacks the small intestines when exposed to gluten products (Parzanese et al., 2017). Celiac disease causes a mucosal impairment of the small intestine, leading to impaired absorption of nutrients and triggering symptoms including diarrhea, constipation, abdominal bloating, or pale, fatty, foul-smelling stool. Individuals with T1D or thyroid disease are at a higher risk of developing celiac disease. Celiac disease increases the risk of cancer.

19.3.4 Inflammatory Bowel Disease

Inflammatory bowel disease (IBD) is an AD that attacks the immune system on the intestinal lining of the bowel, inflicting pain, urgent bowel movements, diarrhea, and weight loss (Richard-Eaglin & Smallheer, 2018). IBD is chronic inflammation of the intestinal tract. Both ulcerative colitis and Crohn's disease are types of IBD. An individual diagnosed with IBD is at increased risk of developing cancer.

19.3.5 Multiple Sclerosis (MS)

MS is an AD that attacks nerve cells causing many debilitating symptoms, including vision loss, weakness, pain, and poor coordination (Ghasemi et al., 2017). The inflammation in MS causes the erosion of the myelin sheath of the nerves, causing a communication disruption between the brain and body (Richard-Eaglin & Smallheer, 2018). The disruption of communication can cause an array of debilitating symptoms, including paresthesias (typically an early symptom), fatigue (70%), pain (30–50%), eye symptoms (33%) that can lead to chronic disability, and decreased quality of life.

19.3.6   TYPE 1 DIABETES (T1D)

T1D is caused by an autoimmune attack on the insulin-producing beta cells in the pancreas and thus requires lifetime insulin for survival (Rojas et al., 2018). T1D is one of the most common ADs. T1D is typically diagnosed in children and young adults. T1D was previously known as juvenile diabetes. Genetic susceptibility and exposure to environmental factors such as vitamin D deficiency, maternal age, exposure to chemicals, infant diet, and gut microbiota may trigger the onset of T1D.

19.3.7   SJOGREN'S SYNDROME

Sjogren's syndrome (SS) is an organ-specific AD (Rojas et al., 2018). SS can affect any endocrine gland. SS primarily affects the lachrymal glands and salivary glands, causing dry mouth and dry eyes. Genetically predisposed susceptibility paired with exposure to viruses such as herpes simplex virus and Epstein-Barr virus may trigger the onset of SS.

19.3.8   AUTOIMMUNE THYROID DISEASES

Autoimmune thyroid disease (ATD) is one of the most common AD. ATDs include Grave's disease (GD), leading to an overproduction of thyroid hormone, and Hashimoto's thyroiditis (HT), leading to an underproduction of thyroid hormone (Richard-Eaglin & Smallheer, 2018). ATD is one of the most prevalent autoimmune disorders. GD can produce various symptoms, including ophthalmopathy (50%), nervousness, weight loss, erectile dysfunction, metrorrhagia, tachycardia, and palpitations. HT can produce a multitude of symptoms, including weight gain, fatigue, dry skin, and constipation. Women are more susceptible to the development of ATDs. Environmental factors such as cigarette smoking, stress, infection, medication, and radiation may trigger ATDs.

19.4   ETIOLOGY

The etiology of ADs is multifactorial (Rosenblum et al., 2015). Possible causes of immune dysfunction include genetics, molecular mimicry, leaky gut, environmental factors, hormone imbalances, chronic infections, mental and emotional stress, specific drugs, and diet (Cohen, 2021; Houghton, 2021). The prevalence of AD is impacted by environmental factors that contribute to 70% of AD development (Leech et al., 2020). Three major environmental factors, which are closely linked to socioeconomic status, include nutrition, ecology, and infections (Lerner et al., 2016).

19.4.1   GENETICS

Most ADs are polygenic and cannot be attributed to one specific gene, with rare exceptions (Okada et al., 2019). Genetics can increase the risk of AD. A combination of genetic susceptibility and exposure to environmental triggers such as smoking and viruses can trigger the onset of autoimmune disease. X chromosomes are also responsible for a greater number of immune responses and immune regulatory genes. Because women have two X chromosomes and men have only one, they are at greater risk for developing ADs (Angum et al., 2020). Siblings are also at an increased risk of developing SLE when compared to the general population (Richard-Eaglin & Smallheer, 2018). SLE risk increases 10 -fold in identical twins.

19.4.2   MOLECULAR MIMICRY

Molecular mimicry involves activation of autoreactive T or B cells by a foreign antigen, such as infections or chemical agents that cause autoimmunity (Rojas et al., 2018). Examples include C. jejuni infection preceding Guillain-Barre syndrome, bovine milk protein butyrophilin preceding MS, and Escherichia coli (E. coli), hepatitis C & B, HIV, or Epstein-Barr virus preceding RA. Molecular mimicry cross-reactivity combines environmental and genetic factors triggering autoimmunity. The molecular mimicry theory may explain why some foods trigger or worsen ADs (Houghton, 2021).

19.4.3   LEAKY GUT

Leaky gut is a dysfunction in the gastrointestinal system (López-Taboada et al., 2020). When the gastrointestinal system has a breach and undigested food, toxins, or bacteria enter the circulatory system, with potential to penetrate the blood–brain barrier. When toxins from the gut leak into the body, the immune system reacts as if invaded and causes inflammation. Healthy gut bacteria benefit from a diet including micronutrients and macronutrients. Neonatal diet is important during the formation of gut microbiota. Infants breastfed have beneficial gut bacteria when compared to formula-fed infants who can develop pathological gut bacteria. A Standard American Diet (SAD) can negatively affect gut bacteria, leading to autoimmune disease, neuropsychiatric disorders, obesity, diabetes, allergies, and metabolic syndrome.

19.4.4   ENVIRONMENTAL FACTORS

Pollutants found in air consist of a mixture of gasses, aerosols, and particulate matter (Gawda et al., 2017). Though the correlation between size and type of the pollutant and development or exacerbation of ADs is unclear, there is evidence to suggest that increased levels of pollutants can result in inflammatory responses that may promote ADs via the production of autoantigens and stimulation of pro-inflammatory cytokines. Studies have shown a link between psychological stress and increased rates of ADs (Dube et al., 2009; Song et al., 2018). Another well-known environmental trigger for ADs is infectious organisms containing fragments of cellular protein or epitopes identical to the self-epitopes of the host (Gershteyn & Ferreira, 2019).

19.4.5   HORMONE IMBALANCES

According to Tsai et al. (2015), T and B cells are found to infiltrate the visceral adipose tissue in obese people, causing an inflammatory status equivalent to the degree of insulin resistance. Furthermore, changes in subclasses of IgGs are also seen in patients with obesity-related insulin resistance. Adaptive immune pathways are believed to contribute to insulin resistance, impact B cell function, and overall metabolism (Tsai et al., 2015).

High levels of estrogen can be helpful or harmful depending on the disease process and patient age (Desai & Brinton, 2019). In ADs such as rheumatoid arthritis and SS, elevated estrogen levels decrease inflammation through increases in regulatory cytokines and transformation of growth factor-B. However, in patients with SLE, higher levels of estrogen can be found in the synovial fluid. It is theorized that in these patients, 17-B-estradiol, the major estrogen secreted by the premenopausal ovary, activates macrophages on immunocompetent cells and promotes pro-inflammatory cytokine production (Angum, 2020).

19.4.6   PATHOGENS

Chronic infections from various pathogens can result in development of ADs (Sherbet, 2009). Bacterial and viral infections are commonly seen in AD. Presence of pathogens over time can result in increased inflammation such as activation of inflammatory cytokines leading to various ADs.

19.4.7 Mental and Emotional Stress

Similar to the body's response to pollutants, psychoneuroimmunology researchers hypothesize that increased psychological stressors result in increased pro-inflammatory cytokines, which promote an overactive immune system and can result in increased rates of ADs (Song et al., 2018). When an individual experiences a stressful situation, an event that exceeds one's perceived ability to cope, the hypothalamic–pituitary–adrenal axis and the sympathetic–adrenal medullary axis are activated, resulting in the release of immune-modulating hormones (Seiler et al., 2020). The presence of stressors has been correlated to slower wound healing, increased risk of viral infection, increased presence of cardiovascular disease, increased risk of type 2 diabetes, and increased risk of specific cancers and progression of immunogenic tumors (Seiler et al., 2020).

19.4.8 Autoimmune Diseases

The most commonly studied and diagnosed drug-induced AD is SLE. Approximately 10 to 15% of SLE cases diagnosed annually are caused by a specific drug (Niklas et al., 2016). Over 90 different drugs have been known to cause drug-induced SLE; however, the greatest risk occurs with procainamide (20% occurrence rate in the first year) and hydralazine (5–8% occurrence rate in the first year; Niklas et al., 2016). Other drug-induced ADs include, but are not limited to, autoimmune hepatitis, systemic sclerosis, and ulcerative colitis.

19.4.9 Diet

Diet has been shown to have a direct impact on the development and progression of ADs.

For the last 6–8 generations, western populations have experienced an epidemic of "civilization diseases" caused by the western diet and lifestyle (Kopp, 2019). Civilization diseases (chronic non-infectious degenerative diseases) include ADs, obesity, cancer, diabetes, and Alzheimer's disease, among others. Civilization diseases like AD are virtually absent in non-westernized populations.

19.4.9.1 A Closer Look at Western Civilization and Diet

At the start of the 20th century, infectious diseases were the most prevalent diseases; however, anti-infectives and vaccinations caused a sharp decline in infectious diseases such as rheumatic fever, hepatitis A, tuberculosis, measles, and mumps (Kopp, 2019). In replacement, westernized civilizations saw a sharp increase in obesity, AD, type 2 diabetes, coronary heart disease, essential hypertension, osteoporosis, and cancer. In non-westernized populations, obesity and "civilization" diseases are virtually absent. The rise of westernized civilizations consuming a Standard American Diet (SAD), also known as Western diet pattern (WPD), has led to non-infectious chronic diseases replacing infectious disease as the major cause of death in the 21st century. The SAD consists of a diet rich in sugar, fat, salt, large amounts of high-glycemic carbohydrates like refined cereals, and a low intake of fiber (López-Taboada et al., 2020). Non-westernized populations such as hunter-gatherers eat a diet obtained naturally from the earth, which includes fruits, vegetables, and honey (a simple carbohydrate) (Pontzer, 2018). Herman Pontzer from Duke Global Health Institute has studied modern-day hunter-gatherers, noting they tend to maintain the same walking speed, body mass, and healthy weight throughout their entire adult lives with virtually no cardiovascular disease, diabetes, or hypertension. Pontzer noted the calories we burn during exercise can decrease the amount of inflammation in the human body. Diets composed of fresh vegetables, fruits, nuts, roots, seeds, and tubers can reduce the risk of civilization non-infectious chronic diseases, including ADs.

Pro-inflammatory foods are foods that stress the immune system potentially triggering AD and worsening symptoms in those already diagnosed with ADs. Examples of pro-inflammatory foods include salt, cow milk, red meat, processed meat, fried foods, margarine, soda, alcohol, and refined carbohydrates such as pastries. Salt may increase the absolute number of cells involved in inflammation and autoimmunity. Large amounts of salt can be found in processed foods, frozen meals, and canned goods. Immune cells attack foreign invaders in the human body. Elevated immune cells specific to a protein found in cow milk have been found in humans with autoimmune type 1 diabetes. In type 1 diabetes, the pancreatic cells that produce insulin are destroyed. Protein in cow milk is similar to the protein found in the human pancreas. The immune system attacks the cow milk protein as foreign and the pancreatic cells that produce insulin. Inflammation in the gut as a result of ingesting pro-inflammatory foods can cause toxins, bacteria, and undigested foods to cross into the bloodstream, which may lead to AD (Leech et al., 2020) and other negative impacts on health.

19.4.9.2   Childhood Trauma and Inflammation

A meta-analysis by Baumeister et al. (2015) examined the impact of childhood trauma and its influence on adult inflammation. Childhood trauma can include neglect, separation from caregivers, physical abuse, sexual abuse, and emotional abuse. The hypothalamic–pituitary–adrenal (HPA) axis is a powerful regulator of inflammation. Pro-inflammatory markers CRP, IL6, and TNF-a have been found to be increased in adults who have experienced childhood trauma. An increase in pro-inflammatory markers can cause inflammation and dysregulation of the inflammatory system. The meta-analysis examined 25 studies with a total sample of 16,870 study participants (Baumeister et al., 2015). The meta-analysis revealed strong evidence linking childhood trauma to dysregulation of the inflammatory system, which increases the risk of multiple adverse health conditions in adulthood, including psychiatric disorders and chronic disease.

19.5   LIFESTYLE BASED THERAPIES TO TREAT AUTOIMMUNE DISEASE

Although traditionally managed with conventional pharmaceuticals, lifestyle therapies are a remarkable preventative and therapeutic approach to reduce inflammation and chronic disease (Bodai, 2017). Lifestyle medicine focuses on prevention, which may improve quality of life, prevent or reverse disease, and extend lives. Nutrition, psychological health, and physical activity all play a crucial role in the development and progression of inflammatory-based autoimmune disease states.

19.5.1   Nutrition

Individuals diagnosed with AD are prescribed a plethora of potent anti-inflammatory medications such as steroids to suppress the immune system (Houghton, 2021). Medications used to suppress the immune system can help reduce symptoms and progression of ADs, but they come with the increased risk of developing infections that can be life-threatening due to immunosuppression. Certain foods have a natural anti-inflammatory effect on the body. A diet that consists of whole plant foods, fruits, and nuts may reduce autoimmune symptoms. Whole plant foods contain phytonutrients and natural antioxidants that have anti-inflammatory effects on the body. Plants are high in fiber, absent of additives, and naturally anti-inflammatory (Alwarith et al., 2019). Flavoring foods with seasoning that includes turmeric and ginger can also decrease inflammation. Adequate intake of vitamin D and omega-3 may reduce the risk of AD. A variety of macronutrients and micronutrients, among other vitamins and minerals, have anti-inflammatory effects related to AD activity. Nutritional management of AD utilizing such food items decreases inflammatory activity, increases antioxidant levels, and positively affects gastrointestinal microbiota, all of which contribute to the immunological pathways that preserve homeostasis (Tsigalou et al., 2020). A variety of macronutrients and micronutrients, among other vitamins and minerals, have anti-inflammatory effects related to AD activity and are described next.

19.5.1.1 Vitamin A

Vitamin A deficiency has been affiliated with ADs such as T1D and RA (Manicassamy et al., 2009; Zunino et al., 2007). Vitamin A decreases the risk for ADs through a mechanism thought to occur on pathogen recognition receptors located on dendritic cells. The presence of Vitamin A induces expression of the retinoic acid (RA) metabolizing enzyme that stimulates T regulatory cells and induces Socs3, a protein that regulates inflammation. T regulatory cells suppress pro-inflammatory lymphocytes Th1 and Th17 and Socs3 suppresses activation of pro-inflammatory cytokines, decreasing the risk for an autoimmune response (Manicassamy et al., 2009).

19.5.1.2 Vitamin D

Several studies have indicated a correlation between Vitamin D deficiency and the presence or exacerbation of multiple ADs (Murdaca et al., 2019). Vitamin D deficiency results in increased risk for ADs as a result of molecular mimicry. Vitamin D deficiency is most prevalent among auto-immune thyroid disease. In patients with SLE and RA, Vitamin D deficiency/insufficiency is affiliated with higher disease activity (Murdaca et al., 2019). Furthermore, in patients with T1D, Vitamin D supplementation appears to improve glycemic control, while Vitamin D deficiency is affiliated with more severe diabetic keto-acidosis presentation (Murdaca et al., 2019). Studies indicate that Vitamin D deficiency correlates with the development and exacerbation of ADs (Skaaby et al., 2015; Murdaca et al., 2019). Adequate levels of Vitamin D appear to decrease risk for AD through inhibition of pro-inflammatory cells Th1, Th9, and Th22 and promotion of anti-inflammatory cells Th2 (Hewison, 2012).

19.5.1.3 Curcumin

Curcumin is the main component of turmeric and has been used for its anti-inflammatory properties in Eastern medicine for hundreds of years. The anti-inflammatory properties of curcumin result from inhibition of the cyclooxygenase and lipoxygenase pathways. Curcumin also decreases inflammation through suppression of the NF-κB pathway (Yang et al., 2019). The anti-inflammatory properties of curcumin appear to have a positive effect on ulcerative colitis; however, more research is needed to determine its efficacy in other ADs such as RA and SLE (Yang et al., 2019).

19.5.1.4 Glutathione

Decreased intracellular glutathione levels have been associated with AD disease severity. ADs exacerbate decreased glutathione levels through a mechanism linked to increased pro-inflammatory Th1 and Th2 cells and results in a cytokine imbalance (Shah & Nath, 2014). The anti-inflammatory properties of glutathione are most effective in the SLE and T1D (Mannucci et al., 2021).

19.5.1.5 Magnesium

Magnesium deficiency has been associated with pro-inflammatory states, increasing risk for AD development and exacerbation (Neilson, 2018). Magnesium deficiency results in increased intracellular calcium ions that promote pro-inflammatory cytokines (Nielson, 2018). Postmenopausal women have declining estrogen levels, which may cause neuroinflammation as a result of reduced intracellular neuronal magnesium (Zhang et al., 2021). Neuroinflammation can lead to magnesium deficiency in postmenopausal women and can lead to cognitive impairment, pain, and depressive symptoms. A study by Zhang et al. examined aged female mice and female mice without their ovaries with neuronal disorders, including depression-like behaviors, pain, and cognitive impairment (2021). The mice were given oral magnesium-L-threonate (L-TAMS). The study concluded that the oral administration of L-TAMS prevented or reversed cognitive impairment, pain, and depressive-like behaviors in both sets of mice. Magnesium supplements may be a treatment option for menopausal symptoms and reduce neuroinflammation.

19.5.1.6   Omega 3s

Omega 3 supplementation results in a decrease of the prostaglandin E2 production and increase of IFN-gamma production and lymphocyte proliferation resulting in a more anti-inflammatory state (Trebble et al., 2013). The anti-inflammatory effects of omega 3 demonstrated an ability to modify and improve clinical presentation in individuals with RA, SLE, and lupus nephritis (Akbar et al., 2017).

19.5.1.7   Selenium

In a review of 32 studies, individuals with collagen vascular ADs exhibited lower selenium plasma levels; however, supplementation with selenium in these individuals resulted in clinical improvement and increased survival rates (Sahebari et al., 2019). Selenium is necessary to preserve the activity of selenoproteins in antioxidative and redox processes. These processes result in inhibition of pro-inflammatory receptors of activated B cells and counteract pro-inflammatory cytokine action, decreasing risk for ADs (Duntas & Hubalewska-Dydejczyk, 2015).

19.5.1.8   Zinc

Zinc has been studied extensively since its importance was recognized in the 1960s, and a meta-analysis of 62 studies has demonstrated the role zinc homeostasis plays in preventing inflammatory disease processes (Sanna et al., 2018). Zinc deficiency has been affiliated with an imbalance between regulatory and pro-inflammatory T cells. Adequate levels of zinc can inhibit Th17 lymphocytes, which have strong inflammatory properties, and make individuals more susceptible to development or exacerbation of ADs (Lee et al., 2015).

19.5.2   Psychological Health

Psychological health is a complex, multi-component area that is affected by a multitude of external and internal factors (Furman et al., 2019); however, the focus of this section is psychological health and its effect on the immune system. Many studies conducted over two decades showed correlations between self-reported mindfulness and psychological health. Several psychological processes are thought to be the cause of the beneficial effects of mindfulness, including increases in mindful awareness, re-perceiving lived experiences, acceptance of oneself and current state, attentional control, memory, values clarification, and behavioral self-regulation (Keng et al., 2011). Based on empirical literature across multiple methodologies, it is clear that mindfulness is a key element that facilitates adaptive psychological functioning. These effects ranged from increased subjective well-being, reduced psychological symptoms, improved emotional reactivity, and improved self-regulation of one's behavior, which could improve compliance to treatment regimens and a healthful diet (Keng et al., 2011).

Many non-communicable and chronic diseases are related to stress. Mindfulness, often in the form of meditation or breathing exercises, is shown to both treat and prevent stress-related physical symptoms (Greeson & Chin, 2018). A current review of evidence-based practices shows a positive correlation between mindfulness being associated with better psychological well-being, coping, and quality of life (Greeson & Chin, 2018). Although there is a paucity of evidence to show the effect of mindfulness practices on the pathological processes of chronic disease, it does appear to reduce subjective symptomatology (Black & Slavich, 2016). One way mindfulness may influence the cellular immune response is via inflammatory proteins produced by immune cells. Some examples of pro-inflammatory proteins include c-reactive protein (CRP), inflammatory cytokines, tumor necrosis factor (TNF), and circulating interleukins. Several studies indicated a decreased measure of serological inflammatory components in those individuals that engaged in mindfulness practices. The activation of supportive immune cells such as T lymphocytes related to mindful awareness practices was also seen in multiple studies. Increased telomerase activity, which indicates improved cellular longevity and augmented antibody secretion related to immune function, was similarly associated with practices of mindfulness meditation (Black & Slavich, 2016). Mindfulness is further discussed in Chapter 31 of this volume.

19.5.3 PHYSICAL ACTIVITY

Physical activity is a modifiable risk factor related to morbidity and mortality in the context of chronic disease (Furman et al., 2019). It is an integral component of health maintenance that improves both physical and mental health. Regular, intentional movement or exercise can contribute to achieving and maintaining healthy body weight and body mass index, strong bone density, and improved muscle strength. There are benefits to mental health as well. Physical activity may promote psychological well-being, lead to stress reduction, and improve overall quality of life. While the aesthetic effects of regular exercise may be well understood, its impact on the immune system and autoimmune disease is more obscure. The general mechanism of immunological activity is related to interleukin release from muscles, which triggers an anti-inflammatory response. The inverse is seen in those individuals that do no exercise (Sharif et al., 2018). Additionally, there is a concomitant release of T-regulatory cells and immunoglobulins that collectively boost the immune response.

Along with immunological improvements, metabolic changes resulting from intentional exercise or physical activity can modify possible development of comorbid conditions. Patients with an autoimmune rheumatic disease (ARD) are at a greater risk for development of cardiovascular diseases. This may be caused by changes in vascular homeostasis, and physical activity is integral to preventing these effects (Pecanha, 2021). ARD patients have accelerated atherosclerotic processes that can be improved with regular physical activity. In patients with ARDs, home-based physical activity improved quality of life (Sieczkowska et al., 2021). Furthermore, patients who participated in greater than 30 minutes of moderate physical activity, three times per week, showed a reduced risk for development of latent autoimmune diabetes (Hjort et al., 2020). Physical activity improved glucose uptake in patients and had beneficial effects on body weight.

19.6 NURSE INTERVENTIONS

Many patients get their nutritional information from media sources (Bodai, 2017). The food industry, pharmaceutical companies, and health care are driven by profit. Chronic disease accounts for more than 70% of health care costs. Most chronic conditions are influenced by lifestyle choices. The primary treatment of disease prevention is lifestyle. Nurses can change the health care landscape by advocating the prioritization of lifestyle recommendations. Nurses can promote healthy lifestyle changes for patients through education, dissemination of information, advocacy, policy change, and promoting change within the health care community. Nurses must address the gap in knowledge pertaining to healthy lifestyle changes to increase the quality of life of those affected by autoimmune disease.

19.7 CONCLUSION

Autoimmune disease is chronic and negatively impacts quality of life. AD remains a complicated disease that evades definitive causation. Genetics combined with environmental factors such as chemicals, infection, and dietary patterns contribute to development of this debilitating disease. Traditional treatment of these disorders can be costly and ineffective due to medication side effects. Strong evidence supports integration of lifestyle therapeutics in the prevention and management of AD. Westernized societies have chosen a lifestyle full of convenience, containing poor food choices, misinformation, and sedentary choices that are negatively impacting health. Consuming a WPD increases risk for developing autoimmune disease. A nutrient-dense diet that includes fruits and vegetables along with healthy fats can promote healing and decrease inflammation. Evidence supports adjunct integration of mindfulness into treatment plans as part of self-care, and in the management of disease states. Physical activity offers additional health advantages by reducing inflammation and is safe for various autoimmune diseases, including SLE, RA, MS, IBD, and psoriasis. Unfortunately, these patients tend to be less active, likely as a result of the symptomatic sequelae of AD. This may be compounded by depression and anxiety that is often experienced in connection with chronic diseases. Diet, physical activity, and mindfulness practices have all proven to ameliorate adverse outcomes secondary to AD and should be a primary therapeutic component to medical care. Nurses are at the forefront of change. Using courage to implement change in health care settings and communities, nurses can disseminate healthy lifestyle information to improve many generations to come.

REFERENCES

Akbar, U., Yang, M., Kurian, D., & Mohan, C. (2017). Omega-3 fatty acids in rheumatic diseases. *JCR: Journal of Clinical Rheumatology*, *23*(6), 330–339. https://doi.org/10.1097/rhu.0000000000000563

Alwarith, J., Kahleova, H., Rembert, E., Yonas, W., Dort, S., Calcagno, M., Burgess, N., Crosby, L., & Barnard, N. D. (2019). Nutrition interventions in rheumatoid arthritis: the potential use of plant-based diets: A review. *Frontiers in Nutrition*, *6*, 141. https://doi.org/10.3389/fnut.2019.00141

Angum, F., Khan, T., Kaler, J., Siddiqui, L., & Hussain, A. (2020). The prevalence of autoimmune disorders in women: A narrative review. *Cureus*, *12*(5), e8094. https://doi.org/10.7759/cureus.8094

Baumeister, D., Akhtar, R., Ciufolini, S., Pariante, C. M., & Mondelli, V. (2015). Childhood trauma and adulthood inflammation: A meta-analysis of peripheral c-reactive protein, interleukin-6 and tumour necrosis factor-α. *Molecular Psychiatry*, *21*(5), 642–649. https://doi.org/10.1038/mp.2015.67

Black, D. S., & Slavich, G. M. (2016). Mindfulness meditation and the immune system: A systematic review of randomized controlled trials. *Annals of the New York Academy of Sciences*, *1373*(1), 13–24. https://doi.org/10.1111/nyas.12998

Bodai, B. (2017). Lifestyle medicine: A brief review of its dramatic impact on health and survival. *The Permanente Journal*, *22*(1). https://doi.org/10.7812/tpp/17-025

Cohen, D. (2021, March 1). *Nine root causes of autoimmune disorders*. Caplan Health. Retrieved November 29, 2021, from www.caplanhealthinstitute.com/nine-root-causes-of-autoimmune-disorders/

Desai, M. K., & Brinton, R. (2019). Autoimmune disease in women: Endocrine transition and risk across the lifespan. *Frontiers in Endocrinology*, *10*. https://doi.org/10.3389/fendo.2019.00265

Dube, S. R., Fairweather, D., Pearson, W. S., Felitti, V. J., Anda, R. F., & Croft, J. B. (2009). Cumulative childhood stress and autoimmune diseases in adults. *Psychosomatic Medicine*, *71*(2), 243–250. https://doi.org/10.1097/psy.0b013e3181907888

Duntas, L. H., & Hubalewska-Dydejczyk, A. (2015). Selenium and inflammation— potential use and future perspectives. *US Endocrinology*, *11*(02), 97. https://doi.org/10.17925/use.2015.11.02.97

Furman, D., Campisi, J., Verdin, E., Carrera-Bastos, P., Targ, S., Franceschi, C., Ferrucci, L., Gilroy, D. W., Fasano, A., Miller, G. W., Miller, A. H., Mantovani, A., Weyand, C. M., Barzilai, N., Goronzy, J. J., Rando, T. A., Effros, R. B., Lucia, A., Kleinstreuer, N., & Slavich, G. M. (2019). Chronic inflammation in the etiology of disease across the life span. *Nature Medicine*, *25*(12), 1822–1832. https://doi.org/10.1038/s41591-019-0675-0

Gawda, A., Majka, G., Nowak, B., & Marcinkiewicz, J. (2017). Air pollution, oxidative stress, and exacerbation of autoimmune diseases. *Central European Journal of Immunology*, *3*, 305–312. https://doi.org/10.5114/ceji.2017.70975

Gershteyn, I. M., & Ferreira, L. M. (2019). Immunodietica: A data-driven approach to investigate interactions between diet and autoimmune disorders. *Journal of Translational Autoimmunity*, *1*, 100003. https://doi.org/10.1016/j.jtauto.2019.100003

Ghasemi, N., Razavi, S., & Nikzad, E. (2017). Multiple sclerosis: Pathogenesis, symptoms, diagnoses and cell-based therapy. *Cell Journal*, *19*(1), 1–10. https://doi.org/10.22074/cellj.2016.4867

Greeson, J. M., & Chin, G. R. (2019). Mindfulness and physical disease: A concise review. *Current Opinion in Psychology*, *28*, 204–210. https://doi.org/10.1016/j.copsyc.2018.12.014

Hewison, M. (2012). An update on vitamin d and human immunity. *Clinical Endocrinology, 76*(3), 315–325. https://doi.org/10.1111/j.1365-2265.2011.04261.x

Hjort, R., Ahlqvist, E., Andersson, T., Alfredsson, L., Carlsson, P.-O., Grill, V., Groop, L., Martinell, M., Sørgjerd, E., Tuomi, T., Åsvold, B., & Carlsson, S. (2020a). Physical activity, genetic susceptibility, and the risk of latent autoimmune diabetes in adults and type 2 diabetes. *The Journal of Clinical Endocrinology & Metabolism, 105*(11), e4112–e4123. https://doi.org/10.1210/clinem/dgaa549

Houghton, T. (2021, July 23). *Autoimmunity and diet: Is there a connection?* Center for Nutrition Studies. Retrieved October 7, 2021, from www.nutritionstudies.org

Keng, S.-L., Smoski, M. J., & Robins, C. J. (2011). Effects of mindfulness on psychological health: A review of empirical studies. *Clinical Psychology Review, 31*(6), 1041–1056. https://doi.org/10.1016/j.cpr.2011.04.006

Kopp, W. (2019). How western diet and lifestyle drive the pandemic of obesity and civilization disease. *Diabetes, Metabolic Syndrome and Obesity: Targets and Therapy, 12*, 2221–2236. https://doi.org/10.2147/dmso.s216791

Lee, H., Kim, B., Choi, Y., Hwang, Y., Kim, D., Cho, S., Hong, S., & Lee, W.-W. (2015). Inhibition of interleukin-1β-mediated interleukin-1 receptor-associated kinase 4 phosphorylation by zinc leads to repression of memory t helper type 17 response in humans. *Immunology, 146*(4), 645–656. https://doi.org/10.1111/imm.12536

Leech, B., McEwen, B., & Sekyere, E. (2020). Diet, digestive health, and autoimmunity: The foundations to an autoimmune disease food pyramid—part 2. *Alternative and Complementary Therapies, 26*(4), 158–167. https://doi.org/10.1089/act.2020.29287.ble

Lerner, A., Jeremias, P., & Matthias, T. (2016). The world incidence and prevalence of autoimmune diseases is increasing. *International Journal of Celiac Disease, 3*(4), 151–155. https://doi.org/10.12691/ijcd-3-4-8

López-Taboada, I., González-Pardo, H., & Conejo, N. (2020). Western diet: Implications for brain function and behavior. *Frontiers in Psychology, 11*, 564413. https://doi.org/10.3389/fpsyg.2020.564413

Manicassamy, S., Ravindran, R., Deng, J., Oluoch, H., Denning, T. L., Kasturi, S., Rosenthal, K. M., Evavold, B. D., & Pulendran, B. (2009). Toll-like receptor 2–dependent induction of vitamin a—metabolizing enzymes in dendritic cells promotes t regulatory responses and inhibits autoimmunity. *Nature Medicine, 15*(4), 401–409. https://doi.org/10.1038/nm.1925

Mannucci, C., Casciaro, M., Sorbara, E., Calapai, F., Di Salvo, E., Pioggia, G., Navarra, M., Calapai, G., & Gangemi, S. (2021). Nutraceuticals against oxidative stress in autoimmune disorders. *Antioxidants, 10*(2), 261. https://doi.org/10.3390/antiox10020261

Murdaca, G., Tonacci, A., Negrini, S., Greco, M., Borro, M., Puppo, F., & Gangemi, S. (2019). Emerging role of vitamin d in autoimmune diseases: An update on evidence and therapeutic implications. *Autoimmunity Reviews, 18*(9), 102350. https://doi.org/10.1016/j.autrev.2019.102350

National Institute of Environmental Health Sciences. (2021, July 12). Autoimmune diseases. National Institute of Environmental Health Sciences. Retrieved October 30, 2021, from https://www.niehs.nih.gov

Nielsen, F. H. (2018). Magnesium deficiency and increased inflammation: Current perspectives. *Journal of Inflammation Research, 11*, 25–34. https://doi.org/10.2147/jir.s136742

Niklas, K., Niklas, A. A., Majewski, D., & Puszczewicz, M. (2016). Rheumatic diseases induced by drugs and environmental factors: The state-of-the-art—part one. *Reumatologia/Rheumatology, 3*(54), 122–127. https://doi.org/10.5114/reum.2016.61212

Okada, Y., Eyre, S., Suzuki, A., Kochi, Y., & Yamamoto, K. (2019). Genetics of rheumatoid arthritis: 2018 status. *Annals of the Rheumatic Diseases, 78*(4), 446-453. http://dx.doi.org/10.1136/annrheumdis-2018-213678

Parzanese, I., Qehajaj, D., Patrinicola, F., Aralica, M., Chiriva-Internati, M., Stifter, S., Elli, L., & Grizzi, F. (2017). Celiac disease: From pathophysiology to treatment. *World Journal of Gastrointestinal Pathophysiology, 8*(2), 27. https://doi.org/10.4291/wjgp.v8.i2.27

Peçanha, T., Bannell, D. J., Sieczkowska, S., Goodson, N., Roschel, H., Sprung, V. S., & Low, D. A. (2021). Effects of physical activity on vascular function in autoimmune rheumatic diseases: A systematic review and meta-analysis. *Rheumatology, 60*(7), 3107–3120. https://doi.org/10.1093/rheumatology/keab094

Pontzer, H., Wood, B. M., & Raichlen, D. A. (2019). Hunter-gatherers as models in public health. *Obesity Reviews, 19*(Suppl 1), 24–35. https://doi.org/10.1111/obr.12785

Ray, S., Sonthalia, N., Kundu, S., & Ganguly, S. (2012). Autoimmune disorders: An overview of molecular and cellular basis in today's perspective. *Journal of Clinical & Cellular Immunology, 01*(S10). https://doi.org/10.4172/2155-9899.s10-003

Richard-Eaglin, A., & Smallheer, B. A. (2018). Immunosuppressive/autoimmune disorders. *Nursing Clinics of North America, 53*(3), 319–334. https://doi.org/10.1016/j.cnur.2018.04.002

Rojas, M., Restrepo-Jiménez, P., Monsalve, D. M., Pacheco, Y., Acosta-Ampudia, Y., Ramírez-Santana, C., Leung, P. S., Ansari, A. A., Gershwin, M., & Anaya, J.-M. (2018). Molecular mimicry and autoimmunity. *Journal of Autoimmunity, 95*, 100–123. https://doi.org/10.1016/j.jaut.2018.10.012

Rosenblum, M. D., Remedios, K. A., & Abbas, A. K. (2015). Mechanisms of human autoimmunity. *Journal of Clinical Investigation, 125*(6), 2228–2233. https://doi.org/10.1172/jci78088

Sahebari, M., Rezaieyazdi, Z., & Khodashahi, M. (2019). Selenium and autoimmune diseases: A review article. *Current Rheumatology Reviews, 15*(2), 123–134. https://doi.org/10.2174/1573397114666181016112342

Sanna, A., Firinu, D., Zavattari, P., & Valera, P. (2018). Zinc status and autoimmunity: A systematic review and meta-analysis. *Nutrients, 10*(1), 68. https://doi.org/10.3390/nu10010068

Seiler, A., Fagundes, C. P., & Christian, L. M. (2020). The impact of everyday stressors on the immune system and health. In Choukèr, A. (Ed.), *Stress challenges and immunity in space* (pp. 71–92). Springer International Publishing. https://doi.org/10.1007/978-3-030-16996-1_6

Shah, D., & Nath, S. K. (2014). Glutathione: A possible link to autophagy in systemic lupus erythematosus. *American Journal of Immunology, 10*(3), 114–115. https://doi.org/10.3844/ajisp.2014.114.115

Sharif, K., Watad, A., Bragazzi, N., Lichtbroun, M., Amital, H., & Shoenfeld, Y. (2018). Physical activity and autoimmune diseases: Get moving and manage the disease. *Autoimmunity Reviews, 17*(1), 53–72. https://doi.org/10.1016/j.autrev.2017.11.010

Sherbet, G. (2009). Bacterial infections and the pathogenesis of autoimmune conditions. *British Journal of Medical Practitioners, 2*(1), 6–13.

Sieczkowska, S., Smaira, F., Mazzolani, B., Gualano, B., Roschel, H., & Peçanha, T. (2021). Efficacy of home-based physical activity interventions in patients with autoimmune rheumatic diseases: A systematic review and meta-analysis. *Seminars in Arthritis and Rheumatism, 51*(3), 576–587. https://doi.org/10.1016/j.semarthrit.2021.04.004

Skaaby, T., Husemoen, L., Thuesen, B., & Linneberg, A. (2015). Prospective population-based study of the association between vitamin D status and incidence of autoimmune disease. *Endocrine, 50*(1), 231–238. https://doi.org/10.1007/s12020-015-0547-4

Song, H., Fang, F., Tomasson, G., Arnberg, F. K., Mataix-Cols, D., Fernández de la Cruz, L., Almqvist, C., Fall, K., & Valdimarsdóttir, U. A. (2018). Association of stress-related disorders with subsequent autoimmune disease. *JAMA, 319*(23), 2388. https://doi.org/10.1001/jama.2018.7028

Trebble, T. M., Wootton, S. A., Miles, E. A., Mullee, M., Arden, N. K., Ballinger, A. B., Stroud, M. A., Burdge, G. C., & Calder, P. C. (2003). Prostaglandin e2 production and t cell function after fish-oil supplementation: Response to antioxidant cosupplementation. *The American Journal of Clinical Nutrition, 78*(3), 376–382. https://doi.org/10.1093/ajcn/78.3.376

Tsai, S., Clemente-Casares, X., Revelo, X. S., Winer, S., & Winer, D. A. (2015). Are obesity-related insulin resistance and type 2 diabetes autoimmune diseases? *Diabetes, 64*(6), 1886–1897. https://doi.org/10.2337/db14-1488

Tsigalou, C., Konstantinidis, T., Paraschaki, A., Stavropoulou, E., Voidarou, C., & Bezirtzoglou, E. (2020). Mediterranean diet as a tool to combat inflammation and chronic diseases. an overview. *Biomedicines, 8*(7), 201. https://doi.org/10.3390/biomedicines8070201

Yang, M., Akbar, U., & Mohan, C. (2019). Curcumin in autoimmune and rheumatic diseases. *Nutrients, 11*(5), 1004. https://doi.org/10.3390/nu11051004

Zhang, J., Mai, C.-L., Xiong, Y., Lin, Z.-J., Jie, Y.-T., Mai, J.-Z., Liu, C., Xie, M.-X., Zhou, X., & Liu, X.-G. (2021). The causal role of magnesium deficiency in the neuroinflammation, pain hypersensitivity and memory/emotional deficits in ovariectomized and aged female mice. *Journal of Inflammation Research, Volume 14*, 6633–6656. https://doi.org/10.2147/jir.s330894

Zunino, S. J., Storms, D. H., & Stephensen, C. B. (2007). Diets rich in polyphenols and vitamin a inhibit the development of type 1 autoimmune diabetes in nonobese diabetic mice. *The Journal of Nutrition, 137*(5), 1216–1221. https://doi.org/10.1093/jn/137.5.1216

20 Cancer

Karen Collins
American Institute for Cancer Research
Arlington, Virginia, USA

CONTENTS

KEY POINTS

- A wide range of lifestyle choices contribute to increasing or decreasing risk of cancer.
- Reaching and maintaining a body composition reduces cancer risk by limiting exposure to adiposity-related hormonal and metabolic pathways that promote cancer development.
- An overall eating pattern focused on a variety of fiber- and nutrient-rich plant foods reduces cancer risk by providing protective compounds and by supporting a healthy weight.
- Limiting red meat, processed meat, sugar-sweetened beverages, highly processed calorie-dense foods, and alcohol are also important lifestyle choices to reduce cancer risk.
- Dietary supplements can help fill identified nutrient gaps, but evidence does not support them as an effective strategy for cancer prevention.
- Regular physical activity and limitation of sedentary time reduce risk of cancer in several ways.
- Avoiding tobacco, regardless of its form, remains a critical lifestyle choice for reducing risk of several cancers.

DOI: 10.1201/9781003178330-23

20.1   INTRODUCTION

20.1.1   EVIDENCE ON CANCER PREVENTION

An estimated 40% of cancers in the US could be prevented through healthful dietary patterns, regular physical activity, a healthy weight (generally a BMI of 18.5 to 24.9 on a population level, though individuals may vary), avoidance of tobacco and excess sun exposure, and use of vaccines and screenings (Islami et al., 2018).

This chapter identifies current recommendations on diet, physical activity, weight, and tobacco; summarizes the evidence behind them; provides practice pearls to assist in their implementation; and addresses common questions on topics not included in these major recommendations.

20.1.2   ETIOLOGIES AND HALLMARKS OF CANCER

Cancer does not develop through any single exposure or insult. Rather, cancer develops through an accumulation of cell damage over time that causes normal processes for controlling cell behavior to fail. This allows reproduction of a rogue cell, along with its abnormal behaviors and capabilities. Damage may occur as a mutation (a permanent change in DNA) or as epigenetic changes that turn gene expression on or off.

Cell damage that leads to cancer can come from exposures in the external environment, from the body's internal environment (including inflammation and certain infections), and from the influence of diet and lifestyle choices (including tobacco, alcohol, physical inactivity, and components of food). Genetic traits may increase some people's vulnerability to these sources of damage.

Genetic and epigenetic changes can alter gene expression and, as they accumulate, enable cells to acquire functional abnormalities known as the hallmarks of cancer (Hanahan & Weinberg, 2011). Current models of cancer development identify eight hallmarks of cancer: Sustained proliferative signaling, evasion of growth suppressors, resistance to cell death/apoptosis, replicative immortality, dysregulated metabolism, immune system evasion, angiogenesis, and invasion and metastasis (World Cancer Research Fund/American Institute for Cancer Research, 2018). Models also incorporate two characteristics—genomic instability and tumor-promoting inflammation—that facilitate cancer's development.

Cells have multiple mechanisms to prevent and repair DNA damage and to remove abnormal cells before cancer can develop. Diet and physical activity support many of these mechanisms. Together, diet, physical activity, and body composition also affect hormone levels and growth factors that influence the promotion and progression of cancer cells.

As research on cancer risk reduction has grown in quantity and quality, evidence has shifted away from a "reductionist" approach focused on individual nutrients. Instead, current evidence supports the importance of overall dietary pattern and lifestyle, and their combined influence on body composition, metabolic health, and gene expression. Of course, a dietary pattern is created by what foods are chosen and in what portions, and which are left for occasional use. Body composition and lifestyle are slowly built by daily choices, often while in an environment that does not make healthy choices the easiest choices.

20.2   IDENTIFYING LIFESTYLE CHOICES TO REDUCE RISK OF CANCER

The American Institute for Cancer Research and the World Cancer Research Fund (AICR/WCRF) established recommendations for cancer prevention based on a structured and systematic analysis of research on nutrition, physical activity, and weight in cancer prevention (World Cancer Research Fund/American Institute for Cancer Research, 2018). These recommendations are aimed at reducing risk of cancer as a whole and are intentionally compatible with major recommendations for overall health. The American Cancer Society (ACS) guidelines on nutrition and physical activity for cancer prevention are based on those recommendations, supplemented by systematic reviews and large pooled analyses published thereafter (Rock et al., 2020).

In addition to the recommendations reviewed in more detail in this chapter, AICR recommendations also include support of breastfeeding (World Cancer Research Fund/American Institute for Cancer Research, 2018). Beyond benefits for overall health of mother and child, evidence shows a modest reduction in risk of both pre- and postmenopausal breast cancer for women who breastfeed. This apparently occurs through effects on lifetime estrogen exposure and effects on cells within the breast. For women who choose to and are able, the longer their total duration of breastfeeding, the greater the reduction in cancer risk. Research also suggests potential for breastfeeding to reduce a mother's risk of ovarian and endometrial cancer (Babic et al., 2020; Ma et al., 2018; World Cancer Research Fund/American Institute for Cancer Research, 2018), although AICR categorizes this evidence as too limited at this time to serve as the basis for breastfeeding recommendations.

20.3   ADIPOSITY AND WEIGHT GAIN

AICR/WCRF and ACS recommendations include achieving and maintaining a healthy body weight throughout life, avoiding weight gain in adult life (Rock et al., 2020; World Cancer Research Fund/American Institute for Cancer Research, 2018). Consistent evidence links greater adiposity with increased risk of at least 12 cancers. Overweight and obesity increase risk of cancers of the esophagus (adenocarcinoma), pancreas, colorectum, breast (postmenopausal), endometrium, liver, kidney, stomach (cardia), gallbladder, ovary, mouth, pharynx, and larynx; and of advanced prostate cancers (World Cancer Research Fund/American Institute for Cancer Research, 2018). Some analyses add thyroid cancer, multiple myeloma, and meningioma (Lauby-Secretan et al., 2016; Rock et al., 2020). Most of the cancers increasing in young adults are obesity-related cancers, and they are increasing at faster rates than in adults over age 50 (Sung et al., 2019).

Several plausible mechanisms can explain adiposity-related cancer risk. Excess body fat is associated with insulin resistance, resulting in elevated levels of insulin and increased bioavailable insulin-like growth factor 1 (IGF-1) (Giovannucci, 2018; World Cancer Research Fund/American Institute for Cancer Research, 2018). Insulin and IGF-1 activate signaling pathways that promote growth and proliferation of cancer cells and inhibit apoptosis (i.e., programmed cell death) (Smith et al., 2018). Excess adiposity can increase release of signaling proteins from adipose tissue that stimulate growth of cancer cells; and it can promote chronic low-grade systemic inflammation that leads to DNA-damaging oxidative stress, heightened local inflammation, and cancer development (Iyengar et al., 2016; Smith et al., 2018). Furthermore, adipose tissue is the primary site of estrogen production in postmenopausal women. Greater adiposity increases bioavailable estrogen, increasing risk of endometrial and postmenopausal breast cancers (Smith et al., 2018; World Cancer Research Fund/American Institute for Cancer Research, 2018). Overweight and obesity may also affect cancer risk through altered immune responses, obesity-linked changes in the gut microbiome, and various organ-specific effects (World Cancer Research Fund/American Institute for Cancer Research, 2018).

The association of metabolic syndrome and cancer is noteworthy in considering the role of adiposity in cancer risk. Metabolic syndrome is defined by the presence of three or more of the following: High blood sugar, high blood pressure, high triglycerides, low HDL cholesterol, and elevated waist circumference. Metabolic syndrome is associated with 20% to more than 60% increased risk of several cancers (Micucci et al., 2016). Metabolic syndrome signals likelihood of dysfunctional adipose tissue, inflammation, insulin resistance, and dysregulated hormones and signaling proteins (Neeland et al., 2019) that could enhance cancer development.

Metabolic syndrome despite a normal BMI tends to occur with higher body fat percentage or with greater distribution in visceral (rather than subcutaneous) adipose tissue depots (Shi et al., 2020). Multiple prospective cohort studies show that besides increased risk of cardiovascular disease, this condition, known as metabolic obesity in the normal weight (MONW), is associated with increased risk of several obesity-related cancers, including postmenopausal breast, endometrial, colorectal, and liver cancers (Liu et al., 2021).

Although BMI is commonly used as a measure of adiposity, especially in large observational studies, it is imperfect, particularly in the elderly and certain other groups. Waist circumference measures abdominal fatness, although it cannot differentiate subcutaneous fat versus the visceral fat linked to hyperinsulinemia and inflammation. AICR recommends a waist circumference no larger than 37 inches (94 cm) in men, and 31.5 inches (80 cm) in women (World Cancer Research Fund/American Institute for Cancer Research, 2018). Waist circumference thresholds signaling risk are lower for people of Asian ethnicity (Alberti et al., 2009; World Cancer Research Fund/American Institute for Cancer Research, 2018), and other ethnicity-related differences in fat distribution and body composition need research. Unintentional adult weight gain can also be a marker of excess body fat, and it is particularly linked with risk of postmenopausal breast cancer (World Cancer Research Fund/American Institute for Cancer Research, 2018).

BOX 20.1   PRACTICE PEARLS ON ADIPOSITY AND WEIGHT GAIN

For people who are overweight or obese, even modest weight loss might reduce cancer risk. Although research on cancer incidence after weight loss is too limited for conclusions (Chlebowski et al., 2019; Look AHEAD Research Group et al., 2020), a 5% to 10% weight loss can produce clinically meaningful changes in biomarkers of the insulin, sex hormone, and inflammatory pathways through which excess adiposity seems to increase cancer risk (Lauby-Secretan et al., 2016; Look AHEAD Research Group et al., 2020; van Gemert et al., 2017).

For people classified with a normal BMI who are experiencing adult weight gain, large waist size, or metabolic syndrome, a **protective first step may be to stop a trend of weight gain**.

20.4   A PREDOMINANTLY PLANT-BASED DIET

AICR/WCRF and ACS recommendations call for a predominantly plant-based dietary pattern (Rock et al., 2020; World Cancer Research Fund/American Institute for Cancer Research, 2018). Growing evidence suggests that this type of diet, which can be implemented in a variety of ways, may provide greater protection than that from any particular nutrients, compounds, or individual foods. Although media sources often use the term "plant-based diet" to refer to a vegetarian diet that includes only plant foods, major evidence-based recommendations for reducing cancer risk use this term in a broader sense to indicate an eating pattern in which whole plant foods constitute the majority of food consumed.

Prospective cohort studies link consumption of non-starchy vegetables and fruits with lower risk of several types of cancer, and whole grains with lower risk of colorectal cancer (World Cancer Research Fund/American Institute for Cancer Research, 2018). Human studies focusing on legumes, such as beans, lentils, and soy foods, and cancer risk are limited and provide inconsistent findings (World Cancer Research Fund/American Institute for Cancer Research, 2018). One reason may be that studies based in the US reflect a population in which few people eat dried beans or soy foods as a regular part of their diet, making comparison between groups that eat high and low amounts difficult.

These plant foods all contribute to creating a diet high in dietary fiber, which is strongly linked to lower risk of colorectal cancer (CRC) (World Cancer Research Fund/American Institute for Cancer

Research, 2018). Different types of dietary fiber can contribute to lower CRC risk through direct protection of cells, help avoiding inflammation and elevations in insulin and related growth factors, and through support for protective, butyrate-producing bacteria in the gut microbiome (O'Keefe, 2016; World Cancer Research Fund/American Institute for Cancer Research, 2018). Women who eat diets higher in fiber may also have lower risk of breast cancer, according to an analysis primarily encompassing large prospective cohort studies (Farvid et al., 2020). In addition to other protective effects, higher fiber intake may act directly or through the gut microbiome to influence systemic estrogen levels (Parida & Sharma, 2019).

Plant foods are rich in vitamins, minerals, and phytochemicals (natural plant compounds) that, as part of the whole food, may protect against cancer through a variety of mechanisms. Studies *in vitro* and *in vivo* demonstrate that certain nutrients and phytochemicals can inhibit or promote activity of carcinogen-metabolizing enzymes, affect cell cycle regulation, and trigger apoptosis (self-destruction of abnormal cells). Some nutrients and compounds may provide direct antioxidant protection; other phytochemicals appear to stimulate endogenous antioxidant systems. Carotenoids show potential to alter cell signaling to inhibit cancer cell growth and promote apoptosis (Li et al., 2016; World Cancer Research Fund/American Institute for Cancer Research, 2018). In laboratory studies, epigenetic changes that in essence either silence or promote expression of genes that regulate cancer progression can be demonstrated from compounds or metabolites of compounds found in cruciferous vegetables, garlic and onion family vegetables, dark green vegetables, grapes, and berries (Bishop & Ferguson, 2015; George et al., 2017). Plant foods also supply fermentable dietary fiber, other types of carbohydrate, and phytochemicals that seem to support a health-protective gut microbiota (Bultman, 2016; O'Keefe, 2016; Sheflin et al., 2017).

Another aspect of the reduction in cancer risk associated with a predominantly plant-based diet is its role in reaching and maintaining a healthy weight (Rock et al., 2020; World Cancer Research Fund/American Institute for Cancer Research, 2018). Such diets tend to be less concentrated in calories, with higher dietary fiber and water content, and thus able to increase satiety without excessive calorie intake.

BOX 20.2   PRACTICE PEARLS REGARDING A PREDOMINANTLY PLANT-BASED DIET

A daily total of at least 30 grams of dietary fiber from food sources is recommended by AICR/WCRF (World Cancer Research Fund/American Institute for Cancer Research, 2018).

Consuming a variety of vegetables and fruits may be advantageous over focusing only on a narrow range of "superfoods," since this provides a broad spectrum of protective nutrients and compounds. A healthful diet can include potatoes and other starchy vegetables if non-starchy vegetables, fruits, and pulses are eaten regularly, too.

Five or more standard servings of non-starchy vegetables and fruits daily (a total of 2.5 cups, though more when this includes raw leafy greens) meet AICR/WCRF recommendations and are associated with lower cancer risk (World Cancer Research Fund/American Institute for Cancer Research, 2018). **Once that habit is established, increasing amounts** to 2.5 to 3 cups of vegetables and 1.5 to 2 cups of fruit each day may further enhance health and weight management and is recommended by ACS (Rock et al., 2020).

A predominantly plant-based diet should also include whole grains daily, and frequent use of legumes (including dried beans and lentils), since these foods expand the variety of fiber types, nutrients, and phytochemicals provided.

20.5   DIETARY COMPONENTS FOR LIMITED USE

20.5.1   RED AND PROCESSED MEATS

AICR/WCRF and ACS recommendations for cancer prevention include limiting consumption of red meat and eating very little, if any, processed meat (Rock et al., 2020; World Cancer Research Fund/American Institute for Cancer Research, 2018).

Excess red meat and processed meat consumption are primarily associated with colorectal cancer. Risk increases approximately 12% for every 100 grams (3.5 ounces) of red meat consumed daily. Evidence is even stronger for processed meat, with a 16% increase in colorectal cancer risk for every 50 grams consumed daily (World Cancer Research Fund/American Institute for Cancer Research, 2018). Association of these meats with increased risk of other cancers has been suggested by some studies, but such findings are preliminary and further research is needed (Rock et al., 2020).

Several plausible mechanisms can account for the association between consumption of red meat or processed meat and colorectal cancer. Risk may stem from red meat's higher content of heme iron, which can increase free radicals that damage DNA and can promote formation of carcinogenic *N*-nitroso compounds (NOCs) within the gut (Demeyer et al., 2016; Hammerling et al., 2016; Rock et al., 2020; World Cancer Research Fund/American Institute for Cancer Research, 2018). Processed meats can increase exposure to compounds such as the polycyclic aromatic hydrocarbons (PAHs) in smoked meats and nitroso-compounds created when nitrites combine with a component of meat protein (Demeyer et al., 2016; Hammerling et al., 2016; Rock et al., 2020; World Cancer Research Fund/American Institute for Cancer Research, 2018).

Red and processed meats may also contribute to development of colorectal cancer through effects on inflammation, possibly through influences on the gut microbiota. Growing evidence suggests that gut microbes can convert protein residues and fat-stimulated bile acids from diets high in meat to substances that are carcinogenic and/or pro-inflammatory (O'Keefe, 2016; Singh et al., 2017).

Cooking meat at high temperatures or over open flames causes production of heterocyclic amines (HCAs) and polycyclic aromatic hydrocarbons (PAHs), both of which are carcinogenic in animals (Demeyer et al., 2016; Hammerling et al., 2016; World Cancer Research Fund/American Institute for Cancer Research, 2018). However, such cooking conditions also produce these compounds in poultry and seafood, and thus cannot account for the greater colorectal cancer risk specifically associated with red and processed meats (Demeyer et al., 2016; World Cancer Research Fund/American Institute for Cancer Research, 2018).

Some literature reviews have used grading systems that emphasize randomized controlled trials (RCTs) and downgrade evidence from observational studies. However, for a disease like cancer that typically develops over decades, a valid and reliable RCT on meat consumption is unlikely (Rock et al., 2020). Therefore, the multiple potential mechanisms and the abundance of prospective cohort studies that consistently find higher amounts of red meat, and especially processed meat, associated with higher risk of colorectal cancer provides strong support for the recommendation to limit their consumption.

BOX 20.3   PRACTICE PEARLS ON RED MEAT AND PROCESSED MEAT

Red meat primarily refers to beef, lamb, and pork, but also includes mutton, goat, and bison. Since cancer-related risk seems to involve components such as heme iron, even lean meats should be kept within recommended limits.

For people who wish to include red meat in their diet, it's best to limit amounts to no more than 12 to 18 ounces (cooked weight) per week. This may be equivalent to about three portions per week for many people. However, if portion size is limited to 3 ounces (deck of cards size), the total limit allows for four to six portions per week.

Processed meat includes meats preserved by smoking, curing, fermenting, salting, or chemical preservatives. Examples include ham, bacon, hot dogs, pastrami, salami, and other sausages prepared by these methods.

Research has not yet demonstrated whether variations in smoking or ingredients can reduce risk posed by processed meat. For now, it is recommended that consumption of all forms of processed meat be minimized.

Predominantly plant-based, cancer-protective diets can include moderate amounts of some animal foods. Evidence does not show any consistent association of poultry or eggs with cancer risk. Limited evidence suggests that fish consumption may be associated with lower risk of liver and colorectal cancers (World Cancer Research Fund/American Institute for Cancer Research, 2018).

20.5.2 SUGAR-SWEETENED BEVERAGES AND PROCESSED FOODS THAT PROMOTE WEIGHT GAIN

AICR/WCRF and ACS recommendations advise limiting consumption of sugar-sweetened beverages (SSBs) as well as "fast foods" and other processed foods high in fat, added sugars, or refined grains (Rock et al., 2020; World Cancer Research Fund/American Institute for Cancer Research, 2018). Because obesity and weight gain exert such a powerful influence, driving metabolic and hormonal pathways that increase cancer risk, limiting consumption of foods and drinks that promote weight gain and excess body fat is an important element in a dietary pattern for cancer prevention.

Frequent consumption of SSBs is a cause of weight gain as well as overweight and obesity in both children and adults (Dietary Guidelines Advisory Committee, 2020; Luger et al., 2017; World Cancer Research Fund/American Institute for Cancer Research, 2018). Emerging research from observational studies suggests that multiple daily servings of SSBs may be associated with increased risk of colorectal cancer, even after accounting for weight. This could relate to effects on sustained elevations of serum insulin, but more research is needed before advising limited SSB consumption to reduce cancer risk through any mechanism other than effects on weight.

Several approaches categorize foods based on the extent and purpose of processing they undergo (Monteiro et al., 2019). Foods designated as "minimally processed" include chopped, frozen, and canned vegetables, fruits, and legumes. Keeping such foods on hand can reduce preparation time and make eating habits consistent with dietary recommendations easier to accomplish.

Foods designated as "ultra-processed" typically employ ingredients (such as high-fructose corn syrup and hydrogenated oils) and processes (such as extrusion into new forms) not typically found in home kitchens. These foods are usually designed to have long shelf-life and include flavorings that make them hyper-palatable (Monteiro et al., 2019).

For reduced cancer risk, the recommendation to limit processed foods targets the influence of these foods on weight gain. Studies show that ultra-processed foods that are high in added sugars, fat, or refined grains promote weight gain, overweight, and obesity when consumed frequently or in large portions (Moradi et al., 2021; Rouhani et al., 2016; World Cancer Research Fund/American Institute for Cancer Research, 2018). Together, these beverages and foods provide concentrated calories, often in portions or forms that don't induce satiety, and negatively influence metabolic risk and tendency toward abdominal adiposity (Monteiro et al., 2019; Mozaffarian, 2016). Limiting these choices helps reduce cancer risk by contributing to reaching and maintaining a healthy body weight.

Limited evidence from prospective cohort studies and RCTs suggests that 100% juice is not consistently associated with adiposity in children or adults (Dietary Guidelines Advisory Committee, 2020). Nutrient intake can be enhanced through 100% fruit juice, especially among those with limited budgets or medical circumstances that pose challenges to eating solid fruit. Most people can include a modest daily portion of fruit juice if desired. However, water is a preferred replacement for SSBs rather than large amounts of even 100% fruit juice, which provides concentrated calories without promoting satiety and without the dietary fiber provided by solid fruit (Rock et al., 2020).

BOX 20.4   PRACTICE PEARLS ON SUGAR-SWEETENED BEVERAGES AND HIGHLY PROCESSED FOODS

Sugar-sweetened beverages (SSBs) include soda, sports and energy drinks, sweetened juice "drinks," and sweet tea and other sweetened tea and coffee beverages.

SSBs can be reduced by gradually replacing them with water as the primary beverage, and including others, such as unsweetened tea or coffee, if desired. Flavored waters without added sweeteners offer another alternative to SSBs and may be produced commercially or by adding herbs or a splash of fruit or juice to tap water.

Artificially sweetened drinks may help some people reduce consumption of SSBs, at least as a transition to increased consumption of water. Evidence does not indicate that artificially sweetened drinks increase cancer risk (Rock et al., 2020; World Cancer Research Fund/American Institute for Cancer Research, 2018). Based on mixed research findings, decisions about whether moderate use supports or detracts from management of weight or other health conditions are best made on an individual basis.

Most foods undergo some form of processing before consumption. Minimally processed foods do not need to be limited. Foods that are highly processed, especially those that are concentrated in calories with high levels of added sugars or unhealthy fats, should be limited to make it easier to reach and maintain a healthy weight.

Diets higher in ultra-processed foods are associated with lower total food expenditures and with lower socioeconomic population groups (Gupta et al., 2021). Therefore, when encouraging reduced use of these foods, it is important to consider specific choices that can be made within individual financial constraints.

Not all high-fat foods need to be avoided. Small servings of oils, nuts, seeds, and avocados, for example, can provide nutrients and phytocompounds in a healthy dietary pattern without providing excessive calories or promoting weight gain (Mozaffarian, 2016; World Cancer Research Fund/American Institute for Cancer Research, 2018).

20.5.3   ALCOHOL

AICR/WCRF and ACS recommendations state that for cancer prevention, it is best to not drink alcohol (Rock et al., 2020; World Cancer Research Fund/American Institute for Cancer Research, 2018). Those who do drink alcohol should limit amounts to no more than one standard drink (equivalent to 14 grams of ethanol) daily for women, or no more than two standard drinks daily for men. Strong evidence identifies alcohol as a cause of cancers; the magnitude of the association varies with the type of cancer and the level of alcohol consumption.

Alcohol-related risk is of special concern to women, since increased breast cancer risk starts at less than one drink per day (LoConte et al., 2018; Rock et al., 2020; Shield et al., 2016; World Cancer Research Fund/American Institute for Cancer Research, 2018). Just 10 grams of ethanol (less than a standard drink) consumed daily raises risk of premenopausal breast cancer 5%, and risk of postmenopausal breast cancer 9%, compared to women who do not drink alcohol (World Cancer Research Fund/American Institute for Cancer Research, 2018). Likewise, risk of oral, pharyngeal, laryngeal, and esophageal (squamous cell) cancers all have a statistically significant increase at less than one drink per day (World Cancer Research Fund/American Institute for Cancer Research, 2018). Risk of head and neck cancers increases two- to five-fold with alcohol consumption beyond three or four drinks per day (LoConte et al., 2018; World Cancer Research Fund/American Institute for Cancer Research, 2018).

Beyond two standard drinks per day, increased risk of colorectal cancer is statistically significant; and beyond three standard drinks per day, risk of liver, stomach, and possibly pancreatic cancer also shows a statistically significant increase in risk.

Recommendations to avoid or limit alcohol might seem contradictory to associations of low-level alcohol consumption with lower cardiovascular and all-cause mortality in some studies. But the effect known as "abstainer bias" (in which people who already have health problems that led them to avoid alcohol are included as non-drinkers) can lead to misinterpretations in which low-volume drinkers appear healthier than non-drinkers (Dietary Guidelines Advisory Committee, 2020; LoConte et al., 2018).

In short, the greatest cancer risk comes from heavy alcohol consumption. Nevertheless, some cancer risk persists even at intake classified as moderate or low.

Alcohol increases cancer risk through several mechanisms (IARC Working Group on the Evaluation of Carcinogenic Risk to Humans, 2012; World Cancer Research Fund/American Institute for Cancer Research, 2018). Alcohol is metabolized to acetaldehyde, which is carcinogenic in humans. In addition, alcohol metabolism increases oxidative stress, and alcohol can increase circulating levels of estrogen, an established risk factor for breast cancer. Further risk can come from alcohol's ability to serve as a solvent, facilitating carcinogen penetration into cells, which is considered a primary explanation for the synergistic increase in risk of mouth and throat cancers for people exposed to both alcohol and tobacco.

BOX 20.5   PRACTICE PEARLS ON LIMITING ALCOHOL

Alcohol's association with cancer risk derives from its ethanol content and is consistent, **regardless** of whether it's beer, wine, or distilled liquor (IARC Working Group on the Evaluation of Carcinogenic Risk to Humans, 2012; LoConte et al., 2018).

Resveratrol is a phytochemical found in red wine that shows anti-carcinogenic effects in laboratory studies. However, human research does not show any difference in cancer risk related to red wine than to other wine or to other alcoholic beverages (IARC Working Group on the Evaluation of Carcinogenic Risk to Humans, 2012; LoConte et al., 2018; Shield et al., 2016).

One standard drink is defined as a portion that provides 14 grams of ethanol. In general, this is 5 ounces of wine, 12 ounces of beer, or 1½ ounces of 80-proof distilled spirits. As beverage glasses have become larger, it's easy to overlook that one drink as served or consumed may be the equivalent of more than one drink in terms of ethanol content and thus cancer risk.

20.6 DIETARY SUPPLEMENTS

Dietary supplements can play a valuable role in promoting health when limited consumption or absorption of a dietary nutrient or compound can't provide amounts that are optimal for a specific individual. AICR/WCRF and ACS recommendations both advise, however, that the overall body of evidence does not support the use of dietary supplements as an effective strategy to reduce cancer risk (Rock et al., 2020; World Cancer Research Fund/American Institute for Cancer Research, 2018).

Since oxidative stress affects genomic instability and tumor-promoting inflammation that facilitate cancer development, there has long been interest in whether antioxidant nutrient supplements could reduce cancer risk. Limited evidence shows low blood levels of some antioxidant nutrients associated with greater risk of some cancers. However, controlled trials have not shown a reduction in cancer risk with antioxidant supplements, and some have even shown increased risk with high doses in some people (Kristal et al., 2014; Rock et al., 2020; Moyer, 2014; World Cancer Research Fund/American Institute for Cancer Research, 2018).

Calcium supplements may help reduce risk of colorectal cancer (World Cancer Research Fund/American Institute for Cancer Research, 2018). Laboratory research shows potential for calcium to decrease cell proliferation and bind unconjugated bile acids, and several prospective cohort studies show an association of calcium supplements with reduced risk. However, since limited evidence links high intake of calcium (including from supplements) with increased risk of prostate cancer, caution is advised regarding dose (Rock et al., 2020; World Cancer Research Fund/American Institute for Cancer Research, 2018).

Vitamin D shows protective effects throughout the cancer process in laboratory studies. Limited evidence from human observational studies links low serum vitamin D levels with greater risk of colorectal cancer, and higher intake from food or supplements with reduced risk (World Cancer Research Fund/American Institute for Cancer Research, 2018). But results are inconsistent in identifying an optimal serum level, and even more inconsistent regarding a level of intake to reach a serum level associated with lower colorectal cancer risk (Zgaga, 2020). RCTs of vitamin D supplements do not currently provide evidence that supplements can reduce cancer risk. A large randomized controlled trial, the VITamin D and OmegA-3 TriaL (VITAL), found no difference in incidence of invasive cancer overall or several specific cancers, except possibly among those with normal BMI, but not those with overweight or obesity (Manson et al., 2019). VITAL identified a potential decrease in metastatic or fatal cancers with 2000 IU of vitamin D supplementation, but again only in those with normal BMI (Chandler et al. 2020). For now, ACS recommendations advise avoiding blood levels categorized as deficient (Rock et al., 2020). Further research is needed on vitamin D's role in reducing risk and how to identify optimal amounts for different individuals.

BOX 20.6   PRACTICE PEARLS ABOUT DIETARY SUPPLEMENTS

Getting nutrients and phytochemicals from food, rather than from supplements, provides a wide range of protectors that may act against cancer development in multiple pathways.

"If some is good, more is better" does not apply to nutrients and cancer risk. For people with low intake or body levels, raising intake with a supplement may be beneficial, but the same supplement for someone else could provide no benefit and, at some point, even be harmful.

20.7   PHYSICAL ACTIVITY

Recommendations for adults are to get at least 150 to 300 minutes of moderate activity, or 75 to 150 minutes of vigorous activity, each week (Rock et al., 2020; World Cancer Research Fund/American Institute for Cancer Research, 2018). The lower end of these ranges meets minimum recommendations for health and lower cancer risk. As fitness improves, participating in at least 45–60 minutes of moderate activity (or at least 30 minutes of vigorous physical activity) every day is optimal (2018 Physical Activity Guidelines Advisory Committee, 2018; Rock et al., 2020; World Cancer Research Fund/American Institute for Cancer Research, 2018).

Research from prospective cohort studies is strongest in support of physical activity (total, recreational, and occupational) to reduce risk of cancers of the colon, endometrium, and breast. Physical activity may also reduce risk of other cancers, including through help reducing weight gain, over-weight, and obesity (Rock et al., 2020; World Cancer Research Fund/American Institute for Cancer Research, 2018).

Both AICR and ACS recommend limiting sedentary behavior such as sitting, lying down, and watching television and other screen-based entertainment (Rock et al., 2020; World Cancer Research Fund/American Institute for Cancer Research, 2018). Increasingly, research is identifying sedentary behavior, which generally reflects time watching television, reading, or at a computer, as a risk factor, especially for cancers of the endometrium, colon, and lung (2018 Physical Activity Guidelines Advisory Committee, 2018; Rock et al., 2020; World Cancer Research Fund/American Institute for Cancer Research, 2018). This association appears to be at least partially independent from physical activity and obesity (Friedenreich et al., 2021).

Mechanisms through which regular physical activity and limitation of sedentary time could reduce cancer risk include reduced weight gain and ectopic body fat. However observational studies and randomized controlled trials (RCTs) provide evidence of effects on serum insulin and insulin sensi-tivity, bioavailable sex steroid hormones, and protection against chronic low-grade inflammation that may occur through effects on body fat and also independently (2018 Physical Activity Guidelines Advisory Committee, 2018; Friedenreich et al., 2021; Rock et al., 2020; World Cancer Research Fund/American Institute for Cancer Research, 2018). Emerging evidence also suggests improved immune function and enhanced endogenous antioxidant defenses that build up with repeated physical activity in response to the reactive oxygen species produced during exercise (Friedenreich et al., 2021).

BOX 20.7   PRACTICE PEARLS ON PHYSICAL ACTIVITY AND SEDENTARY BEHAVIOR

Physical activity "works" regardless of weight and even without weight loss. For people with excess adiposity, weight loss can amplify metabolic benefits of exercise. But physical activity can bring immediate metabolic and hormonal benefits, as well as improved stress management and energy.

The recommended mantra is "move more, sit less." Although accumulating 300 minutes or more of moderate activity weekly (or the equivalent with some or all in vigorous activity) is recommended to maximize cancer protection, the greatest difference in cancer risk is between those who engage in no moderate physical activity and those who get any.

Moderate and vigorous activity are defined based on energy expenditure as defined by METs (metabolic equivalent of task). More easily explained by the "talk test," moderate activity (3.0–5.9 METs) is commonly described as activity during which you can talk, but not sing. Common examples are brisk walking and general gardening. Vigorous activity (≥ 6.0 METs) is often described as activity during which you will not be able to say more than a few words without pausing for a breath. Common examples are jogging, heavy gardening, and aerobics.

Taking regular breaks from sitting for long periods, such as at a computer or watching TV, is recommended to reduce uninterrupted sedentary time.

20.8   TOBACCO

The consistent message across government and non-governmental recommendations for lower risk of cancer and other chronic diseases is for people who don't use tobacco to avoid it, and for people who do use tobacco to quit (Gapstur et al., 2018; Rock et al., 2020; World Cancer Research Fund/American Institute for Cancer Research, 2018). This recommendation pertains to all forms of tobacco. Health consequences of tobacco use increase with both duration and intensity of use.

More than 80% of lung cancers are attributed to **cigarette smoking** (Islami et al., 2018). In addition, major proportions of cancers of the upper aerodigestive tract (larynx, esophagus, oral cavity, and pharynx) and the urinary bladder are also attributed to cigarettes (Islami et al., 2018). Smoking has a smaller, but still significant, relationship to acute myeloid leukemia and to cancers of the cervix, liver, stomach, pancreas, and colorectum. Men with prostate cancer who smoke may have higher mortality rates (American Cancer Society, 2021).

In addition to the cancer risk of cigarette smoking:

- **Cigar** smoking on a regular basis increases risk of cancers of the lung, oral cavity, larynx, and esophagus (American Cancer Society, 2021).
- **Waterpipe** (hookah) smoking is linked in emerging data (currently mostly from case-control studies rather than prospective cohorts) with two to four times increased risk of lung and oral cancers (Waziry et al., 2017).
- **Smokeless tobacco products** marketed in the US include chewing tobacco and snuff. Use of smokeless tobacco increases risk of oral cancer especially, as well as esophageal and pancreatic cancers (Warnakulasuriya & Straif, 2018; Wyss et al., 2016).
- **E-cigarettes** may also be called "e-cigs," "vapes," "e-hookahs," "vape pens," and "electronic nicotine delivery systems." Research is still underway regarding long-term health effects. However, it's well established that e-cigarette aerosol contains nicotine, as well as cancer-causing chemicals and ultra-fine particles that reach deep into lungs (American Cancer Society, 2019; Centers for Disease Control and Prevention (CDC), "About Electronic Cigarettes").

Secondhand smoke includes "mainstream smoke" exhaled by a smoker and "sidestream smoke" that comes directly from the tip of a cigarette. Sidestream smoke burns at a lower temperature than mainstream smoke, and the incomplete combustion results in a high concentration of many carcinogens (Kim et al., 2018). Although cancer risk is not as great as in people who smoke, prospective cohort studies show a significant increase in cancer risk, particularly for lung and breast cancer, associated with secondhand smoke exposure in people who do not smoke (Centers for Disease Control and Prevention (CDC), "Secondhand Smoke"; Kim et al., 2018).

For people who have used tobacco, it's not too late to reduce damage that can lead to cancer. Tobacco cessation leads to increased longevity, reduces the risk of smoking-related cancers and other smoking-related diseases, and improves outcomes for cancer survivors (US Department of Health and Human Services, 2020).

BOX 20.8   PRACTICE PEARLS ABOUT TOBACCO

There is no "safe" form of tobacco.
- **Waterpipe smoking** (often at hookah bars) seems to some people like a safer form of smoking. But hookahs deliver the same or higher levels of toxins as cigarettes. And because of how a hookah is used, people may absorb more of the toxic substances in the smoke than people who smoke cigarettes (American Cancer Society, 2021).
- **Smokeless tobacco** products contain tobacco-specific nitrosamines (TSNAs) and other carcinogenic compounds. In a study of US tobacco users, biomarkers of tobacco-specific nitrosamine exposure were even higher in people who used smokeless tobacco than in people who smoked tobacco (Xia et al., 2021).
- **E-cigarettes** do not have evidence sufficient to recommend them for smoking cessation, and no e-cigarette has currently been FDA-approved as a cessation aid.

With **tobacco cessation**, the earlier the better. But quitting tobacco use improves health at any age, even among people who have smoked for many years or have smoked heavily. The CDC website has in-depth information about tobacco cessation's benefits. As noted in the Surgeon General's report, nicotine is highly addictive, and most people who use tobacco try to quit several times before they succeed (US Department of Health and Human Services, 2020). The report reviews available interventions and concludes that cessation medications approved by the FDA and behavioral counseling increase the likelihood of successfully quitting smoking, particularly when used in combination.

20.9   AFTER A CANCER DIAGNOSIS

AICR/WCRF recommendations advise cancer survivors, unless otherwise advised by a qualified health professional, to follow the cancer prevention recommendations as far as possible after the acute stage of treatment (World Cancer Research Fund/American Institute for Cancer Research, 2018).

During cancer treatment, nutritional needs can differ dramatically. Some people have limited ability to eat or to digest and absorb nutrients. Eating habits that best support their health and ability to continue treatment may differ from the dietary pattern recommended for reducing risk of cancer. For other people, these recommendations can provide a helpful framework for eating habits that support health and health-related quality of life.

Among cancer survivors, higher overall diet quality is associated with lower all-cause mortality and lower cancer mortality, according to a meta-analysis of prospective cohort studies (Morze et al., 2020). Diet quality in this analysis is based on a combination of several different dietary quality index scores. But the consistent thread is a dietary pattern that is high in vegetables, fruits, and whole grains; includes healthy sources of fat; and is low in sodium and added sugars. Evidence quality was rated moderate, which is often considered strong enough to support a recommendation.

Although individual studies may identify associations of single nutrients or specific categories of foods (for example, particular types of vegetables) with better outcomes after a cancer diagnosis, the overall body of research does not support greater protective effects from any single element of a higher-quality diet. Dietary fiber intake is higher in a diet that is categorized as a high-quality dietary pattern, and limited evidence suggests that higher fiber intake may be associated with better outcomes among women after breast cancer (Jayedi et al., 2021; World Cancer Research Fund/American Institute for Cancer Research, 2018). Since different types of fiber could potentially differ in their influence, however, it would be premature to promote dietary fiber intake outside of recommendations for a high-quality, plant-focused dietary pattern.

Overweight and obesity are associated with decreased disease-free and overall survival in several types of cancer (Demark-Wahnefried et al., 2018; Trujillo et al., 2018; World Cancer Research Fund/American Institute for Cancer Research, 2018). But weight is complex, since it reflects body fat, bone, lean muscle tissue, and water balance. Large weight gains (usually referring to gains of at least 5% to 10%) have been linked with increased cancer-specific and all-cause mortality in prostate and breast cancers (McTiernan, 2018; Troeschel et al., 2020).

Intentional weight loss in people with cancer who had overweight or obesity showed improvement in markers of inflammation and metabolic health (Demark-Wahnefried et al., 2018). However, unplanned weight loss among people diagnosed with cancer can reflect loss of lean body mass, result in interruption of treatment, and increase risk of poor outcomes. Sarcopenia is common in people being treated for cancer, and it is associated with poor outcomes even in people with obesity (Trujillo et al., 2018).

To support weight-related recommendations, more research in people after a cancer diagnosis is needed from well-designed studies with repeated measures over time and clarification of the influence of body composition, location of body fat, adiposity-related biomarkers (such as inflammation and insulin resistance), and change in weight and body composition after diagnosis.

More research is also needed regarding the role of physical activity in improving survival after cancer. World Cancer Research Fund/American Institute for Cancer Research (2018) analysis identifies limited evidence suggesting that physical activity could have a protective influence on prognosis for breast cancer survivors.

An expert roundtable concluded that health-related quality of life (including fatigue, anxiety, and physical function) improves with a program combining moderate-intensity aerobic and resistance exercise both during and after treatment (Campbell et al., 2019). Still, it's vital to consider individual differences. Bone fragility, presence of other medical conditions, peripheral nerve damage, and presence or risk of lymphedema don't rule out physical activity, but they can be critical in choosing types of exercise that are safe and comfortable (Campbell et al., 2019; Stout et al., 2020). Health professionals advising individual patients about physical activity after a cancer diagnosis may find recommendations developed by the expert roundtable (Campbell et al., 2019) helpful.

Evidence on the role of lifestyle in cancer survivorship is still limited and provides better insights for a few more common and widely researched cancers. Overall, however, diet and physical activity during and after cancer treatment do seem to improve overall survival and/or health-related quality of life (World Cancer Research Fund/American Institute for Cancer Research, 2018).

BOX 20.9   PRACTICE PEARLS ON RECOMMENDATIONS AFTER A CANCER DIAGNOSIS

Several national organizations have developed lifestyle recommendations specifically for cancer survivors that include achieving and maintaining a weight supportive of individual health, regular physical activity, and a dietary pattern high in vegetables, fruits, and whole grains.

- The American Cancer Society: Nutrition and activity guidelines for cancer survivors (Rock et al., 2012).
- The American College of Sports Medicine roundtable on exercise guidelines for cancer survivors (Campbell et al., 2019).
- National Comprehensive Cancer Network (NCCN) Guidelines for Patients: Survivorship Care for Healthy Living, 2020 (National Comprehensive Cancer Network).

Registered dietitians (RDs) and registered dietitian nutritionists (RDNs), especially those who are Board Certified Specialists in Oncology (CSOs), offer valuable expertise in addressing individual circumstances. For help in finding one, a zip-code based search is available from the website of the Academy of Nutrition and Dietetics (www.eatright.org/).

20.10   COMMON QUESTIONS

The recommendations above identify the lifestyle choices that, in addition to avoiding excess sun exposure, have strongest evidence supporting reduced cancer risk. However, people often have questions about other lifestyle choices not addressed by these major recommendations.

20.10.1   SUGAR

Cancer cells multiply more rapidly than normal cells, and therefore glucose metabolism occurs more rapidly. However, this should not be interpreted to mean that sugar consumption "feeds" cancer. Diets high in added sugars can lead to higher insulin levels, especially in people with insulin resistance. Cancer cells often have an increased concentration of insulin receptors, making them especially responsive to growth signals from elevated insulin. Excessive consumption of added sugars also contributes to calorie intake. This can promote weight gain and obesity and thus indirectly increase cancer risk through adiposity-related pathways.

Research does not support a direct link of added sugars to cancer risk after adjusting for confounding variables (Rock et al., 2020). Limiting consumption of foods and beverages high in added sugars is recommended to limit undesired weight gain and promote metabolic health, as well as to make room for foods that supply protective nutrients and compounds (World Cancer Research Fund/American Institute for Cancer Research, 2018).

20.10.2 DAIRY

Moderate consumption of dairy products and of calcium (calcium intake of 700 to 1000 milligrams per day) show strong links in reducing risk of colorectal cancer and adenomas, possibly reflecting calcium's ability to decrease cell proliferation and bind unconjugated bile acids (Rock et al., 2020; World Cancer Research Fund/American Institute for Cancer Research, 2018). Reduced colorectal cancer linked to dairy consumption could also reflect its vitamin D (Rock et al., 2020; World Cancer Research Fund/American Institute for Cancer Research, 2018). Providing recommendations is complicated by limited evidence suggesting increased risk of prostate cancer with diets high in dairy products or calcium (Rock et al., 2020; World Cancer Research Fund/American Institute for Cancer Research, 2018). Limited evidence suggests that dairy products are associated with reduced risk of premenopausal breast cancer, and diets high in calcium with reduced risk of both pre- and postmenopausal breast cancer (World Cancer Research Fund/American Institute for Cancer Research, 2018). Evidence for dairy and ovarian cancer risk was judged to be too limited for any conclusion. Due to limitations in current evidence, neither AICR nor ACS have included recommendations regarding dairy products (Rock et al., 2020; World Cancer Research Fund/American Institute for Cancer Research, 2018).

20.10.3 COFFEE AND TEA

Coffee consumption is associated with lower risk of liver and endometrial cancers (World Cancer Research Fund/American Institute for Cancer Research, 2018), and one analysis shows a possible reduction in risk of postmenopausal breast cancer (Lafranconi et al., 2018). Possible reductions in risk of other cancers is unclear (Alicandro et al., 2017; World Cancer Research Fund/American Institute for Cancer Research, 2018). Results are generally similar for regular and decaf coffee. Phytochemicals in coffee offer several potential protective mechanisms: Increased support for antioxidant and anti-inflammatory defenses, improved insulin sensitivity and reduced circulating insulin, and reduced bioavailability of estrogen (Hang et al., 2019; World Cancer Research Fund/American Institute for Cancer Research, 2018).

Tea (*Camellia sinensis*) also contains phytochemicals with potential to protect against cancer through support of antioxidant defenses and effects on cell growth and gene expression. Green tea is best known for its EGCG compound; black tea contains some EGCG, with higher levels of other flavonoids. However, lab studies often use amounts of these compounds equivalent to far more than people typically get from drinking tea (Yang et al., 2016). Limited evidence suggests that tea may reduce risk of bladder cancer, but overall, human evidence of cancer risk reduction is inconsistent and too limited for any conclusion (World Cancer Research Fund/American Institute for Cancer Research, 2018; Yang et al., 2016).

20.10.4 ORGANIC FOODS

Occupational exposure to improper use of pesticides may increase risk of some cancers, but it's not clear whether choosing organic foods reduces cancer risk (Rock et al., 2020). Pesticide residue is generally lower in organic foods, yet data from the USDA Pesticide Data Program (PDP) shows many conventionally produced foods with no detectable pesticide residue, and more than 98% with residue levels below EPA tolerances (USDA, 2020). One analysis suggests that selective choice of organic leafy greens and soft-skinned fruit may reduce relevant pesticide exposure (Benbrook & Davis, 2020), whereas another concluded that switching to organic produce does not result in any appreciable reduction of health risks (Winter & Katz, 2011). There is currently no substantiated evidence that foods from genetically engineered crops (such as GMO) increase cancer risk (National Academies of Sciences, 2016; Rock et al., 2020). Since organic foods are generally more expensive than similar conventionally produced choices, it is worth emphasizing that current evidence supports greater reduction in cancer risk by consuming more vegetables, fruits, and whole grains than by choosing organic options (Rock et al., 2020).

20.10.5 SOY FOODS

Questions about soy foods often involve their isoflavones, compounds classified as phytoestrogens based on chemical structure. Early rodent studies suggested potential to increase growth of estrogen receptor-positive (ER+) breast cancer cells. However, later research showed that rodents metabolize isoflavones differently than humans, and their blood levels were much higher than would result from humans consuming soyfoods (Setchell et al., 2011).

Observational studies link soy consumption with lower risk of breast and prostate cancers in Asia, where lifelong consumption is common (Rock et al., 2020; Wu et al., 2016). For breast cancer survivors, some studies show an association of moderate soy consumption a year or more after diagnosis with greater overall survival, and perhaps decreased recurrence (American Institute for Cancer Research, 2021; Nechuta et al., 2012; World Cancer Research Fund/American Institute for Cancer Research, 2018), but evidence is too limited to justify any recommendation (World Cancer Research Fund/American Institute for Cancer Research, 2018). Moderate soy consumption is considered one to two standard servings daily of whole soy foods, such as tofu, soy milk, edamame, or soy nuts. (One serving averages about 7 grams protein and 25 milligrams isoflavones.) AICR and ACS both advise avoidance or caution regarding isoflavone supplements or intake above 100 mg/day (Rock et al., 2020; World Cancer Research Fund/American Institute for Cancer Research, 2018).

20.11 CONCLUSION

The importance of avoiding tobacco to reduce risk of cancer is widely known. Recommendations grounded in thorough analysis of best available research identify additional lifestyle choices to significantly reduce cancer risk: Reach and maintain a healthy weight; move more and sit less; limit alcohol; and create eating habits that limit red and processed meats, highly processed foods, and sugar-sweetened drinks, and emphasize a variety of whole plant foods as the center of delicious eating.

REFERENCES

2018 Physical Activity Guidelines Advisory Committee. (2018). *2018 Physical Activity Guidelines Advisory Committee Scientific Report*. US Department of Health and Human Services.

Alberti, K. G., Eckel, R. H., Grundy, S. M., Zimmet, P. Z., Cleeman, J. I., Donato, K. A., Fruchart, J-C., James, W. P. T., Loria, C. M., & Smith, S. C., Jr. (2009). Harmonizing the metabolic syndrome: A joint interim statement of the International Diabetes Federation Task Force on Epidemiology and Prevention; National Heart, Lung, and Blood Institute; American Heart Association; World Heart Federation; International Atherosclerosis Society; and International Association for the Study of Obesity. *Circulation, 120*(16), 1640–1645. https://doi.org/10.1161/CIRCULATIONAHA.109.192644

Alicandro, G., Tavani, A., & La Vecchia, C. (2017). Coffee and cancer risk: A summary overview. *European Journal of Cancer Prevention*, *26*(5), 424–432. https://doi.org/10.1097/cej.0000000000000341

American Cancer Society. (2019). American Cancer Society position statement on electronic cigarettes. Retrieved November 6, 2021, www.cancer.org/healthy/stay-away-from-tobacco/e-cigarettes-vaping/e-cigarette-position-statement.html

American Cancer Society. (2021). *Cancer facts & figures 2021*. American Cancer Society.

American Institute for Cancer Research. (2021). AICR food facts—foods that fight cancer: Soy. Retrieved from www.aicr.org/cancer-prevention/food-facts/soy/

Babic, A., Sasamoto, N., Rosner, B. A., Tworoger, S. S., Jordan, S. J., Risch, H. A., Harris, H. R., Rossing, M. A., Doherty, J. A., Fortner, R. T., Chang-Claude, J., Goodman, M. T., Thompson, P. J., Moysich, K. B., Ness, R. B., Kjaer, S. K., Jensen, A., Schildkraut, J. M., Titus, L, J., & Terry, K. L. (2020). Association Between Breastfeeding and Ovarian Cancer Risk. *JAMA Oncology*, *6*(6), e200421. https://doi.org/10.1001/jamaoncol.2020.0421

Benbrook, C. M., & Davis, D. R. (2020). The dietary risk index system: a tool to track pesticide dietary risks. *Environmental Health*, *19*(1), 103. https://doi.org/10.1186/s12940-020-00657-z

Bishop, K. S., & Ferguson, L. R. (2015). The interaction between epigenetics, nutrition and the development of cancer. *Nutrients*, *7*(2), 922–947. https://doi.org/10.3390/nu7020922

Bultman, S. J. (2016). The microbiome and its potential as a cancer preventive intervention. *Seminars in Oncology*, *43*(1), 97–106. https://doi.org/10.1053/j.seminoncol.2015.09.001

Campbell, K. L., Winters-Stone, K. M., Wiskemann, J., May, A. M., Schwartz, A. L., Courneya, K. S., Zucker, D. S., Matthews, C. E., Ligibel, J. A., Gerber, L. H., Morris, G. S., Patel, A. V., Hue, T. F., Perna, F. M., & Schmitz, K. H. (2019). Exercise guidelines for cancer survivors: Consensus statement from international multidisciplinary roundtable. *Medicine & Science in Sports & Exercise*, *51*(11), 2375–2390. https://doi.org/10.1249/mss.0000000000002116

Centers for Disease Control and Prevention (CDC). (2021, September 2021). About electronic cigarettes (e-cigarettes). *Smoking & Tobacco Use*. Retrieved from www.cdc.gov/tobacco/basic_information/e-cigarettes/about-e-cigarettes.html

Centers for Disease Control and Prevention (CDC). (2021, March 2). Secondhand smoke. *Smoking & Tobacco Use*. www.cdc.gov/tobacco/basic_information/secondhand_smoke/index.htm

Chandler, P. D., Chen, W. Y., Ajala, O. N., Hazra, A., Cook, N., Bubes, V., Lee, I. M., Giovannucci, E. L., Willett, W., Buring, J. E., Manson, J. E., & VITAL Research Group. (2020). Effect of vitamin D3 supplements on development of advanced cancer: A secondary analysis of the VITAL randomized clinical trial. *JAMA Network Open*, *3*(11), e2025850. https://doi.org/10.1001/jamanetworkopen.2020.25850

Chlebowski, R. T., Luo, J., Anderson, G. L., Barrington, W., Reding, K., Simon, M. S., Manson, J. E., Rohan, T. E., Wactawski-Wende, J., Lane, D., Strickler, H., Mosaver-Rahmani, Y., Freudenheim, J. L., Saquib, N., & Stefanick, M. L. (2019). Weight loss and breast cancer incidence in postmenopausal women. *Cancer*, *125*(2), 205–212. https://doi.org/10.1002/cncr.31687

Demark-Wahnefried, W., Schmitz, K. H., Alfano, C. M., Bail, J. R., Goodwin, P. J., Thomson, C. A., Bradley, D. W., Courneya, K. S., Befort, C. A., Denlinger, C. S., Ligibel, J. A., Dietz, W. H., Stolley, M. R., Irwin, M. L., Bamman, M. M., Apovian, C., M., Pinto, B. M., Wolin, K. Y., … Basen-Engquist, K. (2018). Weight management and physical activity throughout the cancer care continuum. *CA: A Cancer Journal for Clinicians*, *68*(1), 64–89. https://doi.org/10.3322/caac.21441

Demeyer, D., Mertens, B., De Smet, S., & Ulens, M. (2016). Mechanisms linking colorectal cancer to the consumption of (processed) red meat: A review. *Critical Reviews in Food Science and Nutrition*, *56*(16), 2747–2766. https://doi.org/10.1080/10408398.2013.873886

Dietary Guidelines Advisory Committee. (2020). *Scientific report of the 2020 dietary guidelines advisory committee: Advisory report to the secretary of agriculture and the secretary of health and human services*. US Department of Agriculture, Agricultural Research Service.

Farvid, M. S., Spence, N. D., Holmes, M. D., & Barnett, J. B. (2020). Fiber consumption and breast cancer incidence: A systematic review and meta-analysis of prospective studies. *Cancer*, *126*(13), 3061–3075. https://doi.org/10.1002/cncr.32816

Friedenreich, C. M., Ryder-Burbidge, C., & McNeil, J. (2021). Physical activity, obesity and sedentary behavior in cancer etiology: Epidemiologic evidence and biologic mechanisms. *Molecular Oncology*, *15*(3), 790–800. https://doi.org/10.1002/1878-0261.12772

Gapstur, S. M., Drope, J. M., Jacobs, E. J., Teras, L. R., McCullough, M. L., Douglas, C. E., Patel, A. V., Wender, R. C., & Brawley, O. W. (2018). A blueprint for the primary prevention of cancer: Targeting established, modifiable risk factors. *CA: A Cancer Journal for Clinicians*, *68*(6), 446–470. https://doi.org/10.3322/caac.21496

George, V. C., Dellaire, G., & Rupasinghe, H. P. V. (2017). Plant flavonoids in cancer chemoprevention: Role in genome stability. *The Journal of Nutritional Biochemistry*, *45*, 1–14. https://doi.org/10.1016/j.jnutbio.2016.11.007

Giovannucci, E. (2018). A framework to understand diet, physical activity, body weight, and cancer risk. *Cancer Causes &Control: CCC*, *29*(1), 1–6. https://doi.org/10.1007/s10552-017-0975-y

Gupta, S., Rose, C. M., Buszkiewicz, J., Ko, L. K., Mou, J., Cook, A., Aggarwal, A., & Drewnowski, A. (2021). Characterising percentage energy from ultra-processed foods by participant demographics, diet quality and diet cost: Findings from the Seattle Obesity Study (SOS) III. *The British Journal of Nutrition*, *126*(5), 773–781. https://doi.org/10.1017/S0007114520004705

Hammerling, U., Bergman Laurila, J., Grafström, R., & Ilbäck, N.-G. (2016). Consumption of red/processed meat and colorectal carcinoma: Possible mechanisms underlying the significant association. *Critical Reviews in Food Science and Nutrition*, *56*(4), 614–634. https://doi.org/10.1080/10408398.2014.972498

Hanahan, D., & Weinberg, R. A. (2011). Hallmarks of cancer: The next generation. *Cell*, *144*(5), 646–674. https://doi.org/10.1016/j.cell.2011.02.013

Hang, D., Kværner, A. S., Ma, W., Hu, Y., Tabung, F. K., Nan, H., Hu, Z., Shen, H., Mucci, L. A., Chan, A. T., Giovannucchi, E. L., & Song, M. (2019). Coffee consumption and plasma biomarkers of metabolic and inflammatory pathways in US health professionals. *The American Journal of Clinical Nutrition*, *109*(3), 635–647. https://doi.org/10.1093/ajcn/nqy295

IARC Working Group on the Evaluation of Carcinogenic Risk to Humans. (2012). Personal habits and indoor combustions. (IARC Monographs on the Evaluation of Carcinogenic Risks to Humans, No. 100E.) International Agency for Research on Cancer.

Islami, F., Goding Sauer, A., Miller, K. D., Siegel, R. L., Fedewa, S. A., Jacobs, E. J., McCullough, M. L., Patel, A. V., Ma, J., Soerjomataram, I., Flanders, D., Brawley, O. W., Gapstur, S. M., & Jemal, A. (2018). Proportion and number of cancer cases and deaths attributable to potentially modifiable risk factors in the United States. *CA: A Cancer Journal for Clinicians*, *68*(1), 31–54. https://doi.org/10.3322/caac.21440

Iyengar, N. M., Gucalp, A., Dannenberg, A. J., & Hudis, C. A. (2016). Obesity and cancer mechanisms: Tumor microenvironment and inflammation. *Journal of Clinical Oncology: Official Journal of the American Society of Clinical Oncology*, *34*(35), 4270–4276. https://doi.org/10.1200/JCO.2016.67.4283

Jayedi, A., Emadi, A., Khan, T. A., Abdolshahi, A., & Shab-Bidar, S. (2021). Dietary fiber and survival in women with breast cancer: A dose-response meta-analysis of prospective cohort studies. *Nutrition and Cancer*, *73*(9), 1570–1580. https://doi.org/10.1080/01635581.2020.1803928

Kim, A. S., Ko, H. J., Kwon, J. H., & Lee, J. M. (2018). Exposure to secondhand smoke and risk of cancer in never smokers: A meta-analysis of epidemiologic studies. *International Journal of Environmental Research and Public Health*, *15*(9). https://doi.org/10.3390/ijerph15091981

Kristal, A. R., Darke, A. K., Morris, J. S., Tangen, C. M., Goodman, P. J., Thompson, I. M., Meyskens, F. L., Jr., Goodman, G. E., Minasian, L. M., Parnes, H. L., Lippman, S. M., Klein, E. A. (2014). Baseline selenium status and effects of selenium and vitamin e supplementation on prostate cancer risk. *Journal of the National Cancer Institute*, *106*(3), djt456. https://doi.org/10.1093/jnci/djt456

Lafranconi, A., Micek, A., De Paoli, P., Bimonte, S., Rossi, P., Quagliariello, V., & Berretta, M. (2018). Coffee intake decreases risk of postmenopausal breast cancer: A dose-response meta-analysis on prospective cohort studies. *Nutrients*, *10*(2), 112.

Lauby-Secretan, B., Scoccianti, C., Loomis, D., Grosse, Y., Bianchini, F., & Straif, K. (2016). Body fatness and cancer—viewpoint of the IARC Working Group. *New England Journal of Medicine*, *375*(8), 794–798. https://doi.org/10.1056/NEJMsr1606602

Li, W., Guo, Y., Zhang, C., Wu, R., Yang, A. Y., Gaspar, J., & Kong, A. N. (2016). Dietary phytochemicals and cancer chemoprevention: A perspective on oxidative stress, inflammation, and epigenetics. *Chemical Research in Toxicology*, *29*(12), 2071–2095. https://doi.org/10.1021/acs.chemrestox.6b00413

Liu, B., Giffney, H. E., Arthur, R. S., Rohan, T. E., & Dannenberg, A. J. (2021). Cancer risk in normal weight individuals with metabolic obesity: A narrative review. *Cancer Prevention Research*, *14*(5), 509–520. https://doi.org/10.1158/1940-6207.Capr-20-0633

LoConte, N. K., Brewster, A. M., Kaur, J. S., Merrill, J. K., & Alberg, A. J. (2018). Alcohol and cancer: A statement of the American Society of Clinical Oncology. *Journal of Clinical Oncology: Official Journal of the American Society of Clinical Oncology*, *36*(1), 83–93. https://doi.org/10.1200/JCO.2017.76.1155

Look AHEAD Research Group, Yeh, H.-C., Bantle, J. P., Cassidy-Begay, M., Blackburn, G., Bray, G. A., Byers, T., Clark, J. M., Coday, M., Egan, C., Espeland, M. A., Foreyt, J. P., Garcia, K., Goldman, V., Gregg, E. W., Hazuda, H. P., Hesson, L., Hill, J. O., Horton, E. S., ... Yanovski, S. Z. (2020). Intensive weight loss intervention and cancer risk in adults with type 2 diabetes: Analysis of the Look AHEAD randomized clinical trial. *Obesity*, *28*(9), 1678–1686. https://doi.org/10.1002/oby.22936

Luger, M., Lafontan, M., Bes-Rastrollo, M., Winzer, E., Yumuk, V., & Farpour-Lambert, N. (2017). Sugar-sweetened beverages and weight gain in children and adults: A systematic review from 2013 to 2015 and a comparison with previous studies. *Obesity Facts*, *10*(6), 674–693. https://doi.org/10.1159/000484566

Ma, X., Zhao, L. G., Sun, J. W., Yang, Y., Zheng, J. L., Gao, J., & Xiang, Y. B. (2018). Association between breastfeeding and risk of endometrial cancer: a meta-analysis of epidemiological studies. *European Journal of Cancer Prevention: The Official Journal of the European Cancer Prevention Organisation*, *27*(2), 144–151. https://doi.org/10.1097/CEJ.0000000000000186

Manson, J. E., Cook, N. R., Lee, I.-M., Christen, W., Bassuk, S. S., Mora, S., Gibson, H., Gordon, D., Copeland, T., D'Agostino, D., Friedenberg, G., Ridge, C., Bubes, V., Giovannucci, E. L., Willett, W. C., & Buring, J. E. (2019). Vitamin D supplements and prevention of cancer and cardiovascular disease. *New England Journal of Medicine*, *380*(1), 33–44. https://doi.org/10.1056/NEJMoa1809944

McTiernan, A. (2018). Weight, physical activity and breast cancer survival. *Proceedings of the Nutrition Society*, *77*(4), 403–411. https://doi.org/10.1017/S0029665118000010

Micucci, C., Valli, D., Matacchione, G., & Catalano, A. (2016). Current perspectives between metabolic syndrome and cancer. *Oncotarget*, *7*, 38959–38972.

Monteiro, C. A., Cannon, G., Levy, R. B., Moubarac, J. C., Louzada, M. L., Rauber, F., Khandpur, N., Cediel, G., Neri, D., Martinez-Steele., E., Baraldi, L. G., & Jaime, P. C. (2019). Ultra-processed foods: What they are and how to identify them. *Public Health Nutrition*, *22*(5), 936–941.

Moradi, S., Entezari, M. H., Mohammadi, H., Jayedi, A., Lazaridi, A. V., Kermani, M. A. H., & Miraghajani, M. (2021). Ultra-processed food consumption and adult obesity risk: A systematic review and dose-response meta-analysis. *Critical Reviews in Food Science and Nutrition*, 1–12. https://doi.org/10.1080/10408398.2021.1946005

Morze, J., Danielewicz, A., Hoffmann, G., & Schwingshackl, L. (2020). Diet quality as assessed by the healthy eating index, alternate healthy eating index, dietary approaches to stop hypertension score, and health outcomes: A second update of a systematic review and meta-analysis of cohort studies. *Journal of the Academy of Nutrition and Dietetics*, *120*(12), 1998–2031.e1915. https://doi.org/10.1016/j.jand.2020.08.076

Moyer, V. A., & U.S. Preventive Services Task Force. (2014). Vitamin, mineral, and multivitamin supplements for the primary prevention of cardiovascular disease and cancer: U.S. Preventive services Task Force recommendation statement. *Annals of Internal Medicine*, *160*(8), 558–564. http://doi.org/10.7326/M14-0198.

Mozaffarian, D. (2016). Dietary and policy priorities for cardiovascular disease, diabetes, and obesity: A comprehensive review. *Circulation*, *133*(2), 187–225. https://doi.org/10.1161/CIRCULATIONAHA.115.018585

National Academies of Sciences, Engineering, and Medicine. (2016). *Genetically engineered crops: Experiences and prospects*. Washington, DC. Retrieved from https://doi.org/10.17226/23395

National Comprehensive Cancer Network. (2020, July 14). NCCN guidelines for patients: Survivorship care for healthy living, 2020. Retrieved from www.nccn.org/guidelines/guidelines-detail?category=3&id=1466

Nechuta, S. J., Caan, B. J., Chen, W. Y., Lu, W., Chen, Z., Kwan, M. L., Flatt, S. W., Zheng, Y., Zheng, W., Pierce, J. P., & Shu, X. O. (2012). Soy food intake after diagnosis of breast cancer and survival: an in-depth analysis of combined evidence from cohort studies of US and Chinese women. *The American Journal of Clinical Nutrition*, *96*(1), 123–132. https://doi.org/10.3945/ajcn.112.035972

Neeland, I. J., Ross, R., Després, J. P., Matsuzawa, Y., Yamashita, S., Shai, I., Seidell, J., Magni, P., Santos, R. D., Arsenault, B., Cuevas, A., Hu, F. B., Griffin, B., Zambon, A., Barter, P., Fruchart, J-C., & Eckel, R. H. (2019). Visceral and ectopic fat, atherosclerosis, and cardiometabolic disease: A position statement. *Lancet Diabetes & Endocrinology*, *7*(9), 715–725. https://doi.org/10.1016/s2213-8587(19)30084-1

O'Keefe, S. J. (2016). Diet, microorganisms and their metabolites, and colon cancer. *Natural Reviews Gastroenterology & Hepatology*, *13*(12), 691–706. https://doi.org/10.1038/nrgastro.2016.165

Parida, S., & Sharma, D. (2019). The microbiome–estrogen connection and breast cancer risk. *Cells*, *8*(12), 1642.

Rock, C. L., Doyle, C., Demark-Wahnefried, W., Meyerhardt, J., Courneya, K. S., Schwartz, A. L., Bandera, E. V., Hamilton, K. K., Grant, B., McCullough, M., Byers, T., & Gansler, T. (2012). Nutrition and physical activity guidelines for cancer survivors. *CA: A Cancer Journal for Clinicians*, *62*(4), 243–274. https://doi.org/10.3322/caac.21142

Rock, C. L., Thomson, C., Gansler, T., Gapstur, S. M., McCullough, M. L., Patel, A. V., Andrews, K. S., Bandera, E. V., Spees, C. K., Robien, K., Hartman, S., Sullivan, K., Grant, B. L., Hamilton, K. K., Kushi, L. H., Caan, B. J., Kibbe, D., Black, J. D., Wiedt, T. L., … Doyle, C. (2020). American Cancer Society guideline for diet and physical activity for cancer prevention. *CA: A Cancer Journal for Clinicians*, *70*(4), 245–271. https://doi.org/10.3322/caac.21591

Rouhani, M. H., Haghighatdoost, F., Surkan, P. J., & Azadbakht, L. (2016). Associations between dietary energy density and obesity: A systematic review and meta-analysis of observational studies. *Nutrition*, *32*(10), 1037–1047. https://doi.org/10.1016/j.nut.2016.03.017

Setchell, K. D., Brown, N. M., Zhao, X., Lindley, S. L., Heubi, J. E., King, E. C., & Messina, M. J. (2011). Soy isoflavone phase II metabolism differs between rodents and humans: implications for the effect on breast cancer risk. *The American Journal of Clinical Nutrition*, *94*(5), 1284–1294. https://doi.org/10.3945/ajcn.111.019638

Sheflin, A. M., Melby, C. L., Carbonero, F., & Weir, T. L. (2017). Linking dietary patterns with gut microbial composition and function. *Gut Microbes*, *8*(2), 113–129. https://doi.org/10.1080/19490976.2016.1270809

Shi, T. H., Wang, B., & Natarajan, S. (2020). The influence of metabolic syndrome in predicting mortality risk among US adults: Importance of metabolic syndrome even in adults with normal weight. *Preventing Chronic Disease*, *17*, E36. https://doi.org/10.5888/pcd17.200020

Shield, K. D., Soerjomataram, I., & Rehm, J. (2016). Alcohol use and breast cancer: A critical review. *Alcoholism: Clinical and Experimental Research*, *40*(6), 1166–1181. https://doi.org/10.1111/acer.13071

Singh, R. K., Chang, H. W., Yan, D., Lee, K. M., Ucmak, D., Wong, K., Abrouk, M., Farahnik, B., Nakamura, M., Zhu, T. H., Bhutani, T., & Liao, W. (2017). Influence of diet on the gut microbiome and implications for human health. *Journal of Translational Medicine*, *15*(1), 73. https://doi.org/10.1186/s12967-017-1175-y

Smith, L. A., O'Flanagan, C. H., Bowers, L. W., Allott, E. H., & Hursting, S. D. (2018). Translating mechanism-based strategies to break the obesity–cancer link: A narrative review. *Journal of the Academy of Nutrition and Dietetics*, *118*(4), 652–667. https://doi.org/10.1016/j.jand.2017.08.112

Stout, N. L., Brown, J. C., Schwartz, A. L., Marshall, T. F., Campbell, A. M., Nekhlyudov, L., Zucker, D. S., Basen-Engquist, K. M., Campbell, G., Meyerhardt, J., Cheville, A. L., Covington, K. R., Ligibel, J. A., Sokolof, J. M., Schmitz, K. H., … Alfano, C. M. (2020). An exercise oncology clinical pathway: Screening and referral for personalized interventions. *Cancer*, *126*(12), 2750–2758. https://doi.org/10.1002/cncr.32860

Sung, H., Siegel, R. L., Rosenberg, P. S., & Jemal, A. (2019). Emerging cancer trends among young adults in the USA: Analysis of a population-based cancer registry. *The Lancet Public Health*, *4*(3), Pe137–e147.

Troeschel, A. N., Hartman, T. J., Jacobs, E. J., Stevens, V. L., Gansler, T., Flanders, W. D., McCullough, L. E., & Wang, Y. (2020). Postdiagnosis body mass index, weight change, and mortality from prostate cancer, cardiovascular disease, and all causes among survivors of nonmetastatic prostate cancer. *Journal of Clinical Oncology*, *38*(18), 2018–2027. https://doi.org/10.1200/jco.19.02185

Trujillo, E. B., Dixon, S. W., Claghorn, K., Levin, R. M., Mills, J. B., & Spees, C. K. (2018). Closing the gap in nutrition care at outpatient cancer centers: Ongoing initiatives of the oncology nutrition dietetic practice group. *Journal of the Academy of Nutrition and Dietetics*, *118*(4), 749–760. https://doi.org/10.1016/j.jand.2018.02.010

US Department of Health and Human Services. (2020). *Smoking cessation: A report of the surgeon general*. US Department of Health and Human Services, Centers for Disease Control and Prevention, National Center for Chronic Disease Prevention and Health Promotion, Office on Smoking and Health.

US Preventive Services Task Force. (2016). Final recommendation statement: vitamin supplementation to prevent cancer and CVD: Preventive medication.

USDA. (2020). *Pesticide data program annual summary, calendar year 2019*. United States Department of Agriculture, Agricultural Marketing Program.

van Gemert, W. A., Monninkhof, E. M., May, A. M., Elias, S. G., van der Palen, J., Veldhuis, W., Stapper, M., Stellato, R. K., Schuit, J. A., & Peeters, P. H. (2017). Association between changes in fat distribution and biomarkers for breast cancer. *Endocrine-Related Cancer*, *24*(6), 297–305. https://doi.org/10.1530/ERC-16-0490

Warnakulasuriya S., & Straif K. (2018). Carcinogenicity of smokeless tobacco: Evidence from studies in humans & experimental animals. *Indian Journal of Medical Research*, *148*(6), 681–686. https://doi.org/10.4103/ijmr.IJMR_149_18

Waziry, R., Jawad, M., Ballout, R. A., Al Akel, M., & Akl, E. A. (2017). The effects of waterpipe tobacco smoking on health outcomes: An updated systematic review and meta-analysis. *International Journal of Epidemiology*, *46*(1), 32–43. https://doi.org/10.1093/ije/dyw021

Winter, C. K., & Katz, J. M. (2011). Dietary exposure to pesticide residues from commodities alleged to contain the highest contamination levels. *Journal of Toxicology*, *2011*, 589674. https://doi.org/10.1155/2011/589674

World Cancer Research Fund/American Institute for Cancer Research. (2018). *Diet, nutrition, physical activity and cancer: A global perspective. Continuous update project expert report 2018.* Retrieved from dietandcancerreport.org

Wu, J., Zeng, R., Huang, J., Li, X., Zhang, J., Ho, J., & Zheng, Y. (2016). Dietary protein sources and incidence of breast cancer: A dose-response meta-analysis of prospective studies. *Nutrients*, *8*(11), 730.

Wyss, A. B., Hashibe, M., Lee, Y. A., Chuang, S. C., Muscat, J., Chen, C., Schwartz, S. M., Smith, E., Zhang, Z-F., Morgenstern, H., Wei, Q., Li, G., Kelsey, K. T. McClean, M., Winn, D. M., Schantz, S., Yu, G-P., Gillison, M. L., Zevallos, J. P., … Olshan AF. (2016). Smokeless tobacco use and the risk of head and neck cancer: Pooled analysis of US studies in the INHANCE Consortium. *American Journal of Epidemiology*, *184*(10), 703–716. https://doi.org/10.1093/aje/kww075

Xia, B., Blount, B. C., Guillot, T., Brosius, C., Li, Y., Van Bemmel, D. M., Kimmel, H. L., Chang, C. M., Borek, N., Edwards, K. C., Lawrence, C., Hyland, A., Goniewicz, M. L., Pine, B. N., Zia, Y., Bernert, J. T., De Castro, B. R., Lee, J., Brown, J. L., … Wang, L. (2021). Tobacco-specific nitrosamines (NNAL, NNN, NAT, and NAB) exposures in the US population assessment of tobacco and health (PATH) study wave 1 (2013–2014). *Nicotine & Tobacco Research*, *23*(3), 573–583. https://doi.org/10.1093/ntr/ntaa110

Yang, C. S., Chen, J. X., Wang, H., & Lim, J. (2016). Lessons learned from cancer prevention studies with nutrients and non-nutritive dietary constituents. *Molecular Nutrition & Food Research*, *60*(6), 1239–1250. https://doi.org/10.1002/mnfr.201500766

Zgaga, L. (2020). Heterogeneity of the effect of vitamin D supplementation in randomized controlled trials on cancer prevention. *JAMA Network Open*, *3*(11), e2027176–e2027176. https://doi.org/10.1001/jamanetworkopen.2020.27176

21 Cognitive Disorders and Lifestyle Change

Janine Santora

Capital Health Institute for Neurosciences

Pennington, New Jersey, USA

CONTENTS

KEY POINTS

- Cognition is an individual's ability to learn new information, sustain focus and attention, problem solve and reason, maintain short- and long-term memory, and recall information.
- Cognitive function involves four major processes, including receptive function, memory and learning, thinking, and expressive functions.
- Cognitive impairment is when a person's ability to remember, concentrate, learn new things, or make decisions negatively impact their daily life.
- Cognitive assessment screening tools can assess cognitive impairment versus normal age-related changes. Three of the widely used valid, reliable paper screening tools for assessment of impaired cognition include: Mini-Mental State Examination, Saint Louis University Mental Status, and Montreal Cognitive Assessment.

DOI: 10.1201/9781003178330-24

21.1 INTRODUCTION

Cognition utilizes the daily mental processes of thought to learn, form memories, and retrieve information that helps us in our daily lives. Cognition is an individual's ability to learn new information, sustain focus and attention, problem solve and reason, maintain short- and long-term memory, and recall information (*Cognitive Health and Older Adults*, 2020). Cognitive function involves major processes, including receptive function, memory and learning, thinking, and expressive functions (Lezak et al., 2012). Receptive function allows one to select, acquire, classify, and examine information. Memory and learning relate to information storage and retrieval. Thinking involves information organization and reorganization. Thinking is complex and involves calculation, reasoning and judgment, organizing, planning, and problem solving. Thinking is a function of the entire brain. Expressive functions involve how information is communicated or acted upon. Expressive functions include speaking, physical gestures, facial expressions, writing, drawing, and manipulating. All of these systems work together. The brain navigates all the information it receives and decides what to do with it. The prefrontal cortex is responsible for decision making, complex thinking, and information analysis. The prefrontal cortex works along with the hippocampus and surrounding limbic structures such as the amygdala, allowing learning and memory formation. Basic cognitive processes include sensation, perception, attention, and memory.

21.2 MEMORY

Memory processes information and stores memories in the brain. Memory relies on cortical neurons in the brain using an array of connections between neurons in the neocortex, which is the outermost layer of the cerebrum (Lezak et al., 2012). There are three main types of memory: (1) sensory memory, which lasts less than a second involving the five senses of sight, hearing, taste, smell, and touch; (2) short-term memory, also known as working memory; and (3) long-term memory (Camina & Güell, 2017).

21.2.1 SENSORY MEMORY

Sensory memory includes visual memory (iconic memory), aural stimuli (echoic memory), touch (haptic memory), and smell (Camina & Güell, 2017). Children experience sensations even before they can talk. If a young child touches a hot surface, the painful sensation will elicit a perception of pain and then store that painful sensation in their memory. If a child gets an injection, their perception of the pain they experience will be stored in their memory. If the child has a painful experience, they will recall the pain of that experience if they see an injection in the future. The first time a person smells roses, the smell of roses may be perceived as a pleasant smell, and when they smell roses again the person will recall the memory of the smell. When a person sees an object, they will form a perception about the object and remember the object when seen again in the future because it is stored in their memory. If a child hears their mother's voice, they will store the sensory memory, allowing them to remember her voice when heard again.

21.2.2 SHORT-TERM MEMORY

Short-term memory (working memory) is temporary memory storage (Camina & Güell, 2017). Short-term memory can store approximately seven items for up to a minute. Short-term memory (working memory) allows one to use information without losing track of what one is doing. For example, retaining a phone number in short-term memory long enough to dial the number. If the number is dialed often enough, it may be stored in long-term memory. Short-term memory is broken down into two categories:

1. Auditory/Verbal memory is oral information that involves processing, retaining, and recalling.
2. Visual-Spatial memory is visual memory that involves processing, retaining, and recalling. Visual/Spatial memory enables one to remember familiar roads or remember where furniture is located in the dark.

Executive function is a set of mental functions that involve short-term memory (working memory), flexible thinking, and self-control in order to follow directions, focus, and manage emotions.

21.2.3 LONG-TERM MEMORY

Long-term memory involves both explicit (declarative memory), which is conscious, and implicit (non-declarative memory), which is unconscious (Camina & Güell, 2017). Explicit (declarative, conscious memory) has two categories:

1. Episodic memory involves the ability to recall and mentally re-experience specific episodes from a person's unique past, such as a 16th birthday or a first kiss.
2. Semantic memory is the memory for general knowledge such as facts, for example the alphabet or historical facts.

Implicit (non-declarative, unconscious memory) has two categories:

1. Procedural skills are motor skill memory, such as riding a bike, tying shoes, brushing teeth, or swimming.
2. Priming is the activation of concepts associated with memories like feeling joy when remembering a pleasant event, or feeling terror when remembering a scary encounter. For example, every encounter with a spider produces feelings of terror, or every encounter with the ocean produces feeling of joy.

21.2.4 PATHOPHYSIOLOGY

Cognition is dependent on neuroplasticity (Kaliszewska et al., 2021). Neuroplasticity is the brain's ability to adjust to structural and functional changes in response to alterations in the environment. New connections between neurons are formed in response to new experiences and learning, which induce neuronal networks to re-organize and fine-tune brain circuitry. Neurogenesis (growth and development of nervous tissue) is a neurological process supporting cognitive functioning and development. Adult neurogenesis occurs in the hippocampus, which plays a crucial role in memory, mood, and spatial learning. The brain is a complex organ that requires a substantial amount of energy called mitochondrial adenosine triphosphate (ATP). Neurons in the brain require a high level of ATP to process information. The main role of mitochondria is to produce ATP, which is cellular energy (Todorova & Blokland, 2016). Mitochondrial organelles are found in all eukaryotic cells, including neurons. Mitochondrial disorders commonly affect the brain, causing cognitive impairments. It has been shown that an increase in oxidative damage to deoxyribonucleic acid (DNA), proteins, and lipids occurs during aging. One of the major causes of neurodegeneration is neuroinflammation, a process that damages the brain's synaptic plasticity functions (Onyango et al., 2021). The hallmarks of an aging brain include cortical atrophy, synaptic loss, low-grade chronic inflammation, and cerebrovascular pathology. The integrity of blood vessels in the brain allows for adequate cerebral blood flow (CBF). The brain is dependent on adequate CBF for mitochondrial energy metabolism. Brain neurons use 70–80% of mitochondrial energy for functions such as neurogenesis and neuroplasticity, which are important functions to the brain structures involved in cognition. Neuroinflammation, nutrition-induced dysregulation of blood–brain barrier permeability, mitochondrial dysfunction, breakdown of glucose metabolism, and hypoperfusion linked to cerebrovascular dysfunction are factors implicated as underlying causes of cognitive impairment.

21.3 COGNITIVE IMPAIRMENT

Cognitive impairment is a set of symptoms that impair a person's ability to remember, concentrate, interact socially, learn new things, or make decisions, negatively impacting their daily life, caused by an underlying etiology (Jin, 2020). Etiologies of cognitive impairment include Alzheimer's disease, vascular, traumatic brain injury, frontotemporal lobe degeneration, substance abuse, HIV infection, Prion disease, Lewy body disease, Parkinson's disease, Huntington disease, and unspecified causes (Sachdev et al., 2014b). The World Health Organization (WHO) estimates cognitive impairment will affect 75 million people worldwide by the year 2030, and increase to 132 million by the year 2050 (Wallin et al., 2018).

21.3.1 MILD COGNITIVE IMPAIRMENT/MILD NEUROCOGNITIVE DISORDER

Mild cognitive impairment (MCI) individuals become aware of changes in their cognitive function, but it is not severe enough to make a significant impact on an individual's daily life. Mild cognitive impairment (MCI) does not have a single cause or a single outcome (*Mild Cognitive Impairment (MCI)*, 2020). Mild cognitive impairment may progress to dementia, stay stable, or improve back to baseline (Petersen et al., 2017). According to the American Academy of Neurology, MCI prevalence by age group are as follows: 60–64 (6.7%), 65–69 (8.4%), 70–74 (10.1%), 75–79 (14.8%), and 80–84 (25.2%). The strongest risk factors for developing MCI are increasing age and having one or more Apolipoprotein (APOE e4) alleles, which is a genetic risk factor for Alzheimer's disease. The risk of developing Alzheimer's disease increases three-fold if an individual has one APOE e4 allele, and having two APOE e4 alleles increases the risk twelve-fold when compared to non-carriers of the APOE e4 allele (Kadey et al., 2021). Approximately 50% of homozygous APOE e4 allele carriers 80 years or older will never develop Alzheimer's disease. Additional risk factors for developing MCI include smoking, diabetes, elevated cholesterol, obesity, depression, high blood pressure, lack of physical exercise, low education level, and infrequent participation in social or mentally stimulating activities. Individuals with MCI have an increased risk of developing dementia. Per the American Academy of Neurology, the prevalence of individuals with MCI progressing into dementia can be up to 38%, and the prevalence of individuals with MCI reverting back to normal can be up to 55.6%. Depression, aggression, irritability, apathy, and anxiety can occur in individuals with cognitive impairment. MCI is the precursor to dementia.

Practice guidelines by the American Academy of Neurology (Petersen et al., 2017) recommend the avoidance of cholinesterase medications in individuals diagnosed with MCI due to lack of evidence, and instead focus on recommending regular exercise, evaluating modifiable risk factors, assessing functional independence, and treating behavioral symptoms. The evidence shows often MCI develops from similar types of brain changes seen in Alzheimer's disease and other types of dementia. On autopsy and magnetic resonance imaging (MRI), brain changes are seen in the brains of individuals with MCI and dementia (Bangen et al., 2018). Brain changes seen in MCI include:

- Small strokes like lacunar infarcts
- Abnormal clumps of beta-amyloid protein (plaques)
- Microscopic tau changes (tangles)
- Lewy bodies seen in Parkinson's disease and dementia
- Shrinkage of the hippocampus and frontal parietal regions
- Enlargement of the ventricles

- Brain volume loss
- White matter lesions

21.3.2 Dementia/Major Cognitive Disorder

Dementia is a significant decline from baseline that interferes with an individual's ability to complete daily activities, including instrumental activities of daily living (IADLs), such as paying the bills, and/or an impairment with activities of daily living (ADLs), such as remembering to brush their teeth (Petersen et al., 2017). Severe cognitive impairment can cause an individual to become unable to care for themselves. It is important to note that although there are pharmaceutical medications for dementia related to a host of underlying etiologies, including Alzheimer's disease, no medication to date is a cure (Umegaki et al., 2021). Dementia (also known as major neurocognitive disorder) is defined by the American Psychiatric Association's Diagnostic and Statistical Manual of Mental Disorders as a significant decline in one or more cognitive domains (Sachdev et al., 2014a). The six cognitive domains identified in the DSM-5 include:

1. Complex attention (processing speed, selective attention, divided attention, sustained attention).
2. Executive function (decision making, working memory, inhibition, planning, flexibility, responding to feedback).
3. Learning and memory (implicit learning, semantic and autobiographical long-term memory, free recall, cued recall, recognition memory).
4. Language (fluency, grammar and syntax, receptive language, object naming, word finding).
5. Perceptual-motor function (visuo-constructional reasoning, visual perception, perceptual-motor coordination).
6. Social cognition (insight, recognition of emotions, theory of mind).

MCI (also known as mild neurocognitive disorder) differs from dementia because the impairment is not severe enough to interfere with independent functioning. Dementia has a slow, insidious onset as compared to delirium, which has acute and fluctuating onset. Cognitive impairment can adversely impact activities of daily living, such as bathing, dressing, grooming, feeding ourselves, toileting, and work. Cognitive impairment can negatively affect an individual's safety, ability to drive, ability to manage financial affairs, and relationships. Signs of cognitive impairment include:

- Memory loss—forgetting things more often like appointments or social events.
- Asking the same question or repeating the same story.
- Not recognizing familiar places or people.
- Having difficulty exercising judgment—not knowing what to do during an emergency.
- Changes in mood or behavior.
- Becoming more impulsive or showing increasingly poor judgment.
- Difficulty planning and carrying out tasks, such as following a recipe or keeping track of monthly bills.
- Family and friends notice changes in cognition.

21.4　COGNITIVE ASSESSMENT

Cognitive assessment screening tools can assess cognitive impairment versus normal age-related changes. Three of the widely used valid, evidence-based paper screening tools for assessment of impaired cognition include: Mini-Mental State Examination (MMSE), Saint Louis University Mental Status (SLUMS), and Montreal Cognitive Assessment (MoCA) (Ranjit et al., 2020). This section discusses and compares the cognitive assessment screening tools.

21.4.1 MMSE Screening Tool

The MMSE takes 5–10 minutes to administer, testing recall, attention, language, the ability to follow directions, and calculations (Baek et al., 2016). The score range is 0–30. Points. A score of 24–30 indicates normal cognition, 18–23 mild cognitive impairment, and 0–17 severe cognitive impairment. The MMSE advantages include useful in serial testing to monitor cognitive status, ease of use, and useful for testing significant cognitive impairment. MMSE limitations include less efficacious in detecting mild cognitive impairment, lack of usefulness in individuals with lower education, or non-English speakers.

21.4.2 SLUMS Screening Tool

SLUMS has 11 questions with a scoring range of 0–30 points (Howland et al., 2016). SLUMS has the ability to detect mild cognitive impairment (MCI). SLUMS tests memory, attention, orientation, size differentiation, and executive function. The advantage of SLUMS when compared to the MMSE includes special scoring for high school versus less than school education, and the sensitivity to detect mild cognitive impairment. Test interpretation for individuals with high school degree or higher: 27–30 points (normal cognition), 21–26 points (mild neurocognitive disorder), 1–20 points (dementia) versus an individual with less than a high school education: 25–30 points (normal cognition), 20–24 points (mild neurocognitive disorder), 1–19 points (dementia).

21.4.3 MoCA Screening Tool

The MoCA has 13 test items and takes 10–15 minutes to administer (Dautzenberg et al., 2019). The MoCA tests calculations, language, memory, orientation, executive function, visuospatial skills, and conceptual thinking. The score range is 0–30 points. A score of 26 points is considered normal cognition. An extra point is added to the total score for individuals that have a formal education of 12 years or less. Specificity issues involving false-positives have been found when administered in non-clinical environments.

21.5 FACTORS AFFECTING COGNITIVE HEALTH

21.5.1 Food Is Medicine

Per the World Health Organization (WHO) guidelines, a critical component of health and development is nutrition. WHO guidelines state that the intake of optimal nutrition aids the immune system and lowers the risk of non-communicable diseases such as diabetes, stroke, hypertension, and cardiovascular disease. A well-balanced diet includes consuming the necessary micronutrients and macronutrients. A well-balanced diet should include a variety of vegetables, fruits, nuts, whole grains, and legumes. It is highly recommended to avoid processed foods, excess fats, salt, and sugar. Carbohydrates are macronutrients that serve as a main energy source for the body. In the absence of carbohydrates, bodies will use fats or lipids for energy. Proteins are macronutrients that bodies need for immune defense, cell communication, forming of supportive structures, transport of substances, and catalysis of reactions in the body. Vitamins and minerals are micronutrients that are critical to metabolic, regulatory, and biochemical processes. Studies have noted the dietary impact on cognition (Rajaram et al., 2019). A 21-year study examining 15,467 female nurses concluded better overall cognition was associated with increased nut intake (O'Brien et al., 2014). A retrospective eight-year study examined the effect of nut intake on cognitive function in 1866 older men and found better overall cognition in men with a higher nut consumption (Koyama et al., 2015). A five-year prospective cohort study of 2613 men and women ages 40–70 also concluded better cognitive function was associated with higher nut intake (Nooyens et al., 2011). A cross-sectional study of elderly Japanese ages 69–71 concluded plant foods were associated with higher scores on the Japanese MOCA (Okubo et al., 2017). A cohort study of elderly Chinese men (1,926) and women (1,744) over the age of 65 found a diet with higher fruit and vegetable patterns was associated with a reduced risk of cognitive impairment in women (Chan et al., 2013). Giving the body optimal nutrition can increase longevity and quality of life.

21.5.2 GUT HEALTH

Since the 19th century, the effects of gastrointestinal tract on brain function has been recognized (Hirschberg et al., 2019). Around 70–80% of the human body's immune cells are located in the gastrointestinal tract (Yoo & Mazmanian, 2017). Dysbiosis is an imbalance of types of microflora in the gut causing increased gut permeability, causing toxins to leak into the bloodstream, which may contribute to neurodegenerative disorders. The role of the microbiota–gut–brain axis can influence the brain and vice versa. Gut microbiota imbalances have been seen in individuals diagnosed with neurodegenerative disorders such as Alzheimer's disease, Parkinson's disease, Huntington's disease, psychiatric disorders such as anxiety, autoimmune disorders, and neurodevelopmental disorders such as autism. For example, in chronic autoimmune celiac disease (CD), changes in gut micro-biota have been found. Symptoms of CD not only negatively impact the gastrointestinal system but can also cause neurological symptoms, including neuropathy and cognitive impairment. The under-lying causes of dysbiosis include a Westernized diet, antibiotics, chronic stress, and infections. Key nutrients for gut health include: Omega-3 fatty acids (Costantini et al., 2017), vitamin D (Yamamoto & Jørgensen, 2020), vitamin A (Brown & Noelle, 2015), iron (Rusu et al., 2020), zinc (Zackular et al., 2016), and vitamin E (Liu et al., 2021). Interventions to return balance to the gut micro-biota include dietary modifications, reduction of stress, and the use of prebiotics along with further research.

21.5.3 MICRONUTRIENTS FUNCTIONS

Studies have shown micronutrients have an impact on cognition (Melzer et al., 2021). Micronutrients play an essential role in brain function, including oxidation-reduction homeostasis, neurotransmitter synthesis, cellular energy production, cell maintenance, and cell repair.

Clinical evidence supports the role of micronutrients and the role they play on cognition. Thiamine (B1) deficiency has been linked to cognitive impairment (Gibson et al., 2016), intake of pyridoxine (vitamin B6) has been linked to improved cognitive function, and B12 deficiency has been linked to impaired cognition (Smith, 2016). Intake of folic acid (vitamin B6) has been linked with improved cognition (Fortune et al., 2019). Cognitive decline has been linked to decreased vitamin A levels (Shahar et al., 2013). Vitamin A deficiency may be a predictor of mild cognitive impairment. An increased intake of carotenoids was shown to decrease the risk of poor cognitive function. Increased vitamin K intake was associated with better cognitive function in older adults (Soutif-Veillon et al., 2016). Maintaining adequate vitamin D levels during aging may delay the onset of dementia and reduce the risk of cognitive decline (Jia et al., 2019). Additionally, according to the US National Health and Nutrition Examination Survey, better cognitive function was directly correlated to a high intake of magnesium and adequate intake of vitamin D (Peeri et al., 2020). A decrease in mild cog-nitive impairment was seen in individuals with high vitamin C levels (Beydoun et al., 2015). Higher vitamin E levels were associated with higher scores on memory, recall, and better language/verbal fluency (Farina et al., 2017). Circulating and brain selenium concentrations have been noted to be lower in Alzheimer's disease (Varikasuvu et al., 2018).

21.5.4   Physical Activity

There is clear evidence that obesity and a lack of exercise correlate with decreased cognitive perform-ance in children and adults (Wallin et al., 2018). An exploratory study (Treyer et al., 2021) examined 49 individuals between the ages of 84 and 94 years with preserved everyday functioning considered exceptional agers or super-agers. Super-agers are believed to have a high cognitive reserve (factors that preserve cognitive function despite the presence of cerebral pathologies). Clinical dementia, or other disease processes that impair cognition, were included in the exclusion criteria. Of the 49 study participants, the mean MMSE score was 28.35, and the mean BMI was 25.6. Over half of the participants were living independently, still driving, and were also positive for at least one APOE genotype. The study examined associations between pathologies, risk factors, personality traits, and cognition. To examine pathology, every participant underwent an 18-[F]-Flutemetamol-PET scan for estimated cerebral beta-amyloid deposits and Tau accumulation and 3D T1 MRI brain images to assess hippocampal volumetry and brain volume. Hallmarks of pathologic signs of Alzheimer's disease are plaques (large amounts of beta-amyloid deposits) and tangles (misfolded Tau protein). Each participant underwent a battery of tests, including the MMSE, to assess cognitive function. A lifetime experience questionnaire was administered to gather data with regard to education, work experience, leisure, social interactions, and cognitive and physical activity. Data including risk factors for cognitive impairment and cardiovascular risk factors were also obtained. Less than 50% of the study participants reported sleep disturbances (26.5%), never smoked (44.9%) versus former smoker (49%), minimal alcohol use (87.8%), diabetes (8.2%), hypercholesterolemia (40.8%), his-tory of myocardial infarction (18.4%), and first line relatives with dementia (10.2%). The average years of education in the study group was 14.12 years. The Neo-FFI was administered to assess the five domains of personality. The personality domain of neuroticism (an individual's level of emotional stability) was closely examined due to the probable association with impaired cognition. After the data was analyzed, the study noted both high and low amyloid presence in the brains of super-agers. High amyloid presence may have a mild influence on an individual's autonomy and personality. There was a higher incidence of neuroticism in the study of individuals with higher amyloid presence. Low amyloid present in the brain correlated with study individuals who reported high physical activity. Brian and hippocampal volume were average. Extracurricular activities over a lifetime have a positive impact on better executive function, which is a pivotal resource in everyday functioning. There was not a correlation between MMSE scores and amount of amyloid presence. No association was found between brain volume, hippocampal volume, and cerebral amyloid presence in the super-ager/exceptional-ager study participants. Pathologic features of Alzheimer's disease can be seen in aging healthy individuals without the development of the clinical symptoms of dementia. Studying super-agers/exceptional-agers can provide a framework to healthy aging.

A recent narrative review study prompted by the increase of physical inactivity during the COVID-19 pandemic aimed to evaluate the significance of physical activity on brain-derived neuro-trophic factor (BDNF), and its influence on cognition in older adults (Umegaki et al., 2021). During the aging process, cerebral blood flow and cardiac output start to decline, resulting in decreased BDNF levels. The narrative review study noted that several observational studies have found active older adults have higher cerebral blood flow when compared to sedentary older adults (Knight et al., 2021; Li et al., 2021). The narrative study found that physical activity may increase levels of BDNF associated with preserved brain volume. The study also noted studies done in animals have shown that an increase in BDNF has a positive effect on neurogenesis in the hippocampus, also noting that further research is needed in human subjects.

21.5.5   Other Factors

Per the Lancet commission, dementia incidence could be reduced by approximately 30% with pre-ventative interventions focused on cardiovascular risk factors including hypertension, smoking, physical activity, alcohol intake, and diabetes (Juul Rasmussen et al., 2020). A 10-year absolute risk score for dementia examining cardiovascular and genetic risk factors was generated by examining 61,664 individuals aged 20–100 years from two cohort studies, the Copenhagen General Population study and the Copenhagen City Heart Study (Juul Rasmussen et al., 2020). The study found the strongest modifiable risk factors included diabetes, smoking, physical inactivity, midlife hypertension, and education level. The study stressed the importance of reducing an individual's modifiable risk factors for dementia by utilizing interventions to address physical inactivity, diabetes, smoking, education level (fewer than eight years), and cardiovascular risk factors, which was noted to be particularly important in individuals carrying the APOE gene.

Maintaining a healthy body mass index (BMI) in relation to the development of dementia continues to be studied. Data from an English Longitudinal Study of Ageing examined 6582 participants over a 15-year follow-up period to determine if obesity was a risk factor in the development of dementia (Ma et al., 2020). The study found evidence that individuals with a high BMI and increased waist circumference were at higher risk for developing dementia. A large, longitudinal cohort study analyzed data from 36 Alzheimer's Disease Research Centers over a five-year period examining the risk of conversion from MCI to dementia as it relates to carriers versus non-carriers of the APOE e4 allele (Kadey et al., 2021). Of the 1,289 study participants (386 heterozygous APOE e4 carriers and 903 non-carriers with a mean age of 72.1), baseline BMI did not affect conversion outcomes. The baseline mean BMI for non-carriers of the APOE e4 allele was 26.6, and the baseline mean BMI for carriers of the APOE e4 allele was 26.8. The study suggested that individuals with the APOE e4 allele that had significant declines in BMI over time have a greater risk of conversion from MCI to dementia when compared to declines in BMI of non-carriers that did not show an increase in the conversion rate.

21.6 CONCLUSION

A healthy diet of micronutrients, anti-oxidants, and anti-inflammatories and regular physical exercise increases neuroplasticity, life span, and cognition reserve. Nutrition, physical activity, hypertension, smoking, and diabetes are modifiable risk factors to prevent or improve cognitive function. Balanced and adequate nutrition, controlling modifiable risk factors along with exercise, can reduce an individual's risk of cognitive impairment, which decreases the burden and cost on the healthcare system. Further research is needed to further support interventions that decrease the prevalence of cognitive impairment.

REFERENCES

Baek, M., Kim, K., Park, Y., & Kim, S. (2016). The validity and reliability of the mini-mental state examination-2 for detecting mild cognitive impairment and Alzheimer's disease in a Korean population. *PLOS ONE*, *11*(9), e0163792. https://doi.org/10.1371/journal.pone.0163792

Bangen, K. J., Preis, S. R., Delano-Wood, L., Wolf, P. A., Libon, D. J., Bondi, M. W., Au, R., DeCarli, C., & Brickman, A. M. (2018). Baseline white matter hyperintensities and hippocampal volume are associated with conversion from normal cognition to mild cognitive impairment in the Framingham offspring study. *Alzheimer Disease & Associated Disorders*, *32*(1), 50–56. https://doi.org/10.1097/wad.00000 00000000215

Beydoun, M. A., Fanelli-Kuczmarski, M. T., Kitner-Triolo, M. H., Beydoun, H. A., Kaufman, J. S., Mason, M. A., Evans, M. K., & Zonderman, A. B. (2015). Dietary antioxidant intake and its association with cognitive function in an ethnically diverse sample of us adults. *Psychosomatic Medicine*, *77*(1), 68–82. https://doi.org/10.1097/psy.0000000000000129

Brown, C. C., & Noelle, R. J. (2015). Seeing through the dark: New insights into the immune regulatory functions of vitamin A. *European Journal of Immunology*, *45*(5), 1287–1295. https://doi.org/10.1002/eji.201344398

Camina, E., & Güell, F. (2017). The neuroanatomical, neurophysiological and psychological basis of memory: Current models and their origins. *Frontiers in Pharmacology, 8.* https://doi.org/10.3389/fphar.2017.00438

Chan, R., Chan, D., & Woo, J. (2013). A cross sectional study to examine the association between dietary patterns and cognitive impairment in older Chinese people in Hong Kong. *The Journal of Nutrition, Health & Aging, 17*(9), 757–765. https://doi.org/10.1007/s12603-013-0348-5

Cognitive health and older adults. (2020, October 1). National Institute on Aging. www.nia.nih.gov/health/cognitive-health-and-older-adults

Costantini, L., Molinari, R., Farinon, B., & Merendino, N. (2017). Impact of omega-3 fatty acids on the gut microbiota. *International Journal of Molecular Sciences, 18*(12), 2645. https://doi.org/10.3390/ijms18122645

Dautzenberg, G., Lijmer, J., & Beekman, A. (2019). Diagnostic accuracy of the Montreal cognitive assessment (moca) for cognitive screening in old age psychiatry: Determining cutoff scores in clinical practice. avoiding spectrum bias caused by healthy controls. *International Journal of Geriatric Psychiatry, 35*(3), 261–269. https://doi.org/10.1002/gps.5227

Farina, N., Llewellyn, D., Isaac, M., & Tabet, N. (2017). Vitamin e for Alzheimer's dementia and mild cognitive impairment. *Cochrane Database of Systematic Reviews.* https://doi.org/10.1002/14651858.cd002854.pub5

Fortune, N. C., Harville, E. W., Guralnik, J. M., Gustat, J., Chen, W., Qi, L., & Bazzano, L. A. (2019). Dietary intake and cognitive function: Evidence from the Bogalusa heart study. *The American Journal of Clinical Nutrition, 109*(6), 1656–1663. https://doi.org/10.1093/ajcn/nqz026

Gibson, G. E., Hirsch, J. A., Fonzetti, P., Jordan, B. D., Cirio, R. T., & Elder, J. (2016). Vitamin B1 (thiamine) and dementia. *Annals of the New York Academy of Sciences, 1367*(1), 21–30. https://doi.org/10.1111/nyas.13031

Hirschberg, S., Gisevius, B., Duscha, A., & Haghikia, A. (2019). Implications of diet and the gut microbiome in neuroinflammatory and neurodegenerative diseases. *International Journal of Molecular Sciences, 20*(12), 3109. https://doi.org/10.3390/ijms20123109

Howland, M., Tatsuoka, C., Smyth, K. A., & Sajatovic, M. (2016). Detecting change over time: A comparison of the slums examination and the mmse in older adults at risk for cognitive decline. *CNS Neuroscience & Therapeutics, 22*(5), 413–419. https://doi.org/10.1111/cns.12515

Jia, J., Hu, J., Huo, X., Miao, R., Zhang, Y., & Ma, F. (2019). Effects of vitamin d supplementation on cognitive function and blood aβ-related biomarkers in older adults with Alzheimer's disease: A randomised, double-blind, placebo-controlled trial. *Journal of Neurology, Neurosurgery & Psychiatry,* jnnp–2018-320199. https://doi.org/10.1136/jnnp-2018-320199

Jin, J. (2020). Screening for cognitive impairment in older adults. *JAMA, 323*(8), 800. https://doi.org/10.1001/jama.2020.0583

Juul Rasmussen, I., Rasmussen, K., Nordestgaard, B. G., Tybjærg-Hansen, A., & Frikke-Schmidt, R. (2020). Impact of cardiovascular risk factors and genetics on 10-year absolute risk of dementia: Risk charts for targeted prevention. *European Heart Journal, 41*(41), 4024–4033. https://doi.org/10.1093/eurheartj/ehaa695

Kadey, K. R., Woodard, J. L., Moll, A. C., Nielson, K. A., Smith, J., Durgerian, S., & Rao, S. M. (2021). Five-year change in body mass index predicts conversion to mild cognitive impairment or dementia only in apoe ε4 allele carriers. *Journal of Alzheimer's Disease, 81*(1), 189–199. https://doi.org/10.3233/jad-201360

Kaliszewska, A., Allison, J., Martini, M., & Arias, N. (2021). The interaction of diet and mitochondrial dysfunction in aging and cognition. *International Journal of Molecular Sciences, 22*(7), 1–27. https://doi.org/10.3390/ijms22073574

Knight, S. P., Laird, E., Williamson, W., O'Connor, J., Newman, L., Carey, D., De Looze, C., Fagan, A. J., Chappell, M. A., Meaney, J. F., & Kenny, R. (2021). Obesity is associated with reduced cerebral blood flow—modified by physical activity. *Neurobiology of Aging, 105,* 35–47. https://doi.org/10.1016/j.neurobiolaging.2021.04.008

Koyama, A. K., Hagan, K. A., Okereke, O. I., Weisskopf, M. G., Rosner, B., & Grodstein, F. (2015). Evaluation of a self-administered computerized cognitive battery in an older population. *Neuroepidemiology, 45*(4), 264–272. https://doi.org/10.1159/000439592

Lezak, M. D., Howieson, D. B., Bigler, E. D., & Tranel, D. (2012). *Neuropsychological assessment* (5th ed.). Oxford University Press.

Li, L., Wang, J., Guo, S., Xing, Y., Ke, X., Chen, Y., He, Y., Wang, S., Wang, J., Cui, X., Wang, Z., & Tang, L. (2021). Tai chi exercise improves age-associated decline in cerebrovascular function: A cross-sectional study. *BMC Geriatrics, 21*(1), 1–11. https://doi.org/10.1186/s12877-021-02196-9

Liu, K. Y., Nakatsu, C. H., Jones-Hall, Y., Kozik, A., & Jiang, Q. (2021). Vitamin E alpha- and gamma-tocopherol mitigate colitis, protect intestinal barrier function and modulate the gut microbiota in mice. *Free Radical Biology and Medicine, 163*, 180–189. https://doi.org/10.1016/j.freeradbiomed.2020.12.017

Ma, Y., Ajnakina, O., Steptoe, A., & Cadar, D. (2020). Higher risk of dementia in English older individuals who are overweight or obese. *International Journal of Epidemiology, 49*(4), 1353–1365. https://doi.org/10.1093/ije/dyaa099

Melzer, T., Manosso, L., Yau, S., Gil-Mohapel, J., & Brocardo, P. S. (2021). In pursuit of healthy aging: Effects of nutrition on brain function. *International Journal of Molecular Sciences, 22*(9), 1–25. https://doi.org/10.3390/ijms22095026

Mild cognitive impairment (MCI). (2020, September 2). Mayo Clinic. www.mayoclinic.org/diseases-conditions/mild-cognitive-impairment/symptoms-causes/syc-20354578

Nooyens, A. J., Bueno-de-Mesquita, H., van Boxtel, M. J., van Gelder, B. M., Verhagen, H., & Verschuren, W. (2011). Fruit and vegetable intake and cognitive decline in middle-aged men and women: The doetinchem cohort study. *British Journal of Nutrition, 106*(5), 752–761. https://doi.org/10.1017/s0007114511001024

O'Brien, J., Okereke, O., Devore, E., Rosner, B., Breteler, M., & Grodstein, F. (2014). Long-term intake of nuts in relation to cognitive function in older women. *The Journal of Nutrition, Health & Aging, 18*(5), 496–502. https://doi.org/10.1007/s12603-014-0014-6

Okubo, H., Inagaki, H., Gondo, Y., Kamide, K., Ikebe, K., Masui, Y., Arai, Y., Ishizaki, T., Sasaki, S., Nakagawa, T., Kabayama, M., Sugimoto, K., Rakugi, H., & Maeda, Y. (2017). Association between dietary patterns and cognitive function among 70-year-old Japanese elderly: A cross-sectional analysis of the sonic study. *Nutrition Journal, 16*(1). https://doi.org/10.1186/s12937-017-0273-2

Onyango, I. G., Jauregui, G. V., Čarná, M., Bennett, J. P., & Stokin, G. B. (2021). Neuroinflammation in Alzheimer's disease. *Biomedicines, 9*(5), 524. https://doi.org/10.3390/biomedicines9050524

Peeri, N. C., Egan, K. M., Chai, W., & Tao, M.-H. (2020). Association of magnesium intake and vitamin d status with cognitive function in older adults: An analysis of US national health and nutrition examination survey (nhanes) 2011 to 2014. *European Journal of Nutrition, 60*(1), 465–474. https://doi.org/10.1007/s00394-020-02267-4

Petersen, R. C., Lopez, O., Armstrong, M. J., Getchius, T. S., Ganguli, M., Gloss, D., Gronseth, G. S., Marson, D., Pringsheim, T., Day, G. S., Sager, M., Stevens, J., & Rae-Grant, A. (2017). Practice guideline update summary: Mild cognitive impairment. *Neurology, 90*(3), 126–135. https://doi.org/10.1212/wnl.0000000000004826

Rajaram, S., Jones, J., & Lee, G. J. (2019). Plant-based dietary patterns, plant foods, and age-related cognitive decline. *Advances in Nutrition, 10*(Suppl. 4), S422–S436. https://doi.org/10.1093/advances/nmz081

Ranjit, E., Sapra, A., Bhandari, P., Albers, C. E., & Ajmeri, M. S. (2020). Cognitive assessment of geriatric patients in primary care settings. *Cureus, 12*(9). https://doi.org/10.7759/cureus.10443

Rusu, I., Suharoschi, R., Vodnar, D., Pop, C., Socaci, S., Vulturar, R., Istrati, M., Moroşan, I., Fărcaş, A., Kerezsi, A., Mureşan, C., & Pop, O. (2020). Iron supplementation influence on the gut microbiota and probiotic intake effect in iron deficiency—a literature-based review. *Nutrients, 12*(7), 1993. https://doi.org/10.3390/nu12071993

Sachdev, P. S., Blacker, D., Blazer, D. G., Ganguli, M., Jeste, D. V., Paulsen, J. S., & Petersen, R. C. (2014a). Classifying neurocognitive disorders: The DSM-5 approach. *Nature Reviews Neurology, 10*(11), 634–642. https://doi.org/10.1038/nrneurol.2014.181

Sachdev, P. S., Blacker, D., Blazer, D. G., Ganguli, M., Jeste, D. V., Paulsen, J. S., & Petersen, R. C. (2014b). Classifying neurocognitive disorders: The DSM-5 approach. *Nature Reviews Neurology, 10*(11), 634–642. https://doi.org/10.1038/nrneurol.2014.181

Shahar, S., Lee, L., Rajab, N., Lim, C., Harun, N., Noh, M., Mian-Then, S., & Jamal, R. (2013). Association between vitamin A, vitamin E and apolipoprotein e status with mild cognitive impairment among elderly people in low-cost residential areas. *Nutritional Neuroscience, 16*(1), 6–12. https://doi.org/10.1179/1476830512y.0000000013

Smith, A. (2016). Hippocampus as a mediator of the role of vitamin B-12 in memory. *The American Journal of Clinical Nutrition, 103*(4), 959–960. https://doi.org/10.3945/ajcn.116.132266

Soutif-Veillon, A., Ferland, G., Rolland, Y., Presse, N., Boucher, K., Féart, C., & Annweiler, C. (2016). Increased dietary vitamin k intake is associated with less severe subjective memory complaint among older adults. *Maturitas*, *93*, 131–136. https://doi.org/10.1016/j.maturitas.2016.02.004

Todorova, V., & Blokland, A. (2016). Mitochondria and synaptic plasticity in the mature and aging nervous system. *Current Neuropharmacology*, *15*(1), 166–173. https://doi.org/10.2174/1570159x14666160414111821

Treyer, V., Meyer, R. S., Buchmann, A., Crameri, G. G., Studer, S., Saake, A., Gruber, E., Unschuld, P. G., Nitsch, R. M., Hock, C., & Gietl, A. F. (2021). Physical activity is associated with lower cerebral beta-amyloid and cognitive function benefits from lifetime experience–a study in exceptional aging. *PLOS ONE*, *16*(2), e0247225. https://doi.org/10.1371/journal.pone.0247225

Umegaki, H., Sakurai, T., & Arai, H. (2021). Active life for brain health: A narrative review of the mechanism underlying the protective effects of physical activity on the brain. *Frontiers in Aging Neuroscience*, *13*, 1–11. https://doi.org/10.3389/fnagi.2021.761674

Varikasuvu, S., Prasad V, S., Kothapalli, J., & Manne, M. (2018). Brain selenium in Alzheimer's disease (brain sead study): A systematic review and meta-analysis. *Biological Trace Element Research*, *189*(2), 361–369. https://doi.org/10.1007/s12011-018-1492-x

Wallin, A., Kettunen, P., Johansson, P. M., Jonsdottir, I. H., Nilsson, C., Nilsson, M., Eckerström, M., Nordlund, A., Nyberg, L., Sunnerhagen, K. S., Svensson, J., Terzis, B., Wahlund, L.-O., & Georg Kuhn, H. (2018). Cognitive medicine—a new approach in health care science. *BMC Psychiatry*, *18*(1), 1–5. https://doi.org/10.1186/s12888-018-1615-0

Yamamoto, E. A., & Jørgensen, T. N. (2020). Relationships between vitamin D, gut microbiome, and systemic autoimmunity. *Frontiers in Immunology*, *10*. https://doi.org/10.3389/fimmu.2019.03141

Yoo, B. B., & Mazmanian, S. K. (2017). The enteric network: Interactions between the immune and nervous systems of the gut. *Immunity*, *46*(6), 910–926. https://doi.org/10.1016/j.immuni.2017.05.011

Zackular, J. P., Moore, J. L., Jordan, A. T., Juttukonda, L. J., Noto, M. J., Nicholson, M. R., Crews, J. D., Semler, M. W., Zhang, Y., Ware, L. B., Washington, M., Chazin, W. J., Caprioli, R. M., & Skaar, E. P. (2016). Dietary zinc alters the microbiota and decreases resistance to clostridium difficile infection. *Nature Medicine*, *22*(11), 1330–1334. https://doi.org/10.1038/nm.4174

22 Mental Health in Lifestyle Medicine

Carlie M. Felion[1] and Gia Merlo[2]

[1]University of Arizona College of Nursing
Tucson, AZ, USA
Mayo Clinic, Phoenix, AZ, USA

[2]NYU Rory Meyers College of Nursing
New York, New York, USA
NYU Grossman School of Medicine
New York, New York, USA

CONTENTS

DOI: 10.1201/9781003178330-25

KEY POINTS

- Mental health conditions are prevalent worldwide and have an adverse impact on the overall health and well-being of affected individuals.
- The etiologies of mental health conditions are not fully understood, but multiple biological, psychosocial, and environmental factors contribute.
- Lifestyle medicine interventions may be helpful in the prevention and treatment of mental and behavioral health conditions.
- Numerous individual, cultural, social, and systemic factors influence a person's willingness and ability to engage in lifestyle medicine interventions.
- People with mental health conditions are disproportionately affected by social determinants, making it more challenging to adopt and maintain healthy lifestyle changes.
- The stress response plays a crucial role in mental and physical health, and the mechanisms involved in the stress response underlie many of the pillars of lifestyle medicine.

22.1 INTRODUCTION

According to the World Health Organization (2021), mental health can be understood as more than simply the absence of a mental disorder, but as having the ability to think, learn, and understand our own emotions and the reactions of others. The World Health Organization (2001) defines mental health as "a state of well-being in which the individual realizes his or her own abilities, can cope with the normal stresses of life, can work productively and fruitfully, and is able to make a contribution to his or her community." The American Psychiatric Association (2021) defines mental illnesses as health conditions involving changes in emotions, cognition, or behavior (or a combination of these factors) that cause distress, functional impairment, or both. The concept of what constitutes mental health varies across cultures, value systems, and clinical practice settings (Fusar-Poli et al., 2020), but some [GM1] of the domains encompass cognitive capacity, emotions, behaviors, perceptions of self, values, social skills, self-management behaviors, relationships with family members and significant others, physical and sexual health, quality of life, one's attitude toward mental disorders, mental health literacy, and meaning of life (Fusar-Poli et al., 2020). Deficits in one or more of these areas may lead to or indicate problems with mental health.

22.2 DEFINITIONS AND TERMINOLOGY

While the two terms are often used interchangeably, poor mental health and mental illness have different meanings. An individual with poor mental health may not meet diagnostic criteria for a mental illness, and likewise, a person who has a mental illness can experience periods of time where they enjoy physical, mental, and social well-being and can function normally (National Institute of Mental Health, 2021). Poor mental health can occur in any situation where demands placed upon an individual exceed their personal resources and their ability to cope and are subject to change over time depending on a variety of factors and circumstances (Merlo & Vela, 2021).

Mental illnesses present in many forms and include anxiety disorders, depression, substance use disorders, trauma-spectrum disorders, eating disorders, attention deficit hyperactivity disorder, personality disorders, bipolar disorder, and schizophrenia. Mental health conditions (a term that will be used interchangeably with mental illnesses in this chapter) vary in terms of their impact on a person's ability to function and with the degree of impairment occurring on a spectrum from no impairment to mild, moderate, or even severe impairment (National Institute of Mental Health, n.d.).

Serious mental illnesses (SMI) are conditions that cause substantial functional impairment in multiple domains and impair a person's ability to perform one or more major life activities (Evans et al., n.d.). SMIs include psychotic disorders, bipolar disorder, schizophrenia, major depression with psychotic features, and treatment-resistant depression. Eating disorders, anxiety disorders, or personality disorders may be considered SMI if severe impairment in one or more life activities exists (Evans et al., n.d.).

22.3   CAUSES OF MENTAL ILLNESS

There is no single factor that causes mental illnesses, but genetic predisposition, history of stressful life experiences during childhood, chronic medical conditions, traumatic brain injuries, substance misuse or abuse, and social isolation are all contributing factors (Kessler et al., 2007).

The COVID-19 pandemic has profoundly impacted the mental health of Americans, with the number of people experiencing symptoms of depression and anxiety skyrocketing. In a screening conducted by Mental Health America (2020), which surveys people who are looking for support and resources for mental health online, the percentage of people who took the anxiety screen increased by 93% over the total respondents in 2019, and there was a 62% increase in those who took the depression screen (Canady, 2021). The primary reasons cited by those experiencing moderate to severe anxiety or depression symptoms who responded to the questions in the 2020 survey were loneliness or isolation (70%), past trauma (46.18%), and relationship problems (42.56%) (Canady, 2021).

It is essential that nurses and other healthcare professionals remember that the etiologies of mental illnesses are complex, numerous, and diverse and that mental illness will occur and continue regardless of whether people adopt and maintain lifestyle changes (Firth et al., 2020). Nurses and other healthcare professionals must not make assumptions or judgments based on their knowledge of lifestyle medicine regarding the possible associations between a person's lifestyle and their state of mental health (Firth et al., 2020). Those types of biases increase stigma, which has its own negative effects on the physical, mental, and emotional health of individuals and can lead to social isolation, depression, and anxiety (Banerjee & Rai, 2022). Stigma surrounding people who are affected by mental illness may also contribute to reluctance to seek help or treatment or discuss issues or barriers to implementing lifestyle medicine interventions with their nurse or other healthcare professionals.

Due to numerous complex individual, social, and systemic factors, mental illnesses are often underdiagnosed, misdiagnosed, or undertreated. Alarmingly, 57% of adults and 33% of youth affected by mental illness get no treatment (Canady, 2021). Cultural differences, individual health beliefs and preferences, low health literacy, a distrust of healthcare providers and healthcare systems, numerous social determinants, and a nationwide lack of mental health providers and resources are pervasive problems in this vulnerable population.

Social and healthcare disparities are common among people with mental illness, especially those with SMI. People with mental health conditions are at higher risk for living in poverty, being uninsured or underinsured, experiencing food insecurity, living in inadequate or unsafe housing, homelessness, or developing a substance use disorder (Alegria et al., 2018).

22.4   SIGNS AND SYMPTOMS OF MENTAL ILLNESS

Obtaining the signs and symptoms of mental illness are part of the diagnostic evaluation for all patients. Having just one or two of these symptoms does not indicate a person has a mental illness but suggests the need for further evaluation. If several of these signs and symptoms occur at the same time and/or are interfering with a person's daily life or relationships, they should be evaluated by a medical or mental health professional as soon as possible (Parekh, 2018). If a person has thoughts of harming themselves or others or voices the intent to do so, they require emergency attention from a medical or mental health provider. Some of the signs and symptoms include the following:

- Fluctuations of moods.
- Impairment of concentration, speech, and thinking.

- Disturbances in appetite and sleep patterns.
- Altered perceptions, including hallucinations.
- Difficulty completing activities of daily living (ADR).
- Perceptual disturbances with environment.
- Self harm thoughts or actions.
- Substance use concerns.

22.5 PREVALENCE OF MENTAL ILLNESS IN THE UNITED STATES

Mental illnesses are very common. In the United States alone, one in five adults has at least one form of mental illness, and over 50% will develop some form of mental illness during their lifetime (Kessler et al., 2007). Mental illnesses do not discriminate and therefore affect people of all ages and from all walks of life. According to the National Alliance on Mental Illness (2021), the highest prevalence of mental illness exists among those who identify as lesbian, gay, or bisexual (47.4%), non-Hispanic mixed/multiracial individuals (35,8%), and non-Hispanic Whites (22.6%). Additionally, one in twenty adults and one in six youth between the ages of 6 and 17 years old in the US are affected by serious mental illness (National Alliance on Mental Illness, 2021).

22.6 SIGNIFICANCE OF MENTAL ILLNESS

Poor mental health adversely affects individuals, families, communities, and the economy (Hasin & Grant, 2015). Worldwide, nearly 1 billion people are affected by a mental illness, ranging from substance use disorders to dementia to schizophrenia. According to The Lancet Global Health (2020), lost productivity due to the two most common mental health conditions, anxiety and depression, cost the global economy $1 trillion US dollars each year. Total cost to the world economy averages around $2–5 trillion per year in lost productivity alone and does not count costs associated with therapy, prescription drugs, or stays in psychiatric or substance use treatment facilities. Data from 2013 indicates that treatment of mental health and substance abuse disorders cost US $187.8 billion (Winerman, 2017).

Mental health has an enormous impact on a person's overall health and well-being, as it ultimately affects how people respond to stress, relate to other people, and their lifestyle choices. The bidirectional relationship between mental illnesses such as depression and anxiety to physical health outcomes is well known. For example, depression has been associated with an increased risk for numerous chronic health conditions, including heart disease, stroke, and type 2 diabetes mellitus. Conversely, living with a chronic medical illness increases the risk of developing mental illness (National Institute of Mental Health, 2021).

Although some people may die as a direct result of their mental health condition, as is seen in suicide or drug overdose, most premature deaths among people with mental health conditions are caused by preventable, lifestyle-related diseases, such as cardiovascular disease, stroke, diabetes, hypertension, and cancers (Firth et al., 2019). The high prevalence of chronic physical illnesses among people with mental illness is a serious problem that needs to be addressed with increasing awareness and better treatment options (Dandona, 2019), including evidence-based lifestyle medicine interventions. This is especially true given that these chronic physical illnesses are associated with preventable risk factors such as smoking, physical inactivity, obesity, and side effects of psychiatric medications (Merlo & Vela, 2022). Unfortunately, people with mental illness tend not to receive the same amount or quality of treatment for their medical conditions as do those in the general population (Merlo & Vela, 2022). Additionally, the symptoms of the mental health conditions themselves can cause barriers to seeking care, as well as difficulty understanding and following medical advice.

22.7   LIFESTYLE MEDICINE FOR PSYCHIATRIC ILLNESSES

As early as the Middle Ages, physicians have recommended that their patients adopt healthy life-style behaviors, despite lacking a full understanding of the scientific basis for them (Zaman et al., 2019). Fortunately, in modern times, numerous studies have provided supporting evidence for the bidirectional relationship between lifestyle behaviors and mental and physical health (Xu et al., 2010). Each of the six pillars of lifestyle medicine plays an important role not only in the treatment of mental illness but also in supporting good mental health throughout the lifespan.

Historically, lifestyle medicine providers have focused primarily on the prevention, treatment, and cure of chronic lifestyle-related medical conditions, but mounting evidence suggests that lifestyle-based strategies and other non-pharmacological interventions can effectively improve mental health and emotional well-being, often at levels comparable to medications (Morton, 2018).

One reason why lifestyle medicine approaches are especially important for people with mental health conditions, and especially serious mental illnesses, is that these people consistently have higher morbidity and mortality than the general population, mostly due to cardiovascular disease, metabolic disease, diabetes, and respiratory disorders. Although genetic predisposition does con-tribute to the risk for certain physical health problems, modifiable lifestyle and environmental factors such as cigarette smoking, obesity, poor diet, and physical inactivity also play a prominent role (Li et al., 2020). It is important for nurses and healthcare professionals to recognize that the majority of premature and excess deaths in people with psychiatric illnesses are often not caused by the psychi-atric illnesses themselves but are due to chronic, preventable, lifestyle-related medical conditions, such as cancer, diabetes, and cardiovascular disease (Malhi, 2012). It holds true that what is good for the body is good for the brain, and since mental illnesses are brain disorders, it stands to reason that lifestyle medicine interventions are an essential component of the overall treatment of mental health conditions.

In the following paragraphs, supporting evidence and special considerations for each of the six pillars of lifestyle medicine will be discussed. Many people with mental health conditions experi-ence significant barriers to engaging in health-promoting behaviors due to the influence of social determinants of health. Their disease and the effects of certain psychiatric medications also change their appetites (Firth, 2020). There will also be a discussion of some of the common barriers to the implementation of lifestyle medicine interventions in this population and proposed strategies to help overcome them.

22.8   NUTRITION FOR MENTAL HEALTH

Evidence from numerous studies suggests there may be a bidirectional causal relationship between the intake of certain types of foods and mental health and that certain eating patterns can help reduce the risk of developing certain psychiatric conditions (Firth et al., 2020). While more research is needed to expand current understandings of the mechanisms underlying the connections between nutrition and mental health, the topic continues to garner interest from researchers, clinicians, and patients. Poor nutrition has been implicated in the underlying pathophysiology of behavioral health disorders and may hinder the treatment and recovery process (Kris-Etherton et al., 2021). Thus, optimizing nutritional status is a critical, evidence-based part of a multifaceted approach to the prevention and treatment of psychiatric conditions (Beyer & Payne, 2016). Better nutrition can improve psychiatric outcomes while minimizing the risks of comorbid, lifestyle-related chronic health conditions (Beyer & Payne, 2016).

In addition to the adverse effects on brain health and mood, Western dietary patterns have been implicated in the prevalence of obesity, type 2 diabetes mellitus, and cardiovascular disease (Firth et al., 2020). Regularly eating a high-quality diet rich in vegetables, fruits, whole grains, nuts, and legumes with moderate amounts of animal products, and very little red meat, has been linked to a decreased risk for depression (Lasalle et al., 2019) and anxiety (Norowitz, 2021), as well as lowering the risk of metabolic and cardiovascular disorders (Guasch-Ferré et al., 2017). The Mediterranean diet and an anti-inflammatory diet such as a whole-food, plant-centric diet have demonstrated efficacy in the management of metabolic issues among patients affected by severe mental illnesses, including psychotic disorders (Ventriglio et al. 2019a), schizophrenia (Ventriglio et al., 2019b), major depression, and bipolar disorder (Ventriglio et al., 2015).

While a causal relationship between a whole-food, plant-predominant diet and the mechanisms that underlie brain function and mental health has not been firmly established, preliminary studies examining the effects of plant-based diets compared to conventional diets on outcomes such as weight, systemic inflammation, and energy metabolism over a two-year period have shown promising short- and moderate term beneficial effects (Medawar, 2019).

22.8.1 THE FOOD–MOOD CONNECTION

There is a complex bidirectional relationship between food intake and moods. Not only does food intake affect moods and brain health, but the opposite is also true. Psychological state affects appetites as well as food choices and preferences, as evidenced by the common desire for "comfort foods" when feeling stressed or experiencing low moods (Firth et al., 2020). It is widely accepted that humans eat for reasons other than physical hunger, and this behavior can lead to overweight and obesity (Bénard et al., 2018). Emotional eating manifests in several different types and occurs in response to depression (EE-D), anxiety/anger (EE-A), boredom (EE-B), or even in response to experiencing positive emotions (EE-P) (Braden et al., 2018). Researchers have found that distinctive patterns exist between these different types of emotional eating and the resulting psychological outcomes (Braden et al., 2018). The study conducted by Braden et al. (2018) showed that those who ate due to depression, anxiety, and boredom had worse psychological well-being, more disordered eating symptoms, and more difficulties with regulating their emotions. Another study conducted by Camilleri et al. (2014) showed that women who ate in response to depressive symptoms consumed higher amounts of energy-dense snacks, mostly those high in sugar and fat. In men, emotional eating for reasons other than depression was associated with overconsumption of these same foods (Camilleri et al., 2014). Additionally, Bénard et al. (2018) found that impulsivity and consideration of future consequences had a moderating effect on the relationship between emotional eating and body weight. These studies highlight the importance of considering the patient's psychological state when attempting to target unhealthy eating habits.

22.8.2 DIET AND DEPRESSION/ANXIETY

In a recent meta-analysis done by Molendijk et al. (2018), the authors found evidence that a higher quality diet was associated with a lower risk for the onset of depressive symptoms. More recently, Matison et al. (2021) did a systematic review and meta-analysis of associations between nutrition and the incidence of depression in middle-aged and older adults and found that higher consumption of pro-inflammatory diets and Western diets were associated with an increased risk for depression. Additionally, fluctuations in blood sugar caused by the overconsumption of sugars and refined carbohydrates can increase the risk of experiencing symptoms of anxiety and irritability (Towler et al., 1993). Certain types of foods, including added or refined sugars in foods, oils made from industrial seeds (corn oil, grapeseed/canola oil, and soybean oils), and nitrates found in processed foods and meats (hot dogs, bacon, lunch meats), are pro-inflammatory and can induce anxiety symptoms (Naidoo, 2021). Furthermore, recurrent episodes of low blood sugar are associated with the presence of mood disorders (Seaquist et al., 2013) and may therefore increase symptom burden. Additionally, the pro-inflammatory effects of a diet high in calories and saturated fat, as seen in the Western or Standard American Diet, have been implicated in the detrimental effects on brain health, including cognitive deficits and hippocampal dysfunction (Noble et al., 2017). There has also been evidence of a link between the diet-induced changes in the gut microbiome, altered intestinal permeability, and damage to the blood–brain barrier, which allows for increased production of endotoxins by the commensal bacteria and enhanced vulnerability to harmful substances in the bloodstream (Noble et al., 2017). This exposure can lead to neuroinflammation and the development of sickness behaviors seen in depression and alterations in cognition.

22.8.3 DIET AND BIPOLAR DISORDER

Bipolar disorder is a serious mental illness characterized by distinct phases in which people can oscillate between periods of severe depression (and a corresponding increased risk for suicide) followed by intense periods of increased activity, decreased sleep, expansive moods, and irritability/agitation that can have a significant impact on their confidence, perceptions of self-efficacy, and health-related decision making (Tondo, 2003). People with bipolar disorder are more likely to be adversely impacted by poor nutrition and have a mortality gap of up to 20 years as compared to the general population (Malhi, 2012). Studies have found that people with bipolar disorder tend to have comparatively unhealthy diets and may experience periods of increased appetite, which may partially explain their increased risk for obesity and metabolic syndrome (Beyer & Payne, 2016). Another contributing factor is that many medications used to treat bipolar disorder, including mood stabilizers, antipsychotic drugs, and antidepressants, are not only obesogenic but can also promote high cholesterol and triglycerides, high blood sugars, and other cardiometabolic disturbances (Kendall et al., 2014).

22.8.4 DIET AND SCHIZOPHRENIA, MOOD DISORDERS, AND AUTISM SPECTRUM DISORDER

Schizophrenia is a complex and serious mental illness that has a multifactorial etiology and a diverse pattern of symptoms that may include hallucinations, delusions, disorganized speech, disorganized or catatonic behavior, and negative symptoms such as apathy, feeling flat, or lack of speech (Cha & Yang, 2020). An immune-mediated response appears to play a role in the etiology of schizophrenia. It also shares some common immunological features of another immune-mediated condition, celiac disease (Wijarnpreecha et al., 2018).

Celiac disease is a multi-system autoimmune digestive disorder that occurs in genetically susceptible individuals and is triggered by the ingestion of gluten (Cha & Yang, 2020). Gluten is a protein that occurs naturally in wheat, rye, triticale, and barley and is present in many commonly eaten foods, such as cereals, bread, pasta, flour tortillas, baked goods, and as an ingredient or a cross-contaminant in many prepackaged foods (Biesiekierski, 2017). Gluten can also be found in oral care products such as toothpaste and lipstick/lip balm, some medications, and some vitamin and herbal supplements (Biesiekierski, 2017). Ingestion of gluten in a person with celiac disease can cause an inflammatory response that damages the lining of the small intestine. This prevents nutrients from being absorbed properly and can cause vitamin and mineral deficiencies, as well as diarrhea, weight loss, anemia, and a range of neurological and psychiatric symptoms (Cha & Yang, 2020). The inflammatory response to gluten is thought to cause a disruption in the blood–brain barrier, increasing permeability and allowing the influx of substances that could alter mood and behavior (Cha & Yang, 2020). Currently, the only treatment for celiac disease is a strict gluten-free diet for life (Busby et al., 2018). In six out of the nine studies reviewed by Cha and Yang (2020), a strong association was demonstrated between initiating a gluten-free diet and improved outcomes in patients with schizophrenia. Therefore, individuals with schizophrenia and symptoms of celiac disease or gluten intolerance should be tested by a healthcare provider knowledgeable in diagnosing this condition and started on a gluten-free diet if indicated. It is critically important that a person with suspected celiac disease does not start a gluten-free diet prior to testing, which includes blood tests and a biopsy of the duodenum, as this can cause false-negative results (Rubio-Tapia et al., 2013). There is mounting evidence suggesting a potential bidirectional relationship between gluten sensitivity or intolerance and other psychiatric disorders, including mood disorders and autism spectrum disorders (Busby et al., 2018). It is important to note that currently, the evidence for adopting a gluten-free diet to treat or manage conditions other than celiac disease is poor. The diet is difficult to maintain, can be more expensive, carries an increased risk of nutritional deficiencies, and therefore should not be encouraged in the absence of celiac disease (Lerner et al., 2019).

Although further research is needed, a potentially helpful dietary intervention in the treatment of schizophrenia may be the inclusion of Omega-3 fatty acids as an augmentation strategy (Goh et al., 2021). In a meta-analysis of 20 double-blinded randomized control trials, the addition of Omega-3 polyunsaturated fatty acids was well tolerated and associated with significantly improved positive psychiatric symptoms, but not negative symptoms, as well as improvements in serum triglycerides (Goh et al., 2021).

22.9   PHYSICAL ACTIVITY AND MENTAL HEALTH

One of the most effective and accessible ways to improve health, reduce symptoms, and increase function in people with mental illness is to increase physical activity. Regular physical activity improves physical performance, promotes sleep, and reduces the risk for multiple chronic health conditions, such as cardiovascular disease, diabetes, osteoporosis, and depression (Kramer, 2020). Exercise has multiple beneficial effects on the brain. It improves both executive and global functioning in adults, increases cognitive flexibility and reduces impulsivity and inattention in children with attention deficit hyperactivity disorder (ADHD), and improves cognitive function, processing speed, memory, and executive functions, which are often impaired in people with schizophrenia or bipolar disorder (Caponnetto et al., 2021). Exercise has also been shown, in healthy individuals, to increase blood flow to the hippocampus and increase hippocampal volume, stimulate the growth and development of brain cells, modulate synaptic plasticity, and increase the secretion of growth factors such as BDNF (et al., 2011) and orexin-A (Chieffi et al., 2017) that help to optimize brain function and regulate mood.

In a study done by Paolucci et al. (2018), the results indicated that moderate-intensity exercise could improve mental health by reducing levels of the pro-inflammatory cytokine TNF-α, which is associated with depression. Furthermore, positive mental health benefits associated with exercise have been observed for people with pre/post-natal depression, anorexia nervosa, bulimia nervosa, binge eating disorder, post-traumatic stress disorder, and alcohol and substance use disorders, with a low incidence of adverse effects (Ashdown-Franks et al., 2020). Compared to medications, exercise has no harmful side effects, is free or low-cost, and targets many health issues at once, which makes it an ideal treatment for nearly all types of physical and mental illnesses (Kramer, 2020).

22.10   STRESS AND MENTAL HEALTH

Stress is an inescapable aspect of modern life and can be defined as a state of mental, emotional, or physical tension or distress resulting from demanding circumstances that exceed a person's resources or capacity to cope. While a small amount of stress can be beneficial for its effects on human physiology, immunity, motivation, and behavior, exposure to high levels of acute stress or chronic stress (that occurs over a prolonged period) can have detrimental effects on the human body. Chronic stress is especially problematic because it is associated with persistently elevated levels of systemic cortisol, which can promote the development of glucocorticoid receptor resistance and decrease the efficacy of cortisol's anti-inflammatory effects (Bae et al., 2019). Stress influences cognition, emotions, and behavior through various regulatory and reactivity pathways in the brain, potentially affecting adherence to treatment and resulting in greater disease activity (Araki et al., 2020).

22.11   SLEEP AND MENTAL HEALTH

Sleep is more than the absence of wakefulness; it is a complex and dynamic process in which the brain engages in activities that affect the mind and body. According to Blackwelder et al. (2021), one-third of adults living in the United States report sleeping less than the recommended amount, and approximately 20% of US adults are living with a mental illness. The United States National Sleep Foundation recommends that all adults get between seven and nine hours of sleep per night, but around 30% report they get six hours or less.

Inadequate sleep was associated with significantly increased odds of frequent mental distress.

Interestingly, it appears that the single most significant contributing factor to inadequate sleep is exposure to artificial light at night. This artificial light could come from smartphones, televisions, or other electronic devices commonly used by individuals in modern society and disrupts the natural Circadian rhythm (Lunn et al., 2017), which can lead to poor mental health.

Lack of sleep is associated with higher-than-normal levels of pro-inflammatory cytokines, which are small proteins necessary for signaling between cells. In people with poor sleep, increased levels of Interleukin (IL)-6, IL-1β, and Tumor Necrosis Factor (TNF)-α have been noted. These specific cytokines have been implicated in the development of depression and other neuropsychiatric disorders (Felger & Lotrich, 2013). These inflammatory cytokines can enter the brain by several different pathways, such as active transport across the blood–brain barrier, across areas such as the circumventricular organs where the blood–brain barrier is incomplete. Cytokines can also travel to the brain via afferent nerve fibers or by attaching to peripheral monocytes that travel to brain cells and glia. Once there, these cytokines affect mechanisms in the hypothalamus, basal forebrain, and brainstem receptors that can trigger what is known as "sickness behavior." Sickness behavior is a cluster of symptoms including anhedonia, changes in sleep, decreased social interactions, loss of appetite, and low energy, and is thought to be an evolutionary protective response that allows a person who is ill to conserve energy needed for recovery (Felger & Lotrich, 2013).

The deleterious effects of inadequate sleep on mental health are well known to most people, but in people with certain types of mental illness, such as bipolar disorder, it can be dangerous. Some people with a subtype of bipolar disorder are vulnerable to mood elevations in response to sleep deprivation (Lewis, 2017), so it is critically important that they establish and maintain good sleep habits. The importance of sleep is discussed further in Chapter 4 of this volume.

22.12   SOCIAL CONNECTEDNESS AND MENTAL HEALTH

Establishing and maintaining friendships and other social relationships is an important factor in mental health and well-being (Cleary et al., 2018). However, people with mental health conditions such as anxiety, depression, alcohol or substance use disorders, or those who experience SMI can have difficulty connecting with others (Cleary et al., 2018). For people with SMI, and schizophrenia, in particular, barriers to socialization play a role, and they spend less time with friends and family and experience more feelings of loneliness (Weittenhiller et al., 2021). The adverse effects of loneliness and inadequate perceived social support on physical health and mortality are established (Wang et al., 2018), but the effects on mental health have not been well studied. From the study conducted by Wang et al. (2018), people with depression who reported loneliness and low social support had worse outcomes related to symptoms, recovery, and social functioning. Happiness and social connectivity are further explored in Chapter 6 of this volume.

22.13   TOBACCO USE

Tobacco use is the leading preventable cause of death worldwide (Prochaska et al., 2017). People with mental illnesses have an increased prevalence of smoking and, on average, die 25 years earlier due to tobacco use (Prochaska et al., 2017). Smoking in people with mental disorders is known to be an independent risk factor for suicide, and smoking cessation appears to reduce that particular risk (Prochaska et al., 2017). Additionally, people who smoke typically need higher doses of certain psychotropic medications because tobacco smoke induces cytochrome P450 enzymes and alters drug metabolism in the liver (Tsuda et al., 2014). According to Vermeulen et al., 2021), starting to smoke and smoking over the course of a lifetime may be a causal risk factor for developing bipolar disorder. Given that smoking is a modifiable risk factor, there is a need for investment in resources that focus on smoking prevention and treatment to reduce the risk of psychiatric conditions in future generations (Vermeulen et al., 2021). Tobacco use and cessation techniques are discussed in Chapter 23 of this volume.

22.14 POTENTIAL BARRIERS TO ADOPTING LIFESTYLE MEDICINE INTERVENTIONS FOR PEOPLE WITH MENTAL HEALTH CONDITIONS

22.14.1 INDIVIDUAL HEALTH BELIEFS AND PREFERENCES

The Health Belief Model (HBM) is a framework initially developed in the 1950s that has evolved overtime and is widely being used to support health behavior change (Champion & Skinner, 2008). The HBM can help nurses understand how patients with and without mental illness may have difficulty adopting or maintaining lifestyle medicine interventions. The HBM suggests that a person's belief in whether they may be susceptible to an illness or disease combined with their belief in the effectiveness of a specific behavior change or action will predict the degree to which they will adopt the behavior.

The HBM describes certain perceptions that a person may have that could help nurses and other healthcare professionals understand why very few people have fully embraced the principles of lifestyle medicine despite robust evidence of their efficacy and health benefits.

Using the HBM as part of a more comprehensive framework for assessment, nursing diagnosis, care planning, intervention, and evaluation allows for the identification of opportunities for nurses to integrate lifestyle medicine principles seamlessly into patient care. The primary constructs of the Health Belief Model are:

- **Perceived Susceptibility:** A person's belief about their own risk of acquiring a health condition.
- **Perceived Severity:** An individual's beliefs about the seriousness of a disease or the possible consequences if left undiagnosed or untreated.
- **Perceived Benefits:** One's beliefs about the positive aspects of taking action to reduce risk or improve health.
- **Perceived Barriers:** A person's beliefs about the possible negative aspects of taking action or the possible difficulties that could be encountered in doing so.
- **Cues to Action:** The factors that ultimately cause a person to act or change their behavior.
- **Self-Efficacy:** The belief that one can change behavior and achieve the desired outcome.

It is critically important for nurses and other healthcare professionals to remember that a patient's health status reflects their unique biological and genetic attributes as influenced by a unique set of circumstances and life experiences. Much of this patient's history will be unknown to the nurse but exerts a powerful effect on the patient's thoughts, beliefs, and behaviors. As always, for effective therapeutic communication to occur, it is helpful if nurses approach conversations about lifestyle medicine components with their patients from a perspective of curiosity and avoid making judgments.

22.14.2 Cultural Factors

Culture is a term that refers to a set of shared beliefs, norms, and values shared by a group of people. It is critically important that healthcare professionals recognize that significant diversity exists among people from the same culture, depending on age, income, level of acculturation, health status, and other factors. Healthcare providers must avoid stereotyping individuals based on their appearance, racial or ethnic background, socioeconomic status, religion, political affiliation, or other factors. Cultural misunderstandings between patients and healthcare providers can lead to clinician bias and fragmentation of care, which can deter people from accessing, utilizing, and receiving appropriate healthcare services. Not receiving appropriate treatment can have disastrous consequences, including disability in one or more life domains, extreme psychological or emotional distress, self- or other-directed violence, or suicide.

Culture, and health culture, plays a large role in lifestyle choices because it affects people's way of thinking and their behaviors (Jia et al., 2017). This may include food preferences or cooking styles, physical activity patterns, the variety of types of social interactions, sleep habits, stress perception and management, and the amounts and types of substance use. Cultural influences on health and illness can have a significant impact on patient health. They can determine whether a person is willing to engage in lifestyle medicine treatments, how supportive their family or social group is, the type of changes they may be willing to make, and how they fare in treatment (Office of the Surgeon General, 2001).

As nurses, part of the assessment process prior to implementing lifestyle medicine interventions includes a respectful and non-judgmental inquiry into how a person's cultural values, beliefs, and practices may affect their health-related behaviors. It is critical that the assessment takes place in an environment where the patient feels safe sharing information that will help guide the development of a mutually-acceptable plan of care regarding lifestyle changes.

22.14.3 Healthcare Avoidance

Healthcare avoidance is a form of patient disengagement that can have a negative impact on a person's health behaviors, timely access to healthcare services, and overall well-being (Byrne, 2008). Healthcare avoidance is a common and variable phenomenon influenced by demographic, personal, provider-related, and administrative factors (Byrne, 2008). The unfortunate reality is that healthcare avoidance is prevalent among those with mental health conditions. According to the 2007 Health Information Trends Survey, people who were experiencing severe psychological distress (SPD) were more likely to avoid seeking healthcare than those without SPD (Cantor et al., 2007). More recently, Ganson et al. (2020) found that individuals who experienced symptoms common in those with anxiety and depression (feeling nervous, anxious, or on edge; not being able to stop or control worrying; having little interest or pleasure in doing things; feeling down, depressed, or hopeless) in the seven days prior to the study were more likely to avoid having medical care for causes not related to the coronavirus during the COVID-19 pandemic. The fear of being told they had a severe illness, distress at the thought of dying, concerns about revealing personal or sensitive information, and having a physical examination are some factors found to be responsible for healthcare avoidance, even in those who felt it was appropriate to be evaluated (Ye et al., 2012). Additional reasons cited by persons who avoided seeking healthcare included a preference for alternative care or self-care, a stated dislike or mistrust of doctors, aversion to medical treatments, and time or financial constraints (Cantor et al., 2007).

Many people with and without mental health conditions prefer self-care or complementary/alternative treatments to traditional Western medicine approaches. Individuals may elect self-care due to cost, convenience, empowerment, or a closer fit with their beliefs, values, or lifestyle (Narasimhan et al., 2019). Fortunately, for people who prefer self-care or other natural approaches, the six pillars of lifestyle medicine have a great deal to offer. The recommended lifestyle practices of a plant-centric diet, regular physical activity, adequate sleep, stress management, social engagement, and avoidance of risky substance use behaviors do not require medical supervision unless certain comorbid medical problems are present (for example, a person with depression and type 2 diabetes mellitus may need multiple medication adjustments if they significantly change their diet or physical activity levels) once they have been cleared by their healthcare team to participate. Lifestyle medicine interventions are either free or low-cost, making them ideal for people who are disproportionately affected by poverty, have inadequate health insurance coverage, and may face other individual or systemic barriers to achieving optimal whole-person health and wellness.

22.14.4 HEALTH LITERACY

The U. S. Department of Health and Human Services (2010) describes health literacy as the degree to which people can obtain, process, and understand basic health information required to make appropriate health-related decisions. Updated definitions include the ability to use health-related information as opposed to simply understanding it and a focus on a person's ability to make "well-informed" decisions (CDC, 2021b). Health literacy is affected by physical and mental abilities and personal factors, such as age, culture, educational background, and language. In the US, over 90 million adults have low health literacy, which affects their ability to make decisions about behaviors that can be harmful to their health.

Nurses can help assess and improve their patient's health literacy by inquiring how and where they get the information they use to make health decisions. A 2018 study noted that patients with lower health literacy were more likely to rely on sources such as television, social media, and celebrities than from their healthcare providers. Additionally, those with low health literacy often come from marginalized groups, such as immigrants, those living in poverty, people of color, and those who speak English as a second language.

Improving health literacy is a worthy goal and can help empower patients to make sound, health-promoting decisions and improve outcomes. As nurses spend more time with patients than other healthcare team members and develop intimate therapeutic caregiving relationships, they are ideally positioned to help patients access information and resources about lifestyle medicine approaches that benefit their health and their families.

22.14.5 DIFFICULTY WITH ADHERENCE TO LIFESTYLE CHANGES

Adherence is a term that refers to the extent to which a person follows an agreed-upon course of actions. Adherence is a significant health outcome measure for people with mental health conditions because non-adherence is associated with increased morbidity, mortality, and higher healthcare costs (Arbuthnott & Sharpe, 2009). Adherence to treatment plans for people with mental health conditions can be challenging when lifestyle changes are involved. Some people with mental illnesses may lack the cognitive capacity to understand the risk or how their actions or inactions may exacerbate the risk. Some individuals may not have insight into how their behavior may be contributing to how they feel or maybe worsening their condition. They may have trouble with forgetfulness, organization, planning and find it exceedingly difficult to sustain behavioral changes long-term. In some cases, patients with mental illnesses that affect their mood or energy levels may not be able to muster the degree of motivation required to enact lifestyle changes. They may tend to focus on the negative aspects of abandoning a behavior they may enjoy or perceive as beneficial (for example, smoking cigarettes to relieve stress). Establishing a therapeutic alliance and a trusting relationship between the nurse and the patient is essential for identifying and successfully overcoming many of the common issues that may arise when working with patients to implement lifestyle changes.

Disparities may be more pronounced in people from specific groups, such as racial or ethnic minorities, those who are poor, who live in rural areas, who speak English as a second language, and who identify as lesbian, gay, bisexual, transgender, or have other gender-related differences. Discrimination related to immigration status, occupational status, sexual orientation, or race/ethnicity has consistently been shown to adversely affect mental health outcomes in the United States (Alegria et al., 2018).

22.15 POTENTIAL BARRIERS TO DIET CHANGES

Poverty, inadequate access to healthy food options, lack of sufficient food storage or preparation facilities, and inadequate knowledge regarding cooking, nutrition, and how to make healthy food choices are all social and practical issues commonly experienced by people with mental health disorders that may affect their ability to eat an optimal diet. Additionally, not growing up in an environment where healthy eating was practiced or being surrounded by people in a social group who routinely overeat, smoke, use drugs, are physically inactive, or engage in the excessive consumption of junk food, sugar-sweetened, or highly caffeinated beverages can make it challenging to perceive the need for or muster the necessary motivation to make diet and lifestyle changes.

Physical and psychological barriers include poor dental health that may make eating unpleasant or difficult (Chapter 24), not experiencing or responding to satiety cues that tell someone they do not need more food, using food to cope with negative emotions, not being interested in or receptive to health-related messages, the presences of cognitive impairment or cognitive distortions that affect behavior, and poor executive function skills can also present significant challenges.

22.16 CONCLUSION

Lifestyle interventions can improve mental health across the spectrum. Nurses play an important role in addressing the need to implement more lifestyle interventions. The COVID-19 pandemic exacerbated mental health concerns, with the majority of Americans reporting some mental health need, thus highlighting the importance of lifestyle interventions. Tips nurses can use addressing these needs both with themselves and with their patients include:

- Initiating conversations about patients' lifestyles and health behaviors.
- Making reasonable adjustments such as adjusting communication style when discussing lifestyle changes or giving advice to people with learning disabilities, dementia, or mental illness to meet their needs. This includes using and discussing easy-read leaflets where applicable.
- Asking about prior experiences of medication or lifestyle change to identify any problems or barriers to adopting new lifestyle changes.
- Sharing knowledge and responding openly and honestly to questions about interventions, their effectiveness, and possible difficulties along with how they might be managed.
- Helping patients develop strategies to incorporate lifestyle changes or medications into their routines.
- Providing motivational support and trying to understand non-adherence rather than being disappointed.

In working with patients, it is important to remember that consistent little actions done daily can make a significant difference in positive patient outcomes. Lifestyle interventions can have a profound positive impact on both nurses and patients.

REFERENCES

Alegría, M., NeMoyer, A., Falgàs Bagué, I., Wang, Y., & Alvarez, K. (2018). Social determinants of mental health: Where we are and where we need to go. *Current Psychiatry Reports, 20*(11), 95. https://doi.org/10.1007/s11920-018-0969-9

Araki, M., Shinzaki, S., Yamada, T., Arimitsu, S., Komori, M., Shibukawa, N., ... & Takehara, T. (2020). Psychologic stress and disease activity in patients with inflammatory bowel disease: A multicenter cross-sectional study. *PloS One, 15*(5), e0233365.

Arbuthnott, A., & Sharpe, D. (2009). The effect of physician–patient collaboration on patient adherence in non-psychiatric medicine. *Patient Education and Counseling, 77*(1), 60–67. https://doi.org/10.1016/j.pec.2009.03.022

Ashdown-Franks, G., Firth, J., Carney, R., Carvalho, A. F., Hallgren, M., Koyanagi, A., Rosenbaum, S., Schuch, F. B., Smith, L., Solmi, M., Vancampfort, D., & Stubbs, B. (2020). Exercise as medicine for mental and substance use disorders: A meta-review of the benefits for neuropsychiatric and cognitive outcomes. *Sports Medicine (Auckland, N.Z.), 50*(1), 151–170. https://doi.org/10.1007/s40279-019-01187-6

Augystyn, A. (2021). Ramadan. Brittanica. Retrieved January 2 from www.britannica.com/topic/Ramadan

Bae, Y. J., Reinelt, J., Netto, J., Uhlig, M., Willenberg, A., Ceglarek, U., ... & Kratzsch, J. (2019). Salivary cortisone, as a biomarker for psychosocial stress, is associated with state anxiety and heart rate. *Psychoneuroendocrinology, 101*, 35–41.

Banerjee, D., & Rai, M. (2020). Social isolation in Covid-19: The impact of loneliness. *International Journal of Social Psychiatry, 66*(6), 525–527. https://doi.org/10.1177/0020764020922269

Bénard, M., Bellisle, F., Etilé, F., Reach, G., Kesse-Guyot, E., Hercberg, S., & Péneau, S. (2018). Impulsivity and consideration of future consequences as moderators of the association between emotional eating and body weight status. *The International Journal of Behavioral Nutrition and Physical Activity, 15*(1), 84. https://doi.org/10.1186/s12966-018-0721-1

Beyer, J. L., & Payne, M. E. (2016). Nutrition and bipolar depression. *Psychiatric Clinics, 39*(1), 75–86. https://doi.org/10.1016/j.psc.2015.10.003

Biesiekierski, J. R. (2017). What is gluten? *Journal of Gastroenterology and Hepatology, 32*, 78–81. https://doi.org/10.1111/jgh.13703

Blackwelder, A., Hoskins, M., & Huber, L. (2021). Effect of inadequate sleep on frequent mental distress. *Preventing Chronic Disease, 18*, E61. https://doi.org/10.5888/pcd18.200573

Braden, A., Musher-Eizenman, D., Watford, T., & Emley, E. (2018). Eating when depressed, anxious, bored, or happy: Are emotional eating types associated with unique psychological and physical health correlates? *Appetite, 125*, 410–417. https://doi.org/10.1016/j.appet.2018.02.022

Busby, E., Bold, J., Fellows, L., & Rostami, K. (2018). Mood disorders and gluten: It's not all in your mind! A systematic review with meta-analysis. *Nutrients, 10*(11), 1708. https://doi.org/10.3390/nu10111708

Byrne, S. K. (2008). Healthcare avoidance: A critical review. *Holistic Nursing Practice, 22*(5), 280–292. https://doi.org/10.1097/01.HNP.0000334921.31433.c6

Camilleri, G. M., Méjean, C., Kesse-Guyot, E., Andreeva, V. A., Bellisle, F., Hercberg, S., & Péneau, S. (2014). The associations between emotional eating and consumption of energy-dense snack foods are modified by sex and depressive symptomatology. *The Journal of Nutrition, 144*(8), 1264–1273. https://doi.org/10.3945/jn.114.193177

Canady, V. A. (2021). MHA releases largest real-time data from MH help-seekers. *Mental Health Weekly, 31*(6), 7–7. https://doi-org.proxy.library.nyu.edu/10.1002/mhw.32675

Cantor, D., Coa, K., Crystal-Mansour, S., Davis, T., Dipko, S., & Sigman, R. (2009). *Health information national trends survey (HINTS) 2007*. Westat.

Capezuti. (2016). The power and importance of sleep. *Geriatric Nursing (New York), 37*(6), 487–488. https://doi.org/10.1016/j.gerinurse.2016.10.005

Caponnetto, P., Casu, M., Amato, M., Cocuzza, D., Galofaro, V., La Morella, A., ... & Vella, M. C. (2021). The effects of physical exercise on mental health: From cognitive improvements to risk of addiction. *International Journal of Environmental Research and Public Health, 18*(24), 13384. https://doi.org/10.3390/ijerph182413384

Cha, H. Y., & Yang, S. J. (2020). Anti-inflammatory diets and schizophrenia. *Clinical Nutrition Research, 9*(4), 241–257. https://doi.org/10.7762/cnr.2020.9.4.241

Champion, V. L., & Skinner, C. S. (2008). The health belief model. *Health Behavior and Health Education: Theory, Research, and Practice*, *4*, 45–65.

Clark, L. A., Cuthbert, B., Lewis-Fernández, R., Narrow, W. E., & Reed, G. M. (2017). Three approaches to understanding and classifying mental disorder: ICD-11, DSM-5, and the National Institute of Mental Health's Research Domain Criteria (RDoC). *Psychological Science in the Public Interest*, *18*(2), 72–145.

Cleary, M., Lees, D., & Sayers, J. (2018). Friendship and mental health. *Issues in Mental Health Nursing*, *39*(3), 279–281. https://doi.org/10.1080/01612840.2018.1431444

Chieffi, S., Carotenuto, M., Monda, V., Valenzano, A., Villano, I., Precenzano, F., Tafuri, D., Salerno, M., Filippi, N., Nuccio, F., Ruberto, M., De Luca, V., Cipolloni, L., Cibelli, G., Mollica, M. P., Iacono, D., Nigro, E., Monda, M., Messina, G., & Messina, A. (2017). Orexin system: The key for a healthy life. *Frontiers in Physiology*, *8*, 357. https://doi.org/10.3389/fphys.2017.00357

Dandona, R. (2019). Mind and body go together: The need for integrated care. *The Lancet Psychiatry*, *6*(8), 638–639. https://doi.org/10.1016/S2215-0366(19)30251-2

Erickson, K. I., Miller, D. L., & Roecklein, K. A. (2012). The aging hippocampus: Interactions between exercise, depression, and BDNF. *The Neuroscientist*, *18*(1), 82–97. https://doi.org/10.1177/1073858410397054

Evans, T. S., Berkman, N. D., Brown, C., Gaynes, B. N., & Weber, R. P. (2016). Disparities within serious mental illness. *Technical Briefs*, *25*.

Farhud, D., & Aryan, Z. (2018). Circadian rhythm, lifestyle and health: A narrative review. *Iranian Journal of Public Health*, *47*(8), 1068–1076. www.ninds.nih.gov/Disorders/Patient-Caregiver-Education/Understanding-Sleep

Felger, J. C., & Lotrich, F. E. (2013). Inflammatory cytokines in depression: Neurobiological mechanisms and therapeutic implications. *Neuroscience*, *246*, 199–229. https://doi.org/10.1016/j.neuroscience.2013.04.060

Firth, J., Gangwisch, J. E., Borisini, A., Wootton, R. E., & Mayer, E. A. (2020). Food and mood: How do diet and nutrition affect mental wellbeing? *BMJ (Clinical Research Ed.)*, *369*, m2382. https://doi.org/10.1136/bmj.m2382

Firth, J., Siddiqi, N., Koyanagi, A., Siskind, D., Rosenbaum, S., Galletly, C., Allan, S., Caneo, C., Carney, R., Carvalho, A. F., Chatterton, M. L., Correll, C. U., Curtis, J., Gaughran, F., Heald, A., Hoare, E., Jackson, S. E., Kisely, S., Lovell, K., Maj, M., … Stubbs, B. (2019). The Lancet Psychiatry Commission: A blueprint for protecting physical health in people with mental illness. *The Lancet Psychiatry*, *6*(8), 675–712. https://doi.org/10.1016/S2215-0366(19)30132-4

Fusar-Poli, P., Salazar de Pablo, G., De Micheli, A., Nieman, D. H., Correll, C. U., Kessing, L. V., Pfennig, A., Bechdolf, A., Borgwardt, S., Arango, C., & van Amelsvoort, T. (2020). What is good mental health? A scoping review. *European Neuropsychopharmacology: The Journal of the European College of Neuropsychopharmacology*, *31*, 33–46. https://doi.org/10.1016/j.euroneuro.2019.12.105

Ganson, K. T., Weiser, S. D., Tsai, A. C., & Nagata, J. M. (2020). Associations between anxiety and depression symptoms and medical care avoidance during COVID-19. *Journal of General Internal Medicine*, *35*(11), 3406–3408. https://doi.org/10.1007/s11606-020-06156-8

Goh, K. K., Chen, C. Y., Chen, C. H., & Lu, M. L. (2021). Effects of omega-3 polyunsaturated fatty acids supplements on psychopathology and metabolic parameters in schizophrenia: A meta-analysis of randomized controlled trials. *Journal of Psychopharmacology (Oxford, England)*, *35*(3), 221–235. https://doi.org/10.1177/0269881120981392

Guasch-Ferré, M., Salas-Salvadó, J., Ros, E., Estruch, R., Corella, D., Fitó, M., Martínez-González, M. A., & PREDIMED Investigators (2017). The PREDIMED trial, Mediterranean diet and health outcomes: How strong is the evidence? *Nutrition, Metabolism, and Cardiovascular Diseases: NMCD*, *27*(7), 624–632. https://doi.org/10.1016/j.numecd.2017.05.004

Hasin, D. S., & Grant, B. F. (2015). The National Epidemiologic Survey on alcohol and related conditions (NESARC) waves 1 and 2: Review and summary of findings. *Social Psychiatry and Psychiatric Epidemiology*, *50*, 1609–1640. https://doi.org/10.1007/s00127-015-1088-0

Jia, Y., Gao, J., Dai, J., Zheng, P., & Fu, H. (2017). Associations between health culture, health behaviors, and health-related outcomes: A cross-sectional study. *PloS One*, *12*(7), e0178644. https://doi.org/10.1371/journal.pone.0178644

Kendall, T., Morriss, R., Mayo-Wilson, E., & Marcus, E. (2014). Assessment and management of bipolar disorder: Summary of updated NICE guidance. *BMJ*, 349. https://doi.org/10.1136/bmj.g5673

Kessler, R. C., Angermeyer, M., Anthony, J. C., De Graaf, R., Demyttenaere, K., Gasquet, I., De Girolamo, G., Gluzman, S., Gureje, O., Haro, J. M., Kawakami, N., Karam, A., Levinson, D., Medina Mora, M. E., Oakley Browne, M. A., Posada-Villa, J., Stein, D. J., Adley Tsang, C. H., Aguilar-Gaxiola, S., Alonso, J., … Üstün, T. B. (2007). Lifetime prevalence and age-of-onset distributions of mental disorders in the World Health Organization's World Mental Health Survey Initiative. *World Psychiatry: Official Journal of the World Psychiatric Association (WPA)*, *6*(3), 168–176.

Kramer A. (2020). An overview of the beneficial effects of exercise on health and performance. *Advances in Experimental Medicine and Biology*, *1228*, 3–22. https://doi.org/10.1007/978-981-15-1792-1_1

Kris-Etherton, P. M., Petersen, K. S., Hibbeln, J. R., Hurley, D., Kolick, V., Peoples, S., Rodriguez, N., & Woodward-Lopez, G. (2021). Nutrition and behavioral health disorders: Depression and anxiety. *Nutrition Reviews*, *79*(3), 247–260. https://doi.org/10.1093/nutrit/nuaa025

Lassale, C., Batty, G. D., Baghdadli, A., Jacka, F., Sánchez-Villegas, A., Kivimäki, M., & Akbaraly, T. (2019). Healthy dietary indices and risk of depressive outcomes: a systematic review and meta-analysis of observational studies. *Molecular Psychiatry*, *24*(7), 965–986. https://doi.org/10.1038/s41380-018-0237-8

Lerner, B. A., Green, P. H., & Lebwohl, B. (2019). Going against the grains: Gluten-free diets in patients without celiac disease—worthwhile or not? *Digestive Diseases and Sciences*, *64*(7), 1740–1747. https://doi.org/10.1007/s10620-019-05663-x

Lewis, K. S., Gordon-Smith, K., Forty, L., Di Florio, A., Craddock, N., Jones, L., & Jones, I. (2017). Sleep loss as a trigger of mood episodes in bipolar disorder: Individual differences based on diagnostic subtype and gender. *The British Journal of Psychiatry: The Journal of Mental Science*, *211*(3), 169–174. https://doi.org/10.1192/bjp.bp.117.202259

Li, Y., Schoufour, J., Wang, D. D., Dhana, K., Pan, A., Liu, X., … & Hu, F. B. (2020). Healthy lifestyle and life expectancy free of cancer, cardiovascular disease, and type 2 diabetes: Prospective cohort study. *BMJ*, *368*.

Lunn, R. M., Blask, D. E., Coogan, A. N., Figueiro, M. G., Gorman, M. R., Hall, J. E., Hansen, J., Nelson, R. J., Panda, S., Smolensky, M. H., Stevens, R. G., Turek, F. W., Vermeulen, R., Carreón, T., Caruso, C. C., Lawson, C. C., Thayer, K. A., Twery, M. J., Ewens, A. D., … Boyd, W.A. (2017). Health consequences of electric lighting practices in the modern world: A report on the National Toxicology Program's workshop on shift work at night, artificial light at night, and circadian disruption. *Science of the Total Environment*, *607–608*, 1073–1084. doi:10.1016/j.scitotenv.2017.07.056 PMID: 28724246; PMCID: PMC5587396.

Malhi, G. S., Bargh, D. M., McIntyre, R., Gitlin, M., Frye, M. A., Bauer, M., & Berk, M. (2012). Balanced efficacy, safety, and tolerability recommendations for the clinical management of bipolar disorder. *Bipolar Disorders*, *14*(Suppl. 2), 1–21. https://doi.org/10.1111/j.1399-5618.2012.00989.x

Manger, S. (2019). Lifestyle interventions for mental health. *Australian Journal of General Practice*, *48*(10), 670–673. https://doi.org/10.31128/AJGP-06-19-4964

Marx, W., Moseley, G., Berk, M., & Jacka, F. (2017). Nutritional psychiatry: The present state of the evidence. *The Proceedings of the Nutrition Society*, *76*(4), 427–436. https://doi.org/10.1017/S0029665117002026

Matison, A. P., Mather, K. A., Flood, V. M., & Reppermund, S. (2021). Associations between nutrition and the incidence of depression in middle-aged and older adults: A systematic review and meta-analysis of prospective observational population-based studies. *Ageing Research Reviews*, *70*, 101403. https://doi.org/10.1016/j.arr.2021.101403

Medawar, E., Huhn, S., Villringer, A., & Veronica Witte, A. (2019). The effects of plant-based diets on the body and the brain: A systematic review. *Translational Psychiatry*, *9*(1), 226. https://doi.org/10.1038/s41398-019-0552-0

Merlo, G., & Vela, A. (2021). Mental health in lifestyle medicine: A call to action. *American Journal of Lifestyle Medicine*, 1–14. https://doi.org/10.1177/15598276211013313

Merlo, G., & Vela, A. (2022). Mental Health in Lifestyle Medicine: A Call to Action. *American Journal of Lifestyle Medicine*, *16*(1), 7–20. https://doi.org/10.1177/15598276211013313

Molendijk, M., Molero, P., Ortuño Sánchez-Pedreño, F., Van der Does, W., & Angel Martínez-González, M. (2018). Diet quality and depression risk: A systematic review and dose-response meta-analysis of prospective studies. *Journal of Affective Disorders*, *226*, 346–354. https://doi.org/10.1016/j.jad.2017.09.022

Morton D. P. (2018). Combining lifestyle medicine and positive psychology to improve mental health and emotional well-being. American Journal of *Lifestyle Medicine*, *12*(5), 370–374. https://doi.org/10.1177/1559827618766482

Naidoo, U. (2021). Eat to beat stress. *American Journal of Lifestyle Medicine*, *15*(1), 39–42. https://doi.org/10.1177/1559827620973936

Narasimhan, M., Allotey, P., & Hardon, A. (2019). Self-care interventions to advance health and wellbeing: A conceptual framework to inform normative guidance. *BMJ*, *365*, l688. https://doi.org/10.1136/bmj.l688

National Institute of Mental Health. (n.d.) Mental illness. National Institute of Mental Health. Retrieved January 3, 2022 from www.nimh.nih.gov/health/statistics/mental-illness

National Institute of Mental Health. (2021). Chronic Illness and Mental. Retrieved May 7, 2022, from www.nimh.nih.gov/health/publications/chronic-illness-mental-health

National Library of Medicine. (2021). Mental health. National Library of Medicine. Retrieved January 5 from https://medlineplus.gov/mentalhealth.html

Noble, E. E., Hsu, T. M., & Kanoski, S. E. (2017). Gut to brain dysbiosis: Mechanisms linking Western diet Consumption, the microbiome, and cognitive impairment. *Frontiers in Behavioral Neuroscience*, *11*, 9. https://doi.org/10.3389/fnbeh.2017.00009

Norwitz, N. G., & Naidoo U. (2021). Nutrition as metabolic treatment for anxiety. *Front Psychiatry*, *12*, 598119. http://doi.org/10.3389/fpsyt.2021.598119

Office of the Surgeon General (US), Center for Mental Health Services (US), & National Institute of Mental Health (US). (2001). *Mental health: Culture, race, and ethnicity: A supplement to mental health: A Report of the surgeon general*. Substance Abuse and Mental Health Services Administration (US).

Paolucci, E. M., Loukov, D., Bowdish, D., & Heisz, J. J. (2018). Exercise reduces depression and inflammation but intensity matters. *Biological Psychology*, *133*, 79–84. https://doi.org/10.1016/j.biopsycho.2018.01.015

Parekh, R. (2018). Warning Signs of Mental Illness. American Psychiatric Association. Retrieved January 3 from www.psychiatry.org/patients-families/warning-signs-of-mental-illness

Prochaska, J. J., Das, S., & Young-Wolff, K. C. (2017). Smoking, mental illness, and public health. *Annual Review of Public Health*, *38*, 165–185. https://doi.org/10.1146/annurev-publhealth-031816-044618

Rubio-Tapia, A., Hill, I. D., Kelly, C. P., Calderwood, A. H., Murray, J. A., & American College of Gastroenterology (2013). ACG clinical guidelines: Diagnosis and management of celiac disease. *The American Journal of Gastroenterology*, *108*(5), 656–677. https://doi.org/10.1038/ajg.2013.79

Seaquist, E. R., Anderson, J., Childs, B., Cryer, P., Dagogo-Jack, S., Fish, L., Heller, S. R., Rodriguez, H., Rosenzweig, J., Vigersky, R., American Diabetes Association, & Endocrine Society (2013). Hypoglycemia and diabetes: A report of a workgroup of the American Diabetes Association and the Endocrine Society. *The Journal of Clinical Endocrinology and Metabolism*, *98*(5), 1845–1859. https://doi.org/10.1210/jc.2012-4127

Semahegn, A., Torpey, K., Manu, A., Assefa, N., Tesfaye, G., & Ankomah, A. (2020). Psychotropic medication non-adherence and its associated factors among patients with major psychiatric disorders: a systematic review and meta-analysis. *Systematic Reviews*, *9*(1), 17. https://doi.org/10.1186/s13643-020-1274-3

The Lancet Global Health. (2020). Mental health matters. *The Lancet Global Health*, *8*(11), e1352–e1352. https://doi.org/10.1016/S2214-109X(20)30432-0

Tondo, L., Isacsson, G., & Baldessarini, R. (2003). Suicidal behaviour in bipolar disorder: risk and prevention. *CNS Drugs*, *17*(7), 491–511. https://doi.org/10.2165/00023210-200317070-00003

Towler, D. A., Havlin, C. E., Craft, S., & Cryer, P. (1993). Mechanism of awareness of hypoglycemia. Perception of neurogenic (predominantly cholinergic) rather than neuroglycopenic symptoms. *Diabetes*, *42*(12), 1791–1798. https://doi.org/10.2337/diab.42.12.1791

Tsuda, Y., Saruwatari, J., & Yasui-Furukori, N. (2014). Meta-analysis: The effects of smoking on the disposition of two commonly used antipsychotic agents, olanzapine and clozapine. *BMJ Open*, *4*(3), e004216. https://doi.org/10.1136/bmjopen-2013-004216

US Department of Health and Human Services, Office of Disease Prevention and Health Promotion. (2010). *National action plan to improve health literacy*. Washington, DC.

Ventriglio, A., Baldessarini, R. J., Vitrani, G., Bonfitto, I., Cecere, A. C., Rinaldi, A., Petito, A., & Bellomo, A. (2019). Metabolic syndrome in psychotic disorder patients treated with oral and long-acting injected antipsychotics. *Frontiers in Psychiatry*, *9*, 744. https://doi.org/10.3389/fpsyt.2018.00744

Ventriglio, A., Gentile, A., Stella, E., & Bellomo, A. (2015). Metabolic issues in patients affected by schizophrenia: Clinical characteristics and medical management. *Frontiers in Neuroscience*, *9*, 297. https://doi.org/10.3389/fnins.2015.00297

Ventriglio, A., Sancassiani, F., Contu, M. P., Latorre, M., Di Slavatore, M., Fornaro, M., & Bhugra, D. (2020). *Mediterranean diet and its benefits on health and mental health: A literature review. Clinical Practice and Epidemiology in Mental Health: CP & EMH*, *16*(Suppl. 1), 156–164. https://doi.org/10.2174/1745017902016010156

Vermeulen, J. M., Wootton, R. E., Treur, J. L., Sallis, H. M., Jones, H. J., Zammit, S., van den Brink, W., Goodwin, G. M., de Haan, L., & Munafò, M. R. (2021). Smoking and the risk for bipolar disorder: Evidence from a bidirectional Mendelian randomization study. *The British Journal of Psychiatry: The Journal of Mental Science*, *218*(2), 88–94. https://doi.org/10.1192/bjp.2019.202

Wang, J., Mann, F., Lloyd-Evans, B., Ma, R., & Johnson, S. (2018). Associations between loneliness and perceived social support and outcomes of mental health problems: A systematic review. *BMC Psychiatry*, *18*(1), 156. https://doi.org/10.1186/s12888-018-1736-5

Weittenhiller, L. P., Mikhail, M. E., Mote, J., Campellone, T. R., & Kring, A. M. (2021). What gets in the way of social engagement in schizophrenia? *World Journal of Psychiatry*, *11*(1), 13–26. https://doi.org/10.5498/wjp.v11.i1.13

WHO. (2001). Strengthening mental health promotion. Geneva, World Health Organization (Fact sheet, No. 220).

Wijarnpreecha, K., Jaruvongvanich, V., Cheungpasitporn, W., & Ungprasert, P. (2018). Association between celiac disease and schizophrenia: A meta-analysis. *European Journal of Gastroenterology & Hepatology*, *30*(4), 442–446.

Winerman, L. (2017, March). The cost of treatment. *Monitor on Psychology*, *48*(3). www.apa.org/monitor/2017/03/numbers

Xu, Q., Anderson, D., & Courtney, M. (2010). A longitudinal study of the relationship between lifestyle and mental health among midlife and older women in Australia: Findings from Healthy Aging of Women Study. *Health Care for Women International*, *31*(12), 1082–1096. https://doi.org/10.1080/07399332.2010.486096

Ye, J., Shim, R., & Rust, G. (2012). Health care avoidance among people with serious psychological distress: Analyses of 2007 Health Information National Trends Survey. *Journal of Health Care for the Poor and Underserved*, *23*(4), 1620–1629. https://doi.org/10.1353/hpu.2012.0189

Zaman, R., Hankir, A., & Jemni, M. (2019). Lifestyle factors and mental health. *Psychiatria Danubina*, *31*(Suppl. 3), 217–220.

23 Tobacco Products
Risk Reduction and Cessation

Nancy Houston Miller[1] and Karen Laing[2]
[1]Stanford University School of Medicine (Ret)
[2]All Heart Coaching, Inc.
Bon Secours Mercy Health
Cincinnati, Ohio, USA

CONTENTS

KEY POINTS

- Smoking tobacco is the leading cause of preventable death in the United States today.
- Individual, group, and telephone counseling have all been shown to be effective ways to support smokers to quit. Practical counseling, such as problem-solving, skills training, and social support, included in treatment, are especially effective. The use of telephone quitlines is especially useful in reaching diverse populations.
- Success with cessation is increased when numerous healthcare providers offer patients the same message, understand relapses, and follow up with patients throughout the process.
- Whether an individual smokes a traditional cigarette or uses an electronic delivery device, cessation is recommended, and insurance coverage supports these efforts.

23.1 INTRODUCTION

Smoking tobacco is the leading cause of preventable death in the United States today. (NCCDPHP, 2014). In the US, more than 30 million, or 14.1% of Americans, smoke tobacco products (Barua et al., 2018). More than 7 million deaths annually are attributed to tobacco use worldwide (WHO, 2017). Cigarette smoking leads to over 480,000 deaths each year in the US. This includes more than 41,000 deaths due to exposure to secondhand smoke (NCCDPHP, 2014). One-third of all US deaths attributable to smoking are due to cardiovascular disease. Smoking causes endothelial dysfunction, plaque development and destabilization, and imbalances in antithrombotic and prothrombotic factors leading to acute cardiovascular events (Barua et al., 2018).

Smoking tobacco also leads to many different types of diseases and disabilities, harming almost every organ of the body. Currently, over 16 million individuals in the US live with a disease caused by tobacco use. For every person who dies due to smoking-related complications, there are at least 30 living with a serious illness because of smoking (NCCDPHP, 2014). Smoking been shown to cause or increase the risk of cancer, coronary artery disease (CAD), myocardial infarction (MI), stroke, peripheral artery disease (PAD), abdominal aortic aneurysm (AAA), heart failure, atrial and ventricular arrhythmias, lung diseases, diabetes, and chronic obstructive pulmonary diseases (COPD), including emphysema and chronic bronchitis (NCCDPHP, 2014; Barua et al., 2018). It also increases the risk of tuberculosis and, some eye diseases, and causes immune system alterations, such as rheumatoid arthritis. Smoking is also associated with erectile dysfunction (NCCDPHP, 2014). Continued smoking has been shown to increase adverse outcomes following stent placement and coronary artery surgery (Barua et al., 2018). These risks apply to any smoked tobacco product, including hookah tobacco. Smokeless tobacco increases cancer risk, especially cancer of the mouth (NIDA, 2021).

Smoking rates in the United States vary significantly based on geography, race, and sexual orientation. Rates of smoking are highest among those living in the Midwest (22.2%) and the South (22.7%), and lowest in the Northeast (20.1%) and the West (16.3%) (SAMHSA, 2017). The use of cigarettes by U.S adults is also highest in rural areas (28.5%) compared to urban areas (25.1%) (SAMHSA, 2017). Although the rate of smoking among African Americans is only slightly higher (15%) than the overall US population (14%) and they usually start smoking at a later age and smoke fewer cigarettes than White Americans, African Americans are more likely to die of a smoking-related disease (Action on Smoking and Health, 2020). Another disproportionately negatively impacted population who use cigarettes is the lesbian, gay, bisexual, and transgender community. These adults smoke at a rate up to two and a half times higher than straight adults (Action on Smoking and Health, 2020). While tobacco use cessation and risk reduction efforts will be of benefit throughout the US and worldwide, focusing on these higher-risk groups may lead to more significant outcomes.

Tobacco use and the prevalence of nicotine addiction are interlinked. While there are over 4,000 harmful substances found in tobacco products, nicotine is the primary element in tobacco leading to addiction. The main sources of exposure to nicotine are cigarettes and chewing tobacco. Because nicotine readily leads to addiction, it is one of the most difficult substances to give up. Once addicted, individuals use tobacco products regularly to achieve the desired dose of nicotine their body demands. Each person will vary in the intervals between doses and amount of tobacco used. Nicotine is also used as a pharmacologic aide to smoking cessation (Widysanto et al., 2021).

The most severe health effects of tobacco come from chemicals other than nicotine (NIDA, 2021). While, in some ways, nicotine is much more benign than other elements of tobacco, because it is the addictive agent, it is not without risk. When inhaled, tobacco smoke rapidly passes through the pulmonary circulation and enters the bloodstream. Nicotine then easily crosses the blood–brain barrier and enters the brain tissue. This whole process is estimated to take only 2–8 seconds (Widysanto et al., 2021). Newer versions of e-cigarettes use nicotine salts that may be absorbed more quickly, possibly increasing addiction potential (NIDA, 2021). The half-life of nicotine is estimated to be approximately two hours. With repeated exposure, tolerance develops to some of the physiologic effects of nicotine (Widysanto et al., 2021). Each time it is used, nicotine immediately stimulates the adrenal glands to release epinephrine (NIDA, 2021). This then stimulates the sympathetic nervous system, causing an increase in heart rate and cardiac contractility, constricting cutaneous and coronary blood vessels, and leading to a rise in blood pressure (Widysanto et al., 2021).

Nicotine activates the brain's reward circuits, similar to cocaine or heroin, and increases dopamine levels, thus reinforcing this rewarding behavior (NIDA, 2021). It also produces stimulation and decreased feelings of stress and anxiety (Widysanto et al., 2021). Other chemicals in tobacco smoke, such as acetaldehyde, may enhance nicotine's effects on the brain (NIDA, 2021). Tobacco users adjust their intake to experience feelings of arousal and to control their mood throughout the day. Nicotine has been shown to increase concentration, reaction time, and performance in some areas. However, when tobacco use is stopped or is not possible, the individual will experience withdrawal symptoms. These may include irritability, depression, anxiety, increased appetite, and sleeplessness (Widysanto et al., 2021).

23.2 HELPING PATIENTS TO QUIT SMOKING

23.2.1 GUIDELINE RECOMMENDATIONS FOR SUCCESS WITH CESSATION

The guidelines for treating tobacco use and cessation emphasize that tobacco dependence is a chronic disease. Many patients will make multiple attempts to quit and require repeat interventions. Encouragingly, though, the data also support that these interventions can significantly increase long-term quit rates. A key guideline recommendation is that every clinician must consistently identify, document, and treat every tobacco user. Every patient willing to make a quit attempt should be encouraged to use the counseling interventions and medications recommended by the Tobacco Use and Dependence Guideline Panel (2008). (Ref) Many resources exist for information regarding tobacco cessation and medication use. This chapter will focus on the counseling and lifestyle interventions available to the patient and nurse. Even brief tobacco dependence treatment has been shown to be effective and is recommended by the guideline. Individual, group, and telephone counseling have all been shown to be effective ways to support smokers to quit. Practical counseling, such as problem-solving, skills training, and social support, included in treatment, are especially effective. The use of telephone quitlines is especially useful in reaching diverse populations. When a tobacco user is unwilling to make a quit attempt, clinicians should use motivational interventions to increase the possibility and effectiveness of any future quit attempt (Tobacco Use and Dependence Guideline Panel, 2008).

Helping smokers is especially effective within the healthcare system. Seventy percent of smokers see a physician annually. Of those, 70% want to quit, and two-thirds who relapse want to quit again within 30 days. Smokers cite physician advice to quit as an important motivator. Current smokers, those unwilling to quit, and former smokers who recently quit all benefit from brief interventions lasting three minutes or less. Patients are more satisfied if offered smoking interventions, even if they are not ready to quit (Tobacco Use and Dependence Guideline Panel, 2008).

The United States Preventive Services Task Force (USPSTF) gives an A grade to the recommendation that all clinicians ask all pregnant and nonpregnant adults about tobacco use, advise them to stop using tobacco, and provide behavioral interventions for cessation to all persons who use tobacco. US Food and Drug Administration (FDA) approved pharmacotherapy is also part of the recommendation for all adults including nonpregnant women (USPSTF, 2021).

23.2.2 INTERVENTIONS BY NURSES AT EVERY VISIT

23.2.2.1 Strong Personal Advice by Numerous Healthcare Providers

Success with cessation is increased when numerous healthcare providers offer the same message to individuals to quit smoking. Strong credible messages by healthcare professionals increase self-efficacy to quit and should be tailored to the healthcare condition(s) that a patient is encountering (Guideline 2008).

This positive impact of patient smoking cessation counseling in the clinical practice setting can be increased when undertaken by multiple healthcare clinicians (odds ratio [O.R.] 2.5). High-intensity counseling lasting greater than 10 minutes per session for a total time of more than 30 minutes also increases the O.R. to 2.3. The addition of 4–8 follow-up sessions, whether face-to-face or by telephone, increases the O.R. to 1.9–2.3. Finally, when at least 3–4 multiple formats are used, such as self-help materials, individual counseling, and telephone follow-up, the odds ratio of cessation increases to 2.5 (Tobacco Use and Dependence Guideline Panel, 2008).

23.2.2.2 Additional Counseling to Support Individuals

The Agency for Healthcare Research and Quality recommends using the 5As in tobacco cessation counseling.

1. **Ask: Identify tobacco use and document for every patient.** An office-wide system should be implemented to ensure that every patient's tobacco use status is queried and documented at every visit.
2. **Advise: Use a clear, strong, and personalized manner when advising quitting.** Be clear. Make statements such as, "there is no safe level of smoking" or "occasional and light smoking is still dangerous." Be strong. Use words such as, "this is the most important thing you can do for your long-term health." Personalize the message by including the potential impact on any disease or discomfort the patient may be experiencing, such as asthma or shortness of breath.
3. **Assess: Is the tobacco user ready and willing to make a quit attempt?** If they are willing, provide assistance and if needed refer them to an intensive smoking cessation program. Keep a list of available resources for smoking cessation, both locally and on the national level. If they are unwilling to quit, provide motivational interviewing to increase future quit attempts.
4. **Assist: Provide counseling or pharmacotherapy for those ready to make a quit attempt.** Help the patient develop a quit plan. Recommend the patient discuss medication options with their healthcare provider. Set a quit date with the patient normally within one week of the visit or encounter. Encourage the patient to tell family and friends about the quit attempt. Discuss past quit experiences and encourage the patient to remove tobacco from the environment. Anticipate triggers or challenges such as alcohol, other smokers in the home or at work, withdrawal symptoms, high-risk times such as parties, and stress. Connect the patient with resources for further support, such as the national quitline network (1-800-QUIT-NOW), state or local health department, or other available quit resources (AHRQ, 2012).
5. **Arrange: Schedule follow-up, preferably one week following a quit attempt.**

The use of motivational interviewing has been shown to increase future quit attempts for those not ready to quit. Motivational interviewing allows the nurse to express empathy, develop discrepancy, roll with resistance, and support self-efficacy. The nurse can express empathy by exploring through the use of open-ended questions and, through reflective listening, can gain a shared understanding. The expression of empathy allows the patient to normalize their feelings and concerns while supporting the patient's autonomy and right to choose or reject the change. Through motivational interviewing, the nurse can highlight the discrepancy between the patient's values, goals, priorities, and present behavior. This discussion allows the nurse to reinforce and support "change talk" and "commitment language" while building and deepening a commitment to change. The nurse may back off and use reflection when the patient expresses resistance, express empathy, and then ask permission to provide information. The nurse may also support the patient's self-efficacy by identifying and building on past successes. Options may be offered for small achievable steps toward change, such as calling the quitline, reading the handouts, or changing current smoking patterns (USDHHS, 2008).

There are 5Rs of motivational interviewing.

1. **Relevance: Personalize why quitting is relevant.** Ask the patient to identify the negative consequences of smoking. Example: "I understand you aren't ready to quit now, Mrs. Jones but are there any reasons as to why you might want to consider quitting in the future?" The nurse may highlight those that are pertinent to the patient.

2. **Risks: Identify the negative consequences of tobacco use.** Ask the patient to identify potential negative consequences of tobacco use. For Example: "Can you think of any harmful effects if you continue to smoke regularly?" These risks may be acute, such as shortness of breath, asthma exacerbations, or respiratory infections, long-term, such as MI, lung cancers, or COPD, or environmental risks of secondhand smoke to spouses or children.

3. **Rewards: Identify the benefits of stopping smoking.** Ask the patient to identify those benefits. Example: "It sounds like you may have some concerns about the health problems you may face in the future if you continue to smoke. Have you thought of any other benefits if you stop smoking?" The nurse can highlight those that are most relevant to the patient, such as improved health, sense of smell, feeling physically better, saving money, or food that tastes better.

4. **Roadblocks: Identify the barriers to quitting.** Ask the patient to identify the obstacles. Example: "It appears that giving up smoking might be important to you as you want to be around to see your granddaughter go to college. Can you tell me about the real barriers for you now as you think about giving up smoking?" Frequent roadblocks include withdrawal symptoms, fear of failure, weight gain, change of relationships, lack of support, depression, enjoyment of tobacco, limited knowledge on effective treatment options, and being around others who smoke.

5. **Repetition: Repeat this at every visit if the patient is unmotivated.** Encourage patients who have failed attempts that most people must try multiple times before succeeding. (USDHHS, 2008)

Tobacco use cessation occurs over time and frequently includes intermittent lapses. Any attempt to cease an addictive behavior will often end in relapse (Kirchner et al., 2012). A study by Zhou and colleagues (2009) attempted to identify the predictors of relapse in 2,431 smokers from five countries. Those included in the study were smoking five or more cigarettes each day, 35–65 years of age, and followed every three months for 18 months. Items measured in the study included motivation to quit, previous quitting history, smoking dependence, nicotine cues, weight concerns and confidence, chronic conditions, smoking aids, withdrawal, and mood disturbances. The following factors were identified as being associated with relapse: Failed attempt prior to baseline (O.R. 1.61), higher baseline dependence (O.R. 1.16), other smokers in the environment (O.R. 1.38), use of smoking cessation medications (O.R. 0.63), sleep disturbance (O.R. 1.92), mood disturbance (O.R. 1.51), and anxiety/depression (O.R. 1.42; Zhou et al., 2009).

Because lapses to the old behavior of smoking are common, relapse prevention (RP) is an essential component of smoking cessation treatment. One influential model developed by Marlatt and Gordon in 1985 has been widely used with addictive behaviors such as alcohol use and smoking cessation. This model considers what occurs before relapse and the interventions that may be taken to prevent or limit relapse after treatment (Larimer et al., 1999). According to this relapse prevention model (RPM), the primary importance in determining whether a patient who has lapsed will continue toward relapse or cessation is that person's cognitive and emotional responses to the lapse event (Kirchner et al. 2012). The model also suggests that high-risk situations, coping skills, outcome expectations, the abstinence violation effect (AVE), lifestyle factors, urges, and cravings can all contribute to relapse. The AVE focuses on the patient's emotional response to the initial lapse. If the patient attributes the lapse to a personal failure, they are more likely to have feelings of guilt and negative emotions that can lead to further use of the addictive substance, in this case, nicotine, to escape feelings of guilt or failure (Larimer et al., 1999).

The highest relapse rates to return to smoking are associated with negative emotional states such as anger, anxiety, depression, frustration, and boredom. Situations that involve interpersonal conflict such as marital or work-related conflicts can also result in negative emotions and thus lead to relapse. Not all risk-states are negative. Celebrations and other positive emotional states can also precipitate relapse (Larimer et al., 1999).

Although these high-risk situations are considered the lapse trigger, the patient's response to the situation determines whether total relapse will occur. A person with effective coping strategies, such as leaving a high-risk situation or positive self-talk, is less likely to relapse than those lacking these skills. Also, once someone has successfully coped with a high-risk situation, they may experience an increased sense of self-efficacy, a feeling they have mastery over this specific situation (Larimer et al., 1999). Patients can readily tell you their high-risk situations if asked to identify them.

The lifestyle factors identified by Marlatt and Gordon as a supportive intervention involve the balance in the person's life between what they perceive they "should" be doing and fulfilling enjoyable activities. If the individual lives in a constant state of stress due to external demands, negative emotional states may be generated, creating a high-risk situation. Also, the person's desire for pleasure may lead them to feel that an indulgence is justified (Larimer et al., 1999).

The nurse should assist the patient in the identification of high-risk situations. This may include self-monitoring: Recording daily cigarette use, including time of day, description of the situation, and mood rating for 1–2 weeks prior to quitting. This may also consist of a discussion of anticipated actions in high-risk scenarios, or relapse fantasies where the patient will imagine a high-risk situation. The nurse may also provide the patient with a standard 14–28 item self-efficacy rating assessment scale, asking them to rate their ability to withstand the high-risk situations common in smoking cessation (Marlatt & Gordon, 1983).

The patient may also be supported with skills training that includes a problem-solving approach, practice session (behavioral rehearsal, coaching, and feedback), or relapse rehearsal in order to prevent relapse. Relaxation training can be used, including progressive muscle relaxation, meditation, and stress management. Education may be provided regarding the problem of feeling a need for immediate gratification. This can include a discussion of the risks associated with an unbalanced lifestyle mentioned above. It may also include the use of Marlatt and Gordon's decision matrix, which considers the immediate and delayed consequences of remaining abstinent versus resuming substance use (Marlatt & Gordon, 1983).

Another RP intervention strategy may include teaching global self-control strategies. This may involve education regarding the importance of maintaining a balanced daily lifestyle, the "shoulds" versus "wants" mentioned previously. It may also involve the development of positive addictions such as jogging or meditation. The nurse may teach the patient coping imagery and stimulus control techniques (Marlatt & Gordon, 1983).

Finally, the patient should be helped by allowing them to recognize that a lapse is often normal in the process of cessation but to treat this as a lapse rather than a way to resume smoking. This involves focusing on the situation that caused them to lapse, developing both cognitive and behavioral strategies for overcoming the situation should it reoccur, and getting back on track by simply considering the lapse as a slip along the way to cessation.

By increasing our understanding of the relapse process, we may positively impact clinical outcomes. Seen through the lens of RPM, each lapse provides an opportunity to strengthen coping resources and reconfirm commitment to change. Rather than avoiding all negative reactions to lapses, nurses can best serve our patients by encouraging realistic self-evaluation to avoid relapse and get lapsed smokers back on the path to total cessation (Kirchner et al., 2012).

23.2.2.3   Follow-Up

As noted in the Tobacco Use and Treatment Guidelines, follow-up with patients following cessation is important to their overall success with quitting. Nurses have been highly successful in offering support to patients especially in hospital and clinic settings. A Cochrane review of 50 trials from 1990 to 2011 from 13 countries included randomized controlled trials (RCT) and quasi-RCTs involving intensive interventions for smoking cessation in hospitalized patients and one month following discharge. These studies included advice, behavioral therapy, or pharmacotherapy with or without contact after hospital discharge. Advice to quit or behavioral counseling was provided in all 50 studies. Forty-eight of the studies used a nurse or counselor for smoking advice. Forty-two of the studies used follow-up support. Twenty-nine used telephone support ranging from one to 12 months. Thirty-seven studies assessed abstinence at 12 months. Results showed that intensive inpatient intervention with a one-month follow-up increased smoking cessation rates (O.R. 1.37; Rigotti et al., 2012).

In another RCT of 371 hospitalized smokers from the Massachusetts General Hospital, all patients received in-hospital smoking cessation. Those in the treatment arm received sustained care, free medication, and five automated interactive voice recognition (AVR) calls at 2, 14, 30, 60, and 90 days post-hospitalization. Patients in the usual care arm of the study were given a free telephone quitline. The amount of time spent on in-hospital tobacco cessation counseling was equal between the two groups, with a mean time of 25 minutes. Post-discharge medications did not differ between the two groups. The sustained group received four of their five calls via an automated voice recognition (AVR) system. Of the sustained patients, 61% completed at least eight weeks of medical treatment compared to 37% of the standard group. Biochemical confirmation of smoking cessation at six months was 26% in the treatment group versus 15% in those who received standard care (Rigotti et al., 2014).

The effect of telephone support interventions on patient outcomes during cardiac rehabilitation was also evaluated in a Cochrane review of 26 RCTs comparing telephone intervention with standard post-discharge care of patients who had experienced an MI or revascularization. Results showed that telephone versus standard care resulted in fewer hospitalizations (O.R. 0.62) and higher smoking cessation rates (O.R. 1.32). In addition, lower systolic blood pressure and depression/anxiety scores were found through telephone support (Kotb et al., 2014).

Key points for providing smoking interventions to patients:

- Confirm smoking status by asking the appropriate questions.
- Offer strong advice about the need to quit and determine willingness.
- For those willing to quit, take a short smoking history, identify high-risk situations through the use of a self-efficacy scale, and review with the patient.
- Provide the patient with the 1-800 quitline and offer smoking cessation program participation through a hospital- or community-based program; offer self-help materials.
- Make a referral with a tobacco cessation expert if needed.

23.3   OTHER ISSUES RELATED TO TOBACCO USE

23.3.1   OTHER TOBACCO PRODUCTS: ELECTRONIC CIGARETTES AND RISK

E-cigarette use was introduced in the United States in 2007 with and without regulation. By 2014, there were more than 460 brands and over 7,000 flavors. The original e-cigarette devices delivered much less nicotine than a traditional cigarette. The rate of absorption initially was rapid but slower than cigarette smoke. More recent devices have produced an acceleration of heart rate similar to smoking cigarettes with variable effects on blood pressure (Benowitz & Burbank, 2016). Currently, there are multiple ways to deliver and receive nicotine electronically. These include e-cigarettes, vapes, e-hookahs, vape pens, hookah pens, and mods that are customizable and more powerful vaporizers. Compounds in e-cigarette vapors are largely untested but may cause pulmonary injury and chronic inflammation, increasing cardiovascular disease risk (Benowitz & Burbank, 2016).

In May 2016, the US Food and Drug Administration (FDA) included all tobacco products (including e-cigarettes, liquid solutions, cigars, hookah tobacco, and pipe tobacco) in national tobacco regulations. This included restricting the sale of these to minors. In December 2019, the US federal government raised the legal minimum age of sale of tobacco products from 18 to 21 years (NIDA, 2021). Finally, in January 2020, the FDA issued a policy on the sale of flavored vaping cartridges prioritizing enforcement against unauthorized flavored e-cigarette products that appeal to kids, including fruit and mint flavors (USDHHS, 2020).

In 2018, there were 4.9 million youth e-tobacco product users. This total had grown by 1.5 million current youth e-cigarette users in 2018 compared to 2017. The use of any tobacco product by high school students also rose by 38.3% over that same time period, with e-cigarette usage being most responsible for this increase. There was no change found in the use of other tobacco products by this population during this time. Products are now currently being marketed to assist young people in concealing their e-cigarette use, including working pens with vape capability, hoodies with vaping "drawstring," and backpacks built for use with vaping devices (CDC, 2019).

One of the risks associated with the use of electronic nicotine delivery devices is e-cigarette or vaping-associated lung injury or EVALI. As of February 18, 2020, there have been a total of 2,807 hospitalized EVALI cases or deaths across all 50 states, the District of Columbia, and the two US territories of Puerto Rico and the US Virgin Islands. Sixty-eight EVALI-associated deaths have been confirmed. Vitamin E acetate, an additive in some tetrahydrocannabinol (THC)-containing e-cigarettes or vaping products, has also been strongly linked to the outbreak of EVALI (CDC, 2020).

23.3.2 COVERAGE FOR TOBACCO CESSATION

Whether an individual smokes a traditional cigarette or uses an electronic delivery device, cessation is recommended, and insurance coverage supports these efforts. In all 50 states and the District of Columbia, at least some cessation treatments are covered for all Medicaid enrollees. Thirty-three states cover individual counseling, and 10 cover group counseling. Medicare covers four cessation counseling sessions for one attempt to quit, and eight counseling sessions (two quit attempts) are covered every 12 months. Medicare coverage is available for outpatient and hospitalized beneficiaries who use tobacco, whether or not the person has symptoms of tobacco-related illnesses. Medicare counseling sessions can be intermediate (3–10 minutes) or intensive (more than 10 minutes). Over-the-counter treatments are not covered. Most private insurers provide coverage for one or more behavioral interventions (DiGiulio et al., 2020).

23.3.3 NEW RESEARCH RELATED TO TOBACCO USE

While much research has been conducted over the past 50 years with regard to smoking cessation, there remain many opportunities in the field of tobacco use and cessation. The educational methods used may change as new delivery devices are developed and information uncovered regarding how to support specific patient populations in their quit attempts most effectively. Staying abreast of current research ensures awareness of new opportunities and the possible need to offer new interventions to smokers.

Lung cancer screening (LCS) with low-dose computed tomography (LDCT) has been shown to reduce lung cancer mortality. Unfortunately, few individuals eligible for LCS take advantage of this screening opportunity. In a recent study, Raz et al. (2020) showed it is possible to train tobacco cessation educators to include information regarding LCS in their classes. In this study, the information provided was well received and understood by most surveyed smokers. Future research may focus on whether this leads to increased use of the service and, if so, whether that may decrease lung cancer mortality rates by encouraging smokers to quit.

Getting smokers to participate in cessation programs can be a challenge. A recent study done by Moses et al. (2020) evaluated the impact of offering an incentive to employees who took part in a workplace smoking cessation program. When this program was previously offered to employees, participation was voluntary and free, but no incentive was offered. Estimated participation was less than 5%. In this study, participants were offered the incentive of enrollment in an employer-provided health plan that had a 50% lower employee monthly contribution and co-payment than that offered to non-participants. This study experienced a high rate of participation at 72.7%. These findings suggest that using a reward-based incentive can result in smoking cessation program participation rates much higher than the US norms. Further studies could offer other incentives to individuals participating in Medicare or Medicaid programs.

Without significant intervention, long-term smoking success rates remain low. A recent study by Enyoiha et al. (2019) examined the connection between the willingness of adult tobacco cigarette smokers to try different cessation methods depending on their sociodemographics and daily tobacco use. Results showed that non-White participants were more likely to be willing to try counseling, while those with a high school education or less were less likely to be ready to do so. Lower-income participants were less inclined to attempt medication or any counseling. Those who were highly likely to try any evidence-based method were those with high nicotine dependence or a history of quit attempts. Considering a patient's sociodemographics and nicotine dependence level may increase the possibility of success when counseling patients on smoking cessation. Additionally, increased education on evidence-based strategies for smokers attempting to quit can be beneficial and are likely to increase cessation within this population.

There has been much discussion about the possible use of e-cigarettes and tobacco smoking cessation. In a recent study by Kasza and colleagues (2021), 1600 US adult cigarette smokers who were initially smoking daily and had no plans to quit smoking were followed for two years. In this study population, only 6.2% of those who were smoking cigarettes daily at the time of initial evaluation and had no plans to ever quit smoking completely were not smoking cigarettes at the final follow-up. The likelihood of quitting cigarette use was significantly higher (28.0%) among those who were using e-cigarettes daily at the time of the initial evaluation. This study further supports the need for evaluation of the risk–benefit possibilities of e-cigarette use with cigarette smokers who may otherwise not be willing to participate in traditional smoking cessation methods or programs.

23.4 CONCLUSION

Tobacco is the leading preventable cause of death and disability worldwide. Tobacco cessation guidelines indicate that multiple healthcare providers offering advice and behavioral counseling of at least 10 minutes with educational materials in multiple formats increases cessation. Identifying smokers, offering strong advice, and referring to community-based smoking cessation programs will increase the likelihood patients will succeed in quitting smoking.

23.5 RESOURCES

US Department of Health and Human Services
1-800 Quit Now (1-800 784-8669)
Free quit coaching, quit plan, free educational materials, and referral to local resources
BeTobaccoFree.gov
Tobacco prevention and cessation opportunities

National Cancer Institute and National Institutes of Health
Smokefree.gov
Smoke-free treatment and text messaging, apps, and build a quit plan

Centers for Disease Control and Prevention
CDC.gov/tobacco/quit_smoking
Quit smoking
A quit guide and tips from former smokers about how to quit

US Dept. of Defense
ycq2.org
YouCanQuit2
A plan for help US military members quit tobacco use

American Lung Association
lung.org/quit-smoking
Freedom from smoking—a guide to quitting, online support groups, group clinics, and success
stories

American Heart Association
heart.org/en/healthy-living/healthy-lifestyle/quit-smoking-tobacco/help-i-want-to-quit-smoking
Help! I want to quit smoking now—online resources in multiple languages to help individuals
quit smoking

REFERENCES

Action on Smoking and Health. (2020). Tobacco control in the United States: Failure to protect the right to
    health. *Tobacco Prevention & Cessation*, *6*, 34.
Agency for Healthcare Research and Quality. (2012, December). *Five major steps to intervention (The "5
    A's")*. www.ahrq.gov/prevention/guidelines/tobacco/5steps.html
Barua, R. S., Rigotti, N. A., Benowitz, N. L., Cummings, K. M., Jazayeri, M. A., Morris, P. B., Ratchford, E.
    V., Sarna, L., Stecker, E. C., & Wiggins, B. S. (2018). 2018 ACC expert consensus decision pathway
    on tobacco cessation treatment: A report of the American College of Cardiology Task Force on clin-
    ical expert consensus documents. *Journal of the American College of Cardiology*, *72*(25), 3332–3365.
    https://doi-org.ezproxy.hsc.usf.edu/10.1016/j.jacc.2018.10.027
Benowitz, N. L., & Burbank, A. D. (2016). Cardiovascular toxicity of nicotine: Implications for electronic
    cigarette use. *Trends in Cardiovascular Medicine*, *26*(6), 515–523. https://doi-org.ezproxy.hsc.usf.edu/
    10.1016/j.tcm.2016.03.001
Centers for Disease Control and Prevention. (2020, February 25). *Outbreak of lung injury associated with
    the use of e-cigarette, or vaping, products*. Retrieved December 24, 2021 from www.cdc.gov/tobacco/
    basic_information/e-cigarettes/severe-lung-disease.html
Centers for Disease Prevention and Control. (2019, February). *Vitalsigns*. www.cdc.gov/vitalsigns/youth-toba
    cco-use/index.html
DiGiulio, A., Jump, Z., Babb, S., Schecter, A., Williams, K-A. S., Yembra, D., Armour, B. S. (2020). State
    Medicaid coverage for tobacco cessation treatments and barriers to accessing treatments—United
    States, 2008–2018. *MMWR Morbidity and Mortality Weekly Report*, *69*(6), 155–160. http://dx.doi.org/
    10.15585/mmwr.mm6906a2
Enyioha, C., Meernik, C., Ranney, L, Goldstein, A., Sellman, K., & Kistler, C. (2019). Willingness-to-try
    various tobacco cessation methods among US adult cigarette smokers. *Tobacco Prevention & Cessation*,
    5(18). https://doi.org/10.18332/tpc/108555
Kasza, K. A., Edwards, K. C., Kimmel, H. L., Anesetti-Rothermel, A., Cummings, K. M., Niaura, R. S., Sharma,
    A., Ellis, E. M., Jackson, R., Blanco, C., Silveira, M. L., Hatsukami, D. K., & Hyland, A. (2021).
    Association of e-cigarette use with discontinuation of cigarette smoking among adult smokers who were
    initially never planning to quit. *JAMA Network Open*, *4*(12), e2140880. https://doi.org/10.1001/jama
    networkopen.2021.40880
Kirchner, T. R., Shiffman, S., & Wileyto, E. P. (2012). Relapse dynamics during smoking cessation: recurrent
    abstinence violation effects and lapse-relapse progression. *Journal of Abnormal Psychology*, *121*(1),
    187–197. https://doi-org.ezproxy.hsc.usf.edu/10.1037/a0024451

Kotb, A., Hsieh, S., & Wells, G. A. (2014). The effect of telephone support interventions on coronary artery disease (CAD) patient outcomes during cardiac rehabilitation: a systematic review and meta-analysis. *PLoS One, 9*(5), e96581. https://doi.org/10.1371/journal.pone.0096581

Larimer, M. E., Palmer, R. S., & Marlatt, G. A. (1999). Relapse prevention. An overview of Marlatt's cognitive-behavioral model. *Alcohol Research & Health: The Journal of the National Institute on Alcohol Abuse and Alcoholism, 23*(2), 151–160.

Marlatt, F. A., & Gordon, J. R. (1983). Relapse prevention: A self-control strategy for the maintenance of behavior change. In R. B. Stuart (Ed.), *Adherence, compliance and generalization in behavioral medicine*. New York.

Moses, O., Rea, B., Medina, E., Estevez, D., Gaio, J., Hubbard, M., Morton, K., & Singh, P. N. (2020). Participation in a workplace smoking cessation program incentivized by lowering the cost of health care coverage: Findings from the LLUH BREATHE cohort. *Tobacco Prevention & Cessation, 6*, 23. https://doi-org.ezproxy.hsc.usf.edu/10.18332/tpc/118237

National Center for Chronic Disease Prevention and Health Promotion (US) Office on Smoking and Health (NCCDPHP). (2014). *The health consequences of smoking—50 years of progress: A report of the surgeon general*. Centers for Disease Control and Prevention (US).

National Institute on Drug Abuse (NIDA). (2021, April 6). *Cigarettes and other tobacco products drug facts*. Retrieved December 22, 2021, from www.drugabuse.gov/publications/drugfacts/cigarettes-other-tobacco-products

Raz, D. J., Ismail, M. H., Sun, V., Park, S., Alem, A. C., Haupt, E. C., & Gould, M. K. (2020). Incorporating lung cancer screening education into tobacco cessation group counseling. *Tobacco Prevention & Cessation, 6*, 12. https://doi-org.ezproxy.hsc.usf.edu/10.18332/tpc/115166

Rigotti, N. A., Clair, C., Munafò, M. R., & Stead, L. F. (2012). Interventions for smoking cessation in hospitalised patients. *The Cochrane Database of Systematic Reviews, 5*(5), CD001837. https://doi-org.ezproxy.hsc.usf.edu/10.1002/14651858.CD001837.pub3

Rigotti, N. A., Regan, S., Levy, D. E., Japuntich, S., Chang, Y., Park, E. R., Viana, J. C., Kelley, J. H., Reyen, M., & Singer, D. E. (2014). Sustained care intervention and postdischarge smoking cessation among hospitalized adults: a randomized clinical trial. *JAMA, 312*(7), 719–728. https://doi-org.ezproxy.hsc.usf.edu/10.1001/jama.2014.9237

Substance Abuse and Mental Health Services Administration (SAMHSA). (2017). Results from the 2016 National Survey on Drug Use and Health: Detailed tables. Substance Abuse and Mental Health Services Administration, Center for Behavioral Health Statistics and Quality.

Tobacco Use and Dependence Guideline Panel. (2008, May). *Treating tobacco use and dependence*. United States Department of Health and Human Services (USDHHS). www.ncbi.nlm.nih.gov/books/NBK63952/

United States Department of Health and Human Services (USDHHS). (n.d.). *Adolescents and tobacco: Trends*. Retrieved February, 2020 from www.hhs.gov/ash/oah/adolescent-development/substance-use/drugs/tobacco/trends/index.html

United States Preventive Services Task Force (USPSTF). (2021, January 19). *Tobacco smoking cessation in adults, including pregnant persons: Interventions*. www.uspreventiveservicestaskforce.org/uspstf/recommendation/tobacco-use-in-adults-and-pregnant-women-counseling-and-interventions

Widysanto, A., Combest, F. E., Dhakal, A., & Saadabadi, A. (2021). Nicotine addiction. In StatPearls [Internet]. StatPearls Publishing. Retrieved from www.ncbi.nlm.nih.gov/books/NBK499915/

World Health Organization. (2017). WHO report on the global tobacco epidemic. World Health Organization.

Zhou, X., Nonnemaker, J., Sherrill, B., Gilsenan, A. W., Coste, F., & West, R. (2009). Attempts to quit smoking and relapse: Factors associated with success or failure from the ATTEMPT cohort study. *Addictive Behaviors, 34*(4), 365–373. https://doi-org.ezproxy.hsc.usf.edu/10.1016/j.addbeh.2008.11.013

Part IV

Maintaining Health Through Lifestyle Medicine

24 How Often Do You Think About Oral Health as an Essential Part of Wellness and a Healthy Lifestyle?

Judith Haber[1], Erin Hartnett[1], and Jessamin Cipollina[1]
[1]Rory Meyers College of Nursing
New York University
New York, New York, USA

CONTENTS

KEY POINTS

- A healthy lifestyle includes good oral health; oral health plays a pivotal role in advancing positive overall health outcomes.
- Promoting oral health and preventing oral disease is a national population health issue that disproportionally impacts vulnerable populations affected by the social determinants of health.
- The nursing profession is well equipped to integrate oral health assessment, diagnosis, and management as a best wellness and healthy lifestyle practice with patients across the lifespan.

24.1 INTRODUCTION

There is increasing recognition about the important contribution of oral health to overall health. In fact, there are many who say there is no health without oral health (Health Resources and Services Administration [HRSA], 2014; Healthy People 2030, 2020; Hummel et al., 2015; Institute of Medicine [IOM], 2011a; IOM, 2011b; US Department of Health and Human Services [HHS], 2000; Peres et al., 2019; HHS Oral Health Coordinating Committee, 2016; Watt et al., 2019)! Findings from recent

DOI: 10.1201/9781003178330-28

research studies confirm the important relationship between oral health and overall health (American Public Health Association [APHA], 2020; Atchison et al., 2018; Bao et al, 2020; Bissonnette et al., 2020; Cox et al., 2020; Gerontological Society of America [GSA], 2020; Hartnett, 2015; Italiano et al., 2021; Lamster et al., 2021; Lau et al., 2021; MacNeil et al., 2020; Munro & Baker, 2018; Sun et al., 2017). Hundreds of medications and diseases have an impact on the oral cavity, and conversely, poor oral hygiene has a significant negative effect on the body and accelerates pathophysiological changes related to acute and chronic health conditions like diabetes (Lamster et al., 2021; Lau et al., 2021), infections like HPV and COVID-19 (Bao et al., 2020; Cox et al., 2020; Sun et al., 2017), respiratory conditions like pneumonia (Munro & Baker, 2018), and cancer (Bissonnette et al., 2020; Hartnett, 2015). Yet, we see a dearth of nurses, colleagues, and patients considering the role oral health plays in promoting wellness and a healthy lifestyle, thereby promoting health and preventing disease.

Poor oral health is prevalent and has negative outcomes across the lifespan. In the United States, 14% of children have untreated caries (cavities); the prevalence among Hispanic and Black children is double (Dye et al., 2015). Poor oral health in children is reported to be related to school problems and low self-esteem (Long, 2012). Periodontal disease is associated with pregnancy-related complications, poor glycemic control in diabetes, pneumonia, and tooth loss in adults and older adults, thereby affecting mortality (Gil-Montoya et al., 2015; Puertas et al., 2018).

Oral health is one of the top ten health topics in Healthy People 2030 with specific 10-year oral health objectives (Healthy People 2030, 2020). Other national organizations, the Institute of Medicine (IOM) (2011a, 2011b), Health Services Resource Administration (HRSA) (2014), the National Interprofessional Initiative on Oral Health (NIIOH) (2017), American Academy of Pediatric Dentistry (AAPD) (Mitchell-Royston et al., 2014), Oral Health Nursing Education and Practice program (OHNEP) (Haber et al., 2019; Haber et al., 2017; Haber et al., 2020a; Haber et al., 2015; Haber & Hartnett, 2019), and the Santa Fe Group (SFG) (Garcia et al., 2010) have been catalysts in advancing the need for an interprofessional approach to promoting oral health and its links to overall health and oral health training for non-dental providers. The OHNEP program located at New York University's Rory Meyers College of Nursing has proposed replacing the traditional HEENT (head, ears, eyes, nose, and throat) exam with the HEENOT (adding to this exam teeth, gums, mucosa, tongue, and palate) to address oral-systemic health issues (Haber et al., 2015).

While most people have regular contact with a primary care provider, that is, a physician, nurse, nurse practitioner, midwife, or physician assistant, only half of US adults visits the dentist annually (Yarbrough et al., 2014). In fact, that percentage is decreasing, a decline that is greater among communities disproportionately affected by the social determinants of health (Dye et al., 2015; Northridge et al., 2020; Watt et al., 2019). The impact of the COVID-19 pandemic and closure of dental offices for four months, closure of school-based dental programs as well as related anxieties about social distancing and aerosol exposure, has exacerbated the delay and/or decline in obtaining regular appointments for dental health promotion (Benzian et al., 2021). Moreover, a significant number of families have lost health insurance coverage and cannot afford the out-of-pocket dental costs (Dave et al., 2020). With fewer people visiting the dentist, there is more emphasis on the role of other health providers addressing oral health screening, risk assessment, and management within scope of practice including, but not limited to, improving oral health literacy, promoting effective oral hygiene, administering fluoride varnish and HPV vaccinations, conducting smoking cessation groups, managing glycemic control to prevent periodontal disease, and treating xerostomia.

24.1.1 The Oral Microbiome in Health and Disease

The mouth is home to an abundance of microbes. In fact, more than 700 species of bacteria colonize on the hard surfaces of the teeth and the soft tissues of the oral mucosa. There is a complex equilibrium between bacteria responsible for maintaining a healthy oral cavity (mouth, teeth, gums, oral mucosa, tongue, and palate) and bacteria that cause infection and/or inflammation not only in the mouth, but that travel to other parts of the body (Northridge et al., 2020). In health, most of the bacteria have a symbiotic relationship with the host (the mouth). Those bacteria that potentially cause infections or inflammation have been found at low levels in healthy mouths. In diseases of the oral cavity, such as dental caries, periodontal disease, and cancer, there is an increase in the numbers and proportions of bacteria that then become harmful. Across the lifespan, bacterial alterations to this delicate balance occur in the mouth. In particular, early childhood (Hartnett et al., 2015), puberty (Northridge et al., 2020), pregnancy (Hartnett et al., 2016), and old age (GSA, 2020) increase the risk for bacteria to cause conditions like caries (cavities), gingivitis, and periodontal disease.

24.1.2   ETIOLOGY OF TOOTH DECAY

Tooth decay is the breakdown of teeth due to bacteria producing acids from foods or debris. Microbes, like *Streptococcus mutans*, attach to the tooth surface and create a coating of bacteria called a biofilm. As the biofilm grows, it creates an anerobic cariogenic environment from the oxygen being used up. When the normal processes of demineralization and regrowth occur, the bacteria can invade the enamel and dentin of the tooth and cause decay such as cavities, especially when the demineralization rate is faster than the remineralization rate. Another factor contributing to tooth decay is saliva. It is essential in the prevention of caries and infection because it serves to remove food debris, dead cells, and bacteria, and it neutralizes damaging fluids and acids.

- Simple sugars: Foods are the bacteria's primary energy source and a diet high in simple sugar is a risk factor for development of caries.
- Decreased saliva production contributes to a dry mouth condition called *xerostomia*. Xerostomia is associated with chronic conditions such as diabetes and Sjogren syndrome.
- Medications used to treat hypertension, depression, HIV, and cancer and radiation to the head and neck also decrease saliva production.
- Poor oral hygiene associated with accumulation of *plaque*, a soft, sticky film that builds up on teeth and contains bacteria, contributes to decay if not removed through regular brushing and flossing.

24.1.3   ETIOLOGY OF GUM DISEASE

The etiology of gum disease is inflammation caused by bacterial growth in the mouth around the teeth and along the gum line. Plaque buildup related to poor oral hygiene is a major factor that contributes to gum disease infection from bacteria, including *Fusobacterium nucleatum* and *streptococcus mutans*. The bacteria trigger chronic release of inflammatory mediators, including cytokines, prostaglandins, and enzymes from neutrophils and monocytes. This inflammation results in gingivitis and periodontitis, which affect ligaments and bone that support the teeth, leading to bleeding gums, loose teeth, and potential tooth loss. The early stage of gum disease is *gingivitis*. Despite being preventable, three out of four Americans have gingivitis (Peres et al., 2019). Gingivitis, which is reversible, can be treated with intensive dental treatment. Gingivitis can progress to *periodontitis*, which is not reversible due to bone loss and gum recession, and loss of teeth can occur. In more severe cases, bone and gum tissue are destroyed, and loosening and loss of teeth do occur. There is a growing body of evidence that supports the oral-systemic links between oral inflammation and gingivitis and periodontitis:

- Smokers are twice as likely to get gum disease than non-smokers (Centers for Disease Control and Prevention [CDC], 2020c).
- Smoking weakens the immune system, altering the oral microflora and leading to periodontal disease and weakened gums and supporting tooth structures (Borojevic, 2012).

- Smoking causes a lack of oxygen in the bloodstream, meaning infected gums do not heal as well as those of non-smokers (Borojevic, 2012).
- Non-communicable diseases (NCD) with increased risk for gum disease include but are not limited to diabetes, cardiovascular, and respiratory and autoimmune diseases (Bao et al., 2020; CDC, 2020c; Borojevic, 2012; Darling-Fisher et al., 2017; GSA, 2017; Li et al., 2014; Sampson et al., 2020; Seitz et al., 2019).
- Poor oral hygiene contributes to plaque build-up and inflammation of the gums (Borojevic, 2012; CDC, 2020c).

24.2   ORAL HEALTH DURING PREGNANCY

During pregnancy, oral health can affect the health of pregnant persons and their unborn children, as many physiological changes occur in the body during pregnancy. The oral cavity is particularly susceptible to hormonal changes related to pregnancy that increase the likelihood of oral health problems. Periodontitis and gingivitis are especially common among pregnant persons. Gingivitis, the early stage of periodontitis, is when the gums become swollen and red. Periodontitis, the most serious form of periodontal disease, occurs when the gums pull away from the teeth and supporting gum tissues and bone are destroyed (Bobetsis et al., 2020; Corbella et al., 2016; "Periodontal disease fact sheet," 2021). Although these conditions are common among adults in the US and are treatable, findings from several studies show that these oral health issues are associated with negative health outcomes for pregnant preeclampsia, and premature labor (Table 24.1).

A wealth of evidence-based research and policy statements recognize the importance of oral health as an integral part of preventive health care among pregnant persons (APHA, 2020; Azofiefa et al., 2016; Bobetsis et al., 2020; CDC, 2019; Chaparro et al., 2021; Corbella et al., 2016; Figuero et al., 2013; Gogeneni et al., 2015; Haber et al., 2019; Haber et al., 2020b; Hallas et al., 2015; Hartnett et al, 2016; Kruse et al., 2018; Puertas et al., 2018; Skinner, 2016). Despite over a decade of studies and publications emphasizing the need for oral health care for pregnant persons, access to dental care during pregnancy continues to be limited, and integration of oral health competencies are often absent in nursing curricula. The current status of oral health among pregnant persons reflects a need for oral health anticipatory guidance (oral health literacy) and improved access to dental care in this group (Box 24.1). Prevention of periodontal disease is the most important approach to promoting positive birth outcomes: Effective oral hygiene, including brushing and flossing twice a day, minimizing intake of high-sugar and high-carb foods, and visiting the dentist for at least one dental check-up. Treatments for periodontal diseases and preventive dental care are safe for pregnant persons, and there is no evidence of negative health outcomes for parents or infants as a result of receiving dental care during pregnancy (Bobetsis et al., 2020). Preventive dental care is essential for pregnant persons to avoid the long-term consequences of periodontal disease during and after pregnancy, including lasting negative impacts on the oral-systemic health of themselves and their children.

Barriers to accessing dental care include lack of insurance, transportation, and inability to take time off. Even in states with an adult Medicaid dental benefit, it is a challenge to find a dental practice that accepts Medicaid patients, thereby limiting accessible and affordable oral health care. Additionally, there are many myths about dental care being unsafe for pregnant persons that deter them from getting necessary dental cleanings and procedures. Studies have reported that medical professionals may not recommend or may refuse dental services for pregnant patients due to misconceptions about the negative effects of preventive dental care procedures on pregnancy, including but not limited to x-rays, Novocain, and antibiotics, and procedures such as root canals. Many dental and non-dental health care providers are unaware of the oral-systemic connections between oral health and pregnancy, a substantial barrier to pregnant persons' ability to have optimal oral health.

TABLE 24.1

Impact of gingivitis and periodontal disease on pregnancy outcomes

Authors	Title	*Journal*, Year	Strength of Evidence—*strong/ moderate/weak*
Chaparro et al.	Early pregnancy levels of gingival crevicular fluid matrix metalloproteinases-8 and -9 are associated with the severity of periodontitis and the development of gestational diabetes mellitus	*J Periodontol.*, 2021	Findings from a prospective cohort study showed higher concentrations of metalloproteinase (MMP)-8 and -9 in gingival crevicular fluid (GCF) of pregnant women with periodontitis was significantly associated with development of gestational diabetes mellitus (GDM) (Chaparro et al., 2021)—*moderate*
Corbella et al.	Adverse pregnancy outcomes and periodontitis: A systematic review and meta-analysis exploring potential association	*Quintessence Int.*, 2016	Meta-analysis of studies in which researchers controlled for periodontitis as a risk factor associated with negative pregnancy outcomes; found an association between periodontitis and negative consequences in pregnancy including preterm birth and LBW (Corbella et al., 2016)—*strong*
Figuero et al.	Effect of pregnancy on gingival inflammation in systemically healthy women: A systematic review	*J Clin Periodontol.*, 2013	Significant increase in instances of gingivitis throughout pregnancy, as well as higher rates of gingivitis in pregnant versus nonpregnant women (Figuero et al., 2013)—*strong*
Gogeneni et al.	Increased infection with key periodontal pathogens during gestational diabetes mellitus	*J Clin Periodontol.*, 2015	Findings showed that pregnant women with gingivitis and pregnant women with gingivitis and gestational diabetes mellitus (GDM) had high levels of systemic C-reactive protein, demonstrating how gingivitis alone and with GDM can increase risk biomarkers for poor pregnancy outcomes (Gogeneni et al., 2015)—*moderate*
Kruse et al.	Association between high risk for preterm birth and changes in gingiva parameters during pregnancy—a prospective cohort study	*Clin Oral Invest.*, 2018	Gingival inflammation was significantly higher in a sample of women at high-risk for preterm birth compared to their sample of non-risk pregnant women; gingival bacteria was shown to be significantly higher after childbirth in high-risk pregnant women, compared to non-pregnant women (Kruse et al., 2018)—*weak*

BOX 24.1   ORAL HEALTH STATISTICS OF PREGNANT WOMEN

- 40% of pregnant women have some form of periodontal disease (Azofiefa et al., 2016).
- 60–75% of pregnant women have gingivitis (CDC, 2019).
- 41% of pregnant women have dental caries (Azofiefa et al., 2016).
- 56% of pregnant women do not have dental coverage (Skinner, 2016).
- 60% of women did not have their teeth professionally cleaned during their last pregnancy (Skinner, 2016).

Evidence-based oral health literacy products need to align with literacy levels, cultural backgrounds (health beliefs and practices), and linguistic preferences. Oral health literacy needs to be designed to address the needs of different patient populations who access prenatal and child care in a variety of health care settings. Prenatal, postpartum, home visitor, and well-child settings like WIC provide informal opportunities to coach parents about how to integrate oral health strategies in their everyday lives. This ultimately helps prevent a number of oral health conditions that may have severe consequences for both parent and child. Non-dental health care providers—including nurses, nurse practitioners, nurse midwives, doctors, and physician assistants—need to develop their oral health competencies and integrate them into their clinical practice to best serve their pregnant patients. Research findings have demonstrated the effectiveness of oral health education programs for health providers on improving oral health outcomes for pregnant persons during and after pregnancy, as well as improving the oral health of their children (Figuero et al., 2013; Haber et al., 2020b; Hallas et al., 2015). The nursing profession is well equipped to educate and coach patients on oral health care, and improving oral health competencies across the health professions will be an immense contribution to closing the gaps between oral and medical health care to best promote improved overall health for pregnant persons.

24.3   LIFESTYLE ORAL HEALTH FOR CHILDREN AND ADOLESCENTS

Twenty-one years have passed since the landmark Surgeon General's Report Oral Health in America declared early childhood caries (ECC) a "silent epidemic," yet it remains the most common chronic disease of childhood, five times more common than asthma (HHS, 2000). Key findings from the National Health and Nutrition Examination Survey (2015–2016) show that dental caries in children and adolescents age 2–19 increase with age from 21% to 45%, dental caries are higher in populations of color than in White children and adolescents, and higher in populations with lower incomes (National Center for Health Statistics, 2016). Prevalence of treated and untreated dental caries among US youth in this age group was found to be 45.8%, and incidence of caries increased with age with youth age 2–5 at 21.4%, youth age 6–11 at 50.5%, and youth age 12–19 at 53.8% (National Center for Health Statistics, 2016). Non-Hispanic Black youth showed the highest rates of untreated dental caries at 17.1%, followed by Hispanic (13.%), non-Hispanic White (11.7%), and non-Hispanic Asian (10.5%) youth groups (National Center for Health Statistics, 2016). As family income levels increased, the prevalence of treated and untreated dental caries decreased, with 56.3% of youth from families living below the federal poverty level compared to 34.8% of youth from families with income levels greater than 300% of the federal poverty level (National Center for Health Statistics, 2016).

The major socio-behavioral risk factors for the prevalence of dental caries in children and adolescents is related to physical, environmental, behavioral, and lifestyle-related factors. The social determinants of health contribute to oral health disparities, including but not limited to poor nutrition related to food insecurity; insufficient fluoride exposure; poor oral hygiene; inappropriate methods for feeding infants; adolescent use of tobacco and alcohol; and limited availability and accessibility of oral health services.

Health professionals, including nurses, nurse practitioners, and midwives, are well positioned to encourage positive lifestyle behaviors that parents, children and adolescents, and adults can undertake to promote good oral health by promoting oral hygiene practices throughout the lifespan (Table 24.2).

TABLE 24.2
Lifestyle interventions for nutrition and oral health

Age	Feeding Recommendation	Lifestyle Interventions
Newborn–infancy	Breastfeeding until 6 mo.–1 yr.	Educate parent/caregiver on: • Importance of breastfeeding • Breastfeeding techniques • Cleaning gums after feedings for oral hygiene • Monitoring wet diapers and stools for adequate intake
4–6 months	Introduce solids	Educate parent/caregiver on neuro-development for food readiness: • 4 months: Baby has adequate head control and decreased tongue extrusion for solid food readiness • Baby shows interest in food by opening mouth • 6 months: Baby begins to sit up and teeth begin to erupt • Educate parent/caregiver to brush teeth after feedings with infant tooth brush as soon as first tooth appears
	Do not share food or utensils. Do not taste food or clean pacifier in parent/caregiver mouth	Educate parent/caregiver on: • Food and utensil sharing causes saliva exchange which promotes vertical transmission of oral bacteria (*strep mutans*), which causes dental caries
Toddler	Finger foods	Educate parent/caregiver that: • Children often lose interest in food when they become mobile • Important to provide finger foods, nutritious snacks • Avoid foods which are choking hazards, e.g., nuts, grapes, hot dogs
	Avoid walking around with bottles and sippy cups	Educate parents/caregivers that: • Frequent drinks with sugar can increase the time the child's teeth are exposed to sugar, which will cause increased acid and tooth breakdown • Providing milk with meals, water in between meals is best for oral health
Preschooler	Acknowledge children's food preferences	Educate parent/caregiver that: • It is normal for children to become picky eaters at this age • Avoid food fights • Food intolerances are real. The average age of diagnosis for celiac disease is age 3. Celiac disease is associated with dental enamel defects and mouth sores
School-age	Exposure to many new foods	Educate parent/caregiver to: • Be aware of food child is eating outside home to assure adequate nutrition

(continued)

TABLE 24.2 (Continued)
Lifestyle interventions for nutrition and oral health

Age	Feeding Recommendation	Lifestyle Interventions
Adolescence	Awareness of disordered eating patterns	Educate adolescent/parent/caregiver on: • Both obesity and eating disorders • Negative influence of social media and diet culture
Sports	Avoid drinks high in sugar Use of mouth guards	e.g., sports drinks, soda, coffee drinks Educate adolescent/parent/caregiver on: • Importance of using a mouth guard while playing sports to protect mouth and prevent injury
Early/Middle Adulthood	Maintain nutritious diet low in fat and sugar and get plenty of exercise	Educate adult on: • Diet, nutrition, exercise • Preventing diabetes type 2 • Importance of oral hygiene and regular dental care
Older Adulthood	Maintain nutritious diet and healthy mouth	Educate older adult/caretaker on: • Adequate nutrition and weight status • Special diets for health conditions • Importance of ability to chew food • Lack of dental coverage in Medicare • Influence of SDOH • Effects of tooth loss on nutrition, overall health, and social isolation

The increase in dental caries during adolescence can be related to many lifestyle factors, including lack of overall nutritious diet, including the increased intake of sugary beverages and sports drinks. Adolescents are also at increased risk for sports injury to their teeth. Adolescents need age- and media-appropriate oral health literacy that promotes a healthy diet and eating choices and includes information about preventing oral sports injuries through use of mouth guards.

Nurses, nurse practitioners, and midwives can play a significant role in preventing HPV infection and oropharyngeal cancer. According to the Centers for Disease Control and Prevention (CDC), most sexually active American men and women will contract at least one type of HPV virus during their lifetime (2017). This is a particularly important issue in adolescence, as an estimated 55% of male and female teens have had sexual intercourse by age 18 (CDC, 2017).

HPV is a leading cause of oropharyngeal cancer (the very back of the mouth) and a small number of in the front of the mouth (CDC, 2020a; CDC, 2020b). Previously, oral cancers were found in older males who used tobacco and alcohol, but we are seeing this in much younger patients now—non-smoking males age 35–55. Nine strains of HPV are known to cause cancers and another six are suspected of causing cancers. Most HPV infections will be asymptomatic and self-limiting (CDC, 2020b; The Oral Cancer Foundation, 2019). Delayed clearance of an oral/oropharyngeal infection may be a significant risk factor for development of oropharyngeal squamous cell carcinomas (OPSCC) (Pytynia et al., 2014). The HPV-16 strain is associated with more than 70% of all diagnosed OPSCCs and infects 2,600 people each day (CDC, 2020b).

The HPV vaccine, Gardasil, is the first cancer-prevention vaccine. Created in 2006, and a second-generation in 2015, Gardasil 9, protects against HPV genotypes 6, 11, 16, 18, 31, 33, 45, 52, and 58. Findings from current studies suggest that Gardasil provides lifelong protection. To date, studies have followed HPV vaccine recipients for about 10 years; individuals demonstrate high rates of ongoing immunity (Stull et al., 2020; Walker et al., 2018). On June 12, 2020, the FDA approved

TABLE 24.3
HPV vaccine administration recommendation

Age for HPV Vaccine	Administration
9–14 years	2 doses, 6 months apart
15–45 years	3 doses—first 2 doses one month apart, and then 3rd dose 6 months later

Source: FDA expands Gardasil 9 (2020)

the use of Gardasil 9 for prevention of oropharyngeal and head and neck cancer (FDA expands Gardasil 9, 2020).

The HPV vaccine should be administered between ages 9 and 14. The vaccine produces better immunity to fight infection when given at younger ages compared with older ages. Vaccination for HPV is much more effective at preventing disease and cancer if all doses in the series are administered before someone's first sexual contact (Table 24.3). The nursing profession has a long history of health promotion advocacy; continuing this vaccine advocacy role with parents and their children on behalf of increasing HPV vaccination rates is essential.

24.4 LIFESTYLE ORAL HEALTH FOR ADULTS

Few adults think about the connections between oral health and their overall health. Even highly educated interprofessional health care teams sometimes, perhaps often, overlook the need to integrate oral health into whole-person care. Adults of all ages are affected by poor oral health, particularly when they have one or more acute and/or chronic health conditions. A higher prevalence of these conditions is linked to the social determinants of health where a greater burden of oral disease is evident (Yarbrough et al., 2014). Addressing these disparities by integrating oral health in primary and acute care are essential to addressing oral health inequities (Haber et al., 2020a; Petersen, 2003). Diabetes, cancer, cardiovascular disease, and respiratory conditions are among those for which there is a growing body of evidence about links between oral health and overall health.

24.4.1 DIABETES

The prevalence of diabetes is increasing worldwide. By 2030, diabetes is projected to be the seventh leading cause of death globally (Danaei et al., 2011; World Health Organization [WHO], 2021). The majority of adults, 90–95%, have type 2 diabetes (T2DM) (HHS, 2020). In the United States, 10% of the population are affected by diabetes and over 20% of them were unaware of their diabetes diagnosis. Non-Hispanic Blacks, Hispanics, and American Indian/Alaska Natives are at higher risk for T2DM and its complications, which include micro and macro-vascular changes, neuropathy, nephropathy, retinopathy, and susceptibility to infection (HHS, 2020). Addressing oral health needs is an essential component of diabetes prevention and management. The link between diabetes and oral disease can be described as a "2-way street" due to the bi-directionality of how hyperglycemia and oral infection mutually and adversely affect each other (Borgnakke, 2014; Lamster et al., 2021; Preshaw et al., 2012). Hyperglycemia may predispose to or worsen periodontal disease; conversely, periodontal disease and the accompanying inflammation have a negative impact on glycemic control (Zhang et al., 2021). Diabetes can reduce salivary gland function and lead to xerostomia, a dry mouth condition that reduces the bacteria removing function of saliva, thereby predisposing people to dental caries.

Obesity, poor nutrition, and sedentary lifestyle further complicate the situation. Obesity elicits a low grade chronic inflammatory response that can intensify periodontitis and trigger insulin resistance, which in turn increases the risk for prediabetes, subsequent development of T2DM, and poor glycemic control (Deshpande & Amrutiya, 2017). Evidence supports that poorly controlled diabetes increases the risk for periodontal disease; periodontal infection increases blood sugar levels and contributes to diabetic complications (Table 24.4). Management plans for diabetic patients to promote optimal glycemic

---

TABLE 24.4
Oral-systemic Problems of Common Acute and Chronic Health Conditions in Adulthood

Authors	Title	Source, *Year*	Strength of Evidence—*strong/moderate/ weak significance*
Diabetes/Obesity			
Deshpande & Amrutiya	Obesity and oral health—Is there a link? An observational study	*J Indian Soc Periodontol.*, 2017	The prevalence of periodontitis was significantly higher in the obese group compared to the non-obese group. The average gingival index (GI), probing depth, and gingival recession scores were statistically significantly higher among obese participants than their non-obese counterparts (Deshpande & Amrutiya, 2017)—*moderate*
Zhang et al.	Relationship between periodontitis and microangiopathy in type 2 diabetes mellitus: A meta-analysis	*J. Periodontal Res.*, 2021	Periodontitis was associated with increased risk of type 2 diabetic microangiopathy, diabetic retinopathy, and diabetic nephropathy (Zhang et al., 2021)—*strong*
Cancer			
Gomes-Silva et al.	Impact of radiation on tooth loss in patients with head and neck cancer: A retrospective dosimetric-based study	*Oral Surg Oral Med Oral Pathol Oral Radiol Endod.*, 2021	Radiation caries was the most frequent post-HNRT dental adverse event, and maxillary molars ipsilateral to the tumor were lost earlier compared with the other teeth. The odds ratio for post-HNRT tooth extraction risk was approximately three-fold higher for teeth exposed to > 60 Gy followed by an increased risk of delayed healing and osteoradionecrosis (ORN) in sites receiving doses above 50 Gy Gomes-Silva et al., 2021)—*moderate*
Wang et al.	Oral health, caries risk profiles, and oral microbiome of pediatric patients with leukemia submitted to chemotherapy	*BioMed Research International.*, 2021	Prevalence of dental caries, gingivitis, oral mucositis, xerostomia, and candidiasis in children with acute lymphoblastic leukemia (ALL) was higher than that of the healthy control (HC) group. Oral microbiota of ALL groups showed less alpha diversity and significant differences in the composition of the oral microbiome compared to the HC group (Wang et al., 2021)—*moderate*

TABLE 24.4 (Continued)
Oral-systemic Problems of Common Acute and Chronic Health Conditions in Adulthood

Authors	Title	Source, *Year*	Strength of Evidence—*strong/moderate/weak significance*
Cardiovascular Disease			
Li et al.	Periodontal therapy for the management of cardiovascular disease in patients with chronic periodontitis	*Cochrane Database Syst Rev.*, 2014	No studies were identified that assessed primary prevention of CVD in people with periodontitis. No data on deaths (all-cause or CVD-related) were reported. There was insufficient evidence to determine the effect of scaling and root planing (SRP) and community care in reducing the risk of CVD recurrence in patients with chronic periodontitis (Li et al., 2014)—*weak*
Seitz et al.	Current knowledge on correlations between highly prevalent dental conditions and chronic diseases: An umbrella review	*Prev Chronic Dis.*, 2019	Periodontitis was most frequently observed correlations to chronic systemic disease. Type 2 diabetes mellitus (T2DM) had the most frequently observed correlations with a dental condition, and the most dental-chronic disease correlations were found between periodontitis and T2DM, and periodontitis and cardiovascular disease (Seitz et al., 2019)—*moderate*
Respiratory Disease			
Munro & Baker	Reducing missed oral care opportunities to prevent non-ventilator associated hospital acquired pneumonia at the department of veterans' affairs	*Appl Nurs Res.*, 2018	Incidence rate on the geriatric units decreased from 105 to 8.3 cases per 1,000 patient days (by 92%) in the first year. The intervention yielded an estimated cost avoidance of $2.84 million and 13 lives saved in 19 months post-implementation (Munro & Baker, 2018)—*strong*
Behavioral/Mental Health Disorders and Stress			
Kisely et al.	The oral health of people with anxiety and depressive disorders—a systematic review and meta-analysis	*J Affect Disord.*, 2016	All psychiatric diagnoses were associated with increased dental decay on both decayed, missing and filled teeth (DMFT) and surfaces (DMFS) scores, as well as greater tooth loss. There was no association with periodontal disease, except for panic disorder (Kisely et al., 2016)—*weak*
Vasiliou et al.	Current stress and poor oral health	*BMC Oral Health*, 2016	Participants who reported greater perceived current stress were significantly more likely to report progressively poorer oral health and greater oral pain compared to those with less stress. Effects of oral pain were stronger for uninsured participants compared to their insured counterparts (Vasiliou et al., 2016)—*moderate*

control should include oral assessments, including comorbidities, use of motivational interviewing to promote lifestyle changes, including effective oral hygiene, xerostomia management, and ensuring that patients have an accessible and affordable dental home for dental health promotion checkups and periodontal care (Darling-Fisher et al., 2017; "Oral health and diabetes," 2015).

24.4.2 Cancer

Cancer increases risks for oral health complications and impacts quality of life. The oral environment is subject to a wide range of changes during cancer therapy, including immunosuppression, salivary hypofunction, and mucosal ulceration (Bissonnette et al., 2020). As a result, cancer patients are at high risk for oral infections during and after treatment. Yet, oral care is often neglected by health care teams during and after treatment. Over one-third of people treated for cancer develop complications that affect the mouth ("Dental and oral," 2016). Oral health issues that occur during cancer treatment, if left untreated, can lead to severe acute and chronic oral health problems. Prevention, assessment, and treatment of oral problems must be incorporated into cancer care to meet patients' oral care needs. Early detection and prevention of oral health issues is imperative to avoiding serious oral and overall health problems. These oral problems include dental caries, oral candidiasis, mucositis, and xerostomia, among others (Table 24.4; Table 24.5). Patients are more

TABLE 24.5
Oral Health Complications of Cancer Therapy

Oral Complication	Causes	Signs/Symptoms	Lifestyle Interventions
Dental caries	Salivary gland hypofunction and radiation damage to tooth structures that occur during therapy. Patients may use liquid dietary supplements to combat reduced food intake and weight loss; these supplements often contain refined carbohydrates that reduce saliva production.	Patient reports toothache, tooth sensitivity, and/or spontaneous pain, pain when eating or drinking. Visible holes or pits on teeth; brown, black, or white staining on teeth surface.	Make sure that all cancer patients have a dental visit prior to beginning treatment for a cleaning. Refer patients with signs of tooth decay to a dentist prior to and throughout treatment, and educate their patients on best oral health strategies to prevent further decay.
Dysphagia	Difficulty swallowing as a short-term side effect of cancer therapy.	Patient reports difficulty with swallowing.	Refer to speech and language therapist for swallowing therapy. Refer to nutritionist to advise on dietary changes.
Lymphedema	Caused by cancer or by cancer treatment. Cancerous tumors can block the lymph system. Surgery to remove tumors may also remove lymph nodes or vessels that carry the lymph fluid, causing fluid build-up in surrounding tissues.	Patient reports swelling and aching in eyes, face, neck, and/or lips. Stiffness or difficulty moving neck and jaw.	Exercise and limiting sodium in diet can reduce swelling. Maintain diet of soft foods. Refer to physical therapist for assessment and treatment.

TABLE 24.5 (Continued)
Oral Health Complications of Cancer Therapy

Oral Complication	Causes	Signs/Symptoms	Lifestyle Interventions
Mucositis	Cancer treatments break down rapidly divided epithelial cells lining the gastro-intestinal tract, which leaves mucosal tissue vulnerable to painful ulcers and infection.	Patient reports soreness or pain in the mouth or throat, trouble with swallowing or talking, and/or dryness, mild burning, or pain when eating. Red or swollen mouth and gums; blood and/or sores in the mouth.	Lidocaine solutions or sucking on ice chips can provide temporary relief. Use 0.2% morphine or 0.5% doxepin mouth rinses for pain relief. Rinse with salt water or 1% sodium bicarbonate, (chlorhexidine gluconate 0.12%) to reduce impact of mucositis. Refer to physician, oncologist, or dentist as needed.
Osteonecrosis	Poor blood supply due to cancer treatments.	Patient reports mouth pain, swelling, or gum infections. Numbness or a feeling of heaviness in the jaws. Swelling in mouth or signs of infection in gums. Development of exposed bone along jaws.	Frequent saline irrigation and antibiotic medications during infectious periods. Hyperbaric oxygen treatment (HBOT) can be used to accelerate healing. Maintain diet of soft foods. Refer to dentist/dental hygienist for further evaluation. Refer to surgeon for consult.
Ototoxicity	Side effect of cancer therapy and related medications.	Patient reports loss of hearing or difficulty with balance.	Refer to audiologist for assessment and treatment.
Taste Disorders	Hypogeusia (reduced ability to taste), ageusia (loss of taste), or dysgeusia (altered taste) due to nerve damage from cancer therapy.	Patient reports loss of taste or foul or metallic taste in mouth.	Refer to speech and language therapist or nutritionist for further assessment and management.
Thrush (*candidiasis*)	Weakened immune system and xerostomia from therapy and medications often used by patients to reduce treatment side effects.	Patient reports dry mouth, loss of taste, and/or pain while eating or swallowing. White coating on the tongue and tissues, and inflammation in the mouth and throat.	Antifungal medications (e.g., fluconazole itraconazole) and/or topical agents (e.g., clotrimazole), can be used to treat infection. However, these medications may not be as effective in cancer patients due to interactions with other cancer-related medications. Refer to physician or dentist for further treatment as needed.

(continued)

TABLE 24.5 (Continued)
Oral Health Complications of Cancer Therapy

Oral Complication	Causes	Signs/Symptoms	Lifestyle Interventions
Trismus	Caused by scar tissue from cancer therapy or surgery and/or nerve damage.	Patient reports difficulty opening mouth and/or pain when chewing or speaking. Headaches, ear aches, and jaw pain are also common.	Practice jaw-stretching devices and jaw exercises to manage jaw pain and stiffness. Maintain diet of soft foods. Refer to physical therapist or speech and language therapist for ongoing physical therapy.
Xerostomia	Decrease in salivary flow as a side effect of cancer medications, which causes dry mouth.	Patient reports dry mouth, stickiness or thick saliva, bad breath, difficulty speaking and swallowing, dry or sore throat, and/or difficulty wearing dentures.	Sugar-free chewing gum is commonly recommended to increase salivary production, and oral lubricants and saliva substitutes are often used for temporary relief. Refer to pharmacist for consultation as needed.

likely to experience dry mouth due to intake of multiple medications, poor nutrition, and difficulties with food intake, which can greatly impact patients' overall health and wellness during cancer treatment (Hartnett, 2015; Marques et al., 2021).

Before cancer treatment, a comprehensive oral assessment should be performed with the patient to identify oral health issues, administer health promotion interventions like cleanings, and treat severe problems like abscesses. This pre-treatment assessment should include identification of existing oral health issues, stabilization or elimination of potential infection sites and dental trauma, and oral prophylaxis. Nurses can perform an oral exam using the HEENOT approach (Haber et al., 2015) and refer patients to the dentist for treatment, which can reduce the onset of oral complications during and after cancer treatment. Patients undergoing cancer therapy of any kind should receive basic oral health literacy tips and referral to a dentist for cleaning or treatment as needed (Hartnett, 2015).

During treatment, regular oral assessments should be continued using the HEENOT approach (Haber et al., 2015). Oral infections can occur within the first months, and even weeks, of treatment. Continue to advise patients on good oral hygiene practices, which include:

* Brushing teeth with fluoride toothpaste.
* Flossing gently once per day.
* Rinsing with a baking soda and water solution.
* Avoiding mouth rinses with alcohol.
* Sucking on ice chips and/or chewing sugar-free gum to promote salivary flow and relieve dry mouth (Hartnett, 2015).

Oral care assessments should continue as a part of follow-up visits after cancer treatment to monitor oral late-effects that may occur. Patients should be advised to visit their dentist for regular check-ups and report any oral side effects or concerns to their cancer care team for further evaluation. Optimal oral self-care, combined with thorough and consistent assessment of the teeth and gums, is essential to preventing severe oral health problems.

Although many oral health complications are treatable and curable, there are many oral problems that can continue to impact patients' dentition if proper oral care is not provided. Complying with thorough oral hygiene practices and dental check-ups can greatly reduce the incidence of oral complications and can minimize the severity of such oral issues as mucositis and xerostomia. Nurses, nurse practitioners, and the entire health care team must emphasize the importance of maintaining the oral care before, during, and after cancer therapy to prevent long-term oral health problems and improve patients' overall well-being and quality of life.

24.4.3 CARDIOVASCULAR DISEASE

Cardiovascular disease (CVD), including conditions such as ischemic heart disease and ischemic stroke, have been associated with infection and inflammation. Bacteria in the mouth, providing an environment for development of gingivitis and periodontitis, can travel to blood vessels elsewhere in the body, where they cause blood vessel inflammation and damage to the endothelial lining of the blood vessels; tiny blood clots, heart attacks, and stroke may follow (Table 24.4). Evidence supporting this perspective is provided by the remnants of oral bacteria in atherosclerotic blood vessels far from the mouth. Another perspective is that the body's immune response, inflammation in the mouth, sets off a cascade of vascular damage throughout the body, including the heart and the brain. Other potential risk factors include, but are not limited to smoking, poor oral hygiene, obesity, lack of exercise, and poor access to dental and medical health care (GSA, 2017; Li et al., 2014; Seitz et al., 2019). Nurses, nurse practitioners, and interprofessional health team members need to promote oral health literacy about the links between oral health and CVD and emphasize the importance of smoking cessation, oral hygiene, low-carbohydrate diets, weight loss, and exercise in promoting cardiovascular health.

24.4.4 RESPIRATORY DISEASE

Respiratory diseases like pneumonia occur more frequently in patients with poor oral hygiene who have or are at risk for gingivitis or periodontal disease (Table 24.4). The oral pathogens associated with infection and inflammation can travel to the respiratory tract or are aspirated into the lungs, where they release enzymes that modify the oral mucosa surfaces to allow them to adhere to the respiratory epithelium that is altered by the periodontal cytokines to promote infections like ventilator (VAP) or non-ventilator (NVHAP) associated pneumonias. A growing body of evidence links risk for severe COVID-19 with transmission of oral bacteria to the lungs, development of the cytokine storm, pneumonia increasing morbidity and mortality (Bao et al., 2020; Sampson et al., 2020). NVHAP, the most common hospital-acquired infection, increases hospital length of stay and readmissions, as well as mortality, and cost (Munro & Baker, 2018). Integrating oral protocols into patient management to prevent pneumonia is most effective using a team approach developed by Project HAPPEN, a system-wide oral hygiene quality improvement initiative led by nurse practitioners in the Veterans' Administration health system (Munro et al., 2021).

24.4.5 BEHAVIORAL HEALTH

Stress affects the immune system, sleep, and patterns of personal hygiene, which can all affect oral health (Vasiliou et al., 2016). Stress can affect your oral health in a number of ways, damaging teeth and gums (Table 24.6). People with psychological disorders are at risk for oral health problems due to side effects of medications and neglect of oral care at home (Kisely et al., 2016). Early detection, prevention, and treatment of the effect of stress on the oral cavity is essential for a healthy lifestyle.

TABLE 24.6
Stress and oral health complications

Problem	Signs and Symptoms	Lifestyle Interventions
Anti-anxiety medications	Dry mouth (*xerostomia*)	Drink water, limit caffeine intake. Adopt regular oral care practice behaviors: tooth brushing twice per day, flossing once per day.
Cracked teeth	Pain resulting from tooth grinding or jaw clenching	Avoid hard or crunchy foods. Usually requires dental repair.
Dry mouth (*xerostomia*)	Dry, sticky feeling in mouth	Drink water, limit caffeine intake. Adopt regular oral care practice behaviors: tooth brushing twice per day, flossing once per day.
Increased acid reflux	Sour taste in mouth, tooth erosion	Small frequent meals, loose clothing, keep head elevated 45°, avoid spicy foods, alcohol, caffeine, smoking. Establish good elimination pattern. May need weight loss intervention.
Jaw issues (*temporomandibular disorders, TMD*)	Pain around ear and face, popping sound, difficulty chewing or opening mouth	Massage, physical therapy, night guards, pain management; guided imagery, mindfulness meditation
Mouth sores (cancer sores, HSV)	Irritation on lips, gums, tongue	Ice, salt water mouth rinses, topical treatment, anti-viral medication, Avoid sun exposure.
Poor oral hygiene	Plaque build-up, bleeding when brushing, halitosis, periodontitis	Adopt regular oral care practice behaviors: tooth brushing twice per day, flossing once per day.
Teeth grinding (*bruxism*)	May be unaware since grinding occurs during concentration or sleeping. Dull headache, sore jaw, earache	Observe for flattened, fractured, or chipped teeth. Night guard, massage jaw, check Vitamin D levels, avoid chewing gum, deep breathing, guided imagery.
Thrush (*candidiasis*)	White patches on soft tissues of the mouth	Salt water, baking soda rinses, anti-fungal medication.

24.5 CONCLUSION

Promoting oral health is an essential component of overall health. Preventing oral disease is a national population health issue that necessitates advocacy from all health professionals. The burden of oral health problems is particularly severe among vulnerable populations affected by the social determinants of health. The nursing profession, which includes nurses, nurse practitioners, and midwives, is the largest of the health professions. Nurses play a major role in a wide range of health care settings, as many practice in underserved areas and care for large numbers of patients across the lifespan. We play a significant role in coaching patients on their oral health and minimizing the negative impact of poor oral health on overall health.

Oral health integration in clinical nursing education and practice contributes to improved access to screening and preventive oral health services across the lifespan. In an era of health care transformation, it is more important than ever that the nursing profession commit to implementing an interprofessional model of whole person care that includes oral health as a key component of primary, acute, home, and long-term care.

Nurses are perfectly positioned to include oral health assessment, intervention, and appropriate referral in their clinical standards of care. Nurses' scope of practice includes health promotion and illness prevention, and they are qualified to collaborate with nurse practitioners, midwives, physicians, pharmacists, and dentists to assess and manage oral health issues associated with acute and chronic health conditions. Successful integration of oral health care and competencies is key to promoting a healthy lifestyle for all patients.

REFERENCES

American Public Health Association. (2020, October 24). *Improving access to dental care for pregnant women through education, integration of health services, insurance coverage, an appropriate dental workforce, and research.* www.apha.org/Policies-and-Advocacy/Public-Health-Policy-Statements/Policy-Datab ase/2021/01/12/Improving-Access-to-Dental-Care-for-Pregnant-Women

Atchison, K. A., Rozier, J. A., & Weintraub, J. A. (2018). Integration of oral health and primary care: Communication, coordination and referral. *NAM Perspectives*. Discussion Paper. https://doi.org/ 10.31478/201810e

Azofeifa, A., Yeung, L. F., Alverson, C. J., & Beltrán-Aguilar, E. (2016). Dental caries and periodontal disease among U.S. pregnant women and nonpregnant women of reproductive age, National Health and Nutrition Examination Survey, 1999–2004. *Journal of Public Health Dentistry*, *76*(4), 320–329. https:// doi.org/10.1111/jphd.12159

Bao, L., Zhang, C., Dong, J., Zhao, L., Li, Y., & Sun, J. (2020). Oral microbiome and SARS-CoV-2: Beware of lung co-infection. *Frontiers in Microbiology*, *11*, 1840. https://doi.org/10.3389/fmicb.2020.01840

Benzian, H., Beltrán-Aguilar, E., Mathur, M. R., & Niederman, R. (2021). Pandemic considerations on essential oral health care. *Journal of Dental Research*, *100*(3), 221–225. https://doi.org/10.1177/002203452 0979830

Bissonnette, C., McNamara, K., & Kalmar, J. R. (2020). Oral complications in cancer patients: A review of practical interventions in the dental setting. *Journal of the Michigan Dental Association*. www.researchg ate.net/publication/340511491_Oral_Complications_in_Cancer_Patients_A_Review_of_Practical_ Interventions_in_the_Dental_Setting

Bobetsis, Y. A., Graziani, F., Gürsoy, M., & Madianos, P. N. (2020). Periodontal disease and adverse pregnancy outcomes. *Periodontology 2000*, *83*(1), 154–174. https://doi.org/10.1111/prd.12294.

Borgnakke WS. (2014). Hyperglycemia/diabetes mellitus and periodontal infection adversely affect each other. In R. J. Genco & R. C. Williams (Eds.), *Periodontal disease and overall health: A clinician's guide* (pp. 99–122). Professional Audience Communications. https://doi.org/10.13140/RG.2.1.1975.8241

Borojevic T. (2012). Smoking and periodontal disease. *Materia Socio-Medica*, *24*(4), 274–276. https://doi.org/ 10.5455/msm.2012.24.274-276

Centers for Disease Control and Prevention. (2020a). *How many cancers are linked with HPV each year?* www. cdc.gov/cancer/hpv/statistics/cases.htm

Centers for Disease Control and Prevention. (2020b). *HPV and oropharyngeal cancer.* www.cdc.gov/cancer/ hpv/basic_info/hpv_oropharyngeal.htm

Centers for Disease Control and Prevention. (2019). *Pregnancy and oral health.* www.cdc.gov/oralhealth/publi cations/features/pregnancy-and-oral-health.html

Centers for Disease Control and Prevention. (2020c). *Smoking, gum disease, and tooth loss.* www.cdc.gov/toba cco/campaign/tips/diseases/periodontal-gum-disease.html

Centers for Disease Control and Prevention. (2017). *Over half of U.S. teens have had sexual intercourse by age 18, new report shows.* www.cdc.gov/nchs/pressroom/nchs_press_releases/2017/201706_N SFG.htm

Chaparro, A., Realini, O., Hernández, M., Albers, D., Weber, L., Ramírez, V., Param, F., Kusanovic, J. P., Sorsa, T., Rice, G. E., & Illanes, S. E. (2021). Early pregnancy levels of gingival crevicular fluid matrix metalloproteinases-8 and -9 are associated with the severity of periodontitis and the development of gestational diabetes mellitus. *Journal of Periodontology*, *92*(2), 205–215. https://doi.org/10.1002/ JPER.19-0743

Corbella, S., Taschieri, S., Del Fabbro, M., Francetti, L., Weinstein, R., & Ferrazzi, E. (2016). Adverse pregnancy outcomes and periodontitis: A systematic review and meta-analysis exploring potential association. *Quintessence International (Berlin, Germany: 1985)*, *47*(3), 193–204. https://doi.org/10.3290/ j.qi.a34980

Cox, M. J., Loman, N., Bogaert, D., & O'Grady, J. (2020). Co-infections: Potentially lethal and unexplored in COVID-19. *The Lancet Microbe*, *1*(1), e11. https://doi.org/10.1016/S2666-5247(20)30009-4

Danaei, G., Finucane, M. M., Lu, Y., Singh, G. M., Cowan, M. J., Paciorek, C. J., Lin, J. K., Farzadfar, F., Khang, Y. H., Stevens, G. A., Rao, M., Ali, M. K., Riley, L. M., Robinson, C. A., Ezzati, M., & Global Burden of Metabolic Risk Factors of Chronic Diseases Collaborating Group (Blood Glucose) (2011). National, regional, and global trends in fasting plasma glucose and diabetes prevalence since 1980: Systematic analysis of health examination surveys and epidemiological studies with 370 country-years and 2.7 million participants. *Lancet (London, England)*, *378*(9785), 31–40. https://doi.org/10.1016/S0140-6736(11)60679-X

Darling-Fisher, C., Borgnakke, W., & Haber, J. (2017). Oral health and diabetes. *American Nurse Today*, *12*(8), 22–25. www.americannursetoday.com/ana-journal-august-2017/

Dave, M., Seoudi, N., & Coulthard, P. (2020). Urgent dental care for patients during the COVID-19 pandemic. *Lancet (London, England)*, *395*(10232), 1257. https://doi.org/10.1016/S0140-6736(20)30806-0

Dental and oral complications of cancer treatment. (2016, September 1). Leukemia & Lymphoma Society. Retrieved July 9, 2021, from www.lls.org/sites/default/files/National/USA/Pdf/Publications/FS29_Dental_and_Oral_Fact_Sheet_FINAL_9.2016.pdf

Deshpande, N. C., & Amrutiya, M. R. (2017). Obesity and oral health—is there a link? An observational study. *Journal of Indian Society of Periodontology*, *21*(3), 229–233. https://doi.org/10.4103/jisp.jisp_305_16

Dye, B.A., Thornton-Evans, G., Li, X., & Iafolla, T.J. (2015, March 1). Dental caries and sealant prevalence in children and adolescents in the United States, 2011–12. *National Center for Health Statistics*, *191*, 1–8. www.cdc.gov/nchs/data/databriefs/db191.pdf

FDA expands Gardasil 9 approval for head and neck cancer prevention. (2020, June 15). Healio. www.healio.com/news/hematology-oncology/20200615/fda-expands-gardasil-9-approval-for-head-and-neck-cancer-prevention

Figuero, E., Carrillo-de-Albornoz, A., Martín, C., Tobías, A., & Herrera, D. (2013). Effect of pregnancy on gingival inflammation in systemically healthy women: A systematic review. *Journal of Clinical Periodontology*, *40*(5), 457–473. https://doi.org/10.1111/jcpe.12053

Garcia, R. I., Inge, R. E., Niessen, L., & DePaola, D. P. (2010). Envisioning success: The future of the oral health care delivery system in the United States. *Journal of Public Health Dentistry*, *70*(Suppl. 1), S58–S65. https://doi.org/10.1111/j.1752-7325.2010.00185.x

Gerontological Society of America. (2017, July 1) *Oral health: An essential element of healthy aging*. www.geron.org/images/gsa/documents/gsa2017oralhealthwhitepaper.pdf

Gerontological Society of America. (2020). Interrelationships between nutrition and oral health in older adults. *What's Hot*. www.geron.org/images/gsa/documents/whatshotnutritionoralhealth.pdf

Gil-Montoya, J. A., de Mello, A. L., Barrios, R., Gonzalez-Moles, M. A., & Bravo, M. (2015). Oral health in the elderly patient and its impact on general well-being: a nonsystematic review. *Clinical Interventions in Aging*, *10*, 461–467. https://doi.org/10.2147/CIA.S54630

Gogeneni, H., Buduneli, N., Ceyhan-Öztürk, B., Gümüş, P., Akcali, A., Zeller, I., Renaud, D. E., Scott, D. A., & Özçaka, Ö. (2015). Increased infection with key periodontal pathogens during gestational diabetes mellitus. *Journal of Clinical Periodontology*, *42*(6), 506–512. https://doi.org/10.1111/jcpe.12418

Gomes-Silva, W., Morais-Faria, K., Rivera, C., Najas, G. F., Marta, G. N., da Conceição Vasconcelos, K., de Andrade Carvalho, H., de Castro, G., Jr, Brandão, T. B., Epstein, J. B., & Santos-Silva, A. R. (2021). Impact of radiation on tooth loss in patients with head and neck cancer: A retrospective dosimetric-based study. *Oral Surgery, Oral Medicine, Oral Pathology and Oral Radiology*, *132*(4), 409–417. https://doi.org/10.1016/j.oooo.2021.06.021

Haber, J., Dolce, M. C., Hartnett, E., Savageau, J. A., Altman, S., Lange-Kessler, J., & Silk, H. (2019). Integrating oral health curricula into midwifery graduate programs: Results of a US survey. *Journal of Midwifery & Women's Health*, *64*(4), 462–471. https://doi.org/10.1111/jmwh.12974

Haber, J., Hartnett, E., Allen, K., Crowe, R., Adams, J., Bella, A., Riles, T., & Vasilyeva, A. (2017). The impact of oral-systemic health on advancing interprofessional education outcomes. *Journal of Dental Education*, *81*(2), 140–148.

Haber, J., Hartnett, E., Cipollina, J., Allen, K., Crowe, E., Roitman, J., Feldman, L., Fletcher J., & Ng, G. (2020a). Attaining interprofessional competencies by connecting oral health to overall health. *Journal of Dental Education*, *85*(4), 504–512. https://doi.org/10.1002/jdd.12490

Haber, J., Hartnett, E., Allen, K., Hallas, D., Dorsen, C., Lange-Kessler, J., Lloyd, M., Thomas, E., & Wholihan, D. (2015). Putting the mouth back in the head: HEENT to HEENOT. *American Journal of Public Health, 105*(3), 437–441. https://doi.org/10.2105/AJPH.2014.302495

Haber, J., Hartnett, E., Hille, A., & Cipollina, J. (2020b). Promoting oral health for mothers and children: A nurse home visitor education program. *Pediatric Nursing, 46*(2), 70–76.

Haber, J. & Hartnett, E. (2019). The interprofessional role in dental caries management: Impact of the nursing profession in early childhood caries. *Dental Clinics of North America, 63*(4), 653–661. https://doi.org/10.1016/j.cden.2019.05.002

Hallas, D., Fernandez, J. B., Lim, L. J., Catapano, P., Dickson, S. K., Blouin, K. R., Schmidt, T. M., Acal-Jiminez, R., Ali, N., Figueroa, K. E., Jiwani, N. M., & Sharma, A. (2015). OHEP: An oral health education program for mothers of newborns. *Journal of Pediatric Health Care: Official Publication of National Association of Pediatric Nurse Associates & Practitioners, 29*(2), 181–190. https://doi.org/10.1016/j.pedhc.2014.11.004

Hartnett, E., Haber, J., Catapano, P., Dougherty, N., Moursi, A. M., Kashani, R., Osman, C., Chinn, C., & Bella, A. (2019). The impact of an interprofessional pediatric oral health clerkship on advancing interprofessional education outcomes. *Journal of Dental Education, 83*(8), 878–886. https://doi.org/10.21815/JDE.019.088

Hartnett, E., Haber, J., Krainovich-Miller, B., Bella, A., Vasilyeva, A., & Lange Kessler, J. (2016). Oral health in pregnancy. *Journal of Obstetric, Gynecologic, and Neonatal Nursing, 45*(4), 565–573. https://doi.org/10.1016/j.jogn.2016.04.005

Hartnett, E. (2015). Integrating oral health throughout cancer care. *Journal of Clinical Oncology, 19*(5), 615–619. https://doi.org/10.1188/15.CJON.615-619

Health Resources and Services Administration. (2014, February 1). *Integration of oral health and primary care practice.* www.hrsa.gov/sites/default/files/hrsa/oralhealth/integrationoforalhealth.pdf

Healthy People 2030. (2020). Retrieved July 9, 2021, from https://health.gov/healthypeople

Hummel, J., Phillips, K. E., Holt, B., & Hayes, C. (2015, June 1). *Oral health: An essential component of primary care.* Qualis Health. www.safetynetmedicalhome.org/sites/default/files/White-Paper-Oral-Health-Primary-Care.pdf?utm_source=June+2015&utm_campaign=June+2015&utm_medium=archive

Institute of Medicine. (2011a). Advancing oral health in America. *The National Academies Press.* https://doi.org/10.17226/13086

Institute of Medicine. (2011b). Improving access to oral health care for vulnerable and underserved populations. *The National Academies Press.* https://doi.org/10.17226/13116

Italiano, A., Miller, W. H., Jr, Blay, J. Y., Gietema, J. A., Bang, Y. J., Mileshkin, L. R., Hirte, H. W., Higgins, B., Blotner, S., Nichols, G. L., Chen, L. C., Petry, C., Yang, Q. J., Schmitt, C., Jamois, C., & Siu, L. L. (2021). Phase I study of daily and weekly regimens of the orally administered MDM2 antagonist idasanutlin in patients with advanced tumors. *Investigational New Drugs, 39*(6), 1587–1597. https://doi.org/10.1007/s10637-021-01141-2

Kisely, S., Sawyer, E., Siskind, D., & Lalloo, R. (2016). The oral health of people with anxiety and depressive disorders—a systematic review and meta-analysis. *Journal of Affective Disorders, 200*, 119–132. https://doi.org/10.1016/j.jad.2016.04.040

Kruse, A. B., Kuerschner, A. C., Kunze, M., Woelber, J. P., Al-Ahmad, A., Wittmer, A., Vach, K., & Ratka-Krueger, P. (2018). Association between high risk for preterm birth and changes in gingiva parameters during pregnancy—a prospective cohort study. *Clinical Oral Investigations, 22*(3), 1263–1271. https://doi.org/10.1007/s00784-017-2209-9

Lamster, I. B., Malloy, K. P., DiMura, P. M., Cheng, B., Wagner, V. L., Matson, J., Proj, A., Xi, Y., Abel, S. N., & Alfano, M. C. (2021). Dental services and health outcomes in the New York State Medicaid program. *Journal of Dental Research, 100*(9), 928–934. https://doi.org/10.1177/00220345211007448

Lau, P., Tran, A., Chen, M., Boyce, E., Martin, R., & Calache, H. (2021). Interprofessional diabetes and oral health management: what do primary healthcare professionals think? *F1000Research, 10*, 339. https://doi.org/10.12688/f1000research.52297.1

Li, C., Lv, Z., Shi, Z., Zhu, Y., Wu, Y., Li, L., & Iheozor-Ejiofor, Z. (2014). Periodontal therapy for the management of cardiovascular disease in patients with chronic periodontitis. *The Cochrane Database of Systematic Reviews,* (8), CD009197. https://doi.org/10.1002/14651858.CD009197.pub2

Long, S.S. (2012). Children's dental health affects school performance and psychosocial development. *The Journal of Pediatrics, 161*(6), A3. https://doi.org/10.1016/j.jpeds.2012.10.029

MacNeil, R., Hilario, H., Thierer, T. E., & Gesko, D. S. (2020). The case for integrated oral and primary medical health care delivery: Health Partners. *Journal of Dental Education, 84*(8), 932–935. https://doi.org/10.1002/jdd.12288

Marques, J.G., Rozan, C., Proença, L., Peixoto, A., & Manso, C. (2021). Assessment of hyposalivation, xerostomia, and oral health-related quality of life in polymedicated patients. *Medical Sciences Forum, 5*(6). https://doi.org/10.3390/msf5010006

Mitchell-Royston, L., Nowak, A., & Silverman, J. (2014, May 1). Interprofessional study of oral health in primary care. *Pediatric Oral Health Research and Policy Center.* www.aapd.org/assets/1/7/Dentaqu est_Year_1_Final_Report.pdf

Munro, S., & Baker, D. (2018). Reducing missed oral care opportunities to prevent non-ventilator associated hospital acquired pneumonia at the Department of Veterans Affairs. *Applied Nursing Research, 44*, 48–53. https://doi.org/10.1016/j.apnr.2018.09.004

Munro, S. C., Baker, D., Giuliano, K. K., Sullivan, S. C., Haber, J., Jones, B. E., Crist, M. B., Nelson, R. E., Carey, E., Lounsbury, O., Lucatorto, M., Miller, R., Pauley, B., & Klompas, M. (2021). Nonventilator hospital-acquired pneumonia: A call to action. *Infection Control and Hospital Epidemiology, 42*(8), 991–996. https://doi.org/10.1017/ice.2021.239

National Center for Health Statistics. (2016). *Continuous NHANES.* Retrieved July 9, 2021, from wwwn.cdc.gov/nchs/nhanes/continuousnhanes/default.aspx?BeginYear=2015

National Interprofessional Initiative on Oral Health. (2017). *Oral health integration into whole person care.* Retrieved July 9, 2021, from www.niioh.org

Northridge, M. E., Kumar, A., & Kaur, R. (2020). Disparities in access to oral health care. *Annual Review of Public Health, 41*, 513–535. https://doi.org/10.1146/annurev-publhealth-040119-094318

Oral Cancer Foundation. (2019, February 1). *HPV/Oral cancer facts.* Retrieved July 9, 2021, from https://oralc ancerfoundation.org/understanding/hpv/hpv-oral-cancer-facts/

Oral health and diabetes. (2015). Oral Health Nursing Education and Practice. http://ohnep.org/sites/ohnep/files/oral-health-and-diabetes.pdf

Peres, M. A., Macpherson, L., Weyant, R. J., Daly, B., Venturelli, R., Mathur, M. R., Listl, S., Celeste, R. K., Guarnizo-Herreño, C. C., Kearns, C., Benzian, H., Allison, P., & Watt, R. G. (2019). Oral diseases: A global public health challenge. *Lancet (London, England), 394*(10194), 249–260. https://doi.org/10.1016/S0140-6736(19)31146-8

Periodontal disease fact sheet. (2021). American Academy of Periodontology. www.perio.org/newsroom/peri odontal-disease-fact-sheet

Petersen, P. E. (2008). The world oral health report 2003: Continuous improvement of oral health in the 21st century—the approach of the WHO global oral health programme. *Community Dentistry and Oral Epidemiology, 31*, 3–24. https://doi.org/10.1046/j..2003.com122.x

Preshaw, P. M., Alba, A. L., Herrera, D., Jepsen, S., Konstantinidis, A., Makrilakis, K., & Taylor, R. (2015). Periodontitis and diabetes: A two-way relationship. *Diabetologia, 55*(1), 21–31. https://doi.org/10.1007/s00125-011-2342-y

Puertas, A., Magan-Fernandez, A., Blanc, V., Revelles, L., O'Valle, F., Pozo, E., León, R., & Mesa, F. (2018). Association of periodontitis with preterm birth and low birth weight: A comprehensive review. *The Journal of Maternal-Fetal & Neonatal Medicine, 31*(5), 597–602. https://doi.org/10.1080/14767 058.2017.1293023

Pytynia, K. B., Dahlstrom, K. R., & Sturgis, E. M. (2014). Epidemiology of HPV-associated oropharyngeal cancer. *Oral Oncology, 50*(5), 380–386. https://doi.org/10.1016/j.oraloncology.2013.12.019

Sampson, V., Kamona, N., & Sampson, A. (2020). Could there be a link between oral hygiene and the severity of SARS-CoV-2 infections? *British Dental Journal, 228*(12), 971–975. https://doi.org/10.1038/s41 415-020-1747-8

Seitz, M. W., Listl, S., Bartols, A., Schubert, I., Blaschke, K., Haux, C., & Van Der Zande, M. M. (2019). Current knowledge on correlations between highly prevalent dental conditions and chronic diseases: An umbrella review. *Preventing Chronic Disease, 16*, E132. https://doi.org/10.5888/pcd16.180641

Skinner E. (2016). Oral health care and coverage during pregnancy. *National Conference of State Legislatures, 24*(48). www.ncsl.org/research/health/oral-health-care-and-coverage-during-pregnancy.aspx

Stull, C., Freese, R., & Sarvas, E. (2020). Parent perceptions of dental care providers' role in human papillomavirus prevention and vaccine advocacy. *Journal of the American Dental Association, 151*(8), 560–567. https://doi.org/10.1016/j.adaj.2020.05.004

Sun, C. X., Bennett, N., Tran, P., Tang, K. D., Lim, Y., Frazer, I., Samaranayake, L., & Punyadeera, C. (2017). A pilot study into the association between oral health status and human papillomavirus-16 infection. *Diagnostics, 7*(1), 1–11. https://doi.org/10.3390/diagnostics7010011

US Department of Health and Human Services. (2000). *Oral health in America: A report of the Surgeon General.* National Institute of Dental and Craniofacial Research, National Institutes of Health. www.nidcr.nih.gov/sites/default/files/2017-10/hck1ocv.%40www.surgeon.fullrpt.pdf

US Department of Health and Human Services Oral Health Coordinating Committee. (2016). Oral health strategic framework 2014–2017. *US Public Health Service.* www.hrsa.gov/sites/default/files/oralhealth/oral healthframework.pdf

US Department of Health and Human Services (HHS), Centers for Disease Control and Prevention. (2020). *National diabetes statistics report 2020: Estimates of diabetes and its burden in the United States.* www.cdc.gov/diabetes/pdfs/data/statistics/national-diabetes-statistics-report.pdf

Vasiliou, A., Shankardass, K., Nisenbaum, R., & Quiñonez, C. (2016). Current stress and poor oral health. *BMC Oral Health, 16*(1), 88. https://doi.org/10.1186/s12903-016-0284-y

Walker, K. K., Jackson, R. D., Sommariva, S., Neelamegam, M., & Desch, J. (2019). USA dental health providers' role in HPV vaccine communication and HPV-OPC protection: A systematic review. *Human Vaccines & Immunotherapeutics, 15*(7-8), 1863–1869. https://doi.org/10.1080/21645515.2018.1558690

Wang, Y., Zeng, X., Yang, X., Que, J., Du, Q., Zhang, Q., & Zou, J. (2021). Oral health, caries risk profiles, and oral microbiome of pediatric patients with leukemia submitted to chemotherapy. *Biomed Research International*, 6637503. https://doi.org/10.1155/2021/6637503

Watt, R. G., Daly, B., Allison, P., Macpherson, L., Venturelli, R., Listl, S., Weyant, R. J., Mathur, M. R., Guarnizo-Herreño, C. C., Celeste, R. K., Peres, M. A., Kearns, C., & Benzian, H. (2019). Ending the neglect of global oral health: Time for radical action. *Lancet (London, England), 394*(10194), 261–272. https://doi.org/10.1016/S0140-6736(19)31133-X

World Health Organization. (2021). *Diabetes.* Retrieved July 9, 2021, from www.who.int/news-room/fact-she ets/detail/diabetes

Yarbrough, C., Nasseh, K., & Vujicic, M. (2014). Key differences in dental care seeking behavior between Medicaid and non-Medicaid adults and children. *American Dental Association.* www.ada.org/~/media/ADA/Science%20and%20Research/HPI/Files/HPIBrief_0814_4.ashx

Zhang, X., Wang, M., Wang, X., Qu, H., Zhang, R., Gu, J., Wu, Y., Ni, T., Tang, W., & Li, Q. (2021). Relationship between periodontitis and microangiopathy in type 2 diabetes mellitus: A meta-analysis. *Journal of Periodontal Research, 56*(6), 1019–1027. https://doi.org/10.1111/jre.12916

25 Special Considerations for Men's Health

Demetrius J. Porche
School of Nursing
Louisiana State University Health Sciences Center
New Orleans, Louisiana, USA

CONTENTS

KEY POINTS

- A clear, definitive definition and medical specialization boundary does not exist for men's health nor for the special considerations for men's health lifestyle medicine.
- Men's health lifestyle medicine can be defined as the medical practices that impact the essential lifestyle behaviors that produce risk and protective factors that influence a man's physical, mental/psychological, emotional, spiritual, and social health status.
- Gender identity should be a consideration in all interactions with male clients/patients.
- Lifestyle-based interventions for erectile dysfunction are discussed, including ginseng and yohimbine, psychosexual counseling, cognitive behavioral therapy, and penile vacuum devices.

DOI: 10.1201/9781003178330-29

- Lifestyle choices impacting male infertility are explored, including cannabis and other recreational drug consumption, psychological stress, cigarette and alcohol consumption, obesity, diet, advanced paternal age, caffeine consumption, and other lifestyle choices.

25.1 INTRODUCTION

A clear, definitive definition and medical specialization boundary does not exist for men's health nor for the special considerations for men's health lifestyle medicine. Men's health has been characterized, described, and defined as a holistic and comprehensive approach including psychological, mental, emotional, social, and spiritual life experiences and the needs of men in all stages of life (Porche, 2007). Defining men's health serves as the basis for defining the research and practice necessary to improve men's health outcomes. Bardehle et al., (2017) examined the scientific and grey literature using international and national databases from 1990 to 2014 to further explicate a definition of men's health. Bardehle et al. assert that men's health encompasses dimensions of health and disease relevant to men and boys, inclusive of the physical, mental, and social well-being state that results from a balance of both risk and protective factors. Lifestyle can impact the physical, mental/psychological, emotional, spiritual, and social state, thereby influencing men's health outcomes. As a specialized area of men's health lifestyle medicine, the following is offered as a definition or specialization boundary for men's health lifestyle medicine: The medical practices that impact the essential lifestyle behaviors that produce risk and protective factors that influence a man's physical, mental/psychological, emotional, spiritual, and social health status.

This chapter will focus on the following areas of men's health lifestyle medicine—gender identity issues, overweight and obesity, erectile dysfunction, male fertility, chronic prostatitis/chronic pelvic pain syndrome, prostate cancer, testicular dysfunction, and testicular cancer.

25.1.1 GENDER IDENTITY

Gender should be considered a different concept from sex when interacting with male clients/patients. Gender relates to how a person identifies internally and how the person expresses their gender externally. A person can use clothing, physical appearance, and behaviors to express their gender construction. Gender should no longer only be considered along with a binary classification system of man/woman or male/female. Sex is a person's biological factor inclusive of their genetic composition (XX or XY), reproductive organs, and hormone dominance. Sex is also not a binary construction. Gender identity is considered to follow a spectrum of expression. Gender identity can be fluid and not static. A person can also have no gender expression and be considered nonbinary or androgynous. It is important that all clinicians interact with clients/patients with an open mindset regarding gender presentation, gender identity, and gender expression.

25.2 OVERWEIGHT AND OBESITY

Overweight and obesity are known risk factors associated with several acute and chronic illnesses such as but not limited to cardiovascular disease, type 2 diabetes, and osteoarthritis (Robertson et al., 2017). Overweight and obesity are evaluated using the body mass index (BMI). A BMI between 25 to < 30 kg/m^2 is considered overweight and a BMI > 30 kg/m^2 is obese (Campbell et al., 2015). Reduction in total body fat through weight loss is recommended as a men's health strategy to reduce other chronic illnesses. Robertson et al. (2017) suggested that weight loss in men is best achieved through a combination of reducing dietary caloric intake, increased physical activity, and behavior change techniques such as information on diet and exercise and teaching of coping strategies (Robertson et al., 2017).

Lifestyle interventions for overweight and obese men may need adjustments based on race/ethnicity. Griffith et al. (2018) conducted a systematic literature review that identified the need for targeted and tailored interventions for increasing male physical activity among African American and Latino men. Incorporation of male gender and manhood topics into physical activity interventions for African American and Latino men demonstrated more effectiveness with increasing physical activity (Griffith et al., 2018).

25.3 ERECTILE DYSFUNCTION (ED)

Erectile dysfunction is defined as the persistent inability to obtain or maintain sufficient rigidity of the penis to permit satisfactory sexual performance. A common lay term used for erectile dysfunction is "impotence." Erectile dysfunction affects about 30% to 50% of men aged 49 to 70. About 20% of the erectile dysfunction cases have an etiology of psychological causes. Approximately 80% of the erectile dysfunction cases are of organic causes, such as cardiovascular disease or spinal cord injury. Risk factors impacting the presence of erectile dysfunction are age, smoking, and obesity (Khera & Goldstein, 2011).

In addition to medical therapies to treat erectile dysfunction, it is important to consider lifestyle-based interventions that have been demonstrated to influence erectile dysfunction. Lifestyle-based interventions for erectile dysfunction include supplemental nutrients such as ginseng and yohimbine. Psychosexual counseling and cognitive behavior therapy are known to improve sexual functioning in which psychological factors are involved. Other lifestyle-based interventions include penile vacuum devices.

The American Urological Association (AUA) erectile dysfunction clinical guidelines recommend referral for mental health services to promote treatment adherence, reduce performance anxiety, and integrate treatments into sexual relationships. The AUA erectile dysfunction clinical practice guidelines also include recommendations for lifestyle interventions increasing physical activity, vacuum devices, and penile prosthesis implantation (Burnett et al., 2018).

25.3.1 GINSENG AND YOHIMBINE

Red ginseng has limited evidence but has been demonstrated to improve erectile function rates compared to placebo. The red ginseng dosage was 0.5 to 2.0 g daily. Some negative symptoms associated with red ginseng were headache, insomnia, gastric upset, and constipation (Jang et al., 2008).

Yohimbine was identified to improve erectile response as measured by penile rigidity and sexual function. The dosage of yohimbine was 36 mg daily. The adverse effects were agitation, anxiety, headache, a mild increase in blood pressure, increased urinary output, and gastrointestinal upset (Ernst & Pittler, 1998).

25.3.2 PSYCHOSEXUAL COUNSELING

Psychosexual counseling has some demonstrated effectiveness alone and with medical therapies. Psychosexual counseling is considered talk therapy by a "sex therapist." Psychosexual counseling engages the male in discussions about intimacy as a means to improve their sexual satisfaction (Melnik et al., 2008).

25.3.3 COGNITIVE BEHAVIORAL THERAPY

Cognitive behavioral therapy focuses on eliciting and modifying maladaptive thoughts and addressing relationship issues in addition to psychosexual counseling. Both psychosexual and cognitive behavioral therapy are effective alone and in combination with medical therapy (Khera & Goldstein, 2011).

25.3.4 PENILE VACUUM DEVICE

Penile vacuum devices promote engorgement of the penis to increase penile rigidity used alone and in combination with medical therapy and psychosexual and cognitive behavioral therapy. These penile vacuum devices may increase penile rigidity but are less effective in promoting an orgasm. Penile vacuum and other restrictive devices (penile rings) may also result in blocking ejaculation during orgasm (Khera & Goldstein, 2011; Wylie et al., 2003).

25.4 MALE INFERTILITY

Male infertility is the inability to conceive a child with unprotected sexual intercourse between a man and woman for a year or longer. Male infertility is estimated to impact approximately 48.5 million couples, which is about 15% of couples globally. Male infertility frequently results from an etiologic combination of male and female fertility issues. Males are estimated to be the sole etiology in about 20% to 30% of all infertility cases but contribute to about 50% of all cases overall (Agarwal et al., 2015). Agarwal et al. reported that there are at least 30 million men worldwide who are infertile, with the highest rates of infertility in Africa and Eastern Europe.

Male infertility can result from low sperm production, abnormal sperm production, or anatomical blockages that prevent the delivery of sperm into the ejaculate or semen. Semet et al. (2017) reported that cytotoxic drugs along with other medications can impact male fertility through the modification of the hypothalamic–pituitary–gonadal axis hormones or by non-hormonal mechanisms that directly or indirectly precipitate sexual dysfunction and spermatogenesis impairment. Drugs can also cause an alteration of epididymal maturation leading to male infertility (Semet et al., 2017). In addition to drugs impacting male fertility, several lifestyle choices impact male infertility, such as cannabis and other recreational drug consumption, psychological stress, cigarette and alcohol consumption, obesity, diet, advanced paternal age, caffeine consumption, and other lifestyle choices.

25.4.1 CANNABIS AND OTHER RECREATIONAL DRUG CONSUMPTION

Cannabis has been demonstrated to negatively impact male fertility. Cannabis consumption results in reducing sperm count, sperm concentration, inducing abnormalities in sperm morphology, reduction in sperm motility and viability, and inhibiting capacitation and fertilizing capacity (Payne et al., 2019).

Durairajanayagam (2017) indicated that recreational drug usage of cocaine disrupts spermatogenesis and damages the testicular ultrastructure. Men with long term cocaine usage (> 5 years) demonstrated lower sperm concentration and motility and a higher fraction of abnormal sperm morphology. Anabolic-androgenic steroids (AAS) usage is associated with anabolic steroid-induced hypogonadism (ASIH). AAS is associated with reversible suppression of spermatogenesis, testicular atrophy, and infertility. Durairajanayagam suggests discouraging the usage of AAS to improve male fertility.

25.4.2 PSYCHOLOGICAL STRESS

Stress has been indicated as both a primary and independent factor of male infertility. The stress response activates the sympathetic nervous system involving the hypothalamus–pituitary–adrenal axis, which exerts a gonadotropin-inhibitory hormone effect that also impacts the testicular Leydig cells (Durairajanayagam, 2017). Stress is also linked with depression, anxiety, obesity, alcohol, and tobacco consumption. Stress has been associated with low testosterone production and the resultant impact on male spermatogenesis. Lifestyle choices that reduce or facilitate the management of stress, such as counseling to improve coping skills, exercise, and a positive growth mindset, can positively impact psychological stress and male infertility (Hall & Burt, 2012).

25.4.3 CIGARETTE AND ALCOHOL CONSUMPTION

Cigarette smoking exposes the male to over 7,000 chemicals and other hazardous substances, such as tar, nicotine, carbon monoxide, and heavy metals. Cigarette smoking is a known potential factor for decreased male fertility. Smoking is associated with leukocytospermia, reduced sperm count, impaired sperm motility, and abnormal sperm morphology. The reduction in sperm count was associated stronger with heavy (> 20 cigarettes/day) and moderate consumption (10 to 20 cigarettes/day) as compared to mild smoking (< 10 cigarettes/day) (Durairajanayagam, 2017). Positive lifestyle changes of preconception counseling to reduce or eliminate tobacco consumption can improve male fertility.

Alcohol consumption has been associated with reduced semen volume and abnormal sperm morphology. Alcohol consumption also interferes with the HPG axis, production of GnRH, follicle stimulating hormone, luteinizing hormone, and testosterone production. Alcohol consumption also negatively impacts Leydig and Sertoli cells (Durairajanayagam, 2017). Durairajanayagam indicated that the effect of alcohol consumption on male fertility is dependent upon the intake amount; however, a systematic literature review did not indicate a threshold amount beyond which the male becomes at risk for male infertility. Alcohol consumption in moderation can positively impact male fertility.

25.4.4 OVERWEIGHT AND OBESITY

Men who are overweight and obese are at increased risk for a decrease in sperm quality and greater risk for infertility. Weight loss and lowering of the BMI are associated with improved sperm quality in some men (Durairajanayagam, 2017).

25.4.5 DIET

A diet of processed meat, full-fat dairy products, alcohol, coffee, and sugar-sweetened beverages are associated with poor semen quality. In contrast, a diet of vegetables, fruits, fish, poultry, cereals, and low-fat dairy products were associated more positively with sperm quality. A Mediterranean (enriched with omega-3 fatty acids, antioxidants, vitamins, and low saturated and trans-fatty acids) or a Prudent diet (white meat, fruit, vegetables, and whole grains) was more positively associated with positive sperm quality (Durairajanayagam, 2017).

25.4.6 ADVANCED PATERNAL AGE

Advanced paternal age is not well defined for men. Most studies commonly define advanced paternal age as between 35 and 50 years of age. Advanced paternal age is associated with a decline in semen volume, total sperm count, progressive sperm motility issues, and abnormal sperm morphology. Lifestyle decisions about the age at which one pursues parenting are important for fertility.

25.4.7 CAFFEINE CONSUMPTION

There is not a firm association between caffeine consumption and fertility. Some studies have indicated that caffeine consumption through cola consumption may have a greater impact on fertility than through intake from coffee, tea, or cocoa drinks (Durairajanayagam, 2017).

25.4.8 OTHER LIFESTYLE CHOICES IMPACTING FERTILITY

Genital heat stress and sleep disturbances are associated with male fertility issues. Genital heat stress creates scrotal hyperthermia, which increases risk of male infertility. Genital heat stress is associated with prolonged hours of sitting, cycling sports, sauna usage, tight fitting underwear, exposure to radiant heat, and the presence of a hydrocele or cryptorchidism. Men who experience sleep disturbances may also experience issues with fertility. Sleep disturbances have been associated with low semen volume (Durairajanayagam, 2017).

25.5 PROSTATITIS AND PELVIC PAIN SYNDROME

Chronic prostatitis and chronic pelvic pain syndrome (CP/CPPS) are experienced by men together. It is estimated that the prevalence of chronic prostatitis and pelvic pain syndrome is about 2.2 to 9.7% globally. Age greater than 65 years, nightshift work that interferes with circadian rhythms, stress, cigarette smoking, alcohol consumption, imbalanced diet, frequent sexual activity that delays ejaculation, and holding urine are potential lifestyle risk factors for CP/CPPS. Severe pain had a greater association with sedentary lifestyle, drinking caffeinated beverages, and less water intake. Inadequate water intake was associated with both CP and CPPS. Lifestyle modifications recommended to reduce CP and CPPS include regular physical activity, avoidance of caffeinated drinks, and increasing water intake daily (Chen et al., 2016).

25.6 PROSTATE CANCER

The incidence of prostate cancer is higher in the United States than among men in other countries. Several lifestyle factors may have a positive impact on slowing the progression of prostate cancer, mitigating the adverse effects of prostate cancer treatment, and improving quality of life. There is sufficient evidence of the benefit of exercise and pelvic floor muscle training (PFMT) on prostate cancer. Men with prostate cancer reported improvements in physical functioning, quality of life, prostate cancer prognosis, and prostate cancer mortality with exercise that ranged from moderate activity (brisk walking) to vigorous activity (jogging, swimming, or biking). Pelvic floor muscle training improves incontinence, resulting in an improved quality of life. There is limited evidence that dietary lifestyle factors such as pomegranate, soy, or omega-3 fatty acids provide any clinical benefit. A healthy BMI and smoking cessation positively improve clinical outcomes and increase survival of prostate cancer patients. There is limited evidence that diets high in lycopene/tomatoes may improve prostate cancer outcomes (Zuniga et al., 2020).

25.7 TESTICULAR DYSFUNCTION

Testicular dysfunction can include testicular cancer, testicular torsion, and cryptorchidism. Testicular dysfunction can impact spermatogenesis. Testicular function can be impacted by environmental exposure and lifestyle factors. Lifestyle factors that may impact testicular function include heat exposure, estrogens, androgens, alcohol, smoking, ionizing radiations, tadalafil, and prolonged urban automotive driving (Agarwal et al., 2008). Testicular temperature within the scrotum is about 1 to 2 degrees Celsius lower than the core body temperature. An increase in testicular temperature can impact spermatogenesis. Exposure to environmental toxins such as lead and phthalates is harmful and should be avoided (Agarwal et al., 2008).

25.7.1 TESTICULAR CANCER

Testicular cancer is the most prevalent cancer among men aged between 15 and 40 years. Testicular cancer risk factors include cryptorchidism, genitourinary system abnormalities, and endocrine abnormalities and dysfunction (Rovito et al., 2015). The American Cancer Society recommends testicular self-examination (TSE) as an effective strategy for early identification and diagnosis of prostate cancer. TSE should be taught and encouraged as a normal lifestyle practice (ACS, 2014; Rovito et al., 2015).

25.8 MENTAL HEALTH

Depression and anxiety are the leading mental health conditions. Mental health conditions increase the risk of chronic illnesses and can reduce life expectancy by 12 to 15 years (Drew et al., 2020). Drew et al. conducted a systematic literature review and meta-analysis that determined that male-only lifestyle interventions are effective on men's psychological outcomes and mental health. Male-only lifestyle interventions were effective in a variety of settings such as sports clubs, workplaces, universities, or clinics. The male-only lifestyle interventions that were effective consisted of counseling, nutrition education, and physical exercise (Drew et al., 2020).

25.9 CONCLUSION

Lifestyle medicine has the potential to positively impact men's health issues inclusive of male specific disorders involving the male genital and reproductive organs. Common lifestyle medicine strategies include balanced diet low in calories, saturated fat; physical activity, reduction or elimination of alcohol and tobacco consumption, and stress reduction.

REFERENCES

Agarwal, A., Desai, N., Ruffoli, R., & Carpi, A. (2008). Lifestyle and testicular dysfunction: A brief update. *Biomedicine & Pharmacotherapy*, *62*, 550–553.

Agarwal, A., Mulgund, A., Hamada, A., & Chyatte, M. R. (2015). A unique view on male infertility around the globe. *Reproductive Biology and Endocrinology*, *13*(1), 1–9. https://doi.org/10.1186/s12958-015-0032-1

American Cancer Society. (2014). Can testicular cancer be found early? Retrieved from www.cancer.org/cancer/testicular-cancer/detection-diagnosis-staging/detection.html

Bardehle, D., Dinges, M., & White, A. (2017). What is men's health? A definition. *Journal of Men's Health*, *13*, e40–52.

Burnett, A., Nehra, A., Breau, R., Culkin, D. J., Faraday, M. M., Hakim, L. S., Heidelbaugh, J., Khera, M., McVary, K. T., Miner, M. M., Nelson, C. J., Sadeghi-Nejad, H., Seftel, A. D., & Shindel, A. W. (2018). Erectile dysfunction: AUA guideline. *The Journal of Urology*, *200*, 633–641.

Campbell, J., Lane, M., Owens, J., & Bakos, H. (2015). Paternal obesity negatively affects male fertility and associated reproduction outcomes: A systematic review and meta-analysis. *Reproductive Biomedicine Online*, *31*, 593–604.

Chen, X., Hu, C., Peng, Y., Lu, J., Yang, N., Chen, L., Zhang, G., Tang, L., & Dai, J. (2016). Association of diet and lifestyle with chronic prostatitis/chronic pelvic pain syndrome and pain severity: A case-control study. *Prostate Cancer and Prostatic Diseases*, *19*, 92–99.

Drew, R., Morgan, P., Pollock, E., & Young, M. (2020). Impact of male-only lifestyle interventions on men's mental health: A systematic review and meta-analysis. *Obesity Reviews*, *21*, e13104.

Durairajanayagam, D. (2017). Lifestyle causes of male infertility. *Arab Journal of Urology*, *16*, 10–20.

Ernst, E., Pittler, M. (1998). Yohimbine for erectile dysfunction: A systematic review and meta-analysis of randomized controlled clinical trials. *Journal of Urology*, *159*, 433–436.

Griffith, D., Bergner, E., Cornish, E., & McQueen, C. (2018). Physical activity intervention with African American or Latin men: A systematic review. *American Journal of Men's Health*, *12*, 1102–1117.

Hall, E., & Burt, V. (2012). Male infertility: Psychiatric considerations. *Fertility and Sterility*, *97*, 434–439.

Jang, D., Lee, M., Shin, B. Lee, Y-C., & Ernst, E. (2008). Red ginseng for treating erectile dysfunction: A systematic review. *British Journal of Clinical Pharmacology*, *66*, 444–450.

Khera, M., & Goldstein, I. (2011). Erectile dysfunction. *British Medical Journal Clinical Evidence*, *29*, 1803.

Melnik, T., Soares, B., & Nasello, A. (2008). The effectiveness of psychological interventions for the treatment of erectile dysfunction: Systematic review and meta-analysis, including comparisons to sildenafil treatment, intracavernosal injection, and vacuum devices. *Journal of Sex Medicine*, 5, 2562–2574.

Payne, K., Mazur, D., Hotaling, J., & Pastuszak, A. (2019). Cannabis and male fertility: A systematic review. *Journal of Urology*, *202*, 674–681.

Porche, D. (2007). A call for the American Journal of Men's Health. *American Journal of Men's Health*, *1*, 5–7.

Robertson, C., Avenell, A., Stewart, F., Archibald, D., Douglas, F., Hoddinott, P., van Teijlingen, E., & Boyers, D. (2017). Clinical effectiveness of weight loss and weight maintenance interventions for men: A systematic review of men-only randomized controlled trials. *American Journal of Men's Health*, *11*, 1096–1123.

Rovito, M., Cavayero, C., Leone, J., & Harlin, S. (2015). Interventions promoting testicular self-examination (TSE) performance: A systematic review. *American Journal of Men's Health*, *9*, 506–518.

Semet, M., Paci, M., Saias-Magnan, J., Metzler-Guillermain, C., Boissier, R., Lejeune, H., & Perrin, J. (2017). The impact of drugs on male fertility: A review. *Andrology*, *S*, *5*(4), 640–663.

Wylie, K., Jones, R., & Walters, S. (2003). The potential benefit of vacuum devices augmenting psychosexual therapy for erectile dysfunctions: A randomized controlled trial. *Journal of Sex and Marital Therapy*, *29*, 227–236.

Zuniga, K., Chan, J., Ryan, C., & Kenfield, S. (2020). Diet and lifestyle considerations for patients with prostate cancer. *Urology Oncology*, *38*, 105–117.

26 Midwifery Approach to Lifestyle Medicine for Reproductive Health

Susan Altman[1] and Rebecca Feldman[1]
[1]Rory Meyers College of Nursing
New York University
New York, New York, USA

CONTENTS

KEY POINTS

- Midwifery and lifestyle medicine share common goals and core competencies.
- A lifestyle medicine approach has benefits for preconception and pregnancy.
- Eating disorder risk and history must be considered when considering nutritional interventions.
- The perimenopausal and menopausal transition can be assisted by a lifestyle approach.

26.1 INTRODUCTION

The American College of Nurse-Midwives (ACNM), the national professional organization of Certified Nurse-Midwives (CNMs) and Certified Midwives (CMs), defines midwifery as care provided to people that "encompasses a full range of primary health care services … from adolescence beyond menopause" (ACNM, n.d.). Midwives partner with diverse groups of people and their families, utilizing an understanding of social determinants in an effort to work within a model of care that "includes health promotion, disease prevention, and individualized wellness education and counseling" (ACNM, 2012).

DOI: 10.1201/9781003178330-30

ACNM Core Competencies for Basic Midwifery Practice, including the hallmarks of midwifery care, serve as a foundation for this practice. The midwifery model of care incorporates the concepts of

- Evidence-based care.
- Promotion of person-centered care for all.
- Empowerment of those persons seeking midwifery care as partners in their own health care.
- Facilitation of healthy family and interpersonal relationships through communication and counseling.
- Collaboration, consultation, and referral to other members of the interprofessional health care team (ACNM, 2019).

Fundamental core competencies for basic midwifery practice emphasize the midwife's role in providing strategies and therapeutics to facilitate health and promote healthy behaviors in order to prevent disease. Core competencies of lifestyle medicine, established as the minimum guidelines for those practicing lifestyle medicine, include the use of evidence-based care, health promotion, lifestyle changes, relationship building, including family support, and the incorporation of the interdisciplinary team to prevent disease and improve health outcomes (Lianov, 2010). While overlapping with many of the broad-based midwifery competencies, this discipline further concentrates their focus on specific modalities to improve well-being.

26.1.1 INTERSECTION OF MIDWIFERY AND LIFESTYLE MEDICINE

Evaluation and treatment through a holistic lens to promote healthy lifestyle changes and behaviors is key to both midwifery and lifestyle medicine approaches. Building trusting relationships through shared decision making, tenets of both disciplines, fosters a commitment by participants that can ultimately lead to their long-term success. While lifestyle medicine can be and is often considered a newly emerging "stand alone specialty," it has been designed for use by a broad range of providers (Sayburn, 2018), including midwives. Many of its foundational principles, including evidence-based practice, health promotion and education, and interprofessional collaboration, are in alignment with those incorporated in the longstanding midwifery model of care. In addition, the midwifery focus on health care equity and reproductive justice is complementary to the work of lifestyle medicine. Midwives strive to make lifestyle recommendations culturally appropriate, and to view these recommendations through the lens of health equity. Midwives are well positioned to work with women and persons seeking reproductive health care while incorporating a lifestyle medicine approach to improve health care outcomes.

26.2 PRECONCEPTION: PREPARING FOR PREGNANCY THROUGH LIFESTYLE OPTIMIZATION

Ideally, optimal lifestyle preparation begins before pregnancy (Gluckman et al., 2014). Though the definition for this exact timeframe has not been standardized (Dean et al., 2013), preconception has long been considered approximately three months prior to conception (Stephenson et al., 2018). As defined by the World Health Organization (WHO, 2013), preconception care is "the provision of biomedical, behavioral and social health interventions to women and couples before conception occurs." Actively planning and preparing for pregnancy by subscribing to a healthy lifestyle and minimizing behaviors that can negatively impact pregnant persons and their offspring helps ensure positive outcomes.

Developing and fostering habits in the preconception period that help ensure a healthy way of life through the critical periods of conception and the first trimester is crucial for appropriate placental, embryonic, and fetal development. A number of observational studies link health before pregnancy with long-term outcomes extending to future generations, in addition to pregnancy and birth outcomes (Stephenson et al., 2018). Research in the area of epigenetics and "fetal programming" suggests an association between obesity, poor nutrition, and unhealthy lifestyle during the preconception period (Kudesia et al., 2021) and long-term risk of cardiovascular disease in offspring (Steegers, 2014).

Early incorporation of certain lifestyle recommendations into the preconception period has positive impacts on pregnancy and birth outcomes. Daily oral folic acid supplementation (400 micrograms daily) and consumption of foods with folate well before conception (CDC, 2021), both endorsed as standards by the CDC, have been reported to reduce the risk of neural tube defects in newborns by as much as 70% (Stephenson et al., 2018). The role of multivitamin supplementation, inclusive of those with iron and calcium, are documented to have a critical role in fetal development (Wilson et al., 2018). Accordingly, the March of Dimes, recommends that individuals begin taking prenatal multivitamins before pregnancy (March of Dimes, 2020).

Those who intentionally plan a pregnancy may prepare by improving the state of their health prior to pregnancy. Data from one retrospective cross-sectional study of 430 Flemish women, with planned pregnancy ending in birth, revealed that a majority of the participants (83%) stated that they made one or more lifestyle changes in anticipation of pregnancy. Improved nutritional choices, smoking and caffeine reduction or cessation, and achievement of healthier overall body weight were among the changes initiated. Eighty-six percent reported that advice from their professional provider assisted them in making these changes (Goossens et al., 2018).

Despite the wealth of evidence that preconception health is integral to pregnancy success and healthy birth outcomes, there are high rates of poor preconception lifestyle habits throughout the developed world (Kudesia et al., 2021). Though many people are highly motivated to make lifestyle changes before a planned pregnancy (Geyer et al., 2021), approximately half of all pregnancies in the US are unintended (Finer, 2016). This leaves little or no time for individuals to seek formal care regarding lifestyle practices in advance of conception. Due to the high unplanned pregnancy rate, the concept of providing optimal health care throughout the lifespan (King et al., 2019), rather than focusing solely on targeted visits during the time of "preconception," can benefit all individuals of reproductive age. This approach is also in alignment with ACNM's position, which asserts that "improvement in a woman's overall health status and access to healthcare services has the potential to improve her reproductive health" (ACNM, 2013). Preventative care with a focus on a healthy lifestyle approach should be prioritized for those of reproductive age. Prescriptions may include individualized approaches to maintaining optimal nutrition and weight management, adequate physical activity, avoidance of alcohol and tobacco, and stress reduction techniques such as meditation and mindfulness. It is important for clinicians to keep in mind that access to preventative lifestyle measures is not equitable in all populations and communities, and barriers disproportionately affect those who are in greatest need of these interventions. Providers must recognize these barriers and assist patients with obtaining and implementing lifestyle services within their communities to help address racial, ethnic, and socioeconomic inequalities. Midwives are uniquely positioned to support a healthy lifestyle, including the healthy "preconception period," which may occur at any point during the lifespan of a reproductive aged person. As trusted health care providers, clients turn to midwives, who can, in turn, prescribe wellness habits and lifestyle changes supportive of healthy life, healthy preconception, and healthy pregnancy.

26.3 LIFESTYLE PRESCRIPTIONS FOR IMPROVING HEALTH IN PREGNANCY

Pregnancy is a time when many people feel motivated for lifestyle change. Those who may have generally felt less motivated to make healthful choices regarding substance and tobacco use, sleep hygiene and nutrition often find pregnancy a time when these choices feel more feasible.

26.3.1 Exercise

Exercise has numerous, well-documented benefits during pregnancy. Regular exercise of 20 to 30 minutes per day is recommended for healthy pregnant individuals on most days of the week (ACOG, 2020). Strong evidence exists for reduced rates of gestational diabetes and excess weight gain (Dipietro et al., 2019), and evidence also suggests that shorter labors are more likely with regular exercise (Barakat et al., 2018). Incidence of preeclampsia may be reduced with higher rates of exercise (Aune et al., 2014; Kasawara et al., 2012). Currently, 23–28% of United States women meet the minimum recommended amount of daily exercise (Dipietro et al., 2019). Given these low rates for exercise, and the numerous benefits, specific suggestions for exercise from nurses and mid-wives can provide a supportive intervention for overall well-being in pregnancy.

26.3.2 Nutrition

The literature on nutritional changes in pregnancy is limited to prospective or retrospective studies, but these studies confirm that pregnancy is a time when people are more likely to make nutritional modifications (Hillier & Olander, 2017). Clinicians working with preconception or pregnant indi-viduals are more likely to find receptivity and interest in learning about nutrition than in other times in clients' lives. Pregnant individuals also benefit from receiving clear nutritional guidance from nurses and midwives who have sufficient training in providing this information (Forbes et al., 2018).

26.3.3 Mood in Pregnancy and Postpartum

Perinatal mood disorders are the most common complication of pregnancy. These disorders include depression, anxiety, bipolar disorder, PTSD, and postpartum psychosis. Estimates of prevalence range between 10 and 20% of new mothers. Rates of perinatal mood disorders are considerably higher for mothers of color, and rates for screening and treatment are lower. For new fathers, estimates for mood disorders are approximately 10%, but this is an area with considerably less research (Cox et al., 2016; Luca et al., 2020; Meltzer-Brody & Jones, 2015; Sidebottom et al., 2020). Depression during pregnancy is associated with small for gestational age babies and preterm birth. Postpartum depression is associated with poor infant–parent attachment, and learning and cognitive delays in offspring (Santos, 2014). The largest risk factor for perinatal depression is a previous his-tory of depression. The largest risk factor for postpartum depression is depression during pregnancy (Byatt et al., 2016; Wilcox et al., 2018). Other risk factors include family history of depression during or after pregnancy, lack of social support, lower socioeconomic status, lack of a partner, and pregnancy complications (USPSTF, 2019).

There are no clinical guidelines regarding prevention of perinatal mood disorders. Current research has examined a variety of approaches for prevention of perinatal depression. In 2019, the United States Preventative Task Force conducted a systematic review examining the evidence for prevention of peri-natal depression. Cognitive behavioral therapy (CBT) and interpersonal therapy (IPT) approaches have the most robust evidence for prevention of perinatal depression (USPSTF, 2019). A small number of studies looked at exercise as preventative for perinatal depression (Norman et al., 2019; Songøygard et al., 2012; Perales et al., 2015). Two of the three articles included in this review found evidence for exercise as attenuating perinatal depression (Norman et al., 2019; Perales et al., 2015).

Sleep during pregnancy is often impaired by physical discomforts as well as fluctuations in mood. Poor sleep quality can have an adverse effect on mood, leading to greater severity of perinatal mood disturbance (Mindell et al., 2015; Tomfohr et al., 2015). A 2021 systematic review of studies exam-ining sleep strategies as preventative for antenatal and postpartum depression showed the available evidence insufficient to reach conclusions, and further RCTs examining this intervention are needed (Sasaki et al., 2021). Sleep hygiene can be reviewed throughout pregnancy, as well as discussed as a strategy for helping to maintain euthymic mood.

26.4 EATING DISORDERS AND ORTHOREXIA: CONSIDERATIONS FOR LIFESTYLE INTERVENTIONS

Eating disorders include anorexia, bulimia, avoidant restrictive food intake disorder (ARFID), and binge eating disorder (DSM, 2013). Orthorexia nervosa, first described in 1997 by Steven Bratman, is defined as an obsession with healthy eating where a person becomes hyper focused on quality of food (Cena et al., 2019). Though not included in the Diagnostic and Statistical Manual, this disorder has similar qualities to the included eating disorders, with most commonality with ARFID. Occurrence is difficult to measure due to the lack of validated psychometric screening tools. Estimates in the general population of orthorexic eating patterns range from 4.5 to 8% (Niedzielski & Kaźmierczak-Wojtaś, 2021).

As described throughout this book, healthful and wholesome eating has a multitude of benefits. However, for some, healthful eating becomes an all-consuming obsession and can impair their ability to function, enjoy life, and have healthy relationships. Unlike anorexia or bulimia, orthorexia is not largely characterized by a desire to change a person's body; the obsession is mostly related to the quality and perceived healthfulness and purity of food (Barnes & Caltabiano, 2017; Simpson & Mazzeo, 2017).

Risk factors for developing orthorexia include perfectionism, obsessive personality, history of disordered eating, and poor body image (Pauze et al., 2021). Other possible related factors are excessive exercise, being involved in a health-related study, and female gender (McComb & Mills, 2019). In order to guide clinical practice, more research into contributing factors and prevalence of orthorexia is needed (Dunn & Bratman, 2016).

Eating disorders are a mental health issue that tend to persist over the course of a person's lifetime. Puberty and adolescence are recognized as peak times for eating disorder development (Rodgers et al., 2014). While there may be years of remission, recurrence is always possible and can be triggered by life changes, including childbirth or menopause (Knoph et al., 2013), as well as postpartum (Knoph et al., 2013; Thompson et al., 2020). Increasingly, midlife, particularly around menopause, can be a time of new onset (Howard, 2020).

Those who identify as female have double the lifetime risk of eating disorder as those who identify as male, with a lifetime risk of 13% (Stice et al., 2020). These disorders carry lifelong health risks, including malnutrition, electrolyte imbalance, and cardiac arrest (Sachs et al., 2016). Anorexia is the mental illness with the highest mortality rate. Deaths due to anorexia are more than triple the rate of deaths due to bipolar disorder and depression, and approximately 20% of these deaths are due to suicide (Edakubo & Fushimi, 2020; Ward et al., 2015).

Clients with severe eating disorders are the most likely to be diagnosed and treated. However, more common than those with formal diagnosis of an eating disorder are the many people who fit the clinical picture of disordered eating. Many people who are normal weight or in a larger body find themselves fixated on eating perfectly, to the point where this impinges on quality of life (Howard, 2020; Wacker, 2018).

How can clinicians effectively make nutritional recommendations with these key issues in mind? Obtaining a full history is necessary. This history should include asking about personal or family history of eating disorders, obsession with food or quality of food, excessive exercise, or prior struggles with poor body image. Knowing all of this information is helpful to give nuanced dietary advice that considers the full picture of health for each individual.

26.5 PERIMENOPAUSE AND MENOPAUSE

Another season in a person's life in which hormonal influence and changes play a major role is perimenopause and menopause. Perimenopause consists of the years leading up to the loss of menses, and can vary in length considerably, with average length being between four and eight years. Symptoms during this time generally consist of changes in length or timing of menstrual cycle, night sweats, and mood changes. Menopause is defined as the natural event of cessation of menses for a duration of 12 months, and usually occurs between the ages of 45 and 55 (Shifren, 2014). While some find the transition manageable, others may seek treatment and medical intervention for this life phase. Below is a review of the evidence for lifestyle interventions for the perimenopausal or menopausal person.

26.5.1 EXERCISE

Exercise is one of the most frequent recommendations for bothersome symptoms of perimenopause (Nyugen et al., 2020). Forty to sixty percent of people report trying exercise regimens to manage vasomotor symptoms of menopause (Mendoza, 2016). Walking is a commonly prescribed exercise. Preliminary evidence supports its use for the improvement of menopause-related medical issues such as mood changes, sleep problems, and vasomotor symptoms (Sydora et al., 2020). As with other lifestyle interventions specific to women's and reproductive health, more research into the specific role of exercise during perimenopause and menopause is needed. However, available evidence does support routine exercise for its role in potential reduction of symptoms as well as overall health maintenance.

26.5.2 SLEEP HYGIENE

Decreased quality of sleep is a common complaint during menopausal transition. Symptoms of night sweats and hot flashes can be difficult to manage and can interrupt sleep. Women in mid-life may be managing multiple stressors and life changes that may also disrupt sleep. The North American Menopause Society recommends sleep hygiene strategies as means to prevent some of the sleep difficulties of this time of life (Shifren, 2014).

Research regarding lifestyle interventions for sleep quality in perimenopause and menopause is limited. A 2020 report from the Study of Women's Health Across the Nation (SWAN) study examined the experience of 1,407 women enrolled in the study and looked at sleep and vasomotor symptoms over ten years. While the majority of study participants did rate some level of sleep disturbance, the authors note that menopausal transition is not uniform and there is wide variation in the level of sleep disturbances. Therefore, prescriptions for sleep management techniques should take an individualized approach that is tailored to the specific needs of clients (Matthews et al., 2021).

26.5.3 STRESS MANAGEMENT

Menopausal symptoms may be exacerbated by stress, but may be mitigated by stress management strategies (Sood et al., 2019; Velez et al., 2014). Symptom severity may be worse when stress levels are perceived to be higher (Arnot et al., 2021). Mindfulness techniques for management of stress have promising evidence during the menopause transition. A 2019 cross-sectional study looked at mindfulness interventions with 1,744 midlife women. This research suggests that mindfulness techniques help to lower levels of symptom severity (Sood et al., 2019). A 2019 systematic review and meta-analysis examined the evidence for psychological interventions and reduction in hot flash symptoms. Included studies examined mindfulness techniques and cognitive behavioral therapy use during menopause, and the authors concluded that these interventions reduced hot flash severity in the short and medium term (van Driel et al., 2019).

26.6   CONCLUSION

Midwifery and lifestyle medicine are complementary disciplines that provide comprehensive, individualized, and evidence-based reproductive health care throughout the lifespan. Promotion of healthy lifestyle practices during preconception and pregnancy allow individuals to optimize their wellness to achieve positive outcomes. In the postpartum period, the pillars of lifestyle medicine, such as sleep, social support, and reducing stress, are vital for promotion of well-being in a time when many are vulnerable to mood disturbance. Lifestyle interventions such as mindfulness and exercise are approaches that have been found to decrease perimenopausal and menopausal symptoms. Throughout all of a person's reproductive life, the focus on health equity and reproductive justice must be maintained. Intertwining the unique but complementary philosophies of midwifery and lifestyle medicine can help to alleviate barriers that stand in the way of inequitable care.

REFERENCES

American College of Lifestyle Medicine. (n.d.) *JAMA physician competencies for prescribing lifestyle medicine.* www.lifestylemedicine.org/ACLM/About/Core_Competencies/ACLM/About/What_is_Lifestyle_Medicine_/Core_Competencies.aspx?hkey=949ce5f3-757f-4b12-b658-6170fa510390

American College of Nurse Midwives. (n.d.). *About the midwifery profession.* www.midwife.org/About-the-Midwifery-Profession

American College of Nurse Midwives. (2019, October 27). *ACNM core competencies for basic midwifery practice.* www.midwife.org/acnm/files/acnmlibrarydata/uploadfilename/000000000050/ACNMCoreCompetenciesMar2020_final.pdf

American College of Nurse Midwives. (2012, February 6). Definition of midwifery and scope of practice of CNMs and CMs.

American College of Nurse Midwives. (2013). *Position statement: The role of the certified nurse-midwife/certified midwife in preconception health and health care.* www.midwife.org/acnm/files/ACNMLibraryData/UPLOADFILENAME/000000000081/Preconception%20Health%20and%20Health%20Care%20Feb%202013.pdf

American College of Obstetricians and Gynecologists. (2020, March 26). *Physical activity and exercise during pregnancy and the postpartum period.* www.acog.org/clinical/clinical-guidance/committee-opinion/articles/2020/04/physical-activity-and-exercise-during-pregnancy-and-the-postpartum-period

American College of Preventative Medicine. (n.d.). *Lifestyle medicine core competencies program.* www.acpm.org/education-events/continuing-medical-education/2019/lifestyle-medicine-core-competencies-program/

American Psychiatric Association. (2013). *Diagnostic and statistical manual of mental disorders* (5th ed.). https://doi.org/10.1176/appi.books.9780890425596

Arcelus, J., Mitchell, A. J., Wales, J., & Nielsen, S. (2011). Mortality rates in patients with anorexia nervosa and other eating disorders: A meta-analysis of 36 studies. *Archives of General Psychiatry, 68*(7), 724–731. http://doi.org/10.1001/archgenpsychiatry.2011.74

Arnot, M., Emmott, E. H., & Mace, R. (2021). The relationship between social support, stressful events, and menopause symptoms. *PloS One, 16*(1). https://doi.org/10.1371/journal.pone.0245444

Aune, D., Saugstad, O. D., Henriksen, T., & Tonstad, S. (2014). Physical activity and the risk of preeclampsia: A systematic review and meta-analysis. *Epidemiology (Cambridge, Mass.), 25*(3), 331–343. https://doi.org/10.1097/EDE.0000000000000036

Barakat, R., Franco, E., Perales, M., López, C., & Mottola, M. F. (2018). Exercise during pregnancy is associated with a shorter duration of labor: A randomized clinical trial. *European Journal of Obstetrics and Gynecology, 224,* 33–40. https://doi-org.proxy.library.nyu.edu/10.1016/j.ejogrb.2018.03.009

Barnes, M., & Caltabiano, M. (2017). The interrelationship between orthorexia nervosa, perfectionism, body image and attachment style. *Eating and Weight Disorders, 22,* 177–184. h https://doi.org/10.1007/s40519-016-0280-x

Bauer, A., Knapp, M., & Parsonage, M., (2016). Lifetime costs of perinatal anxiety and depression. *Journal of Affective Disorders, 192,* 83–90. https://doi.org/10.1016/j.jad.2015.12.005

Berglund, C., & Bell, R., (2018). Dietary change during pregnancy and women's reasons for change. *Nutrients, 10*(8), 1032. https://doi.org/10.3390/nu10081032

Birmingham, C. L., Su, J., Hlynsky, J. A., Goldner, E. M., & Gao, M. (2005). The mortality rate from anorexia nervosa. *International Journal of Eating Disorders, 38*(2), 143–146. https://doi-org.proxy.library.nyu.edu/10.1002/eat.20164

Bratman, S. (1997, September/October). Health food junkie. *Yoga Journal*, 42–50.

Byatt, N., Xiao, R. S., Dinh, K. H., & Waring, M. E. (2016). Mental health care use in relation to depressive symptoms among pregnant women in the USA. *Archives of Women's Mental Health*, *19*(1), 187–191. https://doi.org/10.1007/s00737-015-0524-1

Cena, H., Barthels, F., Cuzzolaro, M., Bratman, S., Brytek-Matera, A., Dunn, T., Varga, M., Missbach, B., & Donini, L. M. (2019). Definition and diagnostic criteria for orthorexia nervosa: A narrative review of the literature. *Eating and Weight Disorders*, *24*, 209–246. https://doi.org/10.1007/s40519-018-0606-y

Center for Disease Control and Prevention (2021, April 19). *Folic acid*. www.cdc.gov/ncbddd/folicacid/about.html

Cox, E. Q., Sowa, N. A., Meltzer-Brody, S. E., & Gaynes, B. N. (2016). The perinatal depression treatment cascade: Baby steps toward improving outcomes. *The Journal of Clinical Psychiatry*, *77*(9), 1189–1200. https://doi.org/10.4088/JCP.15r10174

Dean, S., Rudan, I., Althabe, F., Webb Girard, A., Howson, C., Langer, A., Lawn, J., Reeve, M. E., Teela, K. C., Toledano, M., Venkatraman, C. M., Belizan, J. M., Car, J., Chan, K. Y., Chatterjee, S., Chitekwe, S., Doherty, T., Donnay, F., Ezzati, M., ... Bhutta, Z. A. (2013). Setting research priorities for preconception care in low- and middle-income countries: aiming to reduce maternal and child mortality and morbidity. *PLoS Medicine*, *10*(9), e1001508. https://doi.org/10.1371/journal.pmed.1001508

Dipietro, L., Evenson, K. R., Bloodgood, B., Sprow, K., Troiano, R. P., Piercy, K. L., Vaux-Bjerke, A., Powell, K. E., & 2018 Physical Activity Guidelines Advisory Committee. (2019). Benefits of physical activity during pregnancy and postpartum: An umbrella review. *Medicine and Science in Sports and Exercise*, *51*(6), 1292–1302. https://doi.org/10.1249/MSS.0000000000001941

Dunn, T. M., & Bratman, S. (2016). On orthorexia nervosa: A review of the literature and proposed diagnostic criteria. *Eating Behaviors*, *21*, 11–17. https://doi-org.proxy.library.nyu.edu/10.1016/j.eatbeh.2015.12.006

Edakubo, S., & Fushimi, K. (2020). Mortality and risk assessment for anorexia nervosa in acute-care hospitals: A nationwide administrative database analysis. *BMC Psychiatry*, *20*(1), 1–8. https://doi-org.proxy.library.nyu.edu/10.1186/s12888-020-2433-8

Finer, L. B., & Zolna, M. R. (2016). Declines in unintended pregnancy in the United States, 2008–2011. *The New England Journal of Medicine*, *374*(9), 843–852. https://doi.org/10.1056/NEJMsa1506575

Forbes, L. E., Graham, J. E., Berglund, C., & Bell, R. C. (2018). Dietary change during pregnancy and women's reasons for change. *Nutrients*, *10*(8), 1032. https://doi.org/10.3390/nu10081032

Geyer, C., McHugh, J., & Tollefson, M. (2021). Lifestyle medicine for women: The time is now! *American Journal of Lifestyle Medicine*, *15*(4), 366–371. https://doi.org/10.1177/15598276211004233

Gluckman, P., Hanson, M., Seng, C., & Bardsley, A. (2014). Nutrition and lifestyle for pregnancy and breastfeeding. Oxford University Press. https://oxfordmedicine.com/view/10.1093/med/9780198722700.001.0001/med-9780198722700

Goossens, J., Beeckman, D., Van Hecke, A., Delbaere, I., & Verhaeghe, S. (2018). Preconception lifestyle changes in women with planned pregnancies. *Midwifery*, *56*, 112–120. https://doi.org/10.1016/j.midw.2017.10.004

Hillier, S. & Olander, E., (2017). Women's dietary changes before and during pregnancy: A systematic review. *Midwifery*, *49*, 19–31. https://doi.org/10.1016/j.midw.2017.01.014

Howard, B. (2020). Not your daughter's eating disorder. *Prevention*, *72*(12), 32–39.

Howard, L. M., Heron, K. E., & Cramer, R. J. (2020). The deliberate denial of disordered eating behaviors scale: Development and initial validation in young women with subclinical disordered eating. *Journal of Psychopathology & Behavioral Assessment*, *42*(4), 774–786. https://doi-org.proxy.library.nyu.edu/10.1007/s10862-020-09819-2

Kasawara, K. T., do Nascimento, S. L., Costa, M. L., Surita, F. G., & e Silva, J. L. (2012). Exercise and physical activity in the prevention of pre-eclampsia: Systematic review. *Acta Obstetricia et Gynecologica Scandinavica*, *91*(10), 1147–1157. https://doi.org/10.1111/j.1600-0412.2012.01483.x

King, T. L., Brucker, M. C., Osborne, K., & Jevitt, C. M. (2019). *Varney's midwifery* (6th ed.). Jones & Bartlett.

Knoph, C., Von Holle, A., Zerwas, S., Torgersen, L., Tambs, K., Stoltenberg, C., Bulik, C. M., & Reichborn-Kjennerud, T. (2013). Course and predictors of maternal eating disorders in the postpartum period. *The International Journal of Eating Disorders*, *46*(4), 355–368. https://doi-org.proxy.library.nyu.edu/10.1002/eat.22088

Kudesia, R., Alexander, M., Gulati, M., Kennard, A., & Tollefson, M. (2021). Dietary approaches to women's sexual and reproductive health. *American Journal of Lifestyle Medicine*, *15*(4), 414–424. https://doi.org/10.1177/15598276211007113

Leung, S. S., Lee, A. M., Wong, D. F., Wong, C. M., Leung, K. Y., Chiang, V. C., Yung, W. K., Chan, S. W., & Chung, K. F. (2016). A brief group intervention using a cognitive-behavioural approach to reduce postnatal depressive symptoms: a randomised controlled trial. *Hong Kong Medical Journal = Xianggang yi xue za zhi*, *22*(Suppl. 2), S4–S8. https://pubmed.ncbi.nlm.nih.gov/26908335/

Lianov L, Johnson M. (2010). Physician competencies for prescribing lifestyle medicine. *JAMA*, *304*(2), 202–203. https://doi.org/10.1001/jama.2010.903

Luca, D. L., Margiotta, C., Staatz, C., Garlow, E., Christensen, A., & Zivin, K. (2020). Financial toll of untreated perinatal mood and anxiety disorders among 2017 births in the United States. *American Journal of Public Health*, *110*(6), 888–896. https://doi.org/10.2105/AJPH.2020.305619

March of Dimes. (2020). *Vitamins and other nutrients during pregnancy.* www.marchofdimes.org/pregnancy/vitamins-and-other-nutrients-during-pregnancy.aspx

Matthews, K. A., Chang, Y., Brooks, M. M., Crawford, S. L., Janssen, I., Joffe, H., Kravitz, H. M., Thurston, R. C., & El Khoudary, S. R. (2020). Identifying women who share patterns of reproductive hormones, vasomotor symptoms, and sleep maintenance problems across the menopause transition: Group-based multi-trajectory modeling in the Study of Women's Health Across the Nation. *Menopause (New York, N.Y.)*, *28*(2), 126–134. https://doi.org/10.1097/GME.0000000000001663

McComb, S. E., & Mills, J. S. (2019). Orthorexia nervosa: A review of psychosocial risk factors. *Appetite*, *140*, 50–75. https://doi.org/10.1016/j.appet.2019.05.005

Meltzer-Brody, S., & Jones, I. (2015). Optimizing the treatment of mood disorders in the perinatal period. *Dialogues in Clinical Neuroscience*, *17*(2), 207–218. https://doi.org/10.31887/DCNS.2015.17.2/smeltzerbrody

Mendoza, N., De Teresa, C., Cano, A., Godoy, D., Hita-Contreras, F., Lapotka, M., Llaneza, P., Manonelles, P., Martínez-Amat, A., Ocón, O., Rodríguez-Alcalá, L., Vélez, M., & Sánchez-Borrego, R. (2016). Benefits of physical exercise in postmenopausal women. *Maturitas*, *93*, 83–88. https://doi.org/10.1016/j.maturitas.2016.04.017

Mindell, J. A., Cook, R. A., & Nikolovski, J. (2015). Sleep patterns and sleep disturbances across pregnancy. *Sleep Medicine*, *16*(4), 483–488. https://doi.org/10.1016/j.sleep.2014.12.006

Niedzielski A, Kaźmierczak-Wojtaś N. (2021). Prevalence of orthorexia nervosa and its diagnostic tools—a literature review. *International Journal of Environmental Research and Public Health*, *18*(10). https://doi.org/10.3390/ijerph18105488

Norman, E., Sherburn, M., Osborne, R. H., & Galea, M. P. (2010). An exercise and education program improves well-being of new mothers: A randomized controlled trial. *Physical Therapy*, *90*(3), 348–355. https://doi.org/10.2522/ptj.20090139

Nguyen, T., Do, T., Tran, T., & Kim, J. (2020). Exercise and quality of life in women with menopausal symptoms: A systematic review and meta-analysis of randomized controlled trials. *International Journal of Environmental Research and Public Health*, *17*(19), 7049, https://doi.org/10.3390/ijerph17197049

Pauzé, A., Plouffe-Demers, M.-P., Fiset, D., Saint-Amour, D., Cyr, C., & Blais, C. (2021). The relationship between orthorexia nervosa symptomatology and body image attitudes and distortion. *Scientific Reports*, *11*(1), 1–15. https://doi.org/10.1038/s41598-021-92569-2

Perales, M., Refoyo, I., Coteron, J., Bacchi, M., & Barakat, R. (2015). Exercise during pregnancy attenuates prenatal depression. *Evaluation & the Health Professions*, *38*(1), 59–72. doi:10.1177/0163278714533566

Rodgers, R., Paxton, S., & McLean, S. (2014). A biopsychosocial model of body image concerns and disordered eating in early adolescent girls. *Journal of Youth & Adolescence*, *43*(5), 814–823. https://doi-org.proxy.library.nyu.edu/10.1007/s10964-013-0013-7

Sachs, K., Harnke, B., Mehler, P., & Krantz, M. (2016). Cardiovascular complications of anorexia nervosa: A systematic review. *International Journal of Eating Disorders*, *49*(3), 238–248. https://doi.org/10.1002/eat.22481

Santos, I. S., Matijasevich, A., Barros, A. J., & Barros, F. C. (2014). Antenatal and postnatal maternal mood symptoms and psychiatric disorders in pre-school children from the 2004 Pelotas Birth Cohort. *Journal of Affective Disorders*, *164*(100), 112–117. https://doi.org/10.1016/j.jad.2014.04.033

Sayburn, A., (2018). Lifestyle medicine: A new medical specialty? *BMJ (Online)*, *363*. https://doi-org.proxy.library.nyu.edu/10.1136/bmj.k4442

Sasaki, N., Yasuma, N., Obikane, E., Narita, Z., Sekiya, J., Inagawa, T., Nakajima, A., Yamada, Y., Yamazaki, R., Matsunaga, A., Saito, T., Imamura, K., Watanabe, K., Kawakami, N., & Nishi, D. (2021). Psycho-educational interventions focused on maternal or infant sleep for pregnant women to prevent the onset of antenatal and postnatal depression: A systematic review. *Neuropsychopharmacology Reports, 41*(1), 2–13. https://doi.org/10.1002/npr2.12155

Shifren, J. L., Gass, M. L., & NAMS Recommendations for Clinical Care of Midlife Women Working Group. (2014). The North American Menopause Society recommendations for clinical care of midlife women. *Menopause, 21*(10), 1038–1062. 10.1097/GME.0000000000000319

Simpson, C. C., & Mazzeo, S. E. (2017). Attitudes toward orthorexia nervosa relative to DSM-5 eating disorders. *The International Journal of Eating Disorders, 50*(7), 781–792. https://doi.org/10.1002/eat.22710

Sidebottom, A., Vacquier, M., LaRusso, E., Erickson, D., & Hardeman, R. (2021). Perinatal depression screening practices in a large health system: Identifying current state and assessing opportunities to provide more equitable care. *Archives of Women's Mental Health, 24*(1), 133–144. https://doi.org/10.1007/s00737-020-01035-x

Stephenson, J., Heslehurst, N., Hall, J., Schoenaker, D., Hutchinson, J., Cade, J., Poston, L., Barrett, G., Crozier, S., Barker, M., Kumaran, K., Yajnik, C., Baird, J., & Mishra, G. (2018). Before the beginning: Nutrition and lifestyle in the preconception period and its importance for future health. *Lancet, 391*(10132), 1830–1841. https://doi.org/10.1016/S0140-6736(18)30311-8

Stice, E., Rohde, P., Shaw, H., & Desjardins, C. (2020). Weight suppression increases odds for future onset of anorexia nervosa, bulimia nervosa, and purging disorder, but not binge eating disorder. *The American Journal of Clinical Nutrition, 112*(1). https://doi.org/10.1093/ajcn/nqaa146

Songøygard, K. M., Stafne, S. N., Evensen, K. A., Salvesen, K. Å., Vik, T., & Mørkved, S. (2012). Does exercise during pregnancy prevent postnatal depression? A randomized controlled trial. *Acta Obstetricia et Gynecologica Scandinavica, 91*(1), 62–67. https://doi.org/10.1111/j.1600-0412.2011.01262.x

Sood, R., Kuhle, C. L., Kapoor, E., Thielen, J. M., Frohmader, K. S., Mara, K. C., & Faubion, S. S. (2019). Association of mindfulness and stress with menopausal symptoms in midlife women. *Climacteric: The Journal of the International Menopause Society, 22*(4), 377–382. https://doi-org.proxy.library.nyu.edu/10.1080/13697137.2018.1551344

Steegers, E., (2014). Embryonale gezondheid en preconceptiezorg: belang voor huidige en toekomstige generaties [Embryonic health and preconception care: Importance for current and future generations]. *Nederlands Tijdschrift voor Geneeskunde, 158*, A7373. https://pubmed.ncbi.nlm.nih.gov/25027216/

Sydora, B.C., Alvadj, T., Malley, A., Mayan, M., Shandro, T., & Ross, S. (2020). Walking together: Women with the severe symptoms of menopause propose a platform for a walking program; outcome from focus groups. *BMC Women's Health*, 20, 165. https://doi.org/10.1186/s12905-020-01037-y

The North American Menopause Society. (2021). *Menopause FAQs: Understanding the symptoms.* www.menopause.org/for-women/expert-answers-to-frequently-asked-questions-about-menopause/menopause-faqs-understanding-the-symptoms

Thompson, K. (2020). An application of psychosocial frameworks for eating disorder risk during the postpartum period: A review and future directions. *Archives of Women's Mental Health, 23*(5), 625–633. https://doi-org.proxy.library.nyu.edu/10.1007/s00737-020-01049-5

Tomfohr, L. M., Buliga, E., Letourneau, N. L., Campbell, T. S., & Giesbrecht, G. F. (2015). Trajectories of sleep quality and associations with mood during the perinatal period. *Sleep*, *38*(8), 1237–1245. https://doi.org/10.5665/sleep.4900

US Preventive Services Task Force. (2019). Interventions to prevent perinatal depression: US Preventive Services Task Force recommendation statement. *JAMA, 321*(6), 580–587. https://doi.org/10.1001/jama.2019.0007

van Driel, C. M., Stuursma, A., Schroevers, M. J., Mourits, M. J., & de Bock, G. H. (2019). Mindfulness, cognitive behavioural and behaviour-based therapy for natural and treatment-induced menopausal symptoms: A systematic review and meta-analysis. *BJOG: An International Journal of Obstetrics and Gynaecology, 126*(3), 330–339. https://doi.org/10.1111/1471-0528.15153

Vélez Toral, M., Godoy-Izquierdo, D., Padial García, A., Lara Moreno, R., Mendoza Ladrón de Guevara, N., Salamanca Ballesteros, A., de Teresa Galván, C., & Godoy García, J. F. (2014). Psychosocial interventions in perimenopausal and postmenopausal women: A systematic review of randomised and non-randomised trials and non-controlled studies. *Maturitas, 77*(2), 93–110. https://doi.org/10.1016/j.maturitas.2013.10.020

Wacker, E. C. (2018). Barriers and facilitators to seeking treatment for subclinical eating disorders: The importance of supportive relationships. *Journal of Family Psychotherapy*, *29*(4), 292–317. https://doi-org.proxy.library.nyu.edu/10.1080/08975353.2018.1471946

Ward, A., Ramsay, R., Russell, G., & Treasure, J. (2015). Follow-up mortality study of compulsorily treated patients with anorexia nervosa. *International Journal of Eating Disorders*, *48*(7), 860–865. https://doi-org.proxy.library.nyu.edu/10.1002/eat.22377

Wilcox, M., McGee, B. A., Ionescu, D. F., Leonte, M., LaCross, L., Reps, J., & Wildenhaus, K. (2018). Perinatal depressive symptoms often start in the prenatal rather than postpartum period: Results from a longitudinal study. *Archives of Women's Mental Health*, *24*(1), 119–131. https://doi.org/10.1007/s00737-020-01017-z

Wilson, R. L., Gummow, J. A., McAninch, D., Bianco-Miotto, T., & Roberts, C. T. (2018). Vitamin and mineral supplementation in pregnancy: Evidence to practice. *Journal of Pharmacy Practice and Research*, *48*, 186–192. https://doi.org/10.1002/jppr.1438

World Health Organization. (2013). Preconception care to reduce maternal and childhood mortality and morbidity: Policy brief. World Health Organization. https://apps.who.int/iris/handle/10665/340533

27 Pediatric Health

Mikki Meadows-Oliver
Rory Meyers College of Nursing
New York University
New York, New York, USA

CONTENTS

KEY POINTS

- Obesity among children and adolescents is increasing. Prevention of obesity through lifestyle behaviors is the preferable approach.
- Since children do not grocery shop, parents play a crucial role in a child's nutritional status.
- There are factors other than what a child eats that affect their overall nutrition, such as their culture, food insecurity, and whether or not a child has special health care needs.
- Physical activity provides health benefits from "tummy time" for infants to organized sports during adolescence.
- Adequate sleep duration and sleep quality are essential to maintaining a healthy lifestyle for children and adolescents. Sleep recommendations vary by age.
- Children and adolescents may be affected by substance use directly (themselves as users) or indirectly (substance use by a family member). Vaping is increasingly popular.
- Children and adolescents experience varying levels of stress as they grow older. Connectedness to family, peers, and school are protective factors.

27.1 INTRODUCTION

Lifestyle medicine is the use of evidence-based lifestyle therapeutic approaches to prevent and treat chronic diseases. This modality includes a focus on a healthy eating pattern, regular activity, sleep, management of stress, avoiding risky substances, and maintaining connectedness (Collings, 2021). These approaches are especially important in pediatrics because the early childhood years may set a foundation for health behaviors later in life. This chapter will review the tenets of lifestyle medicine and its application to the pediatric population.

27.2 HEALTHY EATING AND PHYSICAL ACTIVITY

The overall obesity rate in the United States is increasing and is currently 19% in children and adolescents ages 2–19 years (CDC, 2021a). Children with overweight and obesity are more likely to have high blood pressure and high cholesterol, and be at risk for cardiovascular disease and type

DOI: 10.1201/9781003178330-31

2 diabetes later in life (CDC, 2021b). In children and adolescents, rather than dieting, prevention of obesity through lifestyle behaviors is the preferable approach. Healthy dietary behaviors, along with adequate physical activity, are vital to avoiding excessive pediatric weight gain.

Governmental and professional nursing organizations have issued statements on healthful eating, physical activity, and the treatment and prevention of obesity. The *Dietary Guidelines for Americans* emphasizes the importance of a healthful dietary pattern to prevent diet-related chronic diseases such as cardiovascular disease, type 2 diabetes, and some types of cancer (USDA, 2020). The *Physical Activity Guidelines for Americans* provides recommendations to help people 3 years of age and older improve their health through regular physical activity (US Department of Health and Human Services, 2018). The National Association of Pediatric Nurse Practitioners (NAPNAP) issued a position statement on the prevention of overweight and obesity in the pediatric population (NAPNAP, 2021) that emphasizes promoting healthy eating and active lifestyles for children and families.

Healthy eating and activity patterns in children involve not only the child but parents or caregivers as well. Parents can encourage healthy eating behaviors and act as positive role models by demonstrating healthy eating and physical activity behaviors. Because children do not do their own grocery shopping or cook their own meals, it is important to include family members in any nutritional planning for children (Hagan et al., 2017).

In addition to what a child actually eats, there are other factors that affect a child's nutritional status such as culture, eating environment, experiences, food insecurity, or whether or not the child has special health care needs. A family's cultural practices, such as which foods are eaten and how food is prepared, has an important effect on the feeding practices of infants, children, and adolescents (Chatham & Mixer, 2020). Additionally, a family's culture may influence perceptions of an attractive body image and ideas of a healthy weight (Maezono et al., 2019).

Extra attention may need to be paid to the nutritional status and physical activity of children with special health care needs (CSHN). CSHN may have difficulty with chewing or swallowing foods and/ or be prescribed medications that contribute to weight gain and changes in appetite. They may have physical limitations that reduce their ability to be active and/or they may be faced with a lack of accessible environments that facilitate exercise (Hagan et al., 2017). Depending on the child's particular health condition, they may have specific nutrient demands that need to be met. For example, children with cystic fibrosis are at increased risk for malabsorption of pancreatic enzymes, which places them at risk for undernutrition (McDonald et al., 2021). Another pediatric chronic condition that may affect a child's nutrition and growth is sickle cell disease. Children with sickle cell disease (SCD) may show growth failure in comparison to healthy peers (Mandese et al., 2016). Children and adolescents with mobility limitations and intellectual or learning disabilities may find it difficult to make healthy food choices, control their weight, and be physically active. These factors place them at an increased risk of obesity. As an example, children with Down Syndrome were found to have a higher prevalence of obesity/overweight compared to children in the general population (O' Shea et al., 2018). Due to the increased balance deficits and physical fatigue, children and adolescents with Down Syndrome may adopt a slow walking speed that places them at increased risk for obesity (Chen & Ringenbach, 2018).

Children whose families live in safe and stable places and who have access to a variety of nutritious foods may be more likely to stay healthy and develop optimally. Families with limited financial means may have concerns about their ability to acquire sufficient food. Food insecurity, not having access to sufficient, quality foods, has been associated with malnutrition and greater odds of being overweight or obese (Do et al., 2021). Additionally, families with limited financial means may live in areas where parents are afraid to let their children play—which limits opportunities for physical activity (Hagan et al., 2017).

27.2.1 Promoting Healthy Weight by Age

Healthy nutrition starts before a child is born. Pregnant women need a balanced diet and should also take a prenatal vitamin containing folic acid, vitamin D, choline, and iron in amounts that will help protect the mother's and baby's health. After birth, breastfeeding or bottle feeding with a cow's milk–based, iron-fortified infant formula is recommended to ensure adequate growth. Parents or caregivers should be educated on feeding cues to avoid underfeeding or overfeeding an infant. Other foods or drinks are not advised unless recommended by the health care professional, usually around 6 months of age. At this stage, an infants' physical activity, such as supervised "tummy time," should stimulate motor skill development (Hagan et al., 2017).

During the toddler/preschool period (ages 1–4 years), healthy food choices should be divided into three meals and two to three snacks per day (Hagan et al., 2017). This should provide adequate macronutrients and micronutrients for growth. Children in this age group may display erratic or "picky" eating behaviors. Beginning to participate in food choices may be helpful. For instance, two vegetables can be offered, allowing the child to choose one. Regular physical activity should be encouraged for toddlers and preschoolers. Simple activities such as walking, running, and climbing are important opportunities for physical activity. Toddlers and preschoolers should engage in at least 60 minutes of unstructured physical activity each day and they should not be inactive for more than 60 minutes at a time, except when they are sleeping. Unstructured activities are those that a child chooses for themselves (Hagan et al., 2017).

During the middle childhood years of 5–10 years of age, children are out of the home more and begin to have outside influences on their food choices (Hagan et al., 2017). In addition to peers, media messages strongly influence food choices during middle childhood. Exposure to food advertisements has been associated with poor nutrition among children and adolescents. An analysis of 2,000 social media posts revealed that two-thirds of foods shown were unhealthy, and 61.2% of beverages were sugar sweetened (Bragg et al., 2020).

Children attending school should be offered a healthy breakfast daily. Eating breakfast was associated with higher school attendance and increased test scores (Bartfeld et al., 2019). Similar to guidance for toddlers, school-aged children should engage in at least 60 minutes of unstructured physical activity each day and should not be inactive for more than 60 minutes at a time except when sleeping. Children in this age group have increasing motor skills, which allows them to participate in a wider variety of activities, such as organized sports. It is important for parents to encourage physical activity in the home and community as schools are increasingly limiting the time for physical education classes (Hagan et al., 2017).

Adolescents are increasingly responsible for their own food choices. They often have busy schedules that do not always allow for participation in family meals. Caregivers can support their choices by providing healthy foods at home and providing opportunities for the adolescent to learn about purchasing outside foods that are not high in sugar, fat, or salt. Adolescents who eat vegetarian or vegan diets may require monitoring to ensure that they have adequate intakes of protein, iron, and other nutrients (Hagan et al., 2017). It is important to keep in mind that during this period, adolescents may use practices such as dieting or binge eating to affect their body weight. Such activities can cause an adolescent to develop unhealthy weight control behaviors (Katzman, 2021).

Physical activity often declines during adolescence (Hale et al., 2021). It is important to continue to encourage physical activity as researchers have found that consistent physical activity helps to improve psychological well-being and quality of life in adolescents (Hale et al., 2021). Participating in daily physical activities improves physical health as well. Adolescents who regularly participate in moderate to vigorous physical activity had lower body fat scores than those who did not (Oh et al., 2021). Regular exercise during adolescence has also been associated with increased bone density and increased muscle mass (Hagan et al., 2017).

At every age across the pediatric lifespan, fluids contribute protein, fat, and sugar to a child or adolescent's daily intake (Hagan et al., 2017). Milk is an important source of protein, calcium, and vitamin D for children. A child who does not drink milk will need to have alternative sources of calcium and vitamin D in their diets. Low nutrient foods and drinks that are high in calories, saturated fat, salt, added sugars, and refined grains should be limited. Water should be provided ad lib to children over the age of 1 year. Proteins from sources such as fish, lean meats, legumes, and nuts in addition to fruits and vegetables should be encouraged each day. Foods with whole grains should be chosen over refined grains (Hagan et al., 2017).

27.3 SLEEP

Adequate sleep duration and sleep quality are essential to maintaining a healthy lifestyle for children and adolescents (Hagan et al., 2017). What constitutes proper sleep hygiene in children will vary by age. For infants, sleep discussions have to include information about a safe sleep environment (noting that families from various cultures may view sleep differently). A safe sleep environment, as described by the American Academy of Pediatrics (AAP), is one that reduces the risk of suffocation through the elimination of items such as loose, soft bedding in the crib. Infant sleep position is as important as the sleep environment. Infants should be placed on their backs for every sleep because of the reduction of sudden infant death syndrome (SIDS). Room sharing but not bed sharing is recommended by the AAP. With room sharing, the infant is placed in a separate, but nearby, sleep space (such as a crib) rather than sharing the same bed as their parents. Bed sharing is discouraged as it has been shown to increase the risk of sudden unexpected infant death (SUID) (AAP, 2016).

The average number of hours a child needs for adequate sleep decreases as a child's age increases. Children typically sleep 12 to 14 hours per day by the age of one year (including naps). Nightmares and night terrors may become more common when children are 3–4 years old. Children should sleep an average of 10–11 hours per night in middle childhood and 8–11 hours per night during adolescence (Hagan et al., 2017). However, a majority of middle school students (57.8%) and high school students (72.7%) reported not getting enough sleep on school nights (CDC, 2020a).

Sleep promoting activities during childhood and adolescence include having a consistent bedtime as well as bedtime routine, such as reading or being read to by a parent or sibling. A regular bedtime has been associated with a lower likelihood of having obesity (Do et al., 2021). Inadequate sleep has been associated with factors that increase a child's risk for developing diabetes and hypertension. Shorter sleep duration and lower sleep quality have been associated with a greater risk of developing obesity (Do et al., 2021) and insulin resistance in children and adolescents (Dutil & Chaput, 2017). Subsequent research on sleep duration found that shorter sleep duration was associated with higher blood pressures in childhood (Sparano et al., 2019). Researchers also found that food insecurity may affect sleep patterns in children. Children and adolescents with food insecurity reported having more difficulties staying asleep and a longer average sleep duration compared with those with food security (Do et al., 2021).

Mobile devices are ever-present in the lives of children and adolescents and have been found to negatively affect sleep. Mobile phone usage of greater than four hours per day was associated with nighttime sleep disturbances in adolescents (Liu et al., 2017). An additional factor found to disturb nighttime sleep was the intake of caffeine. Researchers found a significant association between afternoon caffeine use and self-reported sleep problems for adolescents (Cusick et al., 2020). These studies indicate that having a regular bedtime and limiting afternoon caffeine intake and the late-night use of digital mobile devices may help children and adolescents achieve healthy sleep habits and patterns.

27.4 AVOIDANCE OF RISKY SUBSTANCES

Children and adolescents may be affected by substance use directly or indirectly. Direct effects would result from using substances themselves. An indirect effect would be from experiencing the consequences of substance use by family members (Hagan et al., 2017).

In recent years, "vaping," using electronic cigarettes, has become more popular. In children and adolescents, there has been an increase in the use of vaping tobacco products (Gentzke et al., 2019) as well as vaping marijuana products (Patrick et al., 2020). In addition to an increase in vaping, the use of edible marijuana products has increased in the pediatric population (Patrick et al., 2020). Researchers have searched for causes of these increases. Having friends who used substances such as tobacco, marijuana, or alcohol was a predictor of adolescent substance use. Additionally, children are exposed to messaging and images of substance use through media sources. Use of social media platforms has been shown to be associated with vaping in children and adolescents (Lee et al., 2021). Adolescents reported they believed that vaping was safer than smoking cigarettes and vaping was used as a source of stress reduction (Chaplin et al., 2020). When considering substance use as a source of stress reduction, it is important to note that children and adolescents who use substances to cope may have a concurrent mental health problem (Hines et al., 2020). These youth may be more likely to participate in risky behaviors such as unprotected sex, which may put them at risk for sexually transmitted infections and unplanned pregnancy (Bartholomew et al., 2021; CDC, 2020b).

Parents are role models and it is important to understand their attitudes toward drug and alcohol use, as this may determine how they approach the subject with their children (Hagan et al., 2017). Worrying about a family member with a substance use problem may be a source of significant stress for children and adolescents. The use of tobacco, alcohol, and other drugs can have adverse health effects on the entire family. Parental substance use disorder increases the risk of adolescent substance use and the development of mental health disorders (Maina et al., 2021).

Governmental organizations such as the CDC and Food and Drug Administration (FDA) have been working to find ways to reduce substance use in children and adolescents. The CDC encourages schools, families, and communities to work together to reduce high risk drug use. It is recommended that schools connect students to networks of peers and adults in schools and the surrounding community to equip them with the knowledge and skills needed to make informed health decisions regarding substances in their environments. Students should be connected to mental health programs at their schools or in the community (CDC, 2020b).

In an effort to reduce the availability of tobacco products to children and adolescents, the FDA proposed restricting sales of flavored e-cigarettes (other than tobacco, menthol, mint, or non-flavored). Additional strategies to reduce tobacco product use among youths include increasing the price of tobacco products, implementing advertising restrictions, and implementing and enforcing policies that raise the minimum age of purchase for tobacco products to 21 years of age (Gentzke et al., 2019).

Children and adolescents can be made aware of the Smokefree Teen website, which has tools available to help quit or decrease use of nicotine-based products. Smokefree Teen has a free text message program and a quitSTART app that provides tips, advice, and encouragement to help children and adolescents become tobacco free (US Department of Health and Human Services, n.d.). Taken together, these regulatory proposals and access to support resources can help children adolescents reduce or eliminate substance use.

27.5 MANAGING STRESS AND MAINTAINING CONNECTEDNESS

Children and adolescents experience varying levels of stress as they grow older. Major family changes such as parental separation and divorce, illness or death of a parent or other family member, or a move to a new family home can be sources of stress. Additionally, family issues, such as parental substance use disorder, domestic violence, and parental depression, can cause a child to develop a level of stress that may adversely affect their health. In order for children to develop appropriately, they need to live in safe environments that are free of toxic stress (Hagan et al., 2017).

Children and adolescents spend many of their waking hours in school and need to feel safe in their school environment, on their way to and from school, and in their community (Hagan et al., 2017). Something that can make a child feel unsafe in the school environment and interfere with school performance is bullying. Children with special health care needs or developmental differences, such as those with autism spectrum disorder (ASD) or attention-deficit/hyperactivity disorder (ADHD), are at increased risk for bullying victimization (McClemont et al., 2021). Youth who identify as lesbian, gay, bisexual, transgender, or questioning experience higher rates of bullying than do their heterosexual peers (Gower et al., (2018). Another group of children and adolescents who are likely to experience bullying are those who are overweight or obese. Studies have reported that adolescents who are obese are more likely to experience bullying when compared to their healthy weight peers (Rupp & McCoy, 2019). Cyberbullying, also known as online bullying, has become increasingly common and is a source of stress for children and adolescents. Researchers have found that victims of cyberbullying are more at risk for suicide, and school connectedness can reduce the impact of cybervictimization on suicidal behaviors (Kim et al., 2020).

The ability to cope with stress is an important skill for children and adolescents. Mindfulness-based interventions (MBI) have been found to be effective for alleviating stress in a variety of populations. "Mindfulness is the practice of paying attention to what is happening in the present moment without judgment" (Malachowski, 2015, p. 62). Within pediatrics, much of the mindfulness-based research has focused on children at-risk for or who have chronic illnesses. One of the most frequently studied areas of mindfulness in children and adolescents is in the area of weight loss/obesity prevention. This is important because of obesity's link to the future development of heart disease and type 2 diabetes. If obesity can be prevented, children may avoid developing these conditions and the resulting sequelae. When studying MBI in adolescents, researchers have found that mindfulness skills were negatively associated with emotional eating in adolescents with overweight/obesity. This finding is important because emotional eating may contribute to future weight gain, which contributes to continuing obesity (Gouveia et al., 2019). A later study supported these findings. In a sample of pediatric patients, Leung and colleagues (2021) conducted a six-session mindfulness-based pilot intervention comprising three components: Yoga, mindful eating, and stress reduction. Their findings revealed that the intervention increased mindful eating awareness in their study population. Mindful eating has been associated with a lower likelihood of eating in response to stress.

Connectedness, the sense of being cared for, supported, and belonging, is an important protective factor for children and adolescents that can decrease the likelihood of a variety of health risk behaviors. Children and adolescents may feel a sense of connected to their family members, their school, or other important people and organizations in their lives (CDC, 2020c).

Adequate levels of family and school connectedness during adolescence may have long-lasting protective effects across multiple health outcomes (Steiner et al., 2019). Having family connectedness was shown to have protective effects for emotional distress, intimate partner violence, multiple sex partners, and substance use. Similarly, school connectedness was associated with protective effects by reducing emotional distress and odds of suicidal ideation, physical violence victimization and perpetration, multiple sex partners, and substance use (Steiner et al., 2019). Even during remote learning due to the Covid-19 pandemic, a sense of school connectedness was associated with decreased levels of anxiety and depression (Perkins et al., 2021).

Peer connectedness is important and a key factor of mental health wellness in the lives of children and adolescents (Winstone et al., 2021). Peer connectedness may serve as a protective factor for those who lack family connectedness. Peer interactions often occur face to face or through the use of social media platforms. While social media relationships among children and adolescents may be complex, they may offer a source of peer connectedness when in-person socializing is not possible and for youth who find face-to-face interactions difficult.

Families can cultivate connectedness with the children and adolescents in their lives by communicating openly and honestly, being involved with school activities, and spending time together sharing activities. Schools can promote connectedness by supporting student-led clubs, which can offer a safe space for students to socialize with each other and connect with supportive staff. Additionally, schools can implement mentoring programs and connect students to community-based programs that have a network of supportive adults (CDC, 2020c). These are concrete examples of fostering connectedness in children and adolescents that may lead to better health outcomes for this population.

27.6 CONCLUSION

Adhering to the tenets of lifestyle medicine may prevent children and adolescents from becoming overweight or obese. Promoting proper nutrition and regular physical activity provides benefits throughout the pediatric lifespan that will, in turn, influence adult health. Addressing the use of nicotine products may improve long-term outcomes. Helping children and adolescents manage stress and maintain connectedness will enhance their emotional, psychological, and social well-being.

REFERENCES

American Academy of Pediatrics Task Force on Sudden Infant Death Syndrome. (2016). SIDS and other sleep-related infant deaths: Updated 2016 recommendations for a safe infant sleeping environment. *Pediatrics*, *138*(5), e20162938. https://doi.org/10.1542/peds.2016-2938

Bartfeld, J., Berger, L., Men, F., & Chen, Y. (2019). Access to the school breakfast program is associated with higher attendance and test scores among elementary school students. *Journal of Nutrition* , *149*, 336–343.

Bartholomew, R., Kerry-Barnard, S., Beckley-Hoelscher, N., Phillips, R., Reid, F., Fleming, C., Lesniewska, A., Yoward, F., & Oakeshott, P. (2021). Alcohol use, cigarette smoking, vaping and number of sexual partners: A cross-sectional study of sexually active, ethnically diverse, inner-city adolescents. *Health Expectations*, *24*,1009–1014.

Bragg, M., Pageot, Y., Amico, A., Miller, A., Gasbarre, A., Rummo, P., & Elbel. (2020). Fast food, beverage, and snack brands on social media in the United States: An examination of marketing techniques utilized in 2000 brand posts. *Pediatric Obesity*, *15*, 1–10.

Centers for Disease Control and Prevention. (2020a). Sleep in middle and high school students. Retrieved from www.cdc.gov/healthyschools/features/students-sleep.htm

Centers for Disease Control and Prevention (CDC). (2020b). Youth high-risk drug use is linked to risky health behaviors and experiences. Retrieved from www.cdc.gov/healthyyouth/substance-use/hrsu.htm

Centers for Disease Control and Prevention. (2020c). Adolescent connectedness. Retrieved from www.cdc.gov/healthyyouth/protective/youth-connectedness-important-protective-factor-for-health-well-being.htm

Centers for Disease Control and Prevention. (2021a). Childhood obesity. www.cdc.gov/obesity/data/childhood.html

Centers for Disease Control and Prevention. (2021b). Childhood obesity causes and consequences. www.cdc.gov/obesity/childhood/causes.html

Chaplin, M., Brogie, J., Burch, A., Hetzler, J., Hough, D., Gustafson, B., Gray, M., & Gillette, C. (2020). Effectiveness of an educational intervention on health risks of vaping for high school-aged adolescents. *Journal of the American Pharmacists Association*, *60*, e158–e161.

Chatham, R., & Mixer, S. (2020). Cultural influences on childhood obesity in ethnic minorities: A qualitative systematic review. *Journal of Transcultural Nursing*, *31*, 87–99.

Chen, C., & Ringenbach, S. (2018). Walking performance in adolescents and young adults with Down syndrome: The role of obesity and sleep problems. *Journal of Intellectual Disability Research*, *62*, 339–348.

Collings, C. (2021). The power of lifestyle medicine to treat chronic disease. Retrieved from www.lifestylemedicine.org/ACLM/Education/Webinar_Archive_Open_Source/The_Power_of_Lifestyle_Medicine.aspx

Cusick, C., Langberg, J., Breaux, R., Green, C., & Becker, S. (2020). Caffeine use and associations with sleep in adolescents with and without ADHD. *Journal of Pediatric Psychology*, *45*, 643–653.

Do, E., Bowen, G., Ksinan, A., Adams, E., & Fuemmeler, B. (2021). Sleep, food insecurity, and weight status: Findings from the Family Life, Activity, Sun, Health, and Eating Study. *Childhood Obesity*, *17*, 125–135.

Dutil, C., & Chaput, J. P. (2017). Inadequate sleep as a contributor to type 2 diabetes in children and adolescents. *Nutrition & Diabetes*, 7, e266. https://doi.org/10.1038/nutd.2017.19

Gentzke, A., Creamer, M., & Cullen, K. (2019). Vital signs: Tobacco product use among middle and high school student—United States, 2011–2018. *Morbidity and Mortality Weekly Report*, 68, 157–164.

Gouveia, M., Canavarro, M., & Moreira, H. (2019). Associations between mindfulness, self-compassion, difficulties in emotion regulation, and emotional eating among adolescents with overweight/obesity. *Journal of Child and Family Studies*, 28, 273–285. https://doi.org/10.1007/s10826-018-1239-5

Gower, A., Forster, M., Gloppen, K., Eisenberg, M., Borowsky, I., Johnson, A., & Connett, J. (2018). School practices to foster LGBT-supportive climate: Associations with adolescent bullying involvement. *Prevention Science*, 19, 813–821.

Hagan, J., Shaw, J., & Duncan, P. (2017). *Bright futures: Guidelines for health supervision of infants, children and adolescents* (4th ed.) American Academy of Pediatrics.

Hale, G., Colquhoun, L., Lancastle, D., Lewis, N., & Tyson, P. (2021). Review: Physical activity interventions for the mental health and well-being of adolescents—a systematic review. *Child & Adolescent Mental Health*, 26, 357–368.

Hines, L., Freeman, T., Gage, S., Zammit, S., Hickman, M., Cannon, M., Munafo, M., MacLeod, J., & Heron, J. (2020). Association of high-potency cannabis use with mental health and substance use in adolescence. *JAMA Psychiatry*, 77, 1044–1051.

Katzman, D. (2021). The COVID-19 pandemic and eating disorders: A wake-up call for the future of eating disorders among adolescents and young adults. *Journal of Adolescent Health*, 69, 535–537.

Kim, J., Walsh, E., Pike, K., & Thompson, E. (2020). Cyberbullying and victimization and youth suicide risk: The buffering effects of school connectedness. *The Journal of School Nursing*, 36, 251–257.

Lee, J., Tan, A., Porter, L., Young-Wolff, K., Carter-Harris, L., Salloum, R., & Lee, J. (2021). Association between social media use and vaping among Florida adolescents, 2019. *Preventing Chronic Disease*, 18, 1–12.

Leung, M., & Forbes, D. (2021). A mindfulness-based pilot study to reduce childhood obesity risk in underserved Hispanic children: Feasibility, acceptability, and preliminary findings. *Journal of the Academy of Nutrition & Dietetics*, 121, A151–A151.

Liu, S., Zhang, J., Liu, Y., Wing, Y. & Zhang, B. (2017). The associations between long time of mobile phone use and sleep disturbances and emotional distress among youth: A prospective cohort study. *Sleep Medicine*, 40, e197–e198.

Maezono, J., Hamada, S., Sillanmäki, L., Kaneko, H., Ogura, M., Lempinen, L., & Sourander, A. (2019). Cross-cultural, population-based study on adolescent body image and eating distress in Japan and Finland. *Scandinavian Journal of Psychology*, 60, 67–76.

Maina, G., Ogenchuk, M., & Gaudet, S. (2021). Living with parents with problematic substance use: Impacts and turning points. *Public Health Nursing*, 38, 730–737.

Malachowski, M. (2015). Mindfulness for pediatrics: Evidence-based resources. *Journal of Consumer Health on the Internet*, 19, 61–67.

Mandese, V., Marotti, F., Bedetti, L., Bigi, E., Palazzi, G., & Iughetti, L. (2016). Effects of nutritional intake on disease severity in children with sickle cell disease. *Nutrition Journal*, 15, 1–6. https://doi.org/10.1186/s12937-016-0159-8

McClemont, A., Morton, H., Gillis, J., & Romanczyk, R. (2021). Brief report: Predictors of school refusal due to bullying in children with autism spectrum disorder and attention-deficit/hyperactivity disorder. *Journal of Autism & Developmental Disorders*, 51, 1781–1788.

McDonald, C., Bowser, E., Farnham, K., Alvarez, J., Padula, L., & Rozga, M. (2021). Dietary macronutrient distribution and nutrition outcomes in persons with cystic fibrosis: An evidence analysis center systematic review. *Journal of the Academy of Nutrition & Dietetics*, 121, 1574–1574.

National Association of Pediatric Nurse Practitioners. (2021). Position statement on the identification and prevention of overweight and obesity in the pediatric population. *Journal of Pediatric Health Care*, 35, 425–427.

Oh, M., Zhang, D., Whitaker, K., Letuchy, E., Janz, K., & Levy, S. (2021). Moderate-to-vigorous intensity physical activity trajectories during adolescence and young adulthood predict adiposity in young adulthood: The Iowa Bone Development Study. *Journal of Behavioral Medicine*, 44, 231–240.

O' Shea, M., O' Shea, C., Gibson, L., Leo, J., & Carty, C. (2018). The prevalence of obesity in children and young people with Down Syndrome. *Journal of Applied Research in Intellectual Disabilities*, 31, 1225–1229.

Patrick, M., Miech, R., Kloska, D., Wagner, A., & Johnston, L. (2020). Trends in marijuana vaping and edible consumption from 2015 to 2018 among adolescents in the US. *JAMA Pediatrics*, *174*, 900–902.

Perkins, K., Carey, K., Lincoln, E., Shih, A., Donalds, R., Schneider, S., Holt, M., & Green, J. (2021). School connectedness still matters: The association of school connectedness and mental health during remote learning due to COVID-19. *The Journal of Primary Prevention*, *42*, 641–648.

Rupp, K., & McCoy, S. (2019). Bullying perpetration and victimization among adolescents with overweight and obesity in a nationally representative sample. *Childhood Obesity*, *15*, 323–330.

Sparano, S., Lauria, F., Ahrens, W., Fraterman, A., Thumann, B., Iacoviello, L., Marild, S., Michels, N., Molnar, D., Moreno, L. A., Tornaritis, M., Veidebaum, T., & Siani, A. (2019). Sleep duration and blood pressure in children: Analysis of the pan-European IDEFICS cohort. *Journal of Clinical Hypertension*, *21*, 572–578. https://doi.org/10.1111/jch.13520

Steiner, R., Sheremenko, G., Lesesne, C., Dittus, P., Sieving, R., & Ethier, K. (2019). Adolescent connectedness and adult health outcomes. *Pediatrics*, *144*, e20183766. https://doi.org/10.1542/peds.2018-3766

US Department of Agriculture and US Department of Health and Human Services. (2020). *Dietary guidelines for Americans, 2020–2025* (9th ed.). www.dietaryguidelines.gov/resources/2020-2025-dietary-guidelines-online-materials

US Department of Health and Human Services. (2018). *Physical activity guidelines for Americans* (2nd ed.). US Department of Health and Human Services.

US Department of Health and Human Services. (n.d.) Smoke free teen. Retrieved from https://teen.smokefree.gov/

Winstone, L., Mars, B., Haworth, C., & Kidger, J. (2021). Social media use and social connectedness among adolescents in the United Kingdom: A qualitative exploration of displacement and stimulation. *BMC Public Health*, *21*, 1736.

28 Optimizing Function and Physical Health in Frail Adults

Barbara Resnick
University of Maryland School of Nursing
Baltimore, MD, USA

CONTENTS

KEY POINTS

- It has repeatedly been shown that physical activity is associated with the development of frailty and can also help to manage frailty.
- Aerobic activity can result in improvements in muscle mass and thereby decrease frailty. Aerobic activity also promotes optimal cardiovascular status by maintaining lung function and cardiac output.
- Increasing the frail older adult's motivation to engage in physical activity at any level of intensity can be done by using social cognitive theory to address the known barriers to physical activity.
- Although studies show that the benefits of regular exercise for frail older adults are greater than the risks, frail older adults have cardiovascular and musculoskeletal conditions that may lead to a need for modifications in activities.

DOI: 10.1201/9781003178330-32

28.1   FRAILTY DEFINITION

Frailty was first formally defined in 1992 as a syndrome of weakness, impaired mobility, impaired balance, and decreased reserve (Buchner & Wagner, 1992). Subsequent to this, ; and colleagues defined frailty based on a list of symptoms or signs, including unintentional weight loss of 4.5 kilograms or more in the past year, fatigue or exercise intolerance, weakness, decreased motor performance, and decreased physical activity (Fried et al., 2001). It has repeatedly been shown that physical activity is associated with the development of frailty and can also help manage frailty (Huang et al., 2020; Kidd et al., 2019; C. K. Liu & Fielding, 2011; Marcucci et al., 2019). Physical activity is defined by the World Health Organization as any bodily movement that requires energy expended (World Health Organization, 2020). This might be walking, cooking, or even knitting or bed making. Exercise is a subset of physical activity and involves planned, structured, and repetitive activities that are focused on improving or maintaining physical function and fitness. In addition to prevention and management of frailty, additional benefits (Table 28.1) from physical activity include improved bone health, postural stability, flexibility and range of motion (critical for bathing and dressing), reduced fall risk and pain from degenerative joint disease, psychosocial benefits, a positive impact on the cardiovascular system, respiratory system, and maintenance and improvement of function, and provide an overall sense of wellbeing, among others (Arrieta et al., 2019; Garber et al., 2011; Liu-Ambrose et al., 2004; C. J. Liu & Latham, 2009; Williams et al., 2007). Conversely, sedentary behavior and lack of activity promote deconditioning, contractures, pain, pressure ulcers, falls, and exacerbations of chronic illnesses (Biswas et al., 2015).

28.2   IMPACT OF AEROBIC AND RESISTIVE ACTIVITIES ON FRAILTY

Aerobic activity, which is physical activity that involves the use of oxygen to meet energy demands, is performed by repeating activities for extended periods of time. Aerobic activities include walking, jogging, swimming, or bike riding. The intensity of the aerobic activity can vary from:

TABLE 28.1
Benefits of physical activity

System Involved	Benefit
Cardiovascular	Decreased myocardial oxygen cost
	Decrease heart rate and blood pressure
	Increased capillaries in muscles
	Increased threshold for the accumulation of lactate in the blood
	Decreased chest pain or ischemia or claudication
Respiratory	Increased maximum oxygen uptake
	Decreased minute by minute ventilation
Psychological	Decreased anxiety
	Decreased depression
	Optimization of cognition
	Decreased loneliness especially with group activity
	Decreased apathy
	Improved well-being and quality of life
Function	Optimal physical function and maintenance of function over time
	Decreased fall risk and incidence
Syndromes	Improved urinary incontinence particularly for functional incontinence
	Improved bowel function (decreased constipation)
	Improved sleep

(1) low-intensity, which is when the individual works at 40 to 50% of his or her maximum heart rate (most simply calculated as 220—age); (2) moderate intensity, which is working at 50 to 70% of the maximum heart rate; to (3) vigorous exercise, which is working at 70 to 85% of maximum heart rate. Aerobic activity can result in improvements in muscle mass and thereby decrease frailty (Sugawara et al., 2002). Aerobic activity also promotes optimal cardiovascular status by maintaining lung function and cardiac output.

In contrast, resistance activities are activities that result in the muscles contracting against an external resistance. Strength and resistance training offset the loss of muscle mass and strength that are commonly seen with aging and aggravated by disuse. The external resistance can be exercise tubing, one's own body weight, bottles of water, or any size hand-held or applied weight that causes the muscles to contract. Resistance activities can increase muscle mass as well as muscle strength. Multiple studies have shown that resistance activities decrease frailty by increasing strength in older adults (C. J. Liu & Latham, 2009). In addition to increasing muscle strength, aerobic or resistance activities, or a combination of both types of activity, can reduce falls (Liu-Ambrose et al., 2004) and improve grip strength, walking speed (Chen et al., 2020), and other aspects of frailty such as overall physical function (Arrieta et al., 2019; Hsieh et al., 2019; Mañas et al., 2019).

Despite the known benefits of physical activity, for most frail older adults engaging in physical activity may be challenging. Consequently, the intensity and types of physical activity will likely need to be modified. There is evidence, however, that frail older adults can benefit from even limited amounts of physical activity (Mañas et al., 2019). For frail older adults, working at intensity levels as low as 40% of aerobic capacity, or taking as few as 3,000 steps per day, can help improve clinical outcomes and prevent progressive decline (Dohrn et al., 2018; McKinney et al., 2016). Further, increasing physical activity for frail individuals at any level can improve gait and balance, improve appetite, and decrease the risk of hospitalization (Dohrn et al., 2018; Galik et al., 2014; McKinney et al., 2016; Resnick et al., 2011). Thus, there is substantial support to encourage frail older individuals to spend more time engaged in physical activity and less time in bed or sitting.

28.3   MOTIVATING FRAIL OLDER ADULTS TO EXERCISE

Increasing the frail older adult's motivation to engage in physical activity at any level of intensity can be done by addressing a number of the known barriers to physical activity, as shown in Table 28.2. The use of social cognitive theory is helpful to address these barriers. Social cognitive theory (Bandura, 1997) is one of the major theoretical frameworks used to change behavior. Social cognitive theory proposes that the stronger the individual's self-efficacy and outcome expectations, the more likely it is that he or she will initiate and persist with a given activity. Self-efficacy

TABLE 28.2
Factors that influence motivation to exercise in frail older adults

Facilitators	Barriers
New and fun activities	Pain
Stressing the benefits of physical activity	Shortness of breath
Actually performing the activity at any level	Fear of falling or getting hurt or hurting already painful joints
Individualized approaches	Fatigue
Social support	Lack of belief in the benefit of physical activity
Environmental resources	Cognitive challenges to following instructions or remembering
Policies that support physical activity	what to do to be physically active
Identification of goals	

expectations are the individual's beliefs in his or her capabilities to perform a course of action to attain a desired outcome; outcome expectations are the beliefs that certain consequences will be produced by personal action. Efficacy expectations are dynamic and enhanced by four mechanisms: (1) successful performance of the activity; (2) verbal encouragement; (3) seeing how individuals perform the activity; and (4) elimination of unpleasant physiological and affective states associated with the activity.

Examples of ways in which to use self-efficacy–based approaches to motivate individuals to exercise include modeling behavior and providing verbal encouragement to motivate individuals, decrease fear, overcome cultural expectations, and manage cognitive and behavioral challenges. Helping older adults as well as their caregivers to believe in the benefits of physical activity is an important step to engaging frail individuals in physical activity. Encouraging activities in which the individual will be successful and that will not cause discomfort or injury is likewise important. Any unpleasant sensations associated with physical activity will result in decreased motivation and willingness to perform the activity. Interventions such as using heat, positioning, or pain medication (topical or oral) prior to engaging in the activity are helpful.

Social support to participate in physical activity and encouragement provided by others is also critically important to engage frail older adults in physical activity. This encouragement should come from someone who is perceived as knowledgeable and trustworthy to the older individual. Ongoing encouragement is needed to assure adherence to activities even as simple as walking to the dining room or the bathroom. If a frail individual refuses to engage in a physical activity offered, exploring the reason that they do not want to participate, eliminating the barrier, and providing ongoing encouragement to engage in physical activity are helpful approaches and continued sources of motivation. These approaches can improve self-efficacy and help the individual believe in the benefit of physical activity.

Eliminating unpleasant sensations associated with physical activity is also important. It is equally important, however, to ensure that the activity recommended is pleasant and fun. New and varied types of activities, such as dance parties or taking a walk to a favorite destination to get a cup of coffee or favorite food option, are helpful and additional ways to motivate frail individuals in physical activity. Further, setting an individualized goal for the frail older adult makes a statement that others believe he or she has the ability to achieve the goal.

28.4   TYPES OF PHYSICAL ACTIVITY FOR FRAIL OLDER ADULTS TO PERFORM

As noted above, any type of aerobic or resistive physical activity is beneficial for frail older adults. These activities do not require expensive equipment but can be done safely and easily in any setting. Sit-to-stand exercises and balance exercises (Table 28.3) can greatly facilitate maintenance of muscle strength and function. Walking, dancing, a range of motion activities, and engaging in basic functional tasks such as bathing and dressing also serve as easy to do physical activity.

28.5   RISKS OF EXERCISE

Although studies show that the benefits of regular exercise for frail older adults are greater than the risks, frail older adults have cardiovascular and musculoskeletal conditions that may lead to a need for modifications in activities (C. K. Liu & Fielding, 2011). Despite a higher prevalence of comorbidities, there is no evidence to suggest that frail individuals should be screened before engaging in low or moderate levels of physical activity (Min et al., 2020; Resnick et al., 2008). Physical activity actually decreases the risk of mortality associated with comorbidities (Min et al., 2020). In fact, there is a greater risk of exacerbation and worsening of cardiovascular disease from *not* exercising (Biswas et al., 2015) as well as a risk of cardiovascular events during exercise prescreening (Stuart & Ellestad, 1980).

TABLE 28.3
Sit to stand exercise

Steps for a Sit to Stand Exercise

1. Sit on a sturdy chair with your feet flat on the floor.
2. Keep your knees over your heels; bring your chest and arms forward so that your nose is over your toes.
3. Continue to reach your upper body forward until you feel your bottom start to lift off the chair seat. If necessary, use your arms to push up off the chair or chair arms if available.
4. Come forward into a standing position.
5. Stand with the backs of your calves touching the chair seat and **slowly** lower your bottom to the chair. Do not flop back onto the chair rapidly.
6. Repeat this 10 times to start (or less if you feel you become uncomfortably short or breath or fatigued).
7. Identify a goal for you to do a certain amount daily (good examples: three sets of 10 times planned throughout the day; during commercials when watching television).

Balance Exercise
Stand with feet about shoulder-width apart, eyes open, and hold steady for 10 seconds, working your way up to 30 seconds. If you are concerned about falling, do this while holding onto the sink, a sturdy chair, or a sturdy table. You can lift one hand and try the exercise that way. Then drop down to one finger and when comfortable you can do the exercise; this way you can try it without holding on. If you find yourself swaying or reaching for the wall or counter frequently, just keep working on this exercise until you can do it with minimal swaying or support. Once you can hold this position firmly for 30 seconds, move on to the next exercise.

Balance Exercise 2:
Stand with feet together, eyes open, and hold steady for 10 seconds. Work your way up to doing this for 30 seconds.

Balance Exercise 3:
Stand on one foot (flex your knee to 90 degrees) with your eyes open and hold steady for 10 seconds. Work on this till you can hold it for 30 seconds. Do the same thing on the other foot.

Balance Exercise 4:
Once you are comfortable doing all of the exercises above, you can now try and do these exercises without holding onto a chair or table and then with your eyes closed.

Although there is no need for screening, there are some common consequences or risks associated with physical activity that may occur. These risks focus mainly on musculoskeletal injury and cardiovascular disease exacerbations. Musculoskeletal injury is due to the type and intensity of the activity done and the individual's underlying status (e.g., degree of osteoarthritis or osteoporosis). Musculoskeletal events are more likely to occur in individuals who are not physically fit to begin with. Prevention of injury is done by starting at a low level of activity. This means walking for one minute, five minutes, and then building up to ten minutes or starting a resistance exercise against gravity and then increasing to one pound weights and increasing accordingly. Progression to a heavier weight is generally done once the individual can do eight repetitions with the current weight comfortably.

Cardiovascular events are most often associated with vigorous intensity activities and are extremely rare when engaging in mild to moderate level physical activity as occurs with frail older adults. Some ways in which to decrease any possible cardiovascular risks include being aware of underlying comorbidities that may impact endurance and starting at a low intensity and building up slowly. Establishing the intensity of any activity can be done using a subjective assessment on the part of the frail older individual using the Borg Rating of Perceived Exertion (RPE) scale (Table 28.4). The individual is asked to rate, on a scale of 6 (very, very light activity exertion) to 20

TABLE 28.4
Borg measure of perceived exertion

Borg Scale

Scoring	Level of Exertion
6	No exertion
7	Extremely light
8	
9	Very light
10	
11	Light
12	
13	Somewhat hard
14	
15	Hard (heavy)
16	
17	Very hard
18	
19	Extremely hard
20	Maximal exertion

Scoring:
- 9 = "very light" exercise, which equals walking slowly for few minutes at own pace of a healthy individual.
- 13 = "somewhat hard" but the individual is still able to continue the activity.
- 17 = "very hard." A healthy person can continue but must push themselves beyond their comfort of being very fatigued.
- 19 = extremely strenuous exercise. For most people, the hardest they have ever experienced.

(very, very hard physical activity exertion) how they perceive their physical activity. For older adults with cognitive impairment, caregivers should ask how hard the older adult thinks they are working rather than ask them to assign a number to the level of intensity. An RPE score on the Borg measure that falls between 12 and 16 correlates with reaching 60 to 80% of the targeted heart rate, or a moderate intensity of physical activity (Borg Ratings of Perceived Exertion, 2020).

Table 28.5 provides a list of the signs and symptoms staff or caregivers should recognize and teach frail older adults to report as potential danger signs during physical activity. When these signs occur, the activity should be stopped and follow-up by the individual's health care provider arranged.

28.6 EXERCISE PRESCRIPTIONS FOR FRAIL OLDER ADULTS

28.6.1 INDIVIDUAL APPROACHES

Health care providers continue to be challenged and fearful of prescribing physical activity for frail older adults. There are numerous resources (see end of chapter) for engaging older adults in physical activity, although these activities cannot generally be done independently by frail individuals, particularly not those with cognitive impairment or sensory deficits. A more practical and realistic approach is to incorporate physical activity into all routine activities for frail older adults rather than focus on a specific "exercise" program. This allows for an approach that builds from low intensity activity to more and more engagement in physical activity. Integration of physical activity into all activities is done by implementing a *function focused care* approach into whatever setting the individual is living in. Function focused care is a philosophy of care that evaluates the older adult's underlying capability with regard to function and physical activity and develops a plan to engage

TABLE 28.5
Warning signs to recognize during exercise

Warning Signs	Safety Tips to Use When Exercising
• Pale, clammy, cool skin • Sudden change in cognition, such as new confusion or disorientation • Nausea or vomiting • Shortness of breath that does not resolve in 30 minutes • Chest pain • Dizziness • Unusual fatigue • Change in balance or unsteadiness • Acute new onset pain in a joint or muscle • Break out in a cold sweat • Have muscle cramps • Slow down if you have trouble breathing; you should be able to talk while exercising without gasping for breath	• Wear comfortable, loose-fitting clothing and supportive tie shoes/sneakers. • Warm up: Perform a low to moderate intensity warm-up for 5–10 minutes. • Drink water before, during and after physical activity. • Make sure the environment is safe: flat walking area, limited traffic, dry weather that is not too warm or cold. • Wear sunscreen when you are outdoors.

the individual in physical activity at his or her highest level. This philosophy of care is in contrast to what has traditionally been provided to frail older adults, which is to complete all care and tasks for the individual (e.g., bath and dress the individual, provide easy access to a water glass versus having them lift the glass and flex the arm). In task focused care, there tends to be a strong focus on safety and getting tasks completed versus engaging the individual in physical activity. Examples of function focused care activities include such things as providing verbal or visual cues during bathing so the older individual performs the tasks rather than the caregiver; having the individual walk to the bathroom rather than use a commode chair or urinal; and accompanying a resident to an exercise class. Function focused care may engage individuals in independently performing an activity or it may be with the assistance of another individual or at the lowest level with hand-over-hand assistance (the caregiver performs the activity but moves the individual's arms through the motions, as is done with hand over hand help with eating).

Incorporating a function focused care approach for frail older adults requires an individualized approach. There is a tendency to assume that frail older individuals are unable to participate in bathing, dressing, ambulation, or exercise programs. Likewise, there is a tendency to believe that it will be quicker to transport the frail individual from one room to the next if at home or from their room to the dining room for meals within a facility via a wheelchair (Galik et al., 2009; Resnick et al., 2008). There is no known evidence to support this. In fact, caregivers that implement a function focused care approach actually find that they save time as they are not providing unnecessary care to residents (Resnick et al., 2008).

The *Physical Capability Assessment* (Table 28.6) is an easy way in which to identify the underlying ability of the frail older individual and then use this information to establish goals related to physical activity. The Physical Capability Assessment involves evaluating if the frail older individual is able to complete a one, two, or three step command; has upper and lower extremity range of motion, as this will determine if they can do specific functional tasks around bathing, dressing, and eating; can transfer and bear weight bilaterally on lower extremities; and has sufficient standing balance to ambulate. Based on this assessment and input from other members of the health care team as appropriate, a care plan can be developed if in a nursing home or acute care setting, or a service plan if in assisted living, or just set goals if living at home. For example, if the individual has upper

TABLE 28.6
Physical capability scale

Item	Able to Perform	Not Able to Perform	Directions to Participant	Scoring
Upper extremity range of motion			*The evaluator demonstrates the task for the participant and asks them to do the same thing.*	
1. Full flexion (hands over head)	1	0	The evaluator demonstrates and says, "put your hands over your head like this."	1 = range to 160–180 degrees; 0 = inability to range at least to 160–180 degrees.
2. Full external rotation (hands behind head)	1	0	The evaluator demonstrates and says, "put your hands behind your head like this."	1 = ability to put hands behind head; 0 = inability to put hands behind head.
3. Full internal rotation and adduction (hands in small of back	1	0	The evaluator demonstrates and says, "put your hands behind your back like this."	1 = ability to put hands together in small of back; 0 = inability to put hands together in small of back.
Lower extremity range of motion				
4. Able to flex ankle	1	0	When lying or sitting, the participant is asked to point his or her toes to ceiling and to the foot of the bed.	1 = ability to point toes to the ceiling; 0 = inability to point toes to the ceiling.
5. Able to point toe	1	0	When lying or sitting, the participant asked to point his or her toes to ceiling and to the foot of the bed.	1 = ability to point toes to the foot of the bed/ floor; 0 = inability to point toes to the foot of the bed/floor.
6 and 7. Able to flex knees and march	1	0	When sitting, the participant is asked to march with knees flexed at 90 degrees.	1 = ability to march with knees flexed; 0 = inability to march.
Chair rise			*The participant is asked to rise independently (with or without the use of arm strength) from a standard 18-inch hard back chair with arms and stand.*	
8. How many tries does it take	1–3 tries = 1	Unable to rise with 3 tries = 0		A try is defined as any attempt to push up from the chair. 1 = 1–3 attempts to push up from the chair with success occurring by the third try; 0 = unable to rise even on the third try.
9. Does the participant use arms to get up from the chair	1	0		1 = ability to get up without arms; 0 = inability to get up without arms.

TABLE 28.6 (Continued)
Physical capability scale

Item	Able to Perform	Not Able to Perform	Directions to Participant	Scoring
10. Can the participant make it to a full stand and stand independently for 1 minute	1	0		1 = ability to come to stand for a full minute; 0 = inability to come to stand and stay there for a full minute.
Ability to follow commands			*The participant is asked to take a towel, fold it in half, and put it on the table (bedside table or bed or whatever appropriate source is available).*	
11. Follows a one-step verbal command	1	0		1 = picks up the towel; 0 = does not pick up the towel.
12. Follows a two-step verbal command	1	0		1 = picks up the towel and folds it half; 0 = does not pick up the towel or fold it in half.
13. Follows a three-step verbal command	1	0		1 = picks up the towel, folds in half, and puts it on the table; 0 = does not pick up the towel, fold it in half, or put it on the bed.
Follows a three-step visual command			*The evaluator demonstrates for the participant how to take a towel, fold it in half, and put it on the table (bedside table or bed or whatever source is available).*	
14. Follows a one-step visual command	1	0		1 = picks up the towel; 0 = does not pick up the towel.
15. Follows a two-step visual command	1	0		1 = picks up the towel and folds it half; 0 = does not pick up the towel or fold it in half.
16. Follows a three-step visual command	1	0		1 = picks up the towel, folds in half, and puts it on the table; 0 = does not pick up the towel, fold it in half or put it on the bed.

Source: adapted from Capability Assessment, https://functionfocusedcare.wordpress.com/tools-and-materials/

extremity range of motion in all joints and can follow at least a one-step command based on either verbal or visual cues, then he or she should be able to participate in bathing and dressing.

28.6.2 GROUP APPROACHES FOR FRAIL OLDER ADULTS IN LONG-TERM CARE SETTINGS

To increase physical activity among frail older adults in long-term care settings, it can be very helpful and effective to provide opportunities for group-based activities. Examples of group activities include such things as dance related activities, which involve simply providing music that residents can dance to, clap along with, and move to in wheelchairs if not able to stand; physical activity BINGO games from NASCO (2020); wheelchair Tai Chi that individuals can visually follow; or other types of resistance activity with light weights or resistance bands. Ten-minute spurts of physical activity done three times a day will help frail individuals attain the minimum recommendations for physical activity for all adults and can result in clinical benefits (Dohrn et al., 2018). Dance is a terrific way to incorporate group exercise. Set aside 5- or 10-minute periods for putting on fun dance tunes consistent with the cultural preferences of your residents, and dance away to the music. Three to four songs will help the dancers achieve 10 minutes of physical activity. You can make it fun by having dance competitions and giving a prize to whoever dances the longest. Those who are not ambulatory or cannot stand independently can march their feet and swing their arms. Those that need supervision or help with balance can dance with a staff member.

Walking is another cheap and easy to do activity. Residents can be helped to set daily walking goals, or if unable to ambulate, these can be goals for self-propelling for a certain amount of time or to a specific location (e.g., coffee break area or around an outside garden). Musical chairs is another fun activity and can be done by putting on music and having the residents walk or self-propel around a circle of chairs, and sitting or stopping when the music stops.

For residents, particularly some of the female residents, cleaning/caring for their rooms as they did with their homes provides another way to increase physical activity. Give residents the appropriate supplies for them to dust, sweep, clear dining room tables, or set tables for the next meal. Other ways to increase physical activity for frail older adults are to have available horseshoes (foam versions are particularly easy to use), croquet, fly-swatter badminton, shuffleboard, and bean bag tosses (see NASCO.com). Make these activities fun by including groups of participants and engaging families, grandchildren, or outside visitors as appropriate and provide prizes to winners.

28.6.3 CHALLENGES TO OVERCOME TO OPTIMALLY ENGAGE FRAIL OLDER ADULTS IN PHYSICAL ACTIVITY

Potential challenges to engaging frail older adults in physical activity include comorbid conditions that cause symptoms such as pain, shortness of breath or dizziness, fear of injury on the part of the older adults and his or her caregivers, lack of suitable space and resources (e.g., games, music), and lack of knowledge about options for physical activity on the part of formal caregivers within facilities or informal caregivers in home settings. In addition, there may be cognitive, behavioral, and motivational challenges when working with these individuals.

At least 50% of frail older adults in long-term care facilities (nursing homes and assisted living facilities) have some cognitive impairment with associated symptoms of aphasia, motor apraxia, perceptual impairments, and apathy (National Center for Health Statistics, 2020; Sengupta et al., 2020). Further, some individuals may also have behavioral symptoms such as verbal or physical aggression, or resistance to care. Unfortunately, when working with individuals who may be agitated or uncooperative, caregivers tend to focus on maintaining behavioral stability rather than engaging them in functional and physical activities. This leads to a sedentary or passive approach to care and a "just get it done" philosophy with the caregiver completing the functional task for the frail older adult rather than encouraging the individual to participate in care.

Motivational techniques to engage frail older adults with cognitive impairment are available on the Function Focused Care webpage (www.functionfocusedcare.org). This webpage has 12 brief, three-minute video coaching sessions that demonstrate how to engage frail older adults in group as well as individual activities. Written resources and additional ideas for physical activities appropriate for frail older adults are also available at this site. Additional examples include leaving light weights, foam balls, or elastic exercise bands in the dining room and having residents routinely use these prior to meals, placing an exercycle or ergometer in open areas in facilities for frail individuals to use while being supervised if necessary, or implementing group walk to dine programs that gather a group of individuals to walk to meals together.

28.7 CONCLUSION

Engaging frail older adults in physical activity has many advantages to overall physical and mental health and quality of life, and these advantages far outweigh the risks. Physical activity goals and programs should be individualized as the amount and intensity that any individual can do and is willing to do will vary. Evaluating the individual in terms of ability and motivation is an important first step in the process to increasing physical activity. From a practical perspective, it is useful to implement a function focused care philosophy that engages frail older adults in physical activity during all routine care. Without question, physical activity is the best "medicine" for frail older adults as it can help provide individuals with the highest level of health and quality of life as is possible.

28.8 RESOURCES

28.8.1 DEPARTMENT OF HEALTH AND HUMAN SERVICES PHYSICAL ACTIVITY GUIDELINES WEBSITE

- PAG Homepage: www.health.gov/paguidelines/
- Physical Activity Guidelines: https://health.gov/our-work/nutrition-physical-activity/physical-activity-guidelines

28.8.2 NATIONAL INSTITUTES OF HEALTH RESOURCES

- Exercise & Physical Activity: Your Everyday Guide from the National Institute on Aging: www.nia.nih.gov/HealthInformation/Publications/ExerciseGuide/
- NIH Senior Health: www.nia.nih.gov/health

28.8.3 ADMINISTRATION ON COMMUNITY LIVING

- Evidence-Based Prevention Program: https://acl.gov/programs/health-wellness/disease-prevention

28.8.4 PRESIDENT'S COUNCIL ON FITNESS, SPORTS, AND NUTRITION

- Fitness.Gov: www.fitness.gov/

28.8.5 NATIONAL PHYSICAL ACTIVITY PLAN

- National Plan Homepage: http://physicalactivityplan.org/

28.8.6 ACSM/AMA

- Exercise Is Medicine Homepage: www.exerciseismedicine.org/

28.8.7 ONLINE EXERCISE SCREENING TOOL

- EASY Screening Tool: www.easyforyou.info/

28.8.8 NATIONAL COUNCIL ON THE AGING

- Center for Healthy Aging Homepage: www.ncoa.org/

REFERENCES

Arrieta, H., Rezola-Pardo, C., Gil, S., Virgala, J., Iturburu, M., Antón, I., González-Templado, V., Irazusta, J., & Rodriguez-Larrad, A. (2019). Effects of multicomponent exercise on frailty in long-term nursing homes: A randomized controlled trial. *Journal of the American Geriatrics Society, 67*(6), 1145–1151.

Bandura, A. (1997). *Self-efficacy: The exercise of control.* W.H. Freeman and Company.

Biswas, A., Oh, P., Faulkner, G., Bajaj, R. R., Silver, M. A., Mitchell, M. S., & Alter, D. A. (2015). Sedentary time and its association with risk for disease incidence, mortality and hospitalization in adults: A systematic review and meta analysis. *Annals of Internal Medicine, 162*(2), 759–783.

Borg Ratings of Perceived Exertion. (2020). Rating scale. Retrieved November 2020 from www.physio-pedia.com/Borg_Rating_Of_Perceived_Exertion

Buchner, D., & Wagner, E. (1992). Preventing frail health. *Clinics of Geriatric Medicine, 8*(1), 1–17.

Chen, R., Wu, Q., Wang, D., Li, Z., Liu, H., Liu, G., Cui, Y., ^ Song, L. (2020). Effects of elastic band exercise on the frailty states in pre-frail elderly people. *Physiotherapy Theory & Practice, 36*(9), 1000–1008.

Dohrn, I., Kwak, L., Oja, P., Sjöström, M., & Hagströmer, M. (2018). Replacing sedentary time with physical activity—a 15 year follow-up of mortality in a national cohort. *Clinical Epidemiology, 10*, 179–186.

Fried, L., Tangen, C., Walston, J., Newman, A. B., Hirsch, C., Gottdiener, J., Seeman, T., Tracy, R., Kop, W. J., Burke, G., McBurnie, M. A., & Cardiovascular Health Study Collaborative Research Group. (2001). Frailty in older adults: Evidence for a phenotype. *Journal of Gerontology: Biological Sciences Medicine and Science, 56*(3), M146–M156.

Galik, E., Resnick, B., Hammersla, M., & Brightwater, J. (2014). Optimizing function and physical activity among nursing home residents with dementia: Testing the impact of Function Focused Care. *The Gerontologist, 54*(6), 930–943.

Galik, E., Resnick, B., & Pretzer-Aboff, I. (2009). Knowing what makes them tick: Motivating cognitively impaired older adults to participate in restorative care. *International Journal of Nursing Practice, 15*(1), 48–55.

Garber, C., Blissmer, B., & Deschenes, M. (2011). American College of Sports Medicine position stand. The quantity and quality of exercise for developing and maintaining cardiorespiratory, musculoskeletal and neuromotor fitness in apparently healthy adults: Guidance for prescribing exercise. *Medicine Science Sports and Exercise, 43*(7), 1344–1559.

Hsieh, T., Su, S., Chen, C., Kang, Y., Hu, M., & Hsu, L. (2019). Individualized home-based exercise and nutrition interventions improve frailty in older adults: A randomized controlled trial. *International Journal of Behavioral Nutrition & Physical Activity, 16*(1), 1–10.

Huang, C., Umegaki, H., Makino, T., & Uemura, K. (2020). Effect of various exercises on frailty among older adults with subjective cognitive concerns: A randomised controlled trial. *Age and Ageing, 49*, 1011–1019.

Kidd, T., Mold, F., Jones, C., Ream, E., Grosvenor, W., Sund-Levander, M., Tingström, P., & Carey, N. (2019). What are the most effective interventions to improve physical performance in prefrail and frail adults: A systematic review of randomised control trials. *BMC, 19*(184). https://doi.org/10.1186/s12877-019-1196-x

Liu-Ambrose, T., Khan, K., & Eng, J. (2004). Resistance and agility training reduce fall risk in women aged 75 to 85 with low bone mass: A 6 month randomized controlled trial. *Journal of the American Geriatrics Society, 52*(5), 657–665.

Liu, C. K., & Fielding, R. (2011). Exercise as an intervention for frailty. *Clinics of Geriatric Medicine, 27,* 101–110.

Liu, C. J., & Latham, M. (2009). Progressive resistance strength training for improving physical function in older adults. *Cochrane Database Systematic Review, 3*(CD002759).

Mañas, A., del Pozo-Cruz, B., Rodríguez-Gómez, I., Leal-Martín, J., Losa-Reyna, J., Rodríguez-Mañas, L., García-García, F., J, & Ara, I. (2019). Dose-response association between physical activity and sedentary time categories on ageing biomarkers. *BMC Geriatrics, 19*(270).

Marcucci, M., Damanti, S., Germini, F., Apostolo, J., Bobrowicz-Campos, E., Gwyther, H., Holland, C., Kurpas, D., Bujnowska-Fedak, M., Szwamel, K., Santana, S., Nobili, A., D'Avanzo, B., & Cano, A. (2019). Interventions to prevent, delay or reverse frailty in older people: A journey towards clinical guidelines. *BMC, 17*(193).

McKinney, J., Lithwick, D., Morrison, B., Nazzari, A., Isserow, S., Brett Heilbron, B., & Krahn, A. (2016). The health benefits of physical activity and cardiorespiratory fitness. *BCMJ, 58*(3), 131-137.

Min, C., Yoo, D., Wee, J., Lee, H., Byun, S., & Choi, H. (2020). Mortality and cause of death in physical activity and insufficient physical activity participants: A longitudinal follow-up study using a national health screening cohort. *BMC Public Health, 20*(1), 1–9.

NASCO. (2020). NASCO Senior Activities. Retrieved November 2020 from www.enasco.com/c/Senior-Act ivities-Nasco

National Center for Health Statistics. (2020). Alzheimer's Disease national data. Retrieved November 2020 from www.cdc.gov/nchs/fastats/alzheimers.htm

Resnick, B., Galik, E., Gruber-Baldini, A., & Zimmerman, S. (2011). Testing the impact of Function Focused Care in assisted living. *Journal of the American Geriatrics Society, 59*(12), 2233–2240.

Resnick, B., Ory, M., Coday, M., & Riebe, D. (2008). Professional perspectives on physical activity screening practices: shifting the paradigm. *Critical Public Health, 18*(1), 21–32.

Resnick, B., Pretzer-Aboff, I., Galik, E., Russ, K., Cayo, J., Simpson, M., & Zimmerman, S. (2008). Barriers and benefits to implementing a restorative care intervention in nursing homes. *Journal of the American Medical Directors Association, 9*(2), 102–108.

Sengupta, M., Rome, V., Harris-Kojetin, L., & Caffrey, C. (2020). Long-term care providers and services users in the United States-residential care component: National study of long-term care providers, 2015–2016: Weighted national estimates and standard errors. Retrieved November 2020 from www.cdc.gov/nchs/data/nsltcp/2016_NSLTCP_RCC_Weighted_Estimates.pdf

Stuart, R., & Ellestad, M. (1980). National survey of exercise stress testing facilities. *Chest, 77*(1), 94–97.

Sugawara, J., Myachi, M., Moreau, K., Dinenno, F. A., DeSouza, C. A., & Tanaka, H. (2002). Age-related reductions in appendicular skeletal muscle mass: Association with habitual aerobic exercise status. *Clinical Physiology Functional Imaging, 22*(3), 169–172.

Williams, M., Haskell, W., Ades, P., Amsterdam, E. A., Bittner, V., Franklin, B. A., Gulanick, M., Laing, S. T., Stewart, K. J., American Heart Association Council on Clinical Cardiology, & American Heart Association Council on Nutrition, Physical Activity, and Metabolism. (2007). Resistance exercise in individuals with and without cardiovascular disease; 2007 update: A scientific statement from the American Health Association Council on Clinical Cardiology and Council on Nutrition, Physical Activity, and Metabolism. *Circulation, 116*(5), 572–584.

World Health Organization. (2020). Definition of physical activity. Retrieved November 2020 from www.who.int/health-topics/physical-activity#tab=tab_1

Part V

Application and Implementation

29 Spiritual Care
Practice Implications

Elizabeth Johnston Taylor
Loma Linda University
School of Nursing
Loma Linda, California, USA

CONTENTS

KEY POINTS

- Regardless of whether the patient is religious or nonreligious, the attributions of what makes life purposeful, meaningful, worthwhile—or holy and sacred (to use religious wording)—are vital to motivating a patient to live healthfully. Likewise, a patient's spiritual practices can also be harnessed for use in promoting a lifestyle change.
- Empirical evidence and theory suggest linkages between spirituality/religiosity (S/R) and health outcomes; it is characteristically associated with beneficial health outcomes and vital to consider within lifestyle nursing practice.
- Spiritual care, at its essence, is an expression of a nurse's love. Given this, spiritual care will never be prescriptive or forced. It will always reflect the needs and perspectives of the patient.
- Therapeutic communication skills must be implemented when nurses respond to patients' expression of spiritual pain; therapeutics responses are holistic, patient-centered, and follow patient cues.
- Assessment (whether a screening or history) is required for all and must involve more than just an inquiry about religious affiliation.
- Nurses are spiritual care generalists, not experts; thus, collaboration with chaplains or community-based spiritual care experts identified by the patient can be helpful.
- To avoid an inappropriate imposition of one's personal S/R into patient care, it is important to reflect, recognize, and then bracket those beliefs and practices appropriately.

DOI: 10.1201/9781003178330-34

29.1   INTRODUCTION

Consider these nurse–patient encounters:

- Mr. Lee is an outpatient with hypertension who demonstrates difficulty with implementing lifestyle-related interventions (e.g., diet, stress-reduction, and physical exercises). When the nurse asks Mr. Lee "what motivates you?" he responds, "my faith and my family." Follow-up assessment reveals that Mr. Lee is a somewhat observant Christian who occasionally reads the Bible and prays daily. With this information, the nurse recognizes that lifestyle interventions may be more effective if they are framed as methods for honoring the body as a "temple of the living God." The nurse can also explore with Mr. Lee how prayer may afford inner know-ledge about barriers to lifestyle changes and allow petition to God for strength to implement the lifestyle interventions.
- Ms. White is an artist who likewise lives with hypertension and has difficulty implementing lifestyle-related interventions. When the nurse assesses Ms. White's inner resources, she learns she is "not religious, and not even spiritual—a secular humanist." When asked about what gives life purpose, she acknowledges that she wants to "make the world a better place"—and, more specifically, a more aesthetically beautiful place. Thus, the nurse discusses with Miss White how her desire to make the world more beautiful might necessitate a more healthful lifestyle. The nurse also encourages Ms. White to explore how artistic expression could be a means for gaining self-awareness about attitudes and feelings toward health and lifestyle change.

These parallel scenarios both demonstrate how most patients have ideas about what makes their life worthwhile. This sense of purpose can be prompted by religious or secular framings. Regardless of whether the patient is religious or nonreligious, the attributions of what makes life purposeful, meaningful, worthwhile—or holy and sacred (to use religious wording)—are vital to motivating a patient to live healthfully. Likewise, these scenarios illustrate how a patient's spiritual practices can also be harnessed for use in promoting a lifestyle change.

Spiritual care is that aspect of nursing practice that engages and employs the beliefs and practices that emanate from one's worldview or that enliven a person. Before proceeding to discuss nurse-provided spiritual care, a definition of this construct is required to establish a shared perspective. The following definition of spiritual care was developed by a consortium of European nurse educators. Spiritual care:

> recognises and responds to the human spirit when faced with life-changing events (such as birth, trauma, ill health, loss) or sadness, and can include the need for meaning, for self-worth, to express oneself, for faith support, perhaps for rites or prayer or sacrament, or simply for a sensitive listener. Spiritual care begins with encouraging human contact in a compassionate relationship and moves in whatever direction need requires.
>
> *McSherry et al., 2020*

This definition reflects how nurses typically distinguish spirituality (a broad, universal construct) from religiosity (a narrower concept applying to those who ascribe to the beliefs and practices of a community that shares these to some degree) (Taylor, 2012). This definition also illustrates how nurses have elastic boundaries about what spiritual care entails. For some, it includes compassion and what could be simply considered good nursing or psychosocial caring; for others, it is delimited to therapeutics specifically addressing the patient's spiritual or religious needs.

Spirituality and/or religion (S/R) are foundational to a patient's understanding of health, disease, illness, and suffering—and how to relate to and address these (Taylor, 2012). Thus, the purpose of this chapter is to discuss the intersection of spiritual care and lifestyle nursing. After a brief overview of how S/R and health relate, nurse-provided spiritual care will be described. The chapter concludes with implications for lifestyle nursing, including at the end of life.

29.2   SPIRITUALITY, RELIGIOSITY, AND HEALTH

Koenig and colleagues (Koenig, 2012; Koenig et al., 2012) synthesized over 3,300 empirical studies investigating S/R in the context of psychological or physical health. Although the work is a decade old, none other has subsequently been as comprehensive. Koenig et al. observed that in this vast opus of evidence, S/R was usually positively and significantly associated with health outcomes. Eighty percent of the research studies Koenig et al. reviewed measured S/R's impact on psychological outcomes. Prevalent outcomes measured included coping with adversity (n = 344 studies), well-being/happiness (n = 326), self-esteem (n = 69), depression (n = 444), and anxiety (n = 299). For each of these outcomes, the percentage of studies that found that S/R had a positive or beneficial association with the mental health outcome were calculated; most outcomes were found beneficial in about 60–80% of the studies. This synthesis clearly supports the exploration of how S/R practices might contribute to a patient's psychological health.

But how does S/R impact physical outcomes? In the same way, Koenig and collaborators (Koenig, 2012; Koenig et al., 2012) reviewed physical health outcomes associated with S/R. Although the volume of evidence is less and the percentage of studies finding a positive association are fewer, the evidence is still impressive. For example, the impact of S/R on longevity was found to be positively associated in 68% of 121 studies; only 5% observed a harmful association. In 27 studies measuring the association between S/R and immune function, 56% observed a positive association and only 4% observed a negative association. S/R, measured in various ways, was also frequently found to be positively associated with indicators of endocrine function, heart disease, cancer, stroke, hypertension, cancer, dementia, and self-rated health.

Of particular relevance to this chapter, however, are findings about how S/R has been found to be beneficial in lifestyle contexts (Koenig, 2012; Koenig et al., 2012). These included:

- Cigarette smoking (n = 137 studies), 90% observing positive/beneficial association with S/R and none observing a negative/harmful association.
- Exercise (n = 37 studies), 68% finding positive association with S/R and 16% observing a negative association.
- Healthful diet (n = 21), 62% documenting positive association with S/R and 5% documenting a negative association.
- Weight/body mass index (n = 36), 39% finding positive association with S/R and 19% finding a negative association.
- Risky sexual activity (n = 95 studies), 86% observing positive association with S/R and 1% observing a negative association.

In concert, Koenig et al.'s massive synthesis of the research suggests linkages between S/R and health outcomes and that S/R characteristically is associated with beneficial health outcomes and vital to consider within lifestyle nursing practice.

Given the strong pattern suggesting that S/R and health are associated, epidemiologist of religion Levin (2001) proposed a theoretical model for explaining this association. This theoretical perspective will help the lifestyle nurse to understand that there are various mechanisms potentially contributing to the S/R–health linkage. Levin proposed several mechanisms whereby S/R affects health. These are summarized as follows:

- The behavioral or motivational mechanisms, or the religious prescriptions and proscriptions that are now scientifically established to be health-promoting. Indeed, most world faiths advise adherents to do or not do certain activities. For example, most religions discourage inebriation; this reduces accidents and domestic violence. Several religions recommend certain diets (e.g., abstinence from meats or special methods for preparing meats), which can reduce cancer, heart disease, and other diseases. Likewise, most religions advocate monogamy and sexual intercourse only within a marriage. If observed, this admonition prevents sexually transmitted diseases.

- The interpersonal mechanisms of religiosity, or the experiences of social connection with like-minded believers or with spiritual beings (e.g., angels, saints, God), can offer social support, a factor known to be associated with physical and psychological health. These forms of social support, such as membership in a faith community or relationship with a divine Being who is a faithful friend, will minimize isolation and promote a sense of comfort and safety.
- The cognitive mechanism of religiosity refers to the cognitive schema for understanding and explaining the world and its history. Religious stories and beliefs provide a way to make sense of where humans came from, why what happens happens, and where we are going. Religions offer adherents a creation story, beliefs about what happens at death, and ways to make sense of suffering. Although sometimes religious beliefs can be interpreted in ways that are psychologically harmful, they typically provide comfort. Levin asserted that the psychology of these beliefs likely affect the physiology of the believer, thus explaining the religion and health association.
- The psychophysical and affective mechanisms recognize the health-promoting neurochemistry that occurs within a believer's body when they have a spiritual experience. For example, when religious (and nonreligious persons) experience peace, grace, harmony, insight, gratitude, comfort from the divine, and so forth—whether it be during worshipful singing, prayer, yoga, chanting, communion with others, or spontaneously while meditating in a natural setting—such an emotional experience creates health-promoting physiologic outcomes.

Whereas these mechanisms are supported by science, Levin acknowledged that additional unexplainable mechanisms such as "miracles" may exist that account for the faith and health association.

29.3   NURSE-PROVIDED SPIRITUAL CARE

Although there are many interventions that a nurse may implement to promote the spiritual health of a patient, spiritual care is "an intuitive, interpersonal, altruistic, and integrative expression" of the nurse (Sawatzky & Pesut, 2005, p. 23). Spiritual care, at its essence, is an expression of a nurse's love, according to these nurse educators. Given the nature of love, spiritual care will never be prescriptive or forced. It will always reflect the needs and perspectives of the patient.

Although spiritual care ultimately is about *being* (e.g., compassionating, hoping, encouraging, supporting, accompanying), it also involves *doing*. A synthesis of nursing literature identified eight attributes of spiritual care (Ghorbani et al., 2021). These included:

- Exploring the patient's spiritual perspective (e.g., screening and assessing for spiritual distress, needs, resources).
- Being a healing presence (i.e., altruistically and holistically remaining present for a patient, a knowing look, sharing silence).
- Using self therapeutically (e.g., using unconditional positive regard, being non-judgmental, active listening).
- Attuning to the patient (e.g., intuitively sensing patient's spiritual status, experiencing empathy that includes mentalizing or seeing things from the patient's perspective).
- Making care patient centered (i.e., designing therapeutics to address the unique needs and preferences of each patient).
- Using interventions that promote meaningfulness for the patient (e.g., religious support, facilitating meaningful relationships, encouraging the patient to explore and pursue meaningful activities).

- Creating a spiritually nurturing environment (e.g., providing ethical care, safe-guarding patient values).
- Observing healthcare practices related to evaluation and documentation of spiritual care (Ghorbani et al.).

These attributes of spiritual care may still make it seem mysterious. Thus, some examples of spiritual care therapeutics may help to concretize this component of nursing practice. For example, a validated instrument to measure the frequency of nurse-provided spiritual care identified a number of specific spiritual care "therapeutics." These included assessing health-related beliefs and practices, and how these could be supported; listening for spiritual themes within the patient's illness story, or listening to their spiritual concerns; encouraging a patient to talk about how their illness affects spiritual beliefs or challenges amid illness; arranging for a chaplain or patient's clergy to visit; providing information about spiritual resources, offering to pray or read inspiring literature; documenting or discussing spiritual care with colleagues; and being present (Mamier & Taylor, 2015).

Spiritual care ought to vary depending on the patient's needs and preferences; spiritual care therapeutics also ought to reflect the expertise of the provider and the circumstances requiring intervention. Therapeutics could include different ways for helping a patient to ascribe meaningfulness to their situation or to life. For example, Taylor (2002) described how existential psychotherapist Yalom's guidance could be implemented in nurse-provided spiritual care. A patient could be supported to contribute to a cause (e.g., political, artistic, environmental, religious), to pursue pleasurable experiences (e.g., smelling the roses and watching the sunset), to perform an altruistic deed (e.g., a random act of kindness), or to seek experiences that yield increased self-awareness (e.g., meditation, prayer, psychotherapy, dream analysis). Or, prompted by logotherapist and Nazi concentration camp survivor Frankl's observations about how people develop a sense of meaning, the nurse can encourage a patient to reflect on what they take from the world, what they give to the world, and what attitude they choose to adopt in response to suffering (Taylor, 2002).

Recent evidence generated by positive psychologists provides much insight about potential spiritual care therapeutics that can be introduced, taught, or facilitated by nurses (Taylor, 2019a). For instance, maintaining gratitude practices, pursuing awe-inspiring activities, giving altruistically, forgiving self and others, and practicing self-compassion are known to improve health outcomes (see Greater Good Science Center for overviews and tips, https://greatergood.berkeley.edu/key; as well as Kristin Neff's Self-Compassion website at https://self-compassion.org). Likewise, spirit-enhancing practices can also be recommended by the lifestyle nurse when appropriate. Some of these include non-petitionary prayer, meditation, artistic expression (e.g., writing poetry, dancing, or drawing), journal-writing, dream analysis or active imagination, reminiscing about life themes (e.g., dignity therapy), and immersing oneself in nature (Fitchett et al., 2015; Johnson, 1986; Pennebaker & Smyth, 2016; Taylor, 2002). While these therapeutics do have considerable empirical evidence to support their use within healthcare, some spiritual care therapeutics simply are "tried and true" based on decades of modern psychotherapeutic observation or on millennia of ancient religious understanding.

29.4 IMPLICATIONS FOR LIFESTYLE NURSING CARE

Given spiritual and religious beliefs and practices are often associated with health outcomes, and given the nurse can offer spiritual care so as to promote health, a few "basics" about providing spiritual care are in order. In this section, five essential topics are briefly discussed: Guidelines for ethically providing spiritual care; principles for communication about S/R topics; S/R screening and assessment; need for team collaboration; and importance of nurse S/R awareness.

29.4.1 Ethical Spiritual Care

Spiritual care would not be spiritual or care if it were provided unethically. Because spiritual care is often construed with—and indeed often does entail—religious support, there is considerable opportunity for a nurse to unethically impose personal S/R beliefs or practices during a patient encounter. Indeed, a study of 423 rather religious nurses observed that frequency and beliefs about personal prayer among these nurses was positively, albeit weakly, associated with how frequently they offered prayer to a patient (O'Connell-Persaud et al., 2019). Consider the opening scenarios again: A nurse who finds resolve during prayer could potentially unethically impose her prayer beliefs or practice on Mr. Lee or Ms. White, even though they would be well intentioned.

Thus, guidelines for ethical spiritual care are essential. Ethicist Winslow and nurse scholar Wehtje-Winslow (2007) offered the following directions. For a nurse or any clinician to provide ethical spiritual care, they will:

1. Attempt to obtain a basic understanding of the patient's spiritual needs, resources, and preferences. In other words, they will conduct a brief spiritual screening or more detailed history or assessment, as appropriate.
2. Respect the client's expressed desires about receiving spiritual care.
3. Not impose upon a patient spiritual beliefs or practices or pressure the patient to relinquish any spiritual beliefs or practices.

To avoid imposing personal beliefs or practices, the nurse must have some degree of self-awareness about his or her own spirituality and how it can influence caring. For example, a nurse cannot assume that the spiritual orientation that motivates them to live healthfully will be helpful, never mind welcomed, by a patient. Likewise, the religious practices that foster lifestyle change for the nurse cannot be urged on the patient.

29.4.2 Spiritual Care Communication Principles

Therapeutic communication skills are central to spiritual care. While basic communication skills that all nurses learn in their pre-licensure education are essential, these often are forgotten when nurses become witnesses to expressions of spiritual pain (Taylor & Mamier, 2013). It may be that because spirituality and religion are such intimate and socially constrained topics that nurses become tongue-tied when the topics arise. Thus, the application of any communication skills possessed is urged. Some recommendations particularly pertinent to spiritual care, however, are also offered as general guidelines:

- Listen holistically. That is, listen to what the patient says intellectually and emotionally; sometimes, when deeper encounter will be therapeutic, also listen to what is expressed physically (e.g., body language, listening to your own embodied feelings, such as tightness in the neck or gut) and spiritually—attuning to the sacredness within the encounter (e.g., feeling yourself being "on holy ground," exchanging a knowing look or hand squeeze).
- Make your responses patient centered. Name the cutting-edge issues and/or feelings expressed. Link these issues and feelings with the situation so as to help create meaning for it. Formulas such as "feeling bad/sad/mad/glad?" or "guessing you feel X because Y" can be helpful to nurses as they create such responses (Taylor, 2021).
- When a patient discusses S/R intellectually, respond using communication skills that correspond (e.g., restating, paraphrasing, open questioning). When they express S/R themes with emotion, then respond with a skill that recognizes the emotion (e.g., empathic reflection, open question recognizing the affective dimension of their experience). Remember that eyes tearing up, voices becoming coarse, and bodies beginning to tremble are invitations to discuss

a topic "heart to heart." Thus, communicate "head to head" and "heart to heart" for therapeutic encounters that create safety (Taylor, 2007).

- Remember that the patient's spiritual journey is not yours. Remember also that you are not the expert as to how the journey ought to proceed. Rather, you are accompanying, witnessing, or supporting their journey. Thus, unless the purpose is for assessing, avoid pushing the patient to a new topic that they have not yet shown receptivity towards. Follow the patient's cues (Taylor, 2021). Principles of motivational interviewing are most appropriate in the context of spiritual care (see Chapter 30).

- Following the patient's cues also means using their language to discuss S/R concepts instead of imposing your own language—and, to some degree, your own worldview. If, for example, they refer to a Higher Power, then use that terminology rather than Jesus, Allah, or the Divine. Indeed, it is possible that S/R will be discussed without using any overtly S/R language! (Taylor, 2007).

- Avoid responses that tell the patient you are uncomfortable and they are unsafe discussing S/R further with you (if indeed you are able to choose compassion at that moment). Nurse responses that communicate "stop talking about this to me" include changing the topic, inserting humor, minimizing or denigrating the importance of the topic, and asserting quick answers or "preaching" (i.e., having answers to unanswerable questions). Often nurses illustrate these conversation stoppers by self-disclosing without invitation their own S/R stories or beliefs (Taylor, 2007).

Of course, these communication strategies are effective when used in the context of an underlying respect for the patient. Such respect will deter judgmentalism and self-centeredness in the nurse.

29.4.3   Spiritual Screening and Assessment

As the recommendations above about providing ethical and person-centered care mandated, spiritual screening or assessment are paramount to providing spiritual care (Taylor, 2019b). Experts suggest a differentiation between spiritual screening (i.e., to initially determine if spiritual distress exists), history-taking (i.e., to superficially assess needs, preferences, resources), and assessment (i.e., the data collection an expert will complete to obtain in-depth information regarding various dimensions of the patient's S/R experience) (Taylor, 2019b). It is the spiritual screening and history that is appropriate for a lifestyle nurse to complete. This brief discussion will simply provide suggestions for methods that apply to both processes:

- Remember the goal of screening is to determine if distress exists. With a large sample of cancer survivors, King et al. (2017) tested several screening questions against a well-accepted Negative Religious Coping scale to determine their specificity and sensitivity. The strongest items were "do you struggle with the loss of meaning and joy in your life?" and "do you currently have what you would describe as religious or spiritual struggles?" Another screening question is "how much pain do you have deep within your soul/being that is not physical?" More sterile screeners could be an item with a Likert scale response options like "how important is S/R to you?" Or "what is your overall spiritual well-being?" (Taylor, 2019b).

- More in-depth history-taking questions can inquire about what they perceive their needs to be and what their preferences are with regard to healthcare providers giving spiritual support. These questions do not need to use overtly religious language. For example, a nurse could ask:
  - What are the deepest desires your situation has raised for you?
  - What brings inspiration to your life?
  - Where do you get your inner strength and courage to keep going?
  - What is helping you to cope?

- As I've gotten to know you, I've noticed you speak often of (spiritual themes [e.g., betrayal, yearning for love]). How do you think this theme has influenced your life, or will influence your future? How happy are you with your life's theme?
- Tell me about times during your life where you faced a huge challenge. What got you through? Is that resource still available to you now? (Taylor, 2019b)
- Remember that a spiritual screening or assessment may "open a can of worms." Thus, an assessment may quickly lead to spiritual care itself.

Assessment (whether a screening or history) is required for all and must involve more than just an inquiry about religious affiliation. How one Mennonite views health will differ from another's. How one Muslim practices religious dietary proscriptions will differ from another's. Thus, while a general understanding of various faith traditions is helpful, it is incomplete.

29.4.4   TEAM COLLABORATION FOR SPIRITUAL CARE

Lifestyle nurses will do well to remember that they are not spiritual care experts; they are the generalists (Taylor, 2002). At times when more expertise is required, a referral to an expert should be discussed with the patient. Some patients may prefer a Board-Certified Chaplain with extensive training in clinical ministry that is respectful of all S/R traditions and is employed by the healthcare organization. Others, however, may prefer to seek out their own spiritual director or soul friend, guru or shaman, clergy or faith community elder, or other counselor or psychotherapist with spiritual sensitivities. Indeed, it is important to remember that for many patients, the nurse is not perceived or preferred as a spiritual care provider.

29.4.5   NURSE SPIRITUAL SELF-AWARENESS

Nurse personal S/R is associated with the provision of spiritual care (Taylor et al., 2017). It is only natural that who the nurse is as a person will *not* get stuffed in a locker when they go to work; S/R is inherently part of who the nurse is as they give care. Thus, to avoid an inappropriate imposition of one's personal S/R into patient care, it is important to reflect, recognize, and then bracket those beliefs and practices appropriately (Taylor, 2012).

Questions to prompt such reflection might include: What do I believe about health, illness, and suffering? What S/R beliefs do I accept that bring comfort in times of transition? How do these beliefs influence how I practice nursing? How do I relate to persons whose beliefs differ from mine? Do I believe some beliefs are wrong or evil? How does an ultimate value of love (if, for example, that is the ultimate value) influence my interaction with others who view things differently? How do my S/R beliefs influence my being a nurse? While there is potential for a nurse's S/R to hurt the therapeutic relationship, there is also great potential for good. Indeed, S/R germinates compassion, hope, and willingness to provide nursing care.

29.5   SPIRITUAL CARE AT THE END OF LIFE

Although it is easy to assume that lifestyle nursing is about promoting wellness holistically to assist individuals to become more fully alive, it should not be overlooked that it can also be provided to those facing the end of a life. Indeed, patients at the end of their lives and their beloved often have increased spiritual needs (Balboni et al., 2017). Thus, various hospice and palliative care organizations overtly urge clinicians to include spiritual care in their practices (e.g., National Quality Forum, 2006).

As discussed earlier, completing a spiritual screening, history, or assessment is requisite to providing appropriate and ethical spiritual care. Knowing what are often the most salient spiritual needs of patients facing their mortality, however, is helpful. Delgado-Guay et al. (2016) compared various approaches to assessing end of life wishes among 100 American patients with advanced cancer and documented how spiritual needs were most common. The most frequently identified wishes—more frequent than being pain-free—were to be at peace with God (over 70%) and able to pray (over 60%). Other wishes that intersect the spiritual and psychosocial dimensions included having family present, not being a burden to family, and having family prepared for the death, as well as keeping a sense of humor, being able to say goodbyes, and helping others. Indeed, the need to "be at peace" at the end of life was also observed by Steinhauser et al. (2006) as a top need for patients at end of life, and led them to conclude that the assessment question "are you at peace?" was an excellent indicator of overall spiritual well-being. Thus, for the lifestyle nurse wanting to promote spiritual wellness at the end of life, the goal may well be to support patients and their families to be "at peace."

To support persons facing the end of a life to realize inner peace, two therapeutics that lifestyle nurses can introduce or facilitate are offered:

- Dignity therapy is a therapeutic intervention involving asking a set of open questions to solicit life review and foster a sense of meaning. This therapeutic is well researched and known to contribute to various positive outcomes (Fitchett et al., 2015). Dignity therapy questions to prompt meaningful life review include: "Tell me a little about your life history, particularly the parts you either remember most or think are most important? When did you feel most alive? Are there specific things that you would want your family to know about you? What are the most important roles you have played in life? What are your most important accomplishments? Are there particular things that you feel still need to be said? What are your hopes and dreams for your loved ones? What have you learned about life that you would want to pass along? Are there other things that you would like included?" (Fitchett et al.)

- Religious rituals, including prayer, are typically extremely comforting—especially for religious persons (Taylor, 2019c). While some patients will request prayer or another religious ritual, others may benefit from a spontaneously created ritual that is designed to commemorate a salient inner event (e.g., a restored relationship, a changed attitude). Remember that rituals are symbolic behaviors that inherently allow expression of values, help humans to make meaning, and strengthen relationships between participants (Imber-Black & Roberts, 1998). Rituals often involve elements of rhythm or repetition (e.g., music, repeating a prayer), special or stylized behavior (i.e., doing something out of the ordinary), pattern or order (i.e., following a prescribed plan), evocative presentation (e.g., wearing special clothing), and social interaction (e.g., eating together). While encouraging a patient or family member to incorporate these elements into a ritual can support their spiritual health, it is vital that the client desires and directs the planning. For most, existing religious rituals may be preferred. To facilitate these, inquire as to what and how the patient desires. Collaboration with chaplains, patient clergy, or other spiritual care experts will likely be important—especially if the patient is unsure of how the religious ritual is to be performed. Even when a ritual is performed by a religious expert, patients often appreciate their nurse's engagement.

The use of dignity therapy (or any reminiscence work) and rituals (secular or religious) can help persons at the end of life to find wholeness, meaning, peace—spiritual health. A lifestyle nurse can play a key role in advocating for these therapeutics, even if not providing them.

29.6 CONCLUSION

The chapter was introduced with two scenarios illustrating how S/R beliefs and practices could influence a patient's response to lifestyle recommendations. Empirical evidence and theory were presented to posit that lifestyle nurses should therefore include spiritual assessment and care in their practice. By practicing ethical, person-centered spiritual care that is within the scope of nursing, nurses can enable and inspire patients like Mr. Lee and Ms. White to seek wholeness.

REFERENCES

Balboni, T. A., Fitchett, G., Handzo, G. F., Johnson, K. S., Koenig, H. G., Pargament, K. I., Puchalski, C. M., Sinclair, S., Taylor, E. J., & Steinhauser, K. E. (2017, Sep). State of the science of spirituality and palliative care research part ii: Screening, assessment, and interventions. *Journal of Pain and Symptom Management, 54*(3), 441–453. https://doi.org/10.1016/j.jpainsymman.2017.07.029

Delgado-Guay, M. O., Rodriguez-Nunez, A., De la Cruz, V., Frisbee-Hume, S., Williams, J., Wu, J., Liu, D., Fisch, M. J., & Bruera, E. (2016, Oct). Advanced cancer patients' reported wishes at the end of life: A randomized controlled trial. *Supportive Care in Cancer, 24*(10), 4273–4281. https://doi.org/10.1007/s00520-016-3260-9

Fitchett, G., Emanuel, L., Handzo, G., Boyken, L., & Wilkie, D. J. (2015). Care of the human spirit and the role of dignity therapy: A systematic review of dignity therapy research. *BMC Palliative Care, 14*, 8. https://doi.org/10.1186/s12904-015-0007-1

Ghorbani, M., Mohammadi, E., Aghabozorgi, R., & Ramezani, M. (2021). Spiritual care interventions in nursing: An integrative literature review. *Supportive Care in Cancer, 29*(3), 1165–1181. https://doi.org/10.1007/s00520-020-05747-9

Imber-Black, E., & Roberts, J. (1998). *Rituals for our times: Celebrating, healing, and changing our lives and our relationships*. Rowman & Littlefield.

Johnson, R. A. (1986). *Inner work: Using dreams & active imagination for personal growth*. HarperCollins.

King, S. D., Fitchett, G., Murphy, P. E., Pargament, K. I., Harrison, D. A., & Loggers, E. T. (2017). Determining best methods to screen for religious/spiritual distress. *Supportive Care in Cancer, 25*(2), 471–479. https://doi.org/10.1007/s00520-016-3425-6

Koenig, H. G. (2012). Religion, spirituality, and health: The research and clinical implications. *ISRN Psychiatry*, 278730.

Koenig, H. G., King, D., & Carson, V. B. (2012). *Handbook of religion and health* (2nd ed.). Oxford University Press.

Levin, J. (2001). *God, faith, and health: Exploring the spirituality-healing connection*. Wiley.

Mamier, I. & Taylor, E. J. (2015). Psychometric evaluation of the Nurse Spiritual Care Therapeutics Scale. *Western Journal of Nursing Research, 37*(5), 679–694. https://doi.org/10.1177/0193945914530191

McSherry, W., Ross, L., Attard, J., van Leeuwen, R., Giske, T., Kleiven, T., Boughey, A., & EPICC Network. (2020). Preparing undergraduate nurses and midwives for spiritual care: Some developments in European education over the last decade. *Journal for the Study of Spirituality, 10*(1), 55–71. https://doi.org/10.1080/20440243.2020.1726053

National Quality Forum. (2006). *A national framework and preferred practices for palliative and hospice care quality: A consensus report*. N. Q. Forum. www.qualityforum.org/Publications/2006/12/A_National_Framework_and_Preferred_Practices_for_Palliative_and_Hospice_Care_Quality.aspx

O'Connell-Persaud, S., Dehom, S., Mamier, I., Gober-Park, C., & Taylor, E. J. (2019). Online survey of nurses' personal and professional praying. *Holistic Nursing Practice, 33*(3), 131–140. https://doi.org/10.1097/HNP.0000000000000323

Pennebaker, J. W., & Smyth, J. M. (2016). *Opening up by writing it down: How expressive writing improves health and eases emotional pain* (3rd ed.). Guilford Press.

Sawatzky, R., & Pesut, B. (2005). Attributes of spiritual care in nursing practice. *Journal of Holistic Nursing, 23*(1), 19–33. https://doi.org/10.1177/0898010104272010

Steinhauser, K. E., Voils, C. I., Clipp, E. C., Bosworth, H. B., Christakis, N. A., & Tulsky, J. A. (2006, Jan 9). "Are you at peace?": One item to probe spiritual concerns at the end of life. *Archives of Internal Medicine, 166*(1), 101–105. https://doi.org/10.1001/archinte.166.1.101

Taylor, E. J. (2002). *Spiritual care: Nursing theory, research, and practice*. Prentice Hall.

Taylor, E. J. (2007). *What do I say? Talking with patients about spirituality*. Templeton Press.

Taylor, E. J. (2012). *Religion: A clinical guide for nurses*. Springer.

Taylor, E. J. (2019a). Spirituality (Module 30). In *Nursing: A concept-based approach to learning* (3rd ed., vol. 2, pp. 2023–2046). Pearson.

Taylor, E. J. (2019b). Spiritual screening, history, and assessment. In B. R. Ferrell & J.A. Paice (Eds.), *Textbook of palliative nursing care* (5th ed., pp. 432–446). Oxford University Press.

Taylor, E. J. (2019c). *Fast facts about religion: Implications for nursing*. Springer.

Taylor, E. J. (2021). Healing communication: A precision instrument for spiritual care. *Seminars in Oncology Nursing, 37*(5), 151213. https://doi.org/10.1016/j.soncn.2021.151213

Taylor, E. J., & Mamier, I. (2013). Nurse responses to patient expressions of spiritual distress. *Holistic Nursing Practice, 27*(4), 217–224.

Taylor, E. J., Gober-Park, C., Schoonover-Shoffner, K., Mamier, I., Somaiya, C., & Bahjri, K. (2017). Is nurse religiosity associated with spiritual care? An online survey of practicing nurses. *Clinical Nursing Research, 28*(5), 636–652. https://doi.org/10.1177/1054773817725869

Winslow, G. R., & Wehtje-Winslow, B. J. (2007). Ethical boundaries of spiritual care. *Medical Journal of Australia, 186*(10 Suppl.), S63–S66.

30 Empowering Patients Toward Motivation and Maintenance to Change

Lola A. Coke
Rush University College of Nursing
Chicago, Illinois, USA

CONTENTS

KEY POINTS

- Nurses need a toolkit of behavior change theories and communication methods to individualize patient encounters.
- Education alone is not effective in empowering patients toward lifestyle change; it takes a multifaceted approach.
- Motivational interviewing and coaching are proven methods of engaging patients in reducing ambivalence toward lifestyle change.

30.1 INTRODUCTION

A health care paradigm shift by all health providers that focuses on prevention and healthy lifestyle is imperative. Our westernized health care system, steeped in the provider being the expert that "tells the patient what to do," has been clearly shown to be ineffective. Nursing is in a key position to empower patients to take control of their health. All nurses, despite their workplace, can engage their patients in planning healthy lifestyle changes in lifestyle to promote health and well-being. Healthy changes need to occur when patients are both healthy and, in the presence of chronic disease, condition focused on maximal quality of life.

Despite many motivational strategies to empower patients toward lifestyle behavior change, there has been limited impact on improvement in self-care, morbidity and mortality, and, more importantly, quality of life. Many evidence-based strategies have been developed over several decades to empower patients and guide health care providers, including nurses, to partner with patients in the development of effective lifestyle behavior change plans. These strategies focus on important risk

DOI: 10.1201/9781003178330-35

factors in health that include physical activity, dietary habits, smoking cessation, optimal weight, stress management, and medication adherence.

Over the last decade, nursing education has integrated theoretical frameworks for self-care and decision making, social determinants of health and promotion of quality of life, wellness, and lifestyle change for all patients in their teaching. However, the actual tools to operationalize engaging with patients to accomplish this goal are minimal. The nurse must partner with each patient and be armed with a toolkit to engage the patient to create a realistic plan focused on modification of the lifestyle behaviors that need to be changed and able to sustain over time. This toolkit needs to include strategies that include education, support, and follow-up, all of which have been shown to be key elements of successful lifestyle behavior change.

This chapter will provide an overview of key theoretical frameworks in lifestyle behavior change and discuss practical tools for nurses, based on current evidence, that can be used in any clinical setting to motivate and empower patients to set and achieve lifestyle behavior change goals to maximize their quality of life as they live with a chronic health condition or, better yet, prevent a chronic health condition.

30.2   BEHAVIOR CHANGE THEORIES AND FRAMEWORKS

Numerous theories have been used extensively in behavior change research and in the development of effective strategies for facilitating behavior change. Three theories that have been widely used and found effective in helping individuals adopt and maintain healthy behaviors are social learning theory, transtheoretical stages of change, and relapse prevention.

30.2.1   SOCIAL LEARNING THEORY

Social learning theory, or social cognitive theory, developed by Bandura, is the most well-known theory directed at health behavior change (Bandura, 1977). This theory is based on the tenets that behavior change considers personal experience, self and group efficacy in changing behaviors, the importance of a supportive social setting, and the development of skills to maintain new attitudes and practices. This theory emphasizes the concept of self-efficacy as a mediator of change. Self-efficacy is likened to self-confidence and reflects a person's judgment about how successful he or she will be in performing certain tasks. The more confident an individual is that they can change behavior, the more likely the behavior change will occur. The four elements of social learning theory are skill mastery, verbal persuasion from a health care professional, physiologic feedback, and modeling behaviors, which enhance self-efficacy. Measuring self-efficacy can provide practical information for assessing the effectiveness of programs or interventions aimed at health behavior change.

30.2.2   TRANSTHEORETICAL STAGES OF CHANGE

Stages of change were first theorized by Prochaska and DiClemente (Prochaska et al., 1992). This theory posits that the adoption of effective change is based on understanding an individual's *readiness to change*. Individuals progress through five stages of change that include precontemplation, contemplation, preparation, action, and maintenance. An individual's progression through these stages of change requires a collaborative effort with elements of support and follow-up at each stage. These stages also help to define the level of commitment to change. Where an individual is in the process of change can guide the nurse–patient discussion and plan.

30.2.3   RELAPSE PREVENTION

Relapse prevention is an important intervention strategy for reducing the likelihood and severity of relapse following the cessation or adoption of a lifestyle risk behavior. It was first developed by

Marlatt and Gordon in their work with addictive disorders and was published in 1982 (Hendershot et al., 2011). Relapse is strongly contingent on the self-confidence of an individual and the ability to problem solve when in vulnerable situations that would result in engaging in unhealthy behavior. When helping individuals to change lifestyle behavior, it is important that relapse prevention be part of the plan for change and goal setting so individuals can anticipate what barriers they need to overcome in order to continue to maintain goals over time. Overall, the goal of social cognitive therapy is the acquisition of knowledge and skills, while relapse prevention focuses on preventing patients' return to old habits.

30.3   ENGAGING PATIENTS TOWARD BEHAVIOR CHANGE

Theoretical frameworks provide the background and structure to assess an individual's self-efficacy or confidence and readiness to change and can be used to develop education and programs to promote lifestyle behavior change. However, the most critical element for the nurse is to build a rapport and relationship with the patient, truly hearing the patient's story. This involves targeted communication with each patient to motivate and help them set goals and maintain lifestyle changes. Nurses need to have in their toolkit communication techniques shown to be effective in influencing lifestyle change. There are two communication techniques that will be described here.

30.3.1   MOTIVATIONAL INTERVIEWING

Motivational interviewing, rooted in social learning theory, was developed by William Miller in 1983 as a result of working with patients with addictive behaviors (Miller & Rollnick, 2011). He recognized that as long as patients were ambivalent about making a change in behavior, they were resistant to change. Motivational interviewing is defined as "a collaborative, goal-oriented style of communication with particular attention to the language of change." It is designed to strengthen personal motivation for, and commitment to, a specific lifestyle change goal by exploring reasons for change and past experiences with change within a "come alongside" relationship with the nurse. The key tenets of motivational interviewing include partnering with an individual to resolve ambivalence and alleviate resistance toward a lifestyle change. This includes (1) establishing a relationship and rapport with an individual and engaging in communication to discuss reasons for change and prior successful and unsuccessful attempts to change behavior, (2) focusing on the lifestyle behavior that the individual is most motivated to change, (3) evoking intrinsic motivation to develop self-efficacy, a sense of importance to change and developing a personal toolkit for change, and (4) working with the individual to develop a plan and set goals toward the targeted change, including a plan for relapse, support, and follow-up (Miller & Rollnick, 2011).

Change may occur quickly or may take considerable time, depending on the number of lifestyle changes that need to be modified and the patient's willingness to change. Using the transtheoretical stages of change model as a self-efficacy measure can be used until a patient moves to the action stage. Motivational interviewing is used to guide the patient from precontemplation to contemplation to preparation, determining levels of ambivalence and resistance to change in the targeted behavior.

By focusing on one lifestyle change at a time, the patient can develop their own tools for change and use these tools for subsequent lifestyle changes that need to occur. We know from the literature that knowledge alone is not sufficient to motivate change but is essential as a part of the toolkit when planning change (Purath et al., 2014). Patients need to know the importance of a behavior change and what the consequences are if the change doesn't occur. The main goals of motivational interviewing are to engage patients to resolve their ambivalence and determine the reasons why the change is good as well as what the barriers to change will be, essentially developing their own arguments for change. As a patient becomes more confident, the nurse will begin to hear "change talk" that indicates they are ready to make positive changes.

The five core communication skills of motivational interviewing are:

- Asking open-ended questions to help understand the patient's internal frame of reference, strengthen a collaborative relationship, and find a clear direction.
- Affirmation to acknowledge understanding of what the patient is expressing and focusing on the patient's strengths and abilities.
- Reflective listening, which emphasizes the importance of listening carefully to the patient to hear the patient's story.
- Summarizing during each communication session to promote understanding and reinforce progression toward readiness to set and evaluate goals.
- Informing, educating, and advising, which is useful to help patients reach their own conclusions about the relevance of information (Purath et al., 2014).

Motivational interviewing has been used successfully in research as an intervention to promote lifestyle change. It has been used in studies to increase fruit and vegetable intake, increase physical activity, and promote smoking cessation and weight management. Multiple meta-analyses and systematic reviews including the Cochrane databases form the basis for the use of motivational interviewing to promote lifestyle change in persons with diabetes and cardiovascular diseases and for persons at risk for a stroke (Lundahl et al., 2013; Lindson et al., 2019; Morton et al., 2015).

When preparing to use motivational interviewing as a communication strategy, the nurse needs to be strategic in planning each patient encounter. The literature has shown that lifestyle change outcomes are positively correlated with frequency and length of encounters and longer follow-up period for as much as up to a year. Delivering a motivational interviewing conversation face to face has the most positive outcome, although there is emerging literature to support that motivational texts and phone calls can be effective in promoting lifestyle behavior change (Artinian et al., 2010). Literature has shown that patients who engaged in motivational interviewing interventions experienced increased self-efficacy related to diet and exercise, increased physical activity, reduced caloric intake and increased fruit and vegetable consumption, decreased weight, smoking cessation, and medication adherence. This communication technique has been tested with Native Americans, African Americans, Hispanics, women, and adolescents, all with some measure of success (Lundahl et al., 2013; Morton et al., 2015).

30.3.2 COACHING

Health coaching is a second communication technique shown to be effective in lifestyle behavior change. Health coaching is a shortened and more prescriptive way to work with patients toward changing behavior (Miller & Rollnick, 2011). Health coaching is defined as "the practice of health education and health promotion within a coaching context to enhance the well-being of individuals and to facilitate the achievement of their health-related goals." The role of a health coach is to help patients make choices and to plan and identify challenges that will support change for the better. This role involves communication techniques of listening, understanding, facilitating, supporting, motivating, and providing feedback to patients (Kivelä et al., 2014). Motivational interviewing is often the communication technique used by coaches to promote lifestyle behavior change.

Kivelä and colleagues conducted a meta-analysis of coaching strategies used in lifestyle change and found that health coaching for adults with chronic disease showed statistically significant results in physiological, behavioral, psychological, and social outcomes (Kivelä et al., 2014). The results were encouraging for those with diabetes, being overweight, and with chronic diseases such as heart failure and coronary artery disease. However, it was difficult to evaluate how effective treatment was as health coaching varied widely in both the application and methods used in the studies evaluated. Wide variation also occurred in the length of the coaching intervention (i.e., 3 weeks to 12 months) and the type of health coaching (phone, face to face, or web). A combination of methods appeared to show positive results, such as the use of face to face initially followed by telephone or web-based counseling that enhanced adherence motivation.

In a PRISMA review on health and wellness coaching, investigators concluded that coaching was provided primarily by health care professionals (93%), with nurses forming the largest group of coaches (42%). Hours of training varied widely from less than 2 hours to a median between 6 and 40 hours. Behavioral change methods include goal-setting, action-planning, problem-solving, navigating obstacles to goals, finding resources, self-monitoring, and building self-efficacy. Communication techniques include developing rapport, expressing empathy, and providing emotional support. In addition, 61% of coaches were taught communication skills for the change process, including questioning, negotiating, providing feedback, and various forms of reflection (Wolever et al., 2013).

30.4   ELEMENTS OF HEALTH BEHAVIOR CHANGE

While motivational interviewing and coaching are communication strategies to use in helping individuals change behavior, there are additional tools for a nurse's health behavior change toolkit that can be used to ensure success with adopting new or changing behaviors. Theories described earlier also impact health behavior change as they can serve as guiding frameworks for development of educational modules or programs promoting health behavior change in patients. Psychologists and behavioral scientists have spent decades investigating the appropriate elements of health behavior change that form the basis for helping individuals make lifestyle changes such as changing their diet, beginning an exercise program, or maintaining adherence to medicines known to reduce cardiovascular events in secondary prevention of coronary artery disease (Artinian et al., 2010; Van Horn et al., 2016). While each behavior is different, it is the combination of at least two or more elements that allows one to achieve success with health behavior change. Nurses need to understand variation in behaviors and the success of employing different elements related to each behavior. While the use of communication techniques such as motivational interviewing and using elements of health behavior change takes time, the reward comes with seeing successful behavior change in patients. Integrating educational tools that are behaviorally oriented support provider efforts to help individuals with the change process. Self-monitoring logs for exercise, weight loss, and blood pressure can be an effective strategy. Self-monitoring tools such as heart rate monitors, accelerometers, pedometers, and smartphone apps can all support self-monitoring by adding support for change. As credible sources of health information and support to enhance a patient's self-efficacy, nurses play a key role in motivating and coaching individuals to adopt and change behaviors.

30.5   CONCLUSION

In summary, lifestyle behavior change is hard and complex. Each patient needs to be treated individually based on their socioeconomic and personal needs. Health care professionals need a toolkit with a variety of interventions to assist patients with lifestyle behavior change. In working with patients, it is important to target the behavior a patient is most motivated to change and utilize motivational interviewing until there is change talk that signals readiness to change. A plan is developed with goals and appropriate interventions for follow-up of goals. Relapse prevention is part of the planning. All nurses need to consider lifestyle change a priority in the overall health of all their patients to promote wellness and ensure the best quality of life when living with chronic health conditions.

REFERENCES

Artinian, N. T., Fletcher, G. F., Mozaffarian, D., Kris-Etherton, P., Van Horn, L., Lichtenstein, A. H., Kumanyika, S., Kraus, W. E., Fleg, J. L., Redeker, N. S., Meininger, J. C., Banks, J., Stuart-Shor, E. M., Fletcher, B. J., Miller, T. D., Hughes, S., Braun, L. T., Kopin, L. A., Berra, K., ... Burke, L. E. (2010). Interventions to promote physical activity and dietary lifestyle changes for cardiovascular risk factor reduction in adults: A scientific statement from the American Heart Association. *Circulation, 122*(4), 406–441.

Bandura, A. (1977). *Social learning theory.* Englewood Cliffs.

Hendershot, C. S., Witkiewitz, K., George, W. H., & Marlatt, G. A. (2011). Relapse prevention for addictive behaviors. *Substance Abuse Treatment, Prevention, and Policy, 6*(1), 1–17.

Kivelä, K., Elo, S., Kyngäs, H., & Kääriäinen, M. (2014). The effects of health coaching on adult patients with chronic diseases: A systematic review. *Patient Education and Counseling, 97*(2), 147–157.

Lindson, N., Thompson, T. P., Ferrey, A., Lambert, J. D., Aveyard, P. (2019) Motivational interviewing for smoking cessation. *Cochrane Database of Systematic Reviews* 2019, (7), 1–128. Art. No.: CD006936. DOI: 10.1002/14651858.CD006936.pub4.

Lundahl, B., Moleni, T., Burke, B. L., Butters, R., Tollefson, D., Butler, C., & Rollnick, S. (2013). Motivational interviewing in medical care settings: A systematic review and meta-analysis of randomized controlled trials. *Patient Education and Counseling, 93*(2), 157–168.

Miller, W. R., & Rollnick, S. (2012). *Motivational interviewing: Helping people change.* Guilford Press.

Morton, K., Beauchamp, M., Prothero, A., Joyce, L., Saunders, L., Spencer-Bowdage, S., Dancy, B., & Pedlar, C. (2015). The effectiveness of motivational interviewing for health behaviour change in primary care settings: A systematic review. *Health Psychology Review, 9*(2), 205–223.

Prochaska, J. O., DiClemente, C. C., & Norcross John C. (1992). Search of how people change. Applications to addictive behaviors. *American Psychologist, 47*(9), 1102–24.

Purath, J., Keck, A., & Fitzgerald, C. E. (2014). Motivational interviewing for older adults in primary care: A systematic review. *Geriatric Nursing, 35*(3), 219–224.

Van Horn, L., Carson, J. A. S., Appel, L. J., Burke, L. E., Economos, C., Karmally, W., Lancaster, K., Lichtenstein, A. H., Johnson, R. K., Thomas, R. J., Vos, M., Wylie-Rosett, J., & Kris-Etherton, P. (2016). Recommended dietary pattern to achieve adherence to the American Heart Association/American College of Cardiology (AHA/ACC) guidelines: A scientific statement from the American Heart Association. *Circulation, 134*(22), e505–e529.

Wolever, R. Q., Simmons, L. A., Sforzo, G. A., Dill, D., Kaye, M., Bechard, E. M., Southard, M. E., Kennedy, M., Vosloo, J., & Yang, N. (2013). A systematic review of the literature on health and wellness coaching: Defining a key behavioral intervention in healthcare. *Global Advances in Health and Medicine, 2*(4), 38–57.

31 Mindfulness and Meditation Practices

Bhanu Joy Harrison
Choosing Mindfulness
Albuquerque, New Mexico, USA

CONTENTS

KEY POINTS

- Mindfulness is a skill that can be integrated into daily routines.
- Interoception and sensation are vital components of mindfulness practice and self-regulation.
- Mindfulness skills provide tools to build resilience.
- The state of curiosity increases awareness, intuition, and regulation.
- Polyvagal theory is a framework for growing self-regulation and understanding our own and our patients' mental, emotional, and physical states.
- Practitioner *presence* improves and deepens the patient/provider relationship.

DOI: 10.1201/9781003178330-36

31.1   INTRODUCTION

Mindfulness classes and psychotherapy sessions typically begin with an Orienting Practice such as Practice #1 to help participants *arrive* to the present moment.

PRACTICE #1   ORIENTING AND ARRIVING IN THE PRESENT MOMENT

Allow your body to come into a comfortable posture.

With your eyes open, begin to look around your environment, turning your head, neck, and eyes, noticing objects and the space around you.

Become aware of any ambient sounds in your environment.

Notice your sense of touch—your back against the chair, your hands on your thighs or lap.

Are you aware of any fragrances or tastes?

See if you can notice something of interest or beauty in your environment.

Please note: The body is always in present time. This Orienting Practice induces curiosity and the movement of the head and neck stimulates the vagus nerve, which can help us shift to a more parasympathetic state of functioning.

31.1.1   WHAT IS MINDFULNESS?

Mindfulness is paying attention, on purpose, to what is happening in the present moment with curiosity, kindness, and non-judgment. Jon Kabat-Zinn defines mindfulness as "the awareness that arises from paying attention, on purpose, in the present moment and non-judgmentally" (Kabat-Zinn, 2005, p. 4). Ronald Epstein says "meditation is about a sense of presence, balance, and connection with what is most fundamentally important in your life" (Epstein, 2017, p. 8). Diana Winston, Director of UCLA's Mindful Awareness Research Center, defines mindfulness as "a state of consciousness, one characterized by attention to present experience with a stance of open curiosity" (Smalley & Winston, 2010). A common misconception of mindfulness meditation is that it is only successful when the mind is empty of thoughts. Instead, the mind becomes quieter as a result of having more intentional thoughts and being more present with emotions and sensations.

Research into mindfulness practices is still in its infancy, but positive trends are showing up. The challenge in getting statistical data in this field is the sheer variety of mindfulness practices. Also, results are often self-reported by meditators, making them unreliable and difficult to replicate (Goleman & Davidson, 2017). The best research you can do is to enter the laboratory of your own body and mind and experiment with these practices to see what works for you.

31.1.2   HOW DOES MEDITATION DIFFER FROM MINDFULNESS?

Mindfulness can be described as a particular state of consciousness, an open awareness to and curiosity of our present experience. Meditation practices are specific tools that help people become more mindful. While mindfulness and meditation originated from Buddhism, every spiritual and religious tradition has contemplative, meditative practices. The state of mindfulness, therefore, can be integrated into any tradition and be practiced in a secular, nonreligious way. Practitioners are often receptive to secular practices and some choose to integrate the state of mindfulness into their own faith tradition.

31.1.3 PAYING ATTENTION

Mindfulness practices like focused attention or concentration practices can help hone the ability to pay attention. Attention is like a muscle that needs consistent workouts. The more repetitions one does, the stronger the muscle of attention becomes. When one focuses on the breath, for example, one's mind eventually wanders off. Noticing this wandering and returning one's attention to breathing is a repetition. Below is a traditional mindfulness practice on breath awareness.

PRACTICE #2 ATTENTION TO OUR BREATH

Let your body be comfortable in a sitting, standing, or lying down posture.

Turn your attention to your breath, without changing its pace or rhythm.

Where in your body do you feel the sensations of the breath the strongest? Do you notice the cool breath coming into your nostrils, the expansion and contraction of your chest and ribs, or the rise and fall of your abdomen?

Keep noticing these sensations, and when your mind wanders away to another unrelated thought, become aware of this wandering and refocus your attention on the sensations of the breath.

The most important key is not to think about your breath, but to feel the sensations of your breath.

You have just completed one repetition of attention building through noticing your breath!

Please note: People with lung challenges (asthma, COPD) and those with anxiety or PTSD may struggle or be triggered with attention on the breath. It is perfectly fine to choose a different sensation to attend to, such as the feeling of feet in shoes, the touch of hands on clothing, and so forth.

31.2 MINDFUL LIVING

Studies conducted by researchers over the last two decades have shown that there are three pillars of mind training to engage in mental exercises, sometimes called reflective practice, meditation, or mindful awareness practices (MAPs) that include learning to focus attention, opening our awareness, and generating kind intention (Siegel, 2018). These practices can make people feel more comfortable with themselves and increase their presence.

Research suggests that living with such presence:

- Optimizes telomerase levels, which repairs and maintains ends of chromosomes.
- Reduces cardiovascular risk factors.
- Reduces inflammation by altering epigenetic regulation of the inflammatory response.
- Reduces the stress response.
- Enhances immune function.
- Cultivates more integration in the brain, yielding more functional regulation of such processes as emotion, attention, and behavior (Siegel, 2018).

Most health professionals say they do not have time to meditate, which stems from the misconception that mindfulness meditation is only done through a formal sitting practice. In reality, there are many ways to practice informal meditation daily that help promote greater self-regulation and resilience.

Practice #3 is a simple informal mindfulness practice that is like hitting the refresh button on a computer. It can lead to a gentle reset of the nervous system, allowing people to check in and slow down for a moment.

PRACTICE #3   S-T-O-P PRACTICE

S = Stop what you are doing right now.

T = Take a few deep breaths.

O = Observe. Notice something in your environment, a body sensation, a thought, or an emotion. Just be curious about what is present, without the need to change anything.

P = Proceed with what you were doing.

As mindfulness has gained in popularity, many people turn toward mindfulness practices to reap benefits such as reducing anxiety, improving sleep, and lowering blood pressure. However, this goal-oriented focus demonstrates western culture using mindfulness to fix conditions, which contradicts the definition of mindfulness. Mindfulness means paying attention to and accepting the conditions of the present moment, not changing the conditions.

31.3   MINDFULNESS OF THE BODY

Awareness of the body is a foundational mindfulness skill, as the body is always in present time.

One often tunes out the quieter messages their body gives about hunger and fatigue.

Being more mindful or body literate results from learning the language of the body, sensation, which can improve physical and mental well-being. One receives information about the external environment from five senses—sight, sound, touch, taste, and smell. Interoceptive awareness is a sixth sense that allows one to pay "conscious attention to inner body sensations" (Farb et al., 2015) and is critical for homeostasis, physical and emotional regulation, and well-being (Farb et al., 2015). Every body has its own language; hunger for one may be a growling stomach, for another it may be feeling dizzy, and for a third person, it may be hangry (hungry and angry). One's curiosity about their sensations of hunger allows them to learn their body's language and use somatic reappraisal to decide what action to take (Farb et al., 2015).

Mindfulness practices use awareness of one's body as a tool for focus, concentration, and awareness. Tracking sensations and using adjectives to describe them deepens interoceptive skills

---

TABLE 31.1 SENSATION LANGUAGE (INTEROCEPTION SKILL)

We can learn to "track our sensations" by being curious about what we feel inside our bodies. See if you can find 2–3 adjectives that most accurately describe a sensation you are currently feeling. Here is a list to start your creativity … feel free to add more!

hot	shivery	prickly	open	heavy	cold
effervescent	achy	collapsed	jumpy	puffy	icky
nauseated	tense	itchy	dizzy	strong	moist
thready	energized	tingling	smooth	thick	radiating
numb	flaccid	stuck	pulsing	clammy	congested
stabby	empty	dark	electrified	perforated	thin
blocked	flowing	weighted	settled	grounded	agitated
closed	suffocating	calm	foggy	clear	burning

(Gendlin, 1982). Teaching this skill to patients can improve the quality of their care as they become active participants in exploring their body conditions.

Interoception, a perceptual capacity, is introduced in relation to well-being because it is thought to be intimately connected to self-regulation, having likely evolved to help organisms maintain homeostasis (Farb et al., 2015). Practice #4 is about interoception and tracking sensations.

PRACTICE #4   INTEROCEPTION: TRACKING SENSATIONS

Notice a sensation you are currently experiencing. Are you hungry, tired, do you have muscle tension, or perhaps are you feeling relaxed and calm? Then ask yourself questions like:

How do I know I'm hungry? What sensations do I notice that tell me I need food?
    Growling tummy, dizzy, hangry, empty gurgling stomach?
What sensations tell me I'm relaxed?
    Easy breathing, dropped shoulders, soft muscles?
What sensations tell me I'm frustrated?
    Tight jaw, clenched hands, edgy sharp words, muscle bracing?
What sensations do I notice when I feel joy?
    Effervescent, light, giggly, smiling, open, warm?
Where in my body do I feel this?
    Chest, arms, legs, etc.?
What sensations am I aware of right now? How would I describe them?

Please note: Periodically during the day, check in with your body and notice sensations happening right now.

31.4   MINDFULNESS OF EMOTIONS

One learns how to deal with feelings from the modeling of family, friends, and the culture at large. How does one know what emotions they are having? What sensations does one feel when one is joyful, worried, or sad? Becoming mindful of one's emotional experience is key to self-regulation and increased well-being. Not surprisingly, being emotionally literate includes awareness of one's body. Each person has a bio-individuated experience of emotion. For one individual, joy is felt as bubbling in the chest, and for another, an openness in their whole body. Anxiety manifests in many different ways—tight chest, difficulty breathing, racing heart, dry mouth, stomach upset, IBS symptoms, shaking limbs, racing thoughts. Sadness can often be felt as heaviness in the chest, feeling tearful and limp. This demonstrates the interconnectivity between mental and physical experiences where changes in one impact the other (Feldman-Barrett 2020).

When a patient complains that they are feeling worried, asking how they know they are worried and what sensations they are labeling as worried invites curiosity and the possibility of self-reflection on the part of the patient.

Rather than having one's emotions loop around the storyline "he said this, and then I said that, and I'm so mad!," a mindful internal dialogue would be to:

1. Notice I'm angry.
2. Ask myself what sensations am I feeling—hot, tight muscles, set jaw?
3. Take a few breaths.

4. Pause and take a moment to be curious about my body, thoughts, and any underlying emotions.
5. Consciously choose a response, rather than immediately reacting.

Mindfulness practices build skills in learning to pause and respond, rather than immediately reacting. One can become a disentangled participant in the experience of emotions (Smalley & Winston, 2010). Holocaust survivor and author Viktor Frankl (1959) captured this element of mindfulness when he wrote, "everything can be taken from a man but one thing: the last of human freedoms—to choose one's attitude in any given set of circumstances, to choose one's own way" (Frankl, 1959, p. 75).

Thoughts, stories, and imagined events trigger strong emotions, body reactions, and thought processes. Thinking, feeling, and sensing are intimately connected, which can cause pain and suffering, but also offers a doorway to greater regulation. Research has shown that expressing gratitude either in a journal or to others reduces symptoms of depression (Wong et al., 2018). Exercise also helps diminish anxiety and depressive symptoms, and diet affects not only body physiology, but mood as well.

31.4.1 TURNING TOWARD OUR EMOTIONS

Rather than changing or fixing one's uncomfortable and difficult emotions, mindfulness pushes one to be with them, at least for a short time.

Using words to describe emotions increases integration between the brain's left and right hemispheres and down regulates the limbic system, particularly the amygdala (Siegel & Payne Bryson, 2012). This process can help regulate emotions and bring mindful attention to them. Noticing thoughts, feelings, and sensations of emotions allows one to become the *knower* rather than the *owner* of the experience. This meta-awareness demonstrates the idea that one can be a neutral observer of one's experience and opens up the space for presence and kindness (See Figure 31.1).

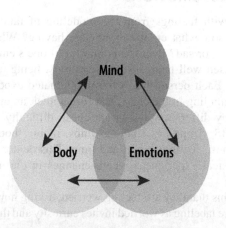

FIGURE 31.1 Mind–body–heart connection—doorways to mindfulness

If your mind is feeling too busy, notice a body sensation or a positive emotion.
If you feel flooded with a difficult emotion, notice a body sensation or a helpful thought.
If you have strong body sensations (pain), remember a neutral to pleasant thought or feeling, remember a positive event, or find a more comfortable area in your body to focus on.

PRACTICE #5   BEING PRESENT WITH EMOTIONS

Become aware of a current emotion. Start with a mild to moderate emotion, or even a positive emotion until you are more familiar with this practice.

What emotion are you feeling?
      Joy, grief, worry, frustration, contentment?
What body sensations are you experiencing that you connect with this emotion?
      Tight, heavy, thick, bouncy, open?
Where in your body do you feel these sensations the strongest?
      Chest, face, jaw, heart, belly, hands?
Now that you have *named it to tame it to frame it*, take a few moments to just be with the sensations. Watch the sensations and see what happens to them next.
Come back to your body sensations if you find yourself lost in the storyline.
What happens to your sensations as you watch them with kindness, curiosity and non-judgment? Do they diffuse a bit or become more consolidated?

Thank yourself for being willing to be present with your emotions!

31.5   MINDFULNESS OF THOUGHTS

The mindfulness skills used with body and emotion can be applied to thoughts. There is a lot of repetition in one's thoughts that can affect one's emotional and physical states, causing pain and suffering. Naming and labeling one's 10 most challenging thoughts in writing as in Table 31.2 can be a helpful practice.

During meditation, one's focus on a breath or sensation, the anchor, gets disrupted by thoughts. Labeling and categorizing these thoughts helps one quickly return to the anchor. The process goes like this:

> I'll notice the cool air coming into my nostrils, then think about my son coming to visit soon. I put that whole storyline into a category or file of "family thoughts". I go back to the sensations of my breath. "I wonder if he was able to get a rental car." Oh ... "worry thought" category. Back to my breath. "Oh I wish my daughter could come visit too." Ah ... "sad thought" category. And on and on.

This is a successful meditation. Success is not having a blank, empty mind. Minds often wander to thoughts. Noticing this wandering of thoughts and returning to the anchor of attention builds the capacity for focus and concentration and disentangles one from a jumble of thoughts.

TABLE 31.2
Common thought loops

I'm no good. (self-criticism)	I'm so worried she'll get sick. (anxiety)
I'm so stupid. (self-criticism)	Why can't he fix this? (angry)
That person is too close. (fear)	It's my fault. (self-criticism)
She's wearing that! (judging)	I can't handle this. (overwhelm)
I'm scared. (traumatic)	I'll never get this done on time. (stress)
Make a list of your most common challenging thoughts.	

TABLE 31.3
Mindfulness tools to work with thoughts

Imagine thoughts floating away in a balloon.	Say to yourself, "This is just a thought, let me return my attention to my anchor."
Labeling thoughts—work thoughts, family thoughts, food thoughts, worry thoughts.	Counting your thoughts (not attending to content, just to quantity).
Can you notice the birth of a thought?	Can you notice the disappearance of a thought?
How fast are your thoughts right now?	Are my thoughts scattered or looping on one topic?
How does this thought affect my body?	How does this thought affect my emotions?
Am I thinking about the past? Let me bring my attention back to right now ideally through noticing a sensation.	Am I thinking about the future? Let me come back to my body by feeling a sensation.

Mindfulness practice changes the structure and function of the brain. People that meditate consistently have thicker brain regions than non-meditators (Holzel et al., 2007; Lazar et al., 2005). Brain waves alter with mindfulness. Theta waves increase in the frontal cortex, consistent with the idea that the front part of the brain is becoming calm (Lazar et al., 2005). EEG patterns reveal increased coherence, suggesting that meditation creates synchronization of various brain regions, from front to back and between the left to right hemispheres (Cahn & Polich, 2006). Practicing mindfulness rewires the brain, changing one's relationship with the present moment. Table 31.3 and Practice #6 present mindfulness tools to work with thoughts.

PRACTICE #6   GETTING OFF THE THOUGHT TRAIN

Use this practice when thoughts keep looping or distracting you from your work, sleep, etc.

Settle into a comfortable position.
Take a few deep breaths.
Become curious about your mental activity.
Are your thoughts going fast, slow, on one topic, jumping around?
Imagine you are on the thought train and you pull the cord to get off the train.
Notice yourself stepping out of the train onto the platform.
Watch your thought train move off into the distance.
What do you feel as you are no longer on this train? A bit of spaciousness? Relief?
Did you ever realize you have the power to get off the train?

Please note: This mindfulness tool takes a lot of practice to develop competency. Don't get discouraged; it will get easier over time.

31.6   AN INTRODUCTION TO POLYVAGAL THEORY

Polyvagal theory, developed by Stephen Porges, is one of the most clinically relevant models of the nervous system. Porges delineates the evolution of the nervous system for one's safety and protection. The dorsal vagal (DV) system, the unmyelinated branch of the 10th cranial vagus nerve, is the most primitive system. It is responsible for the freeze response when one is threatened with little chance for escape. The next evolutionary step is the sympathetic nervous system (SNS), the fight/flight approach to danger. The newest development in the nervous system is the ventral vagal system

(VV), the myelinated ventral branch of our vagus nerve, which allows one to be calm and connected. Interestingly, the ventral vagus is only found in mammals and serves the purpose of helping find safety in alliance with others. The ventral vagal system is neuroprotective and energy efficient, acting as a neural brake by inhibiting the nervous system from going into fight, flight, or freeze states unless it is necessary. The vagus nerve mediates a brain–heart connection, which provides information about the autonomic nervous system, stress levels, and health through heart rate variability (Evans et al., 2013). Respiratory sinus arrhythmia tracks changes in heart rate associated with breath patterns (Sahar et al., 2001).

PRACTICE #7   MODULATING THE BREATH PRACTICE

In this short practice, we will use the science of how to modulate our stress response using the science of respiratory sinus arrhythmias. If you are feeling angry, speedy, or upset (hyperarousal), make your *exhales longer* than your inhales for 5–7 breaths. There should be a tiny slowing of your heart rate and a down regulating effect in your nervous system.

If you are feeling tired, overwhelmed, or collapsed (hypoarousal), make your *inhales longer* than your exhales for 5–7 breaths. This has an effect of slightly increasing your heart rate and "upregulating" your nervous system to give you a tiny boost in energy.

31.6.1   CLINICAL APPLICATIONS OF POLYVAGAL THEORY

Polyvagal theory improves the ability to self-regulate and be present while also giving insight into the neural states of patients. If a nurse is frustrated at an insurance company, for example, they could have a level of upset and dysregulation that may confuse patients. However, if the nurse is mindful that they have gone into a sympathetic nervous system fight response, they can employ mindfulness tools to bring themselves back into the ventral vagal state of calm and connected increasing the ability to be present with patients.

Nurses can also pay attention to the polyvagal state of patients. Perhaps Susan comes in with slumped shoulders and is very quiet. She may be in her dorsal vagal system of freeze or collapse, feeling disconnected, overwhelmed, depressed, or hopeless. If she says "I'm just not feeling like myself these days," a nurse could just respond with "I know, things are so hard lately," which may end the conversation. Or the nurse can become curious and ask what she is noticing. Has her appetite or sleep changed? Was there an event that triggered this feeling? How long has she felt this way? What sensations does she notice in her body? Being curious and interested in her experience will reap many clinical insights that assist with diagnosis or treatment. Most importantly, Susan will feel seen and heard, connected with the nurse as a fellow human being, hopefully leading to increased motivation to comply with treatment and strategies.

The following mindful inquiry practice helps explore the inner landscape of one's nervous system so one can begin to track one's own bio-individuated polyvagal states.

PRACTICE #8   TRACKING OUR POLYVAGAL STATES

Settle for a moment, taking a few breaths.
Ask yourself, "which polyvagal state am I in right now?"
Am I going too fast inside (SNS) or too slow (DV)?
Do I feel angry, worried, anxious, frustrated, scared, or hyperaroused? (SNS)

Do I feel settled and calm, alert and connected? (VV)?
Do I feel shut down, invisible, disconnected, sad, helpless, or hypoaroused? (DV)
What sensations are predominant?
What emotions do I notice in each of these states?
What types of thoughts do I have in these different states?

Please note: Thank yourself for attending and noticing your internal operating state in this moment.

31.6.2 Neuroception

"Neuroception" is a term coined by Stephen Porges (2011) to describe the innate ability of the nervous system to detect safety, danger or life threat (See Figure 31.2).

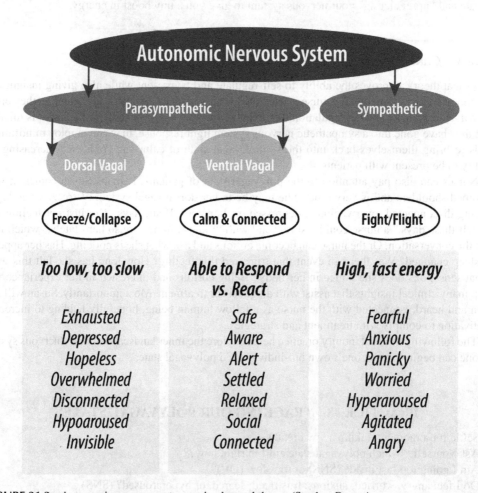

FIGURE 31.2   Autonomic nervous system and polyvagal theory (Stephen Porges)

All nervous systems need three things to feel safe:

Context—the *why, what, and how* of an experience
Choice—offering options to increase self-determination, increases sense of safety
Connection—one needs to be heard and feel like someone is on one's side

Dana, 2021, p. 10

Knowing these three ingredients to enhance safety can transform a nurse's therapeutic alliance with patients. For example, when doing a blood draw, explain why the patient needs it and what will happen during the process (context). Ask if they would like to use their right or left arm (choice). Look at them, say it will hurt just a bit, but you are right there with them (connection).

When a person experiences trauma, their sense of safety is lost and the nervous system can become dysregulated (Levine, 1997). One can get stuck in the fight/flight state or the freeze/collapse state as a means to stay safe. Many patients experience trauma—whether it be relational, medical, developmental, or systemic injustice, to name a few—highlighting the need to be aware of factors that increase the sense of safety.

Understanding how trauma dysregulates the nervous system is helpful to nurses themselves and their patients. Vicarious traumatization happens to those in the caring professions as they hear and see the suffering of those they serve (Halpern, 2011). Being a witness to ongoing, daily traumatic events is taxing, and many professionals push these experiences aside or rather deeper into their physiology, leading to burnout over time.

Mindfulness practices can reconnect one to one's experiences, however difficult, and give the opportunity to metabolize them and hold them with awareness, curiosity, and kindness.

Here is a mindfulness practice to work with traumatic visual experiences:

PRACTICE #9   CAMERA LENS PRACTICE FOR MANAGING TRAUMATIC IMAGES

Acknowledge a difficult image that you can't get out of your mind.

See if you can widen the frame of that image to notice what else you can see. Perhaps you notice a colleague, or a life-saving piece of equipment, or the color of a wall.

Continue to widen the frame of your vision, noticing sounds, other people, or the sky or a tree outside a window.

Notice your body sensations or your breath as the traumatic image takes up less and less space in the frame of your internal image.

Please note: It may take several repetitions of this practice to bring down the intensity or frequency of this image. And please get support from your colleagues if it doesn't resolve.

(Adapted from Levine, 2003)

Trauma narrows one's focus of attention and holds it hostage with the traumatic experience (Levine, 1997). The mindfulness practices shared in this chapter can keep attention flexible and open and help mitigate the effects of vicarious trauma.

31.6.3   THE WINDOW OF TOLERANCE

The window of tolerance, a concept developed by Dan Siegel (1999), is defined as a zone that exists between the extremes of hyper and hypoarousal. It is the zone of optimal arousal or readiness for

TABLE 31.4
Window of tolerance

Hyperarousal zone (Sympathetic nervous system)	Increased sensation Emotional reactivity Hypervigilance Intrusive imagery Disorganized cognitive processing
Optimal arousal zone (Ventral vagal system)	Calm, alert, connected with others Window of tolerance
Hypoarousal zone (Dorsal vagal system)	Relative absence of sensation Numbing of emotions Disabled cognitive processing Reduced physical movement

Source: (Adapted from Ogden et al., 2006, p. 27)

TABLE 31.5
Sample resource list

What activities, environments or people bring me back to my ventral vagal state?

walking	cooking	dancing	singing/laughing
reading	knitting	drawing	being in nature
playing music	talking w/ a friend	journaling	praying
ceremony	gardening	baths	bird watching
church	my children	photography	chopping wood

life or focus on the activity at hand. The levels of arousal change based on the situation and what needs to be done (Treleaven, 2018, p. 88). Dysregulated arousal, swinging uncontrollably between hyper and hypoarousal, is exhausting and occurs when one is overwhelmed or traumatized (See Table 31.4).

The window of tolerance is a helpful mindfulness tool for self-regulation and self-care. One's body provides cues signaling when one is in or out of their window. Understanding these cues and choosing activities to respond helps one stay within their window. For example, one might notice that they are out of their window because they are lying on the couch all day after an intense week of work taking on extra shifts. Recognizing this cue and consciously choosing to take a 30-minute nap and do some stretching exercises can help one move back into one's window.

31.6.4 EMBODYING RESOURCES

Resources help bring one back to the window of tolerance (Levine, 1997). A resource can be any activity, interaction, quality (faith, perseverance, strength) that creates a sense of connection, calm, and safety. Table 31.5 offers a partial list of some resources.

Practicing any of these activities can reduce stress and decrease burnout while adding richness and depth to life experiences. When dysregulated and out of the window, it can be difficult to think

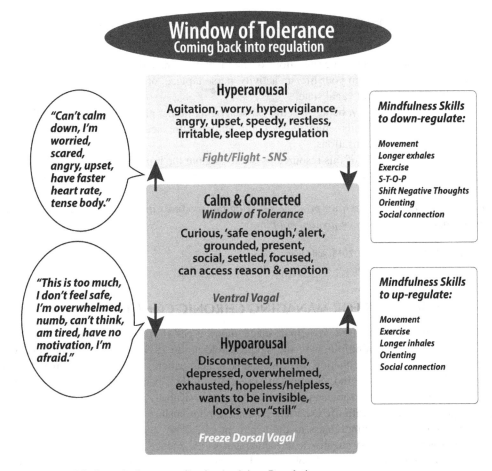

FIGURE 31.3 Window of tolerance—Coming back into Regulation

of resources, so it is good practice to write a personalized list beforehand. For example, a client was overwhelmed with grief over the sudden death of her husband. She was distraught, had difficulty concentrating, and was exhausted from crying. Upon the suggestion of creating a resource list, she wrote down activities she could do when she got too dysregulated from grief. She put these in a mason jar on her dining room table with a taped image of an orange lifejacket. When needed, she would reach in and pull out a strip of paper with a resource and do that activity. Drink some water. Look at the sky. Take a deep breath. Put your hand on your heart. She felt like she put on her lifejacket of resources to ride the tsunami of grief without getting pulled under. This process gave her strength to go through the grieving process and, over time, increased her ability to function.

Embodying internal resources not only builds resilience, it helps bring one back into one's window of tolerance and greater ventral vagal activity, as depicted in Figure 31.3.

Over time, taking in the good can rewire the brain and help override the brain's innate response to attend more to negative or threatening experiences, the negativity bias. The key is to pay attention to sensations, not just think about resources. Paying attention to sensations is the doorway into regulation and balance. Practice #10 helps with savoring and embodying resources and facilitates a return to a more optimal ventral vagal state.

PRACTICE #10   EMBODYING RESOURCES

Allow yourself to settle into a comfortable position, sitting, standing, or lying down.

Take a few breaths, noticing the sensations of the inhalation and exhalation.

Now, think of a resource in your life, an activity, person, place, or object that helps you come back to a calm, ventral vagal state.

Imagine doing this activity, being with this person, being in that place, or sensing that object.

Flesh out the sensory details—movement, color, temperature, etc.—and notice where in your body you feel these sensations.

Now, savor the goodness of this resource by stretching out the remembered sensations of this experience. Stay with the sensations for at least 12–16 seconds or longer if you can.

Please note: The more often we practice savoring the goodness in our life, the more we build neural pathways to embrace joy and happiness.

Source: (Adapted from Hanson, 2013, and Levine, 2003)

31.7   MINDFULNESS FOR MANAGING CHRONIC CONDITIONS

Mindfulness practices are used to help manage many types of physical ailments. Jon Kabat-Zinn introduced secular mindfulness to the medical field in the 1970s. He created the eight-week Mindfulness Based Stress Reduction (MBSR) course to help patients with chronic pain and serious illness. Helping patients be kind, curious, and present with their painful experiences helped them cope better, have greater life satisfaction, and decrease pain (Kabat-Zinn, 2013). Mindfulness practice changes relationships with life experiences, such as relationships with pain.

Judson Brewer brings mindfulness to the treatment of anxiety and addiction treatment. Brewer encourages smokers to be very attentive to the actual sensory experience of smoking, the taste, the smell, the act of inhaling (Brewer, 2021). People often discover that they do not like the taste of cigarettes, which helps them taper their use. In his book, *Unwinding Anxiety*, Dr. Brewer (2021) encourages people to be curious about their sensations of anxiety. Awareness of habitual behaviors and thoughts is key to making change. Mindfulness practices help build such an awareness in all aspects of life.

Clients with chronic pain also use mindfulness practices. Hyperfocusing on the sensation of pain, a signal of danger, builds wider neural pathways and lowers pain threshold (Moseley, 2011). Pain provides a cue that something may be seriously wrong, so it is important to rule out or confirm disease processes that require medical attention. However, "pain is not just a 'body problem', it is a whole system problem. … The systems perspective on pain opens the door for many different possible ways to use your mind intentionally to influence your experience of pain" (Kabat-Zinn, 2013, pp. 367–368). Pain tends to narrow one's focus, just like trauma experiences. Practice #11 shifts attention between areas of discomfort and comfort.

PRACTICE #11   SHIFTING FOCUS PRACTICE FOR PAIN

Settle into as comfortable a position as you can muster. Take a few deep breaths.

Notice an area of discomfort or pain, at a level no more than a 5 on the pain scale.

Where in your body is this pain? How large is the area of discomfort?

What adjectives would you use to describe the pain—hot, stabbing, achy, heavy …?

Now, just watch these uncomfortable sensations for a short bit and be curious to see what happens to them next.

The sensations may stay the same or they may change. If they change, how so? Do the sensations get less intense or spread out? Do you need to find different adjectives to describe the pain now?

Next, shift your focus to a place in your body that has more comfort or is neutral. This area can be small, like the tip of your nose or larger.

As we did with the pain, notice the area and size of this greater comfort.

What adjectives would you use to describe these more comfortable/neutral sensations—light, open, settled, warm?

Keep noticing these sensations and see what happens to them next. Do they expand in size or grow stronger, or do they stay the same? Do you need to find new adjectives?

Take some time to savor these neutral to comfortable sensations.

Now, shift your attention back to the original area of discomfort. Has it changed or stayed the same? Continue to be curious. Take your time.

Begin to pendulate or move your attention slowly from the area of discomfort to the area of comfort, back and forth, back and forth, and notice what happens next.

End this practice with your attention on the area of comfort and thank yourself for being willing to explore all these sensations.

Please note: This practice gets easier over time, especially if you are working with chronic pain. Many people report the pain decreasing or the areas of greater comfort growing larger. Experiment and see what happens for you.

(Adapted from Gendlin, 1982, and Levine, 2003)

This practice helped alleviate some pain for a client suffering from a serious migraine. After showing the area of pain, describing it in adjectives, and shifting her focus to the rest of her body, the client noticed her migraine pain decreased by half. Asking about the rest of her body shifted her attention away from the pain and to her greater area of comfort, allowing her body to come into greater regulation. This quick intervention, of 2–3 minutes, was a profound experience.

31.8 CONTRA-INDICATIONS FOR MINDFULNESS PRACTICE

Unfortunately, mindfulness practices are not helpful to some people. Those with psychosis or dissociative conditions may decompensate when exploring internal body sensations. Also, those with PTSD may find it re-triggering and overwhelming to notice body experiences and discover unacknowledged trauma memories beginning to surface (Treleaven, 2018). Some trauma survivors find meditation instructions to be still or be quiet invoke messages given by their abusers. The key is to find a mindfulness teacher skilled in trauma-sensitive mindfulness tools, offering adaptations to make the practices safer. Keeping eyes open, rather than closed, or using an external anchor (an object, touch, sound, etc.) rather than the breath, helps the student titrate or slowly pace their introduction to mindfulness practices (Treleaven, 2018). Providing referrals for mindfulness education from teachers that are highly skilled (MBSR or UCLA MAPs instructors) and advising patients to ask these teachers if they are trained in trauma-sensitive practice can prevent harm.

31.9 THE GIFT OF PRESENCE

The practice of nursing is a relational one, working daily with doctors, staff, patients, and family members. In many ways, nurses have the closest interactions with patients, and their ability to be present in the moment has a direct impact on the care they deliver (Epstein, 2017). So, what is presence? Epstein defines it as "a quality of listening—without interrupting, interpreting, judging or minimizing" (Epstein, 2017, p. 68). "Deep listening can enhance the quality of care, patient safety, the quality of our professional relationships, and our own sense of meaning and purpose in our work" (Epstein, 2021). Presence depends on creating internal space and quiet, setting aside personal drama and wanderings of the mind. Epstein (2021) suggests a reflective listening practice with patients: At what point in the patients' opening statement do you think of a response? What might you learn if you put your response on pause?

31.9.1 Cultivating Kindness and Compassion

Practicing mindfulness improves attention, self-regulation, and quality of life for many practitioners. Mindfulness practice can also be focused on cultivating particular qualities, such as compassion and kindness. Mindfulness practice has three different components, according to psychologist and mindfulness educator Rick Hanson (2020): Let be, let go, let in. The first is learning to let be with current experiences. Notice the physical pain, or the negative thought just as it is, with kindness and curiosity. The second step, let go, requires recognizing that worries about pain or negative thoughts are unproductive so they should be let go. The third step, let in, cultivates more beneficial qualities, such as kindness and non-judgment (Hanson, 2018, pp. 32–34).

Western culture may foster comparison and criticism of every aspect of life, thus resulting in an inner critic that frequently points out personal failures, stupidities, and flaws. As has become evident through the work on compassion of Kristin Neff, Christopher Germer, and many others, the act of talking with and treating yourself like a very dear friend offers many benefits.

Practicing kindness to oneself elicits one's mammalian care response, allowing the release of oxytocin and endorphins, which decreases stress and increases sense of safety (Neff, n.d.)

Self-compassion involves speaking to oneself in a different way. Regularly practice the following exercise (Practice #12) and see what happens over time.

PRACTICE #12   SELF-COMPASSION PRACTICE

Practice saying a few of the following statements in a friendly, caring way to yourself when you notice you are being critical or unkind toward yourself.

- This is really hard right now.
- I'm here for you. What do you need right now?
- Dear self, slow down and take a breath.
- You won't always feel this way … these hard feelings will eventually pass.
- It's ok to say "no" and set a boundary. This is hard to do, but important to keep you safe.
- Place a hand over your heart. Feel the warmth.
- I'm doing the best I can right now.
- May I have greater ease in my life.
- For whatever it is I am feeling right now, can I hold this, too, with kindness?

Please note: As you speak to yourself in kind words, pay close attention to the sensations in your body. What do you notice? Softening, a deeper breath, slowing down?

Developing clinical empathy for patients can increase tenderness toward oneself. Greater self-compassion results in greater compassion toward others.

31.10   CONCLUSION

This chapter covers mindfulness practices for nurses and patients, with the intention of awakening curiosity for personal experience and providing skills to be a more present, compassionate health practitioner. Furthermore, these mindfulness practices result in greater regulation, resilience, and enjoyment of life. For additional practices by the author go to www.insighttime.com/choosingmindfulness.

> Direct your eye inward, and you'll find
>> A thousand regions in your mind, yet undiscovered.
>> Travel them
> And become an expert in home-cosmography.
>> *Henry David Thoreau*

31.11   RESOURCES

31.11.1   MINDFULNESS APPS

- Buddha's Brain
- Calm
- Craving to Quit
- Headspace
- Ichill
- Inner Strength (teens)
- Insight Timer
- Mindfulness
- Mindfulness for Children
- Ten Percent Happier
- UCLA Mindful
- Waking Up
- www.insighttimer.com/choosingmindfulness

31.11.2   MINDFULNESS TRAINING/EDUCATION PROGRAMS

- UCLA Mindful Awareness Practices classes:
- www.marc.ucla.edu
- MBSR classes/trainings:
- www.brown.edu/public-health/mindfulness/class/mindfulness-based-stress-reduction-mbsr-online-0
- www.mbsrtraining.com
- www.mindfulleader.org
- Mindfulness in Schools:
- www.mindfulschools.org
- www.drchristopherwillard.com
- www.danielrechtschaffen.com

31.11.3   MINDFULNESS TEACHERS/AUTHORS

www.tarabrach.com
www.jackkornfield.com
www.sharonsalzberg.com

www.mindsightinstitute.com (Dan Siegel)
www.rickhanson.net
https://self-compassion.org/ (Kristin Neff)
www.davidtreleaven.com
www.drjud.com (Judson Brewer)
www.rhythmofregulation.com (Deb Dana)
www.stephenporges.com
www.mindfulnesscds.com (Jon Kabat-Zinn)
www.sensorimotorpsyhotherapy.org (Pat Ogden)

31.11.4 MINDFULNESS RETREAT CENTERS

- Insight Meditation Society, Barre, MA—www.dharma.org
- Rocky Mountain Ecodharma Center—www.rmerc.org
- Spirit Rock Meditation Center—www.spiritrock.org

31.11.5 TRAUMA RESOURCES

- Somatic Experiencing Institute—www.traumahealing.org
- Peter Levine, Ph.D.—www.somaticexperiencing.com/
- Pat Ogden, Ph.D.—www.sensorimotorpsychotherapy.org
- David Treleaven—www.davidtreleaven.com

31.11.6 MISCELLANEOUS

- Mindful Magazine—www.mindful.org

REFERENCES

Brewer, J. (2021). *Unwinding anxiety: New science shows how to break the cycles of worry and fear to heal your mind.* Avery-Random House.

Cahn, B. R., & Polich, J. (2006). Meditation states and traits: EEG, ERP, and neuroimaging studies. *Psychology Bulletin, 132*(2), 180–211.

Dana, D. (2021). *Anchored: How to befriend your nervous system using polyvagal theory.* Sounds True.

Epstein, R. (2017). *Attending: Medicine, mindfulness and humanity.* Scribner.

Epstein, R. (2021, May 22). Cultivating compassionate presence and improving patient–provider communication. Mindfulness in healthcare online (summit). www.mindfulhealthcaresummit.com/stream/ron-epstein/

Evans, S., Seidman, L. C., Tsao, J. C., Lung, K. C., Zeltzer, L., & Naliboff, B. (2013). Heart rate variability as a biomarker for autonomic nervous system response differences between children with chronic pain and healthy control children. *Pain Research, 6*, 449–57. https://doi.org/10.2147/JPR.S43849

Farb, N., Daubenmier, J., Price, C., Gard, T., Kerr, C., Dunn, B. D., Klein, A. C., Paulus, M. P., & Mehling, W. E. (2015). Interoception, contemplation and health. *Frontiers of Psychology, 6*, 763.

Feldman-Barrett, L. (2020). *Seven and a half lessons about the brain.* Houghton, Mifflin & Harcourt.

Frankl, V. (1959, 1992). *Man's search for meaning.* Beacon Press.

Gendlin, E. (1982). *Focusing.* Bantam Books.

Germer, C., & Neff, K. (2018). *The mindful self-compassion workbook: A proven way to accept yourself, build inner strength, and thrive.* Guilford Press.

Goleman, D., & Davidson, R. (2017). *Altered traits: Science reveals how meditation changes your mind, brain, and body.* Avery-Random House.

Halpern, J. (2011). *From detached concern to empathy: Humanizing medical practice.* Oxford University Press.

Hanson, R. (2013). *Hardwiring happiness: The new brain science of contentment, calm, and confidence.* Harmony Books.

Hanson R., & Hanson, F. (2018). *Resilient—how to grow an unshakable core of calm, strength, and happiness.* Harmony Books.

Hanson, R. (2020). *Neurodharma: New science, ancient wisdom, and seven practices of the highest happiness.* Harmony Books.

Holzel, B.K., Ott, U., Gard, T., Hempel, H., Weygandt, M., Morgen, K., & Vaitl, D. (2007). Investigation of mindfulness meditation practitioners with voxel-based morphometry. *Social Cognitive and Affective Neuroscience Advances, 3*(1), 55–61.

Kabat-Zinn, J. (2005). *Wherever you go, there you are: Mindfulness meditation in everyday life.* Hachette Book Group.

Kabat-Zinn, J. (2013). *Full catastrophe living: Using the wisdom of your body and mind to face stress, pain and illness.* Bantam Books.

Lazar, S. W., Kerr, C. E., Wasserman, R. H., Gray, J. R, Greve, D. N., Treadway, M. T., McGarvey, M., Quinn, B. T., Dusek, J. A., Benson, H., Rauch, S. L., Moore, C. I., & Fischl, B. (2005). Meditation experience is associated with increased cortical thickness. *Neuroreport, 16*(17), 1893–1897.

Levine, P. (1997). *Waking the tiger—healing trauma.* North Atlantic Books.

Levine, P. (2003). *Adapted techniques from Somatic Experiencing Training Program.* Boulder, CO.

Neff, K. (n.d.). *The chemicals of self-care.* https://self-compassion.org/

Moseley, L. (2011, November 11). *Why things hurt.* [Video]. YouTube. www.youtube.com/watch?v=gwd-wLdIHjs&t=321s

Ogden, P., Minton, K., & Pain, C. (2006). *Trauma and the body: A sensorimotor approach to psychotherapy.* Norton Series on Interpersonal Neurobiology.

Porges, S. (2011). *The polyvagal theory: Neurophysiological foundations of emotions, attachment, communication and self-regulation.* Norton Series on Interpersonal Neurobiology.

Sahar, T., Shalev, A., & Porges, S. (2001). Vagal modulation of responses to mental challenge in posttraumatic stress disorder. *Biological Psychiatry, 49*, 637–643. https://doi.org/10.1016/S0006-3223(00)01045-3

Siegel, D. (1999). *The developing mind: How relationships and the brain interact to shape who we are.* Guilford Press.

Siegel, D., & Payne-Bryson, T. (2012). *The whole brain child: 12 revolutionary strategies to nurture your child's developing mind.* Bantam Books.

Siegel, D. (2018). *Aware: The science and practice of presence—the groundbreaking meditation.* Penguin Random House.

Smalley, S., & Winston, D. (2010). *Fully present: The science, art, and practice of mindfulness.* Da Capo Press.

Thoreau, H. D. (2012). *Walden.* Signet Classics, Penguin Random House.

Treleaven, D. (2018). *Trauma-sensitive mindfulness: Practices for safe and transformative healing.* W.W. Norton & Co.

Wong, J., Owen, J., Gabana, N. T., Brown, J. W., McInnis, S., Toth, P., & Gilman, L. (2018). Does gratitude writing improve the mental health of psychotherapy clients? Evidence from a randomized controlled trial. *Psychotherapy Research, 28*(2), 192–202. DOI: 10.1080/10503307.2016.1169332

32 Promoting Optimal Lifestyle Behaviors

Strategies and Resources

Laura L. Hayman

Robert and Donna Manning College of Nursing & Health Sciences

University of Massachusetts

Boston, Massachusetts, USA

CONTENTS

KEY POINTS

- Lifestyle behaviors are central to optimal health across the life span.
- Health promoting behavioral-lifestyle efforts and interventions must focus on the individual and environments/contexts that influence lifestyle behaviors.
- The social determinants of health affect one's ability and capacity to develop, maintain, and/or modify behavior patterns must be considered in partnering with individuals/patients in prevention and management of chronic conditions.

32.1 INTRODUCTION

The importance of healthy lifestyle behaviors and modification of adverse lifestyle behaviors in health promotion and prevention of chronic conditions is well established. Substantial data generated from clinical and population-based studies have underscored the importance of focusing health-promoting behavioral-lifestyle efforts on the individual and the environments/contexts that influence lifestyle behaviors. Taken together, this evidence and clinical anecdotal

DOI: 10.1201/9781003178330-37

observations have contributed to the emergence of multi-level models and frameworks. Exemplifying this approach is the socio-ecological model (SEM) of health and behavior, which emphasizes the need for healthcare providers to consider the patient's physical, social, and cultural environments in developing and implementing strategies designed to promote the adoption, maintenance, and modification of behavior patterns (Stokols, 1992; Hayman, 2007). Viewed through the SEM lens, the purpose of this chapter is to highlight strategies and resources for nurses to use in partnering with patients to optimize healthy behaviors and lifestyles with emphasis on both primary and secondary prevention of chronic conditions, particularly cardio-vascular disease (CVD).

32.2   OPERATIONALIZING SEM IN PRIMARY AND SECONDARY PREVENTION: FACTORS TO CONSIDER

Primary prevention of chronic conditions focuses on reduction of risk factors and adverse life-style behaviors with the goal of preventing incident events (Arnett et al., 2019). Secondary pre-vention emphasizes interventions designed to reduce the likelihood of events and/or mortality in individuals who have established disease (Smith et al., 2011). Applied to CVD, interventions would target blood pressure, lipids, body weight, blood glucose levels, smoking behaviors and exposures, and patterns of dietary intake, physical activity, and sedentary behaviors. Individual-level, person-centered approaches to reducing these risk factors and changing adverse patterns of behaviors are detailed elsewhere in this text.

Viewed within the SEM, however, nurses and other healthcare providers are strongly encouraged to consider multi-level factors that clearly impact an individual's ability and capacity to adopt and maintain healthy lifestyles. Relatedly, consideration of the social determinants of health is par-ticularly important in developing realistic goals and outcomes that must include the patient/person in development and implementation. The World Health Organization (WHO) defined the social determinants of health broadly as "the circumstances in which people are born, grow, live, work and age and the systems put in place to deal with illness" (WHO, 2008).

Consistent with the SEM perspective and integrating a life course approach, an American Heart Association (AHA) statement presented evidence highlighting socioeconomic position (SEP), race/ethnicity, social support, culture and language, access to care, and residential environment as social determinants of risk and outcomes for CVD (Havranek et al. 2015).

Beyond CVD, substantial data as well as anecdotal observations indicate that social determinants affect physical, psychosocial, and emotional health across the life course (WHO, 2008). Clearly, affordability of and access to safe places for physical activity, outlets for heart-healthy beverages and foods, and healthcare affect health and well-being. Taken together, accumulated evidence has prompted the attention of clinical and public health organizations and advocates supporting action on the potentially modifiable social determinants of health. For example, the US Preventive Services Task Force (USPSTF), an independent, volunteer group of national experts in prevention, behavioral counseling, primary care, and evidence-based medi-cine, offers evidence-based recommendations about clinical preventive services in primary care. The USPSTF issued a position paper on developing primary care-based recommendations for social determinants of health (Davidson et al., 2020). In that statement and after rigorous review of the evidence of effects of screening and interventions on social determinants rele-vant to primary care, the Task Force indicated that this is an evolving area that will continue to be considered in USPSTF recommendations. A framework for identifying additional social determinants of health as well as an analytic framework that identifies the portfolio of research needed to advance the Task Force's efforts is included in the statement. Important to note is the ultimate USPSTF goal of improving the health and well-being of the public and reducing health inequities (Davidson et al., 2020).

32.3 IMPLICATIONS FOR NURSES AND HEALTHCARE PROVIDERS: PROMOTING HEALTHY BEHAVIORS IN PRIMARY AND SECONDARY PREVENTION

Viewed within SEM and considering the social determinants of health, there are numerous implications for nurses and healthcare providers focused on promoting healthy lifestyle behaviors central to primary and secondary prevention. Patient adherence to behavioral-lifestyle as well as pharmacological recommendations for prevention and management of CVD is essential to prevent incident events and reduce the risk of recurring vascular events and mortality. Adherence is a complex process influenced by many factors on the individual, healthcare provider, and healthcare system levels (Ockene et al., 2002; Ockene et al., 2011). Thus, on the individual patient level, and as reaffirmed in recent statements and advisories, age, patient preferences, socioeconomic position and resources, and geographical location are important to consider in developing and implementing adherence-enhancing strategies for both primary and secondary prevention (Havranek et al., 2015; Kris-Etherton et al., 2021). Relatedly, healthcare providers must be aware of and knowledgeable about how these individual factors affect adherence to behavioral-lifestyle as well as pharmacological recommendations. Equally as important, healthcare providers must be informed of the evidence-based interventions known to be effective in modifying adverse behaviors and established risk factors for CVD. Of note, multicomponent interventions that include patient education and counseling, therapeutic patient education, behavioral skills training, motivational techniques and strategies such as motivational interviewing (MI), and eHealth technologies have been shown to be highly effective in maintenance of behavior change as well as in preventing recurring CVD events (Prochaska et al., 2018). These multicomponent interventions are most often provided by multidisciplinary teams of healthcare professionals that include nurses, physicians, behavioral specialists, and social workers. Indeed, as detailed later in this chapter, the efficacy and effectiveness of nurse case-managed, team-based care in the settings of secondary and primary prevention of CVD has been demonstrated (Berra, 2011; Berra et al., 2011).

32.4 STRATEGIES FOR PROMOTING HEALTHY LIFESTYLE BEHAVIORS

32.4.1 PATIENT EDUCATION AND COUNSELING AND THERAPEUTIC PATIENT EDUCATION (TPE)

Patient education and counseling has been a central component of evidence-based guidelines for prevention and management of CVD (Arnett et al., 2019; Stone et al., 2014). A very recent science advisory from the AHA emphasized the importance of healthy lifestyle promotion across the life span and in clinical settings (Kris-Etherton et al., 2021). Specifically, the 5A Model (assess, advise, agree, assist, and arrange) provided the framework for clinical counseling with specific recommendations for lifestyle-related behavior change for patients across the life span. Of note, in all life stages, social determinants of health and unmet social-related health needs as well as overweight and obesity, known to affect CVD risk and outcomes, are highlighted. More attention to healthy lifestyle behaviors during every clinician visit was emphasized with goal of improving cardiovascular health across the life span for population groups.

Recent attention has also focused on TPE interventions with the goal of promoting and optimizing self-management, particularly in patients with established CVD (Barnason et al., 2017). Results of a systematic review of TPE research on cardiovascular self-management interventions pointed to the importance of multiple modes of TPE delivery, including face-to-face, telephone, and telehealth designed to meet the needs of specific CVD patient populations. Team-based, multidisciplinary approaches were affirmed as optimal with the recommendation that a structured protocol for delivery of TPE self-management by various healthcare team members be used to provide a framework for communication among providers, consistent messaging to patients, and a system for tracking the follow-up of patients (Barnason et al., 2017).

32.4.2 Motivational Interviewing (MI)

Motivational interviewing (MI) is a behavior change counseling strategy that emphasizes patient-centered approaches, including eliciting patient priorities, need and values, building rapport (i.e., reflective listening and empathy), and support for self-management (Miller & Rollnick, 2002). MI has been widely used in conjunction with the Transtheoretical Model of Stages of Change (Prochaska et al., 1992) to modify health behaviors in individuals with or at risk for CVD. Of note in the setting of both primary and secondary prevention of CVD, MI has also been used widely as an adjunctive strategy to modify patterns of physical activity and dietary behaviors for overweight and obese individuals (Armstrong et al., 2011; Artinian et al., 2011) (See Chapter 30 in this volume).

32.4.3 Mobile Health (mHealth) and Digital Health (eHealth) Technology

During the past ~two decades, substantial research efforts have focused on development and application of mobile and digital health technologies with emphasis on health behaviors central to both prevention and management of chronic conditions, including CVD (Burke et al., 2016). A systematic review of mobile phone interventions for secondary prevention of CVD supports the promise and potential of text messaging, mobile applications, and telemonitoring in improving outcomes for patients with CVD (Park et al., 2016). The review included observational cohort studies as well as randomized controlled trial (RCT) studies published from January 2002 to January 2016. With the aim of gaining broad coverage of the then emerging mHealth field, studies (n=28) that used text messaging and or/mobile applications with mobile phones for secondary prevention of CVD varied significantly in characteristics of patients, cardiovascular conditions, intervention elements, and measurement of effectiveness. Particularly noteworthy, the majority of studies (n=22; 79%) were efficacious in improving behaviors and clinical outcomes. Key factors associated with successful interventions included personalized messages with individually tailored advice, greater engagement, higher frequency of messages, and use of multiple modalities. Importantly, all studies using text messaging or mobile applications compared with another technology intervention (i.e., Internet or continuous monitoring) found both user adherence and satisfaction to be highest in the text-messaging or mobile application intervention groups. Dale and colleagues (2016), in a review of the effectiveness of mHealth behavior change interventions for CVD self-management, affirmed the potential for this technology to change selected lifestyle behaviors and noted the need for large-scale, longitudinal studies to gain a better understanding of the effects over time and across diverse populations groups.

32.5 SECONDARY PREVENTION: IMPORTANCE OF CARDIAC REHABILITATION PROGRAMS

Cardiac rehabilitation/secondary prevention programs (CR/SPPs) have been in existence for several decades, endorsed by the AHA and the American College of Cardiology (ACC) (Smith et al., 2011) and the American Association of Cardiovascular and Pulmonary Rehabilitation (Balady et al., 2007), and have received more recent renewed attention within the cardiovascular community (Kachur et al., 2017; Rengo et al., 2017; van Halewijin et al., 2017). Accumulated evidence has demonstrated the efficacy and effectiveness of these programs, which include multidisciplinary, multicomponent interventions for behavioral-lifestyle change and risk factor modification. The majority of CR/SPPs programs have three phases; inpatient enrollment, supervised outpatient program, and individual maintenance with the goal of combining education, medical management, dietary modification, individually tailored lifestyle changes, and structured exercise training. In contemporary comprehensive multicomponent programs, patients acquire skills and competencies provided by a multispecialty team including physicians, nurses, exercise physiologists, physical and occupational therapists, dieticians, mental health specialists, and a case manager. Phase II CR/SPPs programs focus on promoting comprehensive lifestyle changes with the goal of long-term behavior modification central to reducing occurring events in patients with CVD. Phase III normally continues outside of a supervised healthcare setting and emphasizes maintenance of behavioral-lifestyle changes with the goal of improving health-related quality of life as well as reducing recurrent CVD events (Kachur et al., 2017). While the efficacy and effectiveness of these CR programs has been demonstrated, referrals and utilization remain less than optimal. Trends over time indicate that specific patient populations, including women, the elderly, ethnic minorities, those with selected comorbidities, and individuals of low socioeconomic status, have low referral rates (Franklin & Brinks, 2015). Disparities in referral rates have prompted exploration of underlying factors and development of alternative models to enhance utilization of CR/SPPs (Arena et al., 2012; Franklin & Brinks, 2015; Sandesara et al., 2015). With systems of healthcare in transition in the US, to be viable and to increase utilization by all eligible CVD patients, alternative models must address known barriers to referral and participation, including associated costs and ease of access. To this end, strategies that include telemedicine and eHealth as well as Internet-based, home-based, and community-based programs have emerged. Available data and anecdotal observations suggest the promise and potential of these alternative models, with outcomes in CVD patients similar to those for conventional hospital-based programs (Clark et al., 2015). Currently, during the COVID-19 pandemic, such alternative models have been and continue to be implemented with evaluation of outcomes to follow.

32.6 MULTICOMPONENT INTERVENTIONS: INTEGRATING BEHAVIORAL-LIFESTYLE CHANGE STRATEGIES WITH MULTIDISCIPLINARY CASE MANAGEMENT

As noted above, multicomponent prevention and management of CVD, similar to other chronic conditions, is a complex process facilitated by multidisciplinary team approaches, multicomponent interventions, and integrated systems of care. Evidence indicates that a multidisciplinary collaborative team model that focuses on individually tailored, guideline-based, patient-centered interventions, family and social support, healthcare providers, community-level factors (i.e., access to CR programs), and systems of care that enable coordination of care providers is highly effective in reducing multiple adverse health behaviors and risk factors and preventing recurring events (Berra et al., 2011; Fletcher et al., 2012; Smith et al., 2011). Of note, these multidisciplinary team-based approaches have shown to be effective across settings, including hospitalized patients, primary care patients, low-income clinics, and community-based healthcare centers (Allen & Dennison, 2010; Berra, 2011). More recently, research focused on multidisciplinary models for both primary and secondary prevention have placed emphasis on inclusion of community health workers (CHWs), also called "promotoras" or "health navigators," who contribute uniquely to community-based healthcare, including behavioral-lifestyle change for individuals with CVD and other chronic conditions. Prompted, in part, by the recognized need to reduce healthcare costs while improving outcomes, integration of CHWs in multidisciplinary teams has demonstrated the potential for extended outreach to vulnerable groups with or at risk for CVD (Allen et al., 2011; Landers & Levinson, 2016). Critically important in optimizing CHWs in behavior change is training and guidance provided by an experienced team member who is often a nurse. As implemented in the Community Outreach and Cardiovascular Health (COACH) Trial, a nurse practitioner (NP/CHW) team intervention focused on promoting therapeutic lifestyle changes (TLC) and adherence to medications and appointments can be an effective model for behavioral change and risk reduction in patients with CVD (Allen et al., 2011).

32.7 RESOURCES FOR PROMOTING OPTIMAL LIFESTYLE BEHAVIORS

Viewed through the lens of the SEM and with consideration of the social determinants of health, evidence-based strategies for optimizing lifestyle behaviors in prevention and management of CVD are highlighted in this chapter. Emphasis is placed on the individual and the contexts that influence the development, maintenance, and modification of adverse patterns of behavior. While nurses are prepared to view patients holistically and to consider and assess physical, psychosocial behavioral, and emotional aspects of health, specialist members of multidisciplinary healthcare teams bring additional expertise in their respective roles and serve as important resources and supports for nurses and patients. For example, in the setting of secondary prevention caring for a patient with multiple adverse behaviors and risk factors for CVD, the nurse case manager, coordinator of patient care, would consult and collaborate with the behavioral specialist on the healthcare team in the development and implementation of evidence-based strategies for modifying adverse behaviors. If the patient has unhealthy patterns of dietary intake and challenges with increasing physical activity and decreasing sedentary behaviors, the dietician and exercise physiologist could be instrumental in developing and implementing a plan of care. As emphasized in this chapter and elsewhere in this text, an individually tailored plan that considers the patient's preferences, sociodemographics (i.e., age, geographical location) resources, culture, and family and social support is critically important and essential for modifying adverse behaviors and sustaining behavior change over time. In addition to the expertise offered by specialist members of the healthcare team, evidence-based resources are available for nurses, healthcare providers, and patients. Resources for nurses as well as patients and healthcare consumers offered by health-promoting organizations are at the end of the chapter. Of note, the sources cited provide evidence-based information that is updated as new evidence becomes available.

32.8 CONCLUSION

Patterns of health behaviors are central to health and well-being across the life span. Interventions and programmatic initiatives designed to promote optimal lifestyle behaviors must consider the contexts and environments that influence those behaviors and the social determinants of health that impact an individual's ability and capacity to adopt, maintain, and/or change behaviors. Evidence-based strategies for promoting health behaviors in the settings of primary and secondary prevention of CVD inform and guide nursing practice. Multicomponent interventions delivered by multidisciplinary teams coordinated by nurses have demonstrated efficacy and effectiveness in modifying adverse behaviors as well as risk factors for CVD.

32.9 RESOURCES

- American College of Lifestyle Medicine: www.lifestylemedicine.org
- American Heart Association: www.americanheart.org
- Centers for Disease Control and Prevention: www.cdc.gov/
- National Institutes of Health: www.nih.gov/
- Preventive Cardiovascular Nurses Association: https://pcna.net/
- Society of Behavioral Medicine: https://sbm.org/

REFERENCES

Allen, J. K., & Dennison, C. R. (2010). Randomized trials of nursing interventions for secondary prevention in patients with coronary artery disease and heart failure: Systematic review. *Journal of Cardiovascular Nursing, 25*(3), 207–220.

Allen, J. K., Dennison-Himmelfarb, C. R., Szanton, S. L., Bone, L., Hill, M. N., Levine, D. M., West, M. Barlow, A., Lewis-Boyer, L., Donnelly-Strozzo, M., Curtis, C., & Andersonet, K. (2011). Community outreach and cardiovascular health (COACH) trial: A randomized controlled trial of nurse practitioner/community health worker cardiovascular disease risk reduction in urban community health centers. *Circulation: Cardiovascular Quality and Outcomes*, *4*, 595–602.

Arena, R., Williams, M., Forman, D. E., Cahalin, L. P., Coke, L., Myers, J., Hamm, L., Kris-Etherton, P., Humphrey, R., Bittner, V., Lavie, C. J., American Heart Association Exercise, Cardiac Rehabilitation and Prevention Committee of the Council on Clinical Cardiology, Council on Epidemiology and Prevention, & Council on Nutrition, Physical Activity and Metabolism (2012). Increasing referral and participation rates to outpatient cardiac rehabilitation: The valuable role of healthcare professionals in the inpatient and home health settings. *Circulation*, *125*, 1321–1329.

Armstrong, M. J., Mottershead, T. A., Ronksley, P. E., Sigal, R. J., Campbell, T. S., & Hemmelgarn, B. R. (2011). Motivational interviewing to improve weight loss in overweight and /or obese patients: A systematic review and meta-analysis of randomized controlled trials. *Obesity Reviews*, *12*(9), 709–723.

Arnett, D., Blumenthal, R. S., Albert, M. A., Buroker, A., Goldberger, Z., Hahn, E., Dennison-Himmelfarb, C., Khera, A., Lloyd-Jones, D., McEvoy, J., Michos, E., Miedema, M., Munoz, D., Smith, S., Virani, S., Williams, K., Yeboah, J., & Ziaeian, B. (2019). 2019 ACC/AHA guideline on the primary prevention of cardiovascular disease: A report of the American College of Cardiology/American Heart Association Task Force on clinical practice guidelines. *Circulation*, *140*(11), e596–e646. https://doi.org/10.1161/cir.0000000000000678

Artinian, N. T., Fletcher, G. F., Mozaffarian, D., Kris-Etherton, P., Van Horn, L., Lichtenstein, A. H., Kumanyika, S., Kraus, W. E., Fleg, J. L., Redeker, N. S., Meininger, J. C., Banks, J., Stuart-Shor, E. M., Fletcher, B. J., Miller, T. D., Hughes, S., Braun, L. T., Kopin, L. A., Berra, K., … Burke, L. E. (2010). Interventions to promote physical activity and dietary lifestyle changes for cardiovascular risk factor reduction in adults: A scientific statement from the American Heart Association. *Circulation*, *122*(4), 406–441.

Balady, G. J., Williams, M. A., Ades, P. A., Bittner, V., Comoss, P., Foody, J. M., Franklin, B., Sanderson, B., Southard, D., American Heart Association Exercise, Cardiac Rehabilitation, and Prevention Committee; the Council on Clinical Cardiology; American Heart Association Council on Cardiovascular Nursing; American Heart Association Council on Epidemiology and Prevention; American Heart Association Council on Nutrition, Physical Activity, and Metabolism; American Association of Cardiovascular and Pulmonary Rehabilitation (2007). Core components of rehabilitation/secondary prevention programs: 2007 update. A scientific statement from the American Heart Association and the Association of Cardiovascular and Pulmonary Rehabilitation. *Circulation*, *115*(20), 2675–2682.

Barnason, S., White-Williams, C., Rossi, L. P., Centeno, M., Crabbe, D. L., Kyoung, S. L., McCabe, N., Nauser, J., Schulz, P., Stamp, K., Wood, K., American Heart Association Council on Cardiovascular and Stroke Nursing; Council on Cardiovascular Disease in the Young; Council on Clinical Cardiology; and Stroke Council. (2017). Evidence for therapeutic patient education interventions to promote cardiovascular patient self-management: A scientific statement from the American Heart Association. *Circulation: Cardiovascular Quality and Outcomes*, *10*, e000025.

Berra, K. (2011). Does nurse case management improve implementation of guidelines for cardiovascular disease risk reduction? *Journal of Cardiovascular Nursing*, *26*(2), 147–167.

Berra, K., Houston Miller, N., & Jennings, C. (2011). Nurse-based models for cardiovascular disease prevention: From research to clinical practice. *Journal of Cardiovascular Nursing*, *26*(4S), 546–555.

Burke, L. E., Ma, J., Azar, K. M., Bennett, G. G., Peterson, E. D., Zheng, Y., Riley, W., Stephens, J., Shah, S. H., Suffoletto, B., Turan, T. N., Spring, B., Steinberger, J., & Quinn, C. C. (2015). Current science on computer use of mobile health for cardiovascular disease prevention. *Circulation*, *132*, 1157–1213.

Berra, K., Franklin, B., & Jennings, C. (2017). Community-based healthy living interventions. *Progress in Cardiovascular Diseases*, *59*, 430–439.

Clark, A. M., Conway, A., & Poulsen, V. (2015). Alternative models of cardiac rehabilitation: A systematic review. *European Journal of Preventive Cardiology*, *22*(1), 35–74.

Dale, L.P., Whittaker, R., Jiang, Y., Stewart, R., Rolleston, A., & Maddison, R. (2016). Text message and internet support for coronary heart disease self-management. Results from the Test4Heart randomized controlled trial. *Journal of Medical Internet Research*, *17*(10), e 237.

Davidson, K. W., Kemper, A. R., Doubeni, C. A., Tseng, C-W., Simon, M. A., Kubik, M., Curry, S. J., Mills, J., Krist, A., Ngo-Metzger, Q., & Borsky, A. (2020, July 14). Developing primary care-based recommendations for social determinants of health: Methods of the U.S. Preventive Services Task Force. *Annals of Internal Medicine*. https://doi.org/10.7326/M20-0730

Fletcher, G. F., Berra, K., Fletcher, B. J., Gilstrap, L., & Wood, M. J. (2012). The integrated team approach to the care of the patient with cardiovascular disease. *Current Problems in Cardiology, 37*, 369–397.

Franklin, B. A., & Brinks, J. (2015). Cardiac rehabilitation: Underrecognized/underutilized. *Current Treatment Options in Cardiovascular Medicine, 17*(62). https://doi.org/10.1007/s11936-015-0422-x

Havranek, E. P., Mujahid, M. S., Barr, D. A., Blair, I. V., Cohen, M. S., Cruz-Flores, S., Davey-Smith, G., Dennison-Himmelfarb, C. R., Lauer, M. S., Lockwood, D. W., Rosal, M., & Yancy, C. W. (2015). Social determinants of risk and outcomes for cardiovascular disease: A scientific statement from the American Heart Association. *Circulation, 132*, 873–898.

Hayman, L. L. (2007). Behavioral medicine across the life course: Challenges and opportunities for interdisciplinary science. *Annals of Behavioral Medicine, 33*(3), 236–241.

Kachur, S., Chongthannakun, V., Lavie, C. J., De Schutter, A., Arena, R., Milani, R. V, & Franklin, B. A. (2017). Impact of cardiac rehabilitation and exercise training programs in coronary heart disease. *Progress in Cardiovascular Diseases, 60*, 103–114.

Kris-Etherton, P. M., Petersen, K. S., Després, J. P., Braun, L., de Ferranti, S. D., Furie, K. L., Lear, S. A., Lobelo, F., Morris, P. B., & Sacks, F. M. (2021). Special considerations for healthy lifestyle promotion across the life span in clinical settings: A science advisory from the American Heart Association. *Circulation, 144*, e515–e532. https://doi.org/10.1161/CIR.0000000000001014

Landers, S., & Levinson, M. (2016). Mounting evidence of the effectiveness of community health workers. *American Journal of Public Health, 106*, 591–592.

Miller, W. R., & Rollnick, S. (2002). *Motivational interviewing: Preparing people for change* (2nd ed.). Guilford Press.

Ockene, I. S., Hayman, L. L., Pasternak, R. C., et al. (2002). Task Force #4—adherence issues and behavior changes: Achieving a long-term solution. *Journal of the American College of Cardiology, 40*(4), 630–640.

Ockene, J. K., Schneider, K. L., Lemon, S. C., & Ockene, I.S. (2011). Can we improve adherence to preventive therapies for cardiovascular health? *Circulation, 124*, 1276–1282.

Park, L. G., Beatty, A., Stafford, Z., & Whooley, M. A. (2016). Mobile phone interventions for the secondary prevention of cardiovascular disease. *Progress in Cardiovascular Disease, 58*, 639–650.

Prochaska, J. O., DiClemente, C. C., & Norcross, J. C. 1992. In search of how people change: Applications to addictive behaviors. *American Psychologist, 47*, 1102–1114.

Rengo, J. L., Savage, P. D., Barrett, T., & Ades, P. A. (2017). Cardiac rehabilitation participation rates and outcomes for patients with heart failure. *Journal of Cardiopulmonary Rehabilitation and Prevention, 38*(1), 38–42. https://doi.org/10.1097/HCR.0000000000000252

Sandersara, P. B., Lambert, C. T., Gordon, N. F., Fletcher, G. F., Franklin, B. A., Wenger, N. K., & Sperling, L. (2015). Cardiac rehabilitation and risk reduction: Time to "rebrand and reinvigorate". *Journal of the American College of Cardiology, 65*(4), 389–395.

Smith, S. C., Benjamin, E. J., Bonow, R. O., Braun, L. T., Creager, M. A., Franklin, B. A., Gibbons, R. J., Grundy, S. M., Hiratzka, L. F., Jones, D. W., Lloyd-Jones, D. M., Minissian, M., Mosca, L., Peterson, E. D., Sacco, R. L., Spertus, J., Stein, J. H., & Taubert, K. A. (2011). AHA/ACCF secondary prevention and risk reduction therapy for patients with coronary and other atherosclerotic vascular disease: 2011 update: A guideline from the American Heart Association and American College of Cardiology Foundation endorsed by the World Heart Federation and the Preventive Cardiovascular Nurses Association. *Circulation, 124*(22), 2458–2473.

Stokols, D. (1992). Establishing and maintaining healthy environments: Toward a social ecology of health promotion. *American Psychologist, 47*(1), 6–22.

Stone, N. J., Robinson, J. G., Lichtenstein, A. H., Merz, C. N. B., Blum, C. B., Eckel, R. H., Goldberg, A. C., Gordon, D., Levy, D., Lloyd-Jones, D. M., McBridge, P., Schwartz, J. S., Shero, S. T., Smith, S. C., Jr., Watson, K., Wilson, P. W. F., American College of Cardiology/American Heart Association Task Force on Practice Guidelines. (2014). 2013 ACC/AHA guideline on the treatment of blood cholesterol to reduce atherosclerotic cardiovascular risk for adults: A report of the American College of Cardiology/ American Heart Association Task Force on Practice Guidelines. *Journal of the American College of Cardiology, 63*, 2889–2934.

Van Halewijn, G., Deckers, J., Tay, H. Y., van Domburg, R., Kotseva, K., & Wood, D. (2017). Lessons from contemporary trials of cardiovascular prevention and rehabilitation: A systematic review and meta-analysis. *International Journal of Cardiology*, *232*, 294–303.

World Health Organization Commission on Social Determinants of Health. (2008). *Closing the gap in a generation: Health equity through action on the social determinants of health*. World Health Organization.

33 Digital Therapeutics

Patricia M. Davidson[1,2], Caleb Ferguson[1], and Michelle Patch[2]
[1]University of Wollongong
Wollongong, Australia
[2]Johns Hopkins School of Nursing
Baltimore, Maryland, USA

CONTENTS

KEY POINTS

- Technology is transforming healthcare models and delivery but should not be exempt from traditional, evidence-based assessment.
- Nurses need to have high levels of digital literacy and competencies.
- Developing an evidence base for digital therapeutics is critical for ensuring targeted and tailored interventions to improve health outcomes.
- Ensuring credibility, validity, and security of patient data is critical for optimizing digital therapeutics.
- Promoting collaboration between government and public and private partnerships is critical to deliver on the promise of digital therapeutics.

33.1 INTRODUCTION

The impact of technology on healthcare has been transformative, and the impact of the COVID-19 pandemic has accelerated uptake and acceptance. COVID-19 has been a catalyst for rapid innovation to develop new ways of caring for patients, through virtual models of healthcare. The Fourth Industrial Revolution, the era of digitization, describes the exponential changes happening to the way we live, work, and relate to one another due the introduction of disruptive technologies and trends such as the Internet of Things (IoT), robotics, virtual and augmented reality, and artificial intelligence (Nagy et al., 2021). The collection and analysis of big data is expected to transform healthcare. Innovations in analytic methods as well as advances in data collection are advancing progress in health care and research. It is also important to consider that not all individuals and

DOI: 10.1201/9781003178330-38

communities may benefit equally from digital advances, and there is concern whether big data research will perpetuate existing health disparities because of the underrepresentation of minority populations leading to biased conclusions.

The cataclysmic global assault of the COVID-19 pandemic on health and society has led to a rapid adoption of telehealth and digital strategies (Fisk et al., 2020) (Baum et al., 2021). The urgency and pressures of the moment have led many individuals reticent about the benefits of telehealth to recognize the huge potential in improving health outcomes. All trends speak to the increased uptake of digital methods in addition to digital therapeutics (DTx). The level of investment in these strategies is also increasing. The benefits of telehealth are decreased cost, improved convenience, and access. Moreover, the computational aspects of DTx have the capacity to improve the tailoring and targeting of health interventions.

Technologies for virtual care, remote monitoring, counselling, and biometric data acquisition are increasingly available and are particularly valuable in providing care in rural and remote areas. These technologies greatly expand the capacity of health systems to meet the needs of the growing numbers of individuals with chronic conditions and the shortage of health care providers in many settings.

In particular, digital strategies are emerging as an important tool in managing conditions where self-management is an important consideration, such as diabetes, heart disease, atrial fibrillation, and chronic obstructive pulmonary disease. The role of DTx for mental health conditions, particularly those employing cognitive behavioral therapy, is increasing (Dang et al., 2020). Many of these conditions have a rich basis of theoretically derived interventions and therapeutics that can be digitized and adapted to engage individuals in self-care.

Increasingly, these devices are embedded within patient care and also marketed to target populations. This chapter seeks to describe the role of therapeutics in healthcare and discuss how nurses can leverage these technologies to improve patient care and incorporate them into care planning and routine care delivery (Ferguson et al., 2018).

33.2   ADOPTION OF DIGITAL HEALTH STRATEGIES AND DIGITAL THERAPEUTICS

There has been an explosion in the uptake of digital health over the last decade with the adoption of social media platforms, smartphones, and implantable and wearable devices for health purposes. The terms telehealth, telemedicine, virtual health, and digital health are used interchangeably, but it is important to differentiate specific applications and target populations. Digital therapeutics (DTx) are defined as evidence-based interventions driven by high-quality software programs to prevent, manage, or treat health conditions (Patel & Butte, 2020). These modalities also have the potential to increase access and effectiveness. Applications using DTx include digital sensors, wearable devices, virtual reality, and artificial intelligence devices where for example, individuals are encouraged to adhere to a particular therapeutic regimen. These applications are differentiated from general wellness applications as they are developed to target specific disease conditions, with an important advantage of being able to personalize messages to precise scenarios and individual attributes. DTx applies algorithmic information management to guide therapeutic approaches. Many of these approaches have been evaluated systematically and endorsed by regulatory agencies, such as the Federal Drug Administration (Dang et al., 2020). The potential of artificial intelligence in refining management and algorithms is increasingly recognized (Palanica et al., 2020). These approaches can be applied as a stand-alone intervention, augment a current approach, or be a complementary strategy for an established therapeutic. Although there can be heterogeneity in the structures of DTx applications, common features include:

- A theoretical basis for behavior change or cognitive behavioral therapy.
- Integration with other electronic platforms such as electronic medical records.
- Aligned with digital sensors and wearable outcomes.

- An evidence-based target with a specific clinical outcome.
- Approval or endorsement by a regulatory agency with a potential for reimbursement.
- Generate data at the level of patient, provider, and health system.

33.3 SPECIFIC EXEMPLARS OF THE USE OF DIGITAL THERAPEUTICS

There are increasing digital solutions to prevent or detect early mental and physical problems (e.g., depression, overweight, and obesity) as well as specific examples of targeted disease management in conditions such as chronic heart failure, chronic obstructive pulmonary disease, chronic pain, and diabetes. The capacity to incorporate virtual reality (VR) technology in DTx enables individuals to learn by experiencing real-world situations. For example, through VR, patients go into situations and learn how to think, feel, and act differently; this approach can be really useful in behavioral management programs. Chatbots, systems that interact with human users using spoken, written, and visual language, have also been adopted (Abd-Alrazaq et al., 2020). Digital technologies and DTx have the potential to increase access and participation in cardiac rehabilitation by mitigating the challenges associated with traditional, facility-based programs (Wongvibulsin et al., 2021). Although many of the interventions have focused primarily on physical activity, there is potential to incorporate more comprehensive and psychodynamic aspects of cardiac rehabilitation. However, issues of prescription and reimbursement remain unclear.

33.3.1 CASE STUDY: DIGITAL HEALTH AND MODELS OF DIGITAL ATRIAL FIBRILLATION MANAGEMENT

Technology is transforming the way in which we manage chronic disease. For example, atrial fibrillation (AF) has been the focus of rapid technological innovation. Technology has transformed methods to screen and detect AF through new devices, including implantables and wearables, enabled better treatment decisions to reduce evidence-practice gaps through the application of clinical decision support tools, and new smartphone apps show promise to increase adherence to anticoagulation therapy for stroke prevention.

Wearables and small portable electronic heart rhythm devices, such as the AliveCor, Omron, and HeartBug devices have, revolutionized capabilities for screening and detection of AF. These small, portable ECG devices allow for single lead ECG monitoring capabilities, allowing providers to capture arrhythmia to document and send to another healthcare provider with ease. Single point in time is a key limitation, but other devices such as wearable adhesive patches can provide continuous readings for 7–14 days. Nurse-delivered iECG has been shown to be more effective that routine 24-hour holter monitoring to detect more AF after stroke, in the in-patient hospital setting (Yan et al., 2020). New ways of working, such as nurses undertaking iECG instead of traditional cardiac monitoring, has the opportunity to disrupt and redefine "nursing work."

Insertable cardiac monitoring (ICM) such as the Reveal LINQ ICM and CONFIRM RX devices show promise in the detection of AF, particularly in ESUS (embolic stroke of unknown source), or cryptogenic stroke (Sanna et al., 2014). Insertable and wearable monitoring cardiac devices continue to show better rates of detection of AF, and this may be partly due to their relative ease of use and increasing availability of such devices. These advanced monitoring capabilities provide smart methods to screen and detect AF in individuals where this may have been previously challenging to capture on a traditional 12-lead ECG.

Electronic decision support (EDS) or clinical decision support (CDS) software is increasingly popular to guide treatment decisions in clinical practice. Evidence-based clinical decision support tools and algorithms can be integrated into existing electronic platforms such as electronic medical records (EMR) or general practice software at point of care. These tools can guide clinicians with risk assessments and treatment decisions and be applied to optimize evidence-based treatment in practice. eHealth tools like CDS can help to enhance guideline-based prescription of evidence-based therapies, such as anticoagulation (Orchard et al., 2019). These tools are especially useful in assisting anticoagulation decision making when combined with patient decision aides to support shared decision making (Ferguson & Hendriks, 2017).

Lastly, smartphone apps, virtual and augmented reality, and gamification are becoming increasingly popular modalities to support patient education and self-management for patients with cardiovascular disease. New technologies warrant new strategies for patient education (Lombardo et al., 2021). Gamification is a broad term used to describe the use of gaming in non-game contexts, such as in healthcare (Ferguson et al., 2015). Immersive learning experiences can be created through gamification, AV, and VR. These strategies may be helpful to drive positive behavior change (Lombardo et al., 2021). While robust evidence to support these interventions is somewhat lacking, these methods are widely available, increasingly popular, and highly acceptable to patients. The lack of high-quality evidence may be partly due to the speed of innovation outpacing the often slow speed of evidence generation through properly conducted randomized controlled trials with quality outcome measures.

Nurses need to be well equipped with the skills to be able to adequately select, appraise, and recommend digital therapeutics in clinical practice. Being equipped with skills in the critical appraisal of new technologies is a skill for the 21st-century nurse, care needs to be taken when recommending technologies to patients, particularly due to the lack of regulation of these therapeutics and their potential to inadvertently cause harm. In this context, harm could include addiction, data and privacy concerns or breaches, or the potential to reinforce misinformation related to self-management.

Nurses have a key role in supporting patients to make choices and in providing recommendations about which digital therapeutic tools to apply, particularly in the context of self-management for chronic disease (Ferguson & Jackson, 2017).

33.4 EXPANDING ACCESS TO HEALTHCARE AND A POPULATION-BASED APPROACH

Data generated through DTx applications and integrated data systems have the potential to manage health on a population level and to integrate other technologies such as social network analysis. For example, in March 2020, the Mount Sinai Health System Inflammatory Bowel Disease Center in New York City reported an increase in telephone call volume, with many IBD patients expressing anxiety about being on immunosuppressive agents during the COVID-19 pandemic. Rapidly, they designed and delivered a population-based digital navigation program to provide support, symptom monitoring, triage, and telehealth (Atreja et al., 2021).

33.5 TOWARD A PERSON-CENTERED APPROACH IN DIGITAL THERAPEUTICS

Often the use of technology is perceived to be less personal than traditional methods of clinical interaction. However, like most devices and interventions, quality and utility are based upon the quality of the design and the acceptability to end users. Often, the design and development of clinical information systems are carried out with minimal engagement of end-users in respect of both content and interface. Images used in applications can be potentially alienating to a diverse society and potentiate stereotypes. Partnering with communities, particularly those who are linguistically and socially diverse, can help to overcome this challenge. Involving patients, clinicians, and researchers (technology end-users) in the innovation and development process optimizes the likelihood of the intervention being effective and can increase adoption and decrease risks of abandonment or non-adoption (Ferguson et al., 2018).

Health literacy is recognized as a potent social determinant of health. The ability to seek, find, understand, and appraise health information from electronic sources and apply the knowledge gained to addressing or solving a health problem is termed electronic health literacy or e-health literacy (Eysenbach, 2001). The 10 core principles of e-health have relevance and salience to DTx. These are briefly summarized below:

1. **Efficiency:** Increase efficiency through enhanced communication and promoting patient and consumer involvement.
2. **Enhancing quality:** Through involving consumers as partners and accessing evidence-based care from the best quality providers.
3. **Evidence based:** e-health interventions should be evidence-based and promote best practice.
4. **Empowerment:** Promoting patient engagement opens possibilities for person-centered approaches.
5. **Encouragement** of a new relationship between the individual and health professional, through shared decision making.
6. **Education** of health providers through online sources and consumers through digital access.
7. **Enabling** information exchange and communication in a standardized way between health care establishments.
8. **Extending** the scope of health care beyond conventional geographical boundaries.
9. **Ethics:** e-health involves new forms of patient–provider interaction and, despite benefits, presents challenges and threats to professional practice such as informed consent, privacy, and equity issues.
10. **Equity:** To make health care more equitable, we need to ensure digital access (Eysenbach, 2001).

33.6 BARRIERS TO THE ADOPTION OF DIGITAL THERAPEUTICS

Individual, provider, and system issues can serve as barriers to the adoption of DTx (Williams et al., 2020). Telehealth and DTx challenge the traditional boundaries of regulatory and approval agencies, demanding a need for new paradigms that transcend professional, regional, and national boundaries. As in many areas of healthcare, technology has overtaken social norms, laws, and regulations.

Although DTx interventions have the capacity to address existing barriers to health care, such as geographical distance and access to expertise, this model of care delivery can render a unique set of challenges related to both the digital interface and monitoring and governance. At the front of mind are the risks of security and privacy as well as partnerships with private vendors (Olivier et al., 2021). We should be concerned about not only the protection of personal data but also issues of biosecurity. Other important considerations include:

- Standardizing approaches for regulatory approval as well as post-approval surveillance.
- Differentiating evidence based DTx interventions within a crowded market of wearable and off-the-shelf devices.
- Enabling operability across multiple information systems.
- Ensuring insurers and payers recognize the benefit of reimbursement.
- Monitoring standards and outcomes within an agreed framework.
- Ensuring health professionals have the knowledge, skills, and competencies to work in a digital environment.
- Promoting adequate reimbursement and incentive for health professionals to engage in DTx strategies.

33.7   THE ROLE OF NURSES IN DIGITAL THERAPEUTICS

Digital therapeutics have the potential to improve health outcomes. Ensuring nurses have the knowledge, skills, and competencies to create, apply, and evaluate DTx is critical for advancing healthcare. Moreover, it is critically important that nurses generate research questions and are actively engaged in research.

Frequently nurses are asked "is there an app for that?" or "what's the best app for managing my condition?"; informal caregivers seek advice on where to seek virtual support post-hospitalization of a loved one. While these questions may seem almost trivial, these are complex questions to which nurses have professional obligations to adopt an ethical and professional stance. Selecting, appraising, and recommending a smartphone app is a skill that is required of all nurses, be it novice to expert. Ferguson and Jackson (2017) offer an appraisal framework and suggest six criteria for appraising apps. These include (1) purpose, description, and audience; (2) app development and production; (3) content and evidence; (4) endorsement and credibility; (5) usability, review, and rank; and (6) patient centered-ness. Ferguson and Jackson (2017) provide a series of 23 individual questions to support clinical nurses to appraise apps and provide an overall assessment of quality. These steps are important to undertake prior to recommending apps to patients. Importantly, patient level factors—such as considering a patient's health status and well-being, frailty, cognitive abilities, and health literacy, along with digital literacy—are important to consider. Consideration of the role of the family caregiver is important, to address if the app is suitable for them. While issues of data security and safety are not well described in Ferguson and Jackson's framework of assessment, these are fundamental issues to assess and communicate with patients.

Various nursing professional organizations and regulatory bodies include DTx-related competencies in their education and practice guidelines. These competencies are increasingly recognized across all areas of nursing practice. For example, the National Association of Clinical Nurse Specialists, representing over 90,000 CNSs across North America, emphasizes technology selection, evaluation, and application as a core advanced practice competency supporting nursing practice and patient outcomes (National Association of Clinical Nurse Specialists, 2019). Given increasing healthcare complexity and rapidly evolving digital therapeutic options, CNSs bring their unique skill set to bear by:

- Assessing new and cutting-edge DTx for safety, effectiveness, integration with existing technologies and workflows, ease of patient and/or staff use, and cost–benefit determinations.
- Considering equity and ethical implications of DTx use in specific and generalized care applications.
- Educating and coaching patients, families, and staff on DTx use.
- Consulting on procurement and implementation planning.
- Providing feedback to technology and healthcare organizations on DTx use within their specialty.
- Partnering with other disciplines to lead and develop novel DTx applications.
- Evaluating DTx adoption and influence on processes and outcomes.

As wearables become more readily available, less expensive, and sophisticated, nurses need to consider how we integrate these new technologies into our everyday work. Additionally, the implications of these devices on patient assessment, monitoring, and care needs to be evaluated. For example, in the future—if nurses are no longer required to manually obtain vital signs due to highly effective wearable monitoring capabilities, how will nurses take advantage of this time and how will this impact the delivery of care?

33.8 CONCLUSION

Technological advances have shaped not just modern health care but the world in which we live. We will experience an increasing interface between humans and machines. Across the globe, health care systems are struggling with escalating demands, rising costs, and increasing accountability. Health information and digital technologies can help meet these challenges, support population health goals, improve consumer experience, and drive discovery and innovation. Although the focus of these approaches has been predominantly chronic conditions, many companies are now looking at acute considerations and pharmacological indications. However, we cannot consider technology isolated from the human experience and the values we uphold as health professionals. Nurses have an important role in not only supporting individuals in the uptake of DTx and undertaking rigorous research but also promoting governance measures to support privacy and confidentiality of data.

REFERENCES

Abd-Alrazaq, A. A., Rababeh, A., Alajlani, M., Bewick, B. M., & Househ, M. (2020). Effectiveness and safety of using Chatbots to improve mental health: Systematic review and meta-analysis. *Journal of Medical Internet Research*, *22*(7), e16021.

Atreja, A., Fasihuddin, F., Garge, S., Davidoff, L., Rubin, J., Kakkar, S., Wedel, N., Madisetty, D., Singhania, R., Jain, C. M., Kurra, S., … Sands, B. (2021). A population-based approach to digital outreach, triage, and monitoring of IBD patients during the COVID-19 pandemic. *Gastroenterology, 160*(3), S7.

Baum, A., Kaboli, P. J., & Schwartz, M. D. (2021). Reduced in-person and increased telehealth outpatient visits during the COVID-19 pandemic. *Annals of Internal Medicine*, *174*(1), 129–131.

Dang, A., Arora, D., & Rane, P. (2020). Role of digital therapeutics and the changing future of healthcare. *Journal of Family Medicine and Primary Care*, *9*(5), 2207.

Eysenbach, G. (2001). What is e-health? *Journal of Medical Internet Research*, *3*(2), e20.

Ferguson, C., & Hendriks, J. (2017). *Partnering with patients in shared decision-making for stroke prevention in atrial fibrillation*. Oxford University Press.

Ferguson, C., Hickman, L., Wright, R., Davidson, P. M., & Jackson, D. (2018). *Preparing nurses to be prescribers of digital therapeutics*. Taylor & Francis.

Ferguson, C., & Jackson, D. (2017). Selecting, appraising, recommending and using mobile applications (apps) in nursing. *Journal of Clinical Nursing*, *26*(21–22), 3253–3255.

Ferguson, C., Davidson, P. M., Scott, P. J., Jackson, D., & Hickman, L. D. (2015). Augmented reality, virtual reality and gaming: An integral part of nursing. *Contemporary Nurse*, *51*(1), 1–4.

Fisk, M., Livingstone, A., & Pit, S. W. (2020). Telehealth in the context of COVID-19: Changing perspectives in Australia, the United Kingdom, and the United States. *Journal of Medical Internet Research*, *22*(6), e19264.

Lombardo, L., Wynne, R., Hickman, L., & Ferguson, C. (2021). New technologies call for new strategies for patient education. *European Journal of Cardiovascular Nursing*, *20*(5), 399–401.

Nagy, M., Abbad, H. M., Darwish, A., & Hassanien, A. E. (2021). The 4th Industrial Revolution in coronavirus pandemic era. In A. E. Hassanien & A. Darwish (Eds.), *Digital Transformation and Emerging Technologies for Fighting COVID-19 Pandemic: Innovative Approaches* (pp. 219–231). Springer.

National Association of Clinical Nurse Specialists. (2019). *Statement on clinical nurse specialist practice and education*. NACNS.

Olivier, C. B., Middleton, S. K., Purington, N., Shashidhar, S., Hereford, J., Mahaffey, K. W., & Turakhia, M. P. (2021). Why digital health trials can fail: Lessons learned from a randomized trial of health coaching and virtual cardiac rehabilitation. *Cardiovascular Digital Health Journal*, *2*(2), 101–108.

Orchard, J., Neubeck, L., Freedman, B., Li, J., Webster, R., Zwar, N., Gallagher, R., Ferguson, C., & Lowres, N. (2019). eHealth tools to provide structured assistance for atrial fibrillation screening, management, and Guideline-Recommended therapy in metropolitan general practice: The AF-SMART study. *Journal of the American Heart Association*, *8*(1), e010959.

Palanica, A., Docktor, M. J., Lieberman, M., & Fossat, Y. (2020). The need for artificial intelligence in digital therapeutics. *Digital Biomarkers*, *4*(1), 21–25.

Patel, N. A., & Butte, A. J. (2020). Characteristics and challenges of the clinical pipeline of digital therapeutics. *NPJ Digital Medicine*, *3*(1), 1–5.

Sanna, T., Diener, H.-C., Passman, R. S., Di Lazzaro, V., Bernstein, R. A., Morillo, C. A., Rymer, M. M., Thijs, V., Rogers, T., Beckers, F., Lindborg, K., & Brachman, J. (2014). Cryptogenic stroke and underlying atrial fibrillation. *New England Journal of Medicine*, *370*(26), 2478–2486.

Williams, M. G., Stott, R., Bromwich, N., Oblak, S. K., Espie, C. A., & Rose, J. B. (2020). Determinants of and barriers to adoption of digital therapeutics for mental health at scale in the NHS. *BMJ Innovations*, *6*(3).

Wongvibulsin, S., Habeos, E. E., Huynh, P. P., Xun, H., Shan, R., Rodriguez, K. A. P., Wang, J., Gandapur, Y. K., Osuji, N., Shah, L. M., Spaulding, E. M., Hung, G., Knowles, K., Yang, W. E., Marvel, F. A., Levin, E., Maron, D. J., Gordon, N. F., & Martin, S. S. (2021). Digital health interventions for cardiac rehabilitation: Systematic literature review. *Journal of Medical Internet Research*, *23*(2), e18773.

Yan, B., Tu, H., Lam, C., Swift, C., Ho, M. S., Mok, V. C., Sui, Y., Sharpe, D., Ghia, D., Jannes, J., Davis, S., Liu, X., & Freedman, B. (2020). Nurse led smartphone electrographic monitoring for atrial fibrillation after ischemic stroke: SPOT-AF. *Journal of Stroke*, *22*(3), 387.

Index

Note: Figures are indicated by *italics* and tables by **bold type**. Endnotes are indicated by the page number followed by "n" and the endnote number e.g., 126n1 refers to endnote 1 on page 126.

A

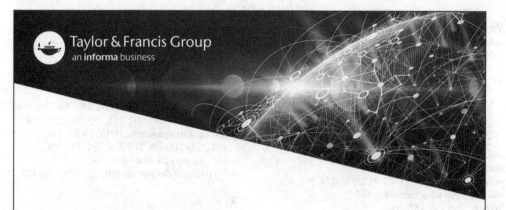
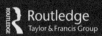
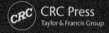